Handbook of Family and Marital Therapy

Edited by Benjamin B. Wolman and George Stricker

Family and marital therapy is rapidly becoming the choice method of treatment for mental disorders. The last few decades have brought about an increasing awareness of the fact that, excluding those of organic origin, practically all mental disorders are caused, fostered, and/or related to faulty interpersonal relations. This handbook presents current ideas and techniques in the area of family and marital therapy, showing that it is effective not only in treatment but in prevention of disorders as well.

The editors have collected papers from leading experts in this area of psychotherapy. Their papers offer an up-to-date and wide-ranging survey of the field. The introductory chapter written by Dr. Wolman explores the changing vistas in marriage and parenthood and discusses the basic reasons and rationale for marital and family therapy. Subsequent papers analyze the main conceptual issues related to communication, research, and training in family and marital therapy. A number of papers discuss the major therapeutic systems currently practiced. The volume also includes several papers that deal with such special problems and issues as treating one-parent families, stepfamilies, sex therapy for couples, and therapy with minority groups.

A groundbreaking work in a most important area of psychotherapy, *Handbook of Family and Marital Therapy* will be an indispensable guide for clinical psychologists, psychiatrists, and social workers.

Jacket design by R. B. Goldgraben

Handbook of Family and Marital Therapy

Handbook of Family and Marital Therapy

Edited by
Benjamin B. Wolman
and
George Stricker

Consulting Editors
James Framo, Joseph W. Newirth,
Max Rosenbaum, and Harl H. Young

Plenum Press · New York and London

Library of Congress Cataloging in Publication Data

Main entry under title:

Handbook of family and marital therapy.

Bibliography: p.
Includes index.
1. Family psychotherapy. 2. Marital psychotherapy. I Wolman, Benjamin B. II. Stricker, George. [DNLM: 1. Family therapy. 2. Marital Therapy. WM 430.5.F2 H2355]
RC488.5.H327 1983 616.89′156 83-9650
ISBN-13: 978-1-4684-4444-5 e-ISBN-13: 978-1-4684-4442-1
DOI: 10.1007/978-1-4684-4442-1

Softcover reprint of the hardcover 1st edition 1983

A Division of Plenum Publishing Corporation
233 Spring Street, New York, N.Y. 10013

Contributors

Charles P. Barnard, Ed. D.
School of Education and Human Services
University of Wisconsin-Stout
Menomonie, Wisconsin

Janet Beavin Bavelas, Ph.D.
Department of Psychology
University of Victoria
Victoria, British Columbia
Canada

John Elderkin Bell, Ed.D.
751 De Soto Drive
Palo Alto, California

Bryan D. Brook
3185 South Dahlia Street
Denver, Colorado

Ruth E. Clifford, Ph.D.
Department of Psychiatry & Behavioral Sciences
Stanford University School of Medicine
Stanford, California

Stanley N. Cohen, Ph.D.
Department of Psychiatry
The Oregon Health Sciences University
Portland, Oregon

Herbert Goldenberg, Ph.D.
Department of Psychology
California State University
Los Angeles, California

Irene Goldenberg, Ed. D.
Department of Psychiatry
University of California at Los Angeles
School of Medicine
Los Angeles, California

Paula Hollins Gritzer, M.S.W.
243 President Street
Brooklyn, New York

F. Nolan Jones, Ph.D.
Clackamas County Family Court Service
Oregon City, Oregon

Les Katz, Psy. D.
2993 S. Peoria
Suite 302
Aurora, Colorado

David V. Keith, M.D.
Department of Psychiatry
University of Wisconsin
Clinical Sciences Center
Madison, Wisconsin

Jodie Kliman, Ph.D.
New England Center for the Study of the Family
Newton, Massachusetts

Robert C. Kolodny, M.D.
Masters and Johnson Institute
24 S. Kingshighway
St. Louis, Missouri

Gayla Margolin, Ph.D.
Department of Psychology—SGM 923
University of Southern California
Los Angeles, California

Joseph W. Newirth, Ph.D.
Institute of Advanced Psychological Studies
Adelphi University
Garden City, New York

Helen S. Okun, M.S.W.
243 President Street
Brooklyn, New York

Daniel V. Papero, Ph.D.
Veterans Administration Medical Center
Nashville, Tennessee

Jo-Ann M. Rivera, Ph.D.
Family Studies Section
Albert Einstein College of Medicine
Bronx Psychiatric Center
Bronx, New York

John B. Rosenberg, Ed.D.
Philadelphia Child Guidance Clinic
Philadelphia, Pennsylvania

Bonnie M. Ruth
Bonnie Ruth and Associates, Ltd.
Lakewood Medical Center
Lakewood, Colorado

Lynn Segal, L.C.S.W.
Mental Research Institute
555 Middlefield Road
Palo Alto, California

M. Duncan Stanton, Ph.D.
University of Pennsylvania School of Medicine and
Philadelphia Child Guidance Clinic
Philadelphia, Pennsylvania

Janice M. Steil, Ph.D.
Institute of Advanced Psychological Studies
Adelphi University
Garden City, New York

Sharon Stein, M.S.W.
Department of Behavioral Sciences
Children's Hospital
Denver, Colorado

George Stricker, Ph.D.
Institute of Advanced Psychological Studies
Adelphi University
Garden City, New York

Thomas C. Todd, Ph.D.
Harlem Valley Psychiatric Center and
Philadelphia Child Guidance Clinic
Philadelphia, Pennsylvania

David W. Trimble, Ph.D.
North Shore Professional Associates
Lynn, Massachusetts

David N. Ulrich, Ph.D.
337 Thornridge Drive
Stamford, Connecticut

Jandyra Velazquez, M.S.
Child, Adolescent, and Family Services
Fordham Tremont Community Mental Health Center
Bronx, New York

Paula Walker
3185 South Dahlia Street
Denver, Colorado

Gwen Kathleen Weber, Ph.D.
Department of Psychiatry
C. Louis Meyer Children's Rehabilitation Institute
Omaha, Nebraska

Carl A. Whitaker, M.D.
Department of Psychiatry
University of Wisconsin
Clinical Sciences Center
Madison, Wisconsin

Benjamin B. Wolman, Ph.D.
International Encyclopedia of Psychiatry, Psychology, Psychoanalysis, and Neurology
10 West 66th Street
Suite 6D
New York, New York

Robert Henley Woody, Ph.D., Sc.D.
Department of Psychology
University of Nebraska at Omaha
Omaha, Nebraska

Harl H. Young
School of Professional Psychology
University of Denver
Denver, Colorado

Preface

Family and marital therapies are rapidly becoming highly used methods of treatment of mental disorders and are no longer ancillary methods to individual psychotherapy. The last few decades have brought about an increasing awareness of the fact that, excluding organic etiology, practically all mental disorders are caused, fostered, and/or related to faulty interpersonal relations. As a rule, the earlier in life one is exposed to noxious factors, the more severe is the damage. Thus, early child–parents' and child–siblings' interactions are highly relevant determinants of mental health and mental disorder.

Moreover, parents themselves do not live in a vacuum. Their marital interaction significantly contributes to their own mental health or to its decline, and parent–child relationships are greatly influenced by the nature of intraparental relationships. Parental discord, conflicts, and abandonment affect the child's personality development. Thus, family and marital therapy is more than therapy; it is an important contribution to the prevention of mental disorder.

The present volume is comprised of three parts. The first, primarily theoretical, analyzes the fundamental aspects of marital and family therapy. The second part describes the various therapeutic techniques and the last deals with several specific issues.

It gives me great pleasure to acknowledge my gratitude to my coeditor, Dr. George Stricker. Without his thorough and devoted efforts, this volume could not have come into being. I am also profoundly indebted to our consulting editors, Dr. James Framo, Dr. Joseph Newirth, Dr. Max Rosenbaum, and Dr. Harl Young, and to Ms. Hilary Evans, senior medical editor of Plenum, for their wise and friendly help.

BENJAMIN B. WOLMAN

Contents

I Foundations

II Therapeutic Systems

III Special Problems and Issues

I

Foundations

1

Marriage and Parenthood

THE CHANGING SCENE

BENJAMIN B. WOLMAN

Institutions based on subjugation usually have been more stable than those based on equal rights. Those who subjugate are unmistakably conservative, and social inequality always has been associated with continuous efforts to preserve the status quo. Privileged classes and/or individuals oppose change; thus, slavery always has claimed more stability than freedom.

Traditional family has been based on male supremacy, on subjugation of females, and the conservation of both. The male–female relationship has been influenced by the relative power positions of the sexes; their display of force, dependence, aggression; and persistent brainwashing. There is no evidence for the Upanishad myth that assumed that

> the first human being on earth, Atman, felt no delight. Therefore a man who is lonely feels no delight. He wished for a second. He was so large as man and wife together. He then made this his self to fall in two, and hence arose husband and wife. (Quoted after Freud, 1920/1957, p. 58)

According to the Indian myth, it was the *man* who had the need for a companion, thus the male superiority was clearly stated.

The biblical story of Adam and Eve confirms male superiority. According to the Bible, Adam was created first, despite the well-known fact that all men were born by women. Eve was a part of his body. Mediaeval Christian philosophers argued that women have no soul, for the Old Testament did not mention God having given a soul to Eve. When the time for the expulsion from the Garden of Eden had come, the Lord said to Eve: "He shalt rule over thee." Apparently, Adam needed an outside authority to impose his rule over the woman.

According to Freud, "From the earliest times it was the muscular strength which decided who owned things or whose will shall prevail. Muscular strength was soon supplemented by the use of tools; the winner was the one who had the better weapons or who used them more skillfully. From the moment at which weapons were introduced, intellectual superiority already began to replace brute muscular strength; but the first purpose of the fight remained the same" (1932, pp. 272–275).

BENJAMIN B. WOLMAN • International Encyclopedia of Psychiatry, Psychology, Psychoanalysis, and Neurology, 10 West 66th Street, Suite 6D, New York, New York 10023.

With rare exceptions, described by Evans-Pritchard (1967), Mead (1949), Murdock (1949), and others, men subjugated women in practically all prehistorical ancient societies. Women were a property to be robbed or bought, used or abused. In the underpopulated areas of the ancient world children-producing women were a useful commodity. The ancient Romans raped the Sabinian women and practiced *ius vitae necisque* (the right of life and death) over their women and children. In ancient Hebrew the word *baal* stands for both owner and husband.

There were two main sources for male supremacy. First, the male superior physical strength. This muscular superiority has nothing to do with the alleged superiority of sexual organs. Alfred Adler wrote volumes on sexual "organ inferiority" of women; the superiority I am referring to is the sheer, brute, physical force. In infrahuman primitive societies as well as today most males grow bigger and stronger than females. Strong males have used their force and subjugated women, children, and lesser males. Men could rape women, beat them, and even kill them for insubordination. With very few exceptions, the male physical domination was the general rule in primitive societies.

At all times survival has been the preoccupation of mankind. Hunting and fighting against other human beings required maximum physical strength. It is, therefore, not surprising that men assumed or usurped domineering positions in primitive societies where physical prowess was the most relevant factor in the struggle for survival.

In ancient times, in the shepherd-type and early farming economies, having children was one of the most relevant aspects of the economy. In the poorly populated lands only those who had many children had enough labor for tending the herds, tilling the soil, and fighting off the neighbors. According to the Bible, the Lord promised Abraham that his progeny will be numerous. In lack of labor power and prior to the system of mass slavery, production of children was one of the fundamental factors in an economy. With the advent of mass slavery in the times of decline of the Roman Empire the size of the family shrank and the incidence of homosexuality rose sharply.

Moreover, an average woman can bear 10 to 15 children in her lifetime, but hardly any woman can provide adequate care for all of them. A man can fertilize several women and, if he possesses a large number of women, he can produce an army. Polygamy was not determined by the alleged male superiority but by economic reasons and by the difference in the respective roles of males and females in the reproductive process. The subjugation of women by men was a product of the socioeconomic system where physical force was at a premium and the child-bearing women could not provide food and shelter for themselves and their offspring.

Power has thus become the symbol of masculinity. The Latin word *virtus* ("virtue") is derived from the *vir* which means a man. The Hebrew *gibbor* ("Hero") and *g'vurah* ("courage") are derivatives of *gever* ("male"). In practically all languages *homo* ("human being") is synonymous with an adult male. Wisdom, courage, and responsibility have been ascribed to men despite the obvious fact that such a generalization flies in the face of evidence. Rationalizations are more common and older than rational thinking, for cowardly, sheepish, and stupid men by far outnumber the brave, self-assured, and wise ones.

The innumerable cases of heroic women have been played down, partly silenced, and often totally denied by male-dominated historiography. Psychological traits praised in men were discouraged and ridiculed in women; brave, aggressive, and wise women were branded as being pushy and arrogant and therefore nonfeminine. As usual, slave owners preferred submissive, subservient, and dull slaves.

1. The Penis Pride

The male sexual organ, besides being a source of sensual pleasure, has become a symbol of masculine power. Although penises never have played any significant role in the struggle for survival, they have enjoyed a unique status related to the feeling of power. The so-called virility, he-man feeling and the men's ability to sleep with women and produce children have been glorified as spectacular symbols of power.

In their earliest hungry and danger-fraught origins human beings had some reasons for fostering the myth of male pride and male supremacy. Eunuchs, impotents, and sexually passive males were ridiculed and ostracized because they were of little help to tribes that needed workers and warriors. Male sexual productivity was admired for economic and military reasons and some primitive religions prayed to the God-Father with an erected penis.

2. Brainwashing

Male domination greatly depended on brainwashing of the females. In peace or at war men felt free to "conquer" (physically) any women they could lay a hand on, but women were supposed to be faithful to their permanent or temporary users. Promiscuity in men was hailed as a great virtue and a noble sign of virility. Poets and troubadours glorified the splendid conquests of Don Juans, and every king and ruler was surrounded by a host of courtesans and ladies-in-waiting.

Women were not only subjugated but also brainwashed into a willing acceptance of their subordinated role. They were told that to be feminine meant not to display intelligence, initiative, maturity, and courage. The ideal woman as prescribed by men was supposed to represent a mixture of an obedient infant and a caring mother. When men were in their artificially fanned, domineering, or heroic mood, women were expected to be as gentle, as submissive, and as obedient as infants. Whenever men were tired, defeated, and hurt, women were expected to act the compassionate, affectionate, and caring mothers.

This brainwashing encompassed every aspect of a girl's life from cradle to grave. A little girl was told she must not act in a free self-expressive manner as her brothers did. As she was growing up, the male-controlled educational systems trained her for her future role as man's slave and toy.

Pregnancy, childbirth, and child care have made women weaker than men and thus facilitated their subjugation. Pregnant women and mothers of infants have been dependent on their keepers. The need to stay around the house and take care of the children substantially reduced women's working ability and forced them to perform household chores and whatever was believed to be less important. Men were hunters and fishermen, shepherds and farmers who went out to the fields with herds or plows, while women had to stay home to cook and to mind the children, waiting for men to provide food.

The Christian civilization has been notoriously unfair in dealing with male and female sexuality. Although the medieval church fathers believed that sexuality as such was sinful, they never persecuted promiscuous men but put all the blame on women. Only women were accused of witchcraft, and pious monks wrote volumes describing the forbidden sexual pleasures that female witches had with devils. The persecution of witches was a strange combination of sadism with pornography. Apparently, the "holy" fathers and monks derived some vicarious pleasure from shaving off the pubic hair of women accused of fornication with the devil. The knights and nobles never missed an opportunity to rape farm girls and the daughters and wives of heretics and Jews, but they never forgot to attach chastity belts to their sweethearts and wives at home.

Even in modern times, young men were allowed to seek premarital sexual satisfaction, while a pregnant single girl was exposed to ostracism and persecution. The discrimination against women and mental and physical abuse of them did not come to an end.

3. Penis Envy

Freud discovered what others tried to hide. In the prudish, bigoted Victorian times many girls wished that they were boys, for it was the only, though imaginary way of escaping discrimination and subservience. Boys could go wherever they pleased, talk to whomever they wished, and choose the occupation they preferred, but a girl was her father's slave until he agreed to transfer her to her future husband. Marriage was, in a way, the only way of escaping father's tyranny, but the marital oath committed the woman to love, cherish, and *obey* her new master. Most women preferred new masters to old ones, and some of them somehow managed to outsmart their marital partners.

In the Victorian era, marriage was the only socially acceptable avenue for women. Unmarried women were ridiculed and blamed for remaining single. When a girl preferred an active and independent life, she was called tomboy, amazon, and masculine. To be feminine meant to be a sort of hybrid between infantile dependence and motherly worries. All women were expected to accept the great "feminine" K: *Küche, Kirche, Kinder* (kitchen, church, and children).

In Freud's time masculine and feminine behavior could have been defined as follows:

> When you say masculine, you mean as a rule "active," and when you say "feminine" you mean passive. . . . The male sexual cell is active and mobile; it seeks out the female one, while the latter is stationary and waits passively. This behavior of the elementary organism of sex is more or less a model of the behavior of the individuals of each sex in sexual intercourse. The male pursues the female for the purpose of sexual unity, seizes her and pushes his way into her. (Freud, 1932, p. 156)

Freud did not invent "penis envy" but discovered this culturally determined phenomenon. The more restrictions were imposed on girls, the more frequently they wished to escape by changing their gender. Forty years ago, in the early days of my clinical practice, some of my female patients who came from conservative families dreamed about "switching the railroad tracks," clearly indicating their wish to be males.

Penis envy was not, however, a universal phenomenon common to all women at all times. For instance, the Tschambuli and Arapesh women did not experience penis envy. In Arapesh, men and women shared household and child rearing responsibilities, and among the Tschambuli, women were the dominating sex (Murdock, 1949).

Freud's observations of penis envy in women who were reared in an atmosphere of discrimination and subjugation should be related to the tendency of children to identify with the "strong aggressor." In patriarchal families, where the father was the absolute ruler, both male and female children were proud to identify with the father rather than with the mother. It is not surprising that Freud noticed the preference for a masculine, father-based superego (Freud, 1938).

Apparently penis envy in girls was not directed to the male organ of their playmates or brothers but, probably, it was an expression of a wish for the possession of the father's penis and with it the *fatherly power*. The penis was envied by women not because of its sexual significance, for vaginas can undoubtedly procure as much and often more sensual pleasure than penises; it was the penis as the *power symbol* that elicited the well understood envy feelings.

4. Discrimination

One can readily understand the socioeconomic reasons for the subjugation of women in olden times and explain their current rebellion in terms of technological development. There is, however, an important aspect of the male–female relationship that defies such an interpretation, namely the "mother–whore complex," that is, the idealization and debasement of women by men.

For every human being, male and female alike, the mother is the prototype of a *friendly power*. The mother is the main, if not the only, source of life and the main protector. The adoration of mother is ontogenetically typical for all infants, and phylogenetically typical for periods of oppression and despair. The adoration of the Holy Mother is a case in point.

One seeks support of a friendly power as long as one feels weak and expects to receive unconditional support, but such an ideal relationship may not last long. Infants "love" the "good" mother who unconditionally satisfies their wishes, but they hate the same mother when she refuses to meet their demands. Ambivalent feelings toward powerful protectors often carry the seeds of a rebellion against being weak and dependent. Welfare recipients do not love their benefactors and poor relatives often resent their wealthy supporters.

The boys' ambivalent feelings toward the mother often has been channeled into the mother–whore complex. Even cowardly and ineffectual men often discharge brute force toward someone weaker than themselves. Women were the choice target, and the male-controlled public opinion has been and partially still is in favor of the "masculine assertion" toward women and children.

The possession of a penis has given men an additional tool to use for the humiliation of women and for self-aggrandizement. The sexual act as such is neither beautiful nor ugly and, as with almost everything else in human life, it can be practiced in a most lofty or a most base manner. However, the allegedly aggressive and domineering insertion of the penis in intercourse has been often described in vulgar language. Quite often the male dominated manners and norms have distinguished between the birth-giving and caring motherly women and the allegedly base, sexy women, thus combining admiration and disrespect for the sexual behavior that they enjoy and debase.

The male–female relationship is not just a sexual one. There are a great many other aspects of interaction, and it would be patently absurd to reduce all human relations to sexual intercourse. There are, however, distinct psychological traits that are conducive to the male discrimination against women.

I had the opportunity to treat several men who discriminated against women. Apparently, some people need to discriminate against others. They seem to feel that they acquire importance by assuming their superiority in regard to others and displaying their hostile superiority feelings. Some people ridicule children, look down upon people of other races, and hurt them in an apparent pursuit of an easy self-aggrandizement.

It seems that the need to discriminate hinges upon one's self-esteem and the feeling of one's own power. Consider somebody strong and self-confident. Such a person would have little need for putting others down and enhancing his own value by undermining the value of other people. Self-confident and self-assured men and women tend to be considerate and magnanimous. The more powerful one is, the less one has the need to show power at the expense of others. Some men, aware of their own inadequacy, tend to act in a manner that gives them the feeling of power. Self-aggrandizement is easily accomplished at the expense of other people.

Several years ago I conducted a study in social relations in a classroom situation. In this study I observed teachers in their relationship to children. I also tested the teachers' and students' attitudes toward one another using a rating tool called *statogram*. Teachers who had a great deal of self-esteem and self-assuredness did not ridicule the children and were not hostile toward them. Being sure of themselves, they easily controlled the children and did not need to show their power. Insecure teachers displayed an exaggerated amount of power, as if trying to show how great they were (Wolman, 1974).

Men who doubt their masculine prowess tend to boast about their true or imaginary sexual achievements. Women who doubt their femininity throw themselves on men and tend to be exceedingly promiscuous, as if trying to prove that they are "real" women. The proverbial Don Juan or Don Giovanni is usually a man who is unable to relate to women and is afraid of them. He attempts to "win over" one after another, as if trying to prove to himself and others how virile he is. Actually, a Don Juan does not run after women, but *runs away* from them. As soon as he succeeds in a relationship with a woman, he begins to destroy it out of fear that he may lose his penis.

In my clinical practice I noticed that insecure men, underachievers, men who are pushed around on their jobs and are not respected by their colleagues and associates, are *prone* to discriminate against women. It seems that this is the only area where they can show their nonexistent power. Feeling inferior to other men, they tend to assert themselves against whomever they feel somewhat superior to, and they display brutal force against their wives and daughters. The men who need to beat their wives and daughters (I had a great many cases of this kind in my practice), were cowards who would never stand up to other men. When things went wrong at their jobs, they used their wives or daughters as scapegoats. I had in treatment a man who, whenever rebuffed by superiors, went home and provoked his wife into a conflict to "show her" who was the boss. I once had in treatment a man who was subservient and subdued in relationships with his colleagues and superiors, but at home acted like an adolescent bully, cursed his wife and two daughters, and occasionally hit them.

There are probably some general psychological reasons for this kind of attitude toward women. One is that all men were brought into the world by women and, for several years, their very survival depended upon their mothers' approval. In my clinical studies, I have found that children of rejecting parents develop a peculiar attitude toward their future mates, male or female. Men who in childhood felt that their mothers did not love them, tend to relate in an ambivalent manner to women in the future. On one hand, they are exceedingly dependent on women and try very hard to please them and win them over. They are usually generous to their girl friends and overpolite to their secretaries. However, as soon as they feel that they have established themselves in the eyes of the courted woman, they turn from the sweet Dr. Jekyll into the hostile Mr. Hyde. Some of my patients initially were meek and subservient to their girl friends, but as soon as they won them over, they turned into brutal tyrants. They often broke up the relationship, rejecting the woman whose love they had vied for. It seems as if they were driven by an unconscious mechanism and took revenge on all women for the rejection they suffered from their mothers in childhood. In childhood, they needed and craved their mothers' approval, and as adults they desired women as long as they *did not have* their approval.

Discrimination against women follows fundamentally the same rules as any other discrimination. People discriminate against others for self-aggrandizement at the expense of others. Those who feel inadequate are prone to discriminate against others. As a rule, however, people *do not discriminate against those who have the power to retaliate.*

Whenever one follows the history of humanity with its conflicts, clashes, international wars, and fratricidal murders, the message is always the same. Nations fight one another, but *they discriminate against and persecute only those who cannot defend themselves.* In the times of the Crusades, the Christian nations *fought* the Moslem nations. But the Crusaders on their way to the Holy Land *persecuted* the Jews. The Turks had a great many wars with other nations, but they persecuted Greeks and Armenians. Persecution is a particular type of hostility related not to competition and fighting among equals, but to the *desire to destroy those who can be easily destroyed.* There was never persecution of majority groups, of powerful individuals, or of strong political organizations. The persecution always was directed against those who could be easily persecuted.

5. Emancipation of Women

Errors die hard and the owl of wisdom is a notorious latecomer. The emancipation of women was started by men for not too noble reasons: men needed women to work for them.

The Industrial Revolution with its insatiable need for working hands pulled out thousands of women from behind hearths and cribs. The decline of the feudal system and the rapidly diminished role played by agriculture forced masses of women into the open labor markets of the budding capitalist economy.

Women's participation in the production and distribution of goods has irrevocably changed their psychosocial roles. The privileged and respected role of the sole provider that was the backbone of the traditional male-dominated family structure began to crack and presently is heading toward a hitherto unknown crisis.

The erosion of the traditional male–female relationship first started in the lowest and then the highest socioeconomic classes. The middle classes have been notoriously the bulwark of conservatism, and in conservative middle class families in the nineteenth century the fathers exercised an absolute power despite the Industrial Revolution.

The present-day family constellation deprived the father of his authority but did not replace it with any other authority. One cannot help wondering what is going to happen in our times to the Oedipus complex, the latency period, and the whole area of male–female relationships. Modern women successfully have destroyed the myth of their alleged intellectual inferiority and denied, in vivo, the legends of their either angel or witch personality.

The three factors in male supremacy, namely, physical force, economic life, and sexual behavior, have lost their validity. The male's physical force is no longer a relevant factor in success in life. Neither economic, political, nor hardly any other success in life depends on how many pounds one can lift; a tiny and skinny factory owner controls thousands of husky, heavy, strong menial workers. Even in warfare there is no longer room for the giant Goliath and agile David; a machine gun, a guided missile, and the A-bomb can kill an entire army of muscular warriors.

A professional or a business woman can be a leader and control the lives of a great many men. The lives of male patients may depend on a female doctor (in the Soviet Union the vast majority of physicians are women); a woman lawyer or politician can determine the fate of scores of men. Women in leading economic and governmental positions easily can afford bodyguards to protect themselves against "male supremacy." In olden times, a man could beat up his wife; the only thing she could do was to run to her father or brother who would then probably blame her for being insubordinate to her husband. Today, hoodlums who attack women, regardless of whether they are married to them or not, are punished by law.

The Industrial Revolution did not bring equal rights for women, but it provided the first dent in their economic dependence. It took almost two centuries, and more and more women have become gainfully employed and more and more women have entered occupations hitherto jealously guarded by men for men. Women fight for equal rights and, as soon as their income equals that of men, their economic dependence and marital slavery disappears. Today 45% of mothers are gainfully employed, almost all single and married childless women hold jobs, and there are more dual-earner couples than those in which the husband is the sole provider.

In the past men could divorce women and engage in extramarital relations, but a married woman was buried with no hope of ever breaking the marital yoke. Having no occupation, no money of her own, and no place to go, a woman was doomed to stay married even when her marriage was totally unsatisfactory. Today, a great many young women do not intend to get married. They see no reason for it and prefer to stay alone or to live with a man they love without accepting legal commitment.

The sexual revolution of our time is an additional factor that undermines the traditional marriage. The fear of pregnancy was instrumental in a totally different approach to education of boys and girls. Boys were supposed to be self-assertive, but girls were brought up to be passive and submissive and to hold on to their virginity.

The invention of anticonception methods used by women, especially the pill, reduced the chances of conception to a minimum, thus allowing women to get rid of their fear of pregnancy and, subsequently, to disregard the man's demand for virginity. Sexual freedom put an end to one of the worst inequalities between the two halves of mankind. A modern woman can say to her partner, lover, or husband, "It is either freedom for *both* of us or commitment for both of us." Planned parenthood put the responsibility on both parents, and several civilized countries make men share the responsibility regardless of whether the child is legitimate or illegitimate.

Not such a long time ago, a young man was practically forced to marry if he wanted to have a regular supply of sexual gratification. He could go to prostitutes, of course, but the "nice girls" with whom he associated would turn down his sexual advances unless they were backed up by engagement and wedding rings. Sexual equality and freedom make marriage less urgent and hardly anyone would marry today solely for sexual reasons.

A great many women rebel against male supremacy, and it is difficult to continue slavery without brainwashing the slaves. Social and political movements of all kinds support the demands of women; our democratic system has a built-in 50% female vote. There are few people in the world who could question the fact that there are no intellectual differences between men and women and there are no special intelligence tests for women.

6. Decline in Marital Stability

Today more men and women prefer to remain single longer than ever before. Between 1960 and 1978 the median age at first marriage rose from 22.8 to 24.2 for males and from 20.3 to 21.8 for females. The number of never-married 29-year-old women grew by 51% between 1960 and 1980.

A growing number of young people live together without getting married. In 1981 there were an estimated 1.2 million "unmarried-couple" households, a 120% increase since 1970. However, according to Macklin (1978), in most cases after a few years cohabitation ends in marriage or it breaks up.

Many contemporary women face the difficult dilemma of choosing between career and family life. Quite often they regret either choice. Ms. R., a 45-year-old successful and highly intelligent physician who diligently pursued her career, envied her 47-year-old sister, Mrs. S., who married soon after graduating from college and had three children; but Mrs. S. came to my office seeking psychological help. She was resentful of her life and envious of her successful sister. Mrs. S. regretted her own "lack of ambition," and having abandoned her career for her "selfish husband and ungrateful children."

Rosenfield (1980) studied depressive symptoms in women. He found a high level of depression in those who did not work outside the home; working women had lower depression scores than their husbands.

As mentioned above, marital relationships were quite stable as long as they were based on subjugation of women. Contemporary marriages are democratic and men and women have equal rights. There is, however, no majority vote in marriage and all decisions must be negotiated and agreed upon, which is by no means easily accomplished. Quite often one of the marital partners tries to impose his or her will on the other; quite often the disagreement causes both of them to act in a disagreeable manner, and no less often the unresolved conflicts cause serious damage to the marital relationships and lead to separation and divorce. In some instance the conflicts lead to physical violence and wife abuse (Hartik, 1982; Hofeller, 1982).

Success in contemporary marriage depends on mutual consideration, tactfulness, understanding of the other person, and willingness to adjust and compromise. According to Burgess, Locke, and Thomes, (1963) marriage

> has been in transition from an institutional to a companionship form. This transition is in part the result of major social changes which have placed families in a radically different environment from that of the past. Important changes are the shift from a rural to an urban society, from stability of residence to mobility, from familism to individualism, and from a relatively short family life cycle to one which continues for years after the children have established homes of their own. All of these changes have occurred in the United States, and most of them have taken place in other countries. Most of the changes result in situations in which impersonal, secondary associations predominate, and the small-family unit becomes the major area of intimate, affectional association. This has resulted in the growth of the companionship family, characterized by the mutual affection, sympathetic understanding, and comradeship of its members. (1963, p. vii)

Apparently, contemporary marital roles make historically unprecedented demands on the adult's personal resources. According to Gadlin (1977), the burden of self-fulfillment was placed on marital relationships. The last 50 years have witnessed an increase in personal fulfillment in marriage as a counterbalancing value to that of marital stability. The male–female equality in marriage has democratized the expectation of personal growth, the burden of which is borne by the companionship aspects of marriage. It is small wonder that contemporary marriage is more intense and more fragile than was traditional marriage.

Contemporary marriage requires a mutual understanding and agreement to support each other's self-perception and self-esteem. However, since the choice of a mate is largely a matter of unconscious, many marital conflicts stem from the spouses' difficulty in accepting their partner's real personality traits. As Bowen (1976) pointed out, often, in the early stage of marriage, the spouses see each other through the glasses of their unconscious wishes. As time passes, the unconscious distortions become untenable and the spouses face each other as *real persons* instead of idealized images. The difficulty in demystification of the spouse and accepting him or her for what he or she really is may lead to conflicts. Distressed spouses tend to overreact to the negative behavior of their partners and the resulting intramarital conflicts become serious and jeopardize the future of the marriage (Gottman, 1979).

7. Divorce

According to Doherty and Jacobson (1982, p. 669), the most striking change in the 1970s was the upsurge of the divorce rate. In 1970 there were 708,000 divorces, a rate of 15 divorces for every 1,000 married couples; 1.5% of existing marriages ended in divorce during 1970. In 1978 divorces numbered 1,122,000, a rate of 22 divorces per 1,000 married couples, indicating that 2.2% of marriages ended in divorce. The divorce rate increased 48% from 1970 to 1978. Data for 1979 and 1980 indicate that the rate of divorces is continuing to climb. The greatest upturn during the 1970s was in the age group 25 to 39 years. If current divorce rates persist, some demographers estimate that future generations of married couples will experience greater than 50% probability of divorce. These figures imply that a considerable proportion of American adults experience marital distress sufficient to cause a complete breakdown of their marriage. Along with this increase in marital disruption is the increase in single parenthood. Single-parent families headed by the mother increased 55% during the 1960s and another 78% from 1970 to 1978, and single parenthood is an increasingly common life role for female adults in our society.

According to Kelly's review of research literature (1982),

> there are clear gender differences in the nature and frequency of complaints described by men and women. Women had more complaints about the marriage than did men. Two-thirds of the women complained of *feeling unloved* (compared to 37 percent of the men). This complaint ranked first in mentioned frequency for women and third for men. Most women associated these feelings with a gradual erosion of affectionate feelings for their spouse and a corresponding feeling of *emptiness* that led many finally to initiate divorce.
>
> For the men the complaint mentioned most frequently (by 53 percent) was of the wife's being "inattentive," of neglecting or slighting what husbands saw as their needs and wishes.
>
> The second most commonly voiced complaint of the men was that of major incompatibility in interests, values, and goals from the very beginning of the marriage. Three times as many men (39 percent) as women (13 percent) complained of such longstanding incompatibility. When recent change in interests or goals is included with the longer-term incompatibility complaints, 72 percent of the men and 44 percent of the women were dissatisfied with the dissimilarity in interests and values.

> One-third of the women complained that their competence and intelligence were constantly belittled by their spouses, resulting not just in resentment but in the eventual feeling that they could do nothing right. One-third also reported that their spouses were hypercritical of everything about them, including their manner, clothing, physical appearance, ideas, conversations, and child-rearing practices.
>
> Beyond these most common complaints there were few differences in the rankings for the next cluster of complaints. Sexual deprivation figured prominently for 34 percent of the men and for almost as many women. Men blamed their spouse's disinterest or frigidity; the women blamed the husband's disinterest or extramarital affairs for the sexual deprivation. Considering that 71 percent of the men had one or more extramarital affairs during the marriage (versus 15 percent of the women), it is surprising that infidelity did not rank higher. A number of couples had not had sexual intercourse for three to five years prior to separation.
>
> Thirty-three percent of the men and 24 percent of the women complained that their spouse was chronically "bitchy" or extremely angry. Complaints of excessive nagging, of frequent outbursts of excessive anger, or an inability to enjoy anything were included in this category. Some spouses struggled along in marriages dominated by the real mental illness of their husband or wife. (pp. 739ff.)

In 40 years of psychotherapeutic experience I dealt with numerous cases of separation and divorce. In some instances mental disorder of one of the spouses was the cause of divorce, but it was not the major nor the most frequent cause. Disappointment in each other and a failure to meet the partner's exaggerated expectations have been the main reasons for the breakdown of marriage among my patients. Quite often they expected to receive from their partner all the love, affection, and protection they did not receive in childhood from their parents.

In most instances sadness was the main symptom before divorce; in most cases depression and bitterness followed the divorce. On some occasions they entered bitter and prolonged legal battles that profited no one except the divorce lawyers.

Wallerstein and Kelly (1980) arrived at a similar conclusion. Kelly (1982) described the situation as follows:

> The intense *anger* of the separating spouses found expression in a wide range of behaviors around a limited number of issues. Money was one such issue, and the intense hostility which accompanied the economic division of property was a reflection not just of the marital conflict but was related just as strongly to the psychology of the divorce itself for each spouse. The abandoned spouse felt not only devastated and angry at being left but also viewed his/her spouse's ability to take one-half of the community property as a final insult. Such outraged spouses were more likely to fight about every dollar or every piece of furniture in the property settlement and expend thousands of dollars in legal fees in the process. The second issue was the children. Angry parents withheld the children as a punishment or attempted to form an alliance with the child which, if successful, hostilely excluded the other parent from the child's life. Embittered fathers childnapped, used physical violence, and entered into custody battles for children with whom they may have had previously inadequate relationships. They attempted to convince the children and the courts that the mothers were morally bankrupt and unfit. Despite their angry dènials embittered vengeful mothers were intent on destroying the father–child relationship through frequent tirades aimed at convincing the children that the father no longer loved them and by blocking visitings through any means possible. These embittered parents were more likely to turn to the court to seek redress for real or imagined grievances than were the less angry men and women. The endless litigation served to refuel and consolidate their rage, maintaining the anger at a high level of intensity for several years.
>
> On the basis of spouse and cross-spouse descriptions, ratings of presence, severity, and duration of depression *during* the marriage as well as *after separation* were made for each adult participating in the California Divorce Study. There were significant sex differences, with depression more common in the marriage for women, of greater severity and of longer duration. None of the men had attempted suicide during the marriage, contrasted to 14 percent of the women making one or several attempts. Fifty-four percent of the men and 21 percent of the women were

> essentially free of depression throughout the marriage. Of the remaining men 10 percent experienced severe, disabling depressions, some requiring hospitalization, and 36 percent experienced moderate depression. Among the women 31 percent were severely depressed, again with some recurrent hospitalizations in this group, and nearly half were moderately depressed at some time in their marriage. Of the women 42 percent (versus 16 percent of the men) had chronic depressions of more than five years' duration, often accompanied by psychosomatic symptoms, including numbness, vague pains, and severe and recurring migraines. (p. 742)

8. The Traditional Family

In the past the parents spent most of their time at home or near the home and even fathers did not go too far away and not for too long a time. Whether the father was a farmer or an artisan, he worked most of the time at home or near his home and had all or most of his meals with his family. Father was the unquestioned head of the household and no child could challenge his authority.

The fact that the parents were at home or near the home all the time gave them a good opportunity to set an example for appropriate behavior, and their attitude toward their children, although authoritarian, was usually more guidance than reprisal. An important factor was the size of the family. Every child had brothers and sisters to whom he could relate and develop close friendships. Families were large and comprised of several generations, with grandparents, uncles and aunts, and a multitude of cousins. A pouting child was not doomed to suffer in isolation; he or she could be cheered up by the multitude of peers and adults around him and the family clan offered many opportunities for release of energy and relief from tension. The conflict between parents and children rarely if ever turned into an unbearable burden, and often a good-natured grandparent offered moral support to an unjustly treated child, thus contributing to a more wholesome emotional climate in the family.

Public opinion and the prevailing set of values have contributed to the stability of the traditional family. For centuries the family was believed to be the natural and indispensable social unit and the very foundation of society at large. All religious denominations praised the family and made the marital contract into a sacred bond. Children's obedience to the parents was believed to be one of the holy Ten Commandments that reads, "Thou shalt honor thy father and mother." Philosophers and statesmen, clergymen and public leaders have offered an unswerving support to the traditional family structure and the prevailing educational concepts have caused parents and children to believe that this was the only way society could survive. The self-preservation of authoritarian forms of life is a self-fulfilling prophecy and self-perpetuating mechanism; the generally accepted set of cultural values was made to prevent cracks in the traditional social structure and its bulwark, the traditional, authoritarian family (Evans-Pritchard, 1965; Frazer, 1945; Parsons, 1955).

9. Ambivalent Parental Attitudes

The traditional family, although definitely more stable than the contemporary one, was by no means a child's paradise. Child abuse is not a new phenomenon and parental cruelty is as old as parenthood.

According to Charles Darwin the dawn of human civilization was associated with infanticide. He wrote: "Our early semi-human progenitors would not have practiced infanticide. . . . The instincts of the lower animals are never so perverted as to lead them regularly to destroy their own offspring'' (1936, p. 430). And further: infanticide ''originated in savages recognizing the difficulty or rather the impossibility of supporting all the infants that are born'' (1936, p. 430).

Frazer (1945) reported child killing as a regular occurrence among aborigine Polynesians. According to Sumner (1906) the Australian aborigines killed one of their children when they did not have enough food or water for all of them. According to the Bible infanticide was a frequent occurrence. Children were sacrificed to the pagan God Moloch and were burnt alive. The king Ahaz burnt alive the children of Hinom. Moses was saved from death by his mother who put the infant in the river, disobeying Pharaoh's order of slaughter of children. The ancient Canaanites often killed their first born child as a sacrifice to their gods (Leach, 1949). In ancient Rome the father had the right to kill his children; the *ius vitae necisque* (the law of life and death) allowed men to give life and to take it away at will (Lee, 1956). The ancient Spartans and Romans murdered weak, sickly, and defective newborns.

One cannot draw clear-cut conclusions concerning the allegedly ''instinctual'' origins of maternal and paternal love. Mother nature does not speak unequivocal language, and animal paternal care does not follow a uniform path (Rheingold, 1963).

Apparently human parenthood is a mixed bag of positive and negative feelings. Most parents care for their children and take care of them and even sacrifice their own needs for the sake of children. However, even caring and self-sacrificing parents are torn by ambivalent feelings of love and resentment toward their children, and many parents feel that children are a burden. Often a woman experiences the fear of losing her personality in favor of the child or ''an oppressive fear of loss of professional and intellectual values,'' or loss of beauty, and so on (Deutsch, 1945, vol. 2, p. 47). Childbirth involves injury to the mother and great pain. Thus it ''may well arouse aggressive impulses in the mother toward the child'' (Bakan, 1971, p. 96).

Child rearing often requires a good deal of parental patience and tolerance, for the children's behavior can be quite annoying and sometimes exasperating. It is not surprising that many parents experience hostile feelings toward a child. Most parents control their anger, but quite often they harbor hostile and abusive fantasies (Helfer & Kempe, 1968). Some parents, unconsciously or consciously, have death wishes against their children. Tired, overtaxed, depressed parents often experience infanticide wishes (D. Block, 1965), and some parents act out their wishes. (Child abuse will be discussed at a later point.)

10. From Marriage to Parenthood

Although marriage usually leads to parenthood, the psychological issues of parenthood are quite different and sometimes diametrically opposed to marriage. For one thing, there is no evidence that having children improves the intramarital relationship. In my clinical experience I came across marital couples who related to one another in a quite friendly manner as long as they had no children; but with the arrival of the first child everything changed. The women invested their entire love and devotion in the infant with an apparent neglect of the husband. Sometimes they treated their husbands as ''mother's helpers'' and expected a total subordination of marital life to the child-rearing tasks. The arrival of the first child changed the household from husband-centered to child-centered, and most husbands resented the change. Quite often both the husband and the wife resented each other; they did not blame the child but blamed each other for being selfish, bossy, and uncaring.

Some men developed a sort of a "fatherhood neurosis," competing with the children for their wives' affection. Pregnancy and childbirth usually reduce the frequency of sexual relations and some men and women who were disappointed in each other have become overinvolved with their children. There also has been an increase in the incidence of marital infidelity.

Many women and men who expected to find enjoyment in parenthood become disappointed when they have to face the new obligations and occasional discomfort and stress. A decrease in marital satisfaction associated with parenthood has been noticed by several authors, among them Nock (1982) and Rossi (1968).

Parenthood imposes new obligations that compete for time that the couple used to spend leisurely. This especially affects the woman (Rossi, 1968). The advanced phase of pregnancy and childbirth reduce the income of the average family. Most often the new mother drops out of the labor force.

The last few decades have brought an increase in the numbers of childless marriages. Apparently more people avoid having children. According to Glick (1977, 1979), in 1967 only 3.1% of married women age 18 to 39 did not wish to have children, whereas in 1977 5.4% of married women the same age decided to have no children. In the 1920s, 1930, and 1940s marrying adults planned to have three or four children; in the seventies they planned to have one or two children. In 1960s the average couple waited 14 months from the day of wedding to the first childbirth; in 1979 the average waiting period was 24 months.

11. Motherhood

Motherhood is biology, but is mothering also biologically determined? A female who gives birth to an offspring is a mother. Is mothering, that is, taking care of the child, therefore a universal, innate drive or a culturally determined behavior?

According to Wilson, the pattern of parental care, being a biological trait like any other, is genetically programmed and varies from one species to the next (1975, p. 336). Most psychoanalysts also believe that child care is a deeply rooted, innate psycholocical need.

There is, however, very little data concerning the genetic origins of parental child care (Schaffer, 1977) and, as mentioned above, nature does not provide an unequivocal guidance. The tree shrews do not care too much for their offspring and sometimes kill and eat them, but chimpanzee and baboon mothers protect and nurse their infants. India's hanuman langur (the sacred monkey) mothers neglect their offspring and allow wounded or malformed infants to starve or to be killed (Rheingold, 1963).

Pregnancy usually is a difficult period of life and not only from the physiological viewpoint. Many women worry about their own appearance and, moreover, are concerned with the physical and mental well-being of the children they will give birth to. Maternal anxiety during pregnancy could affect adversely the child's physical and mental development (Davids & DeVault, 1962; Shainess, 1977).

Emotional support from the woman's mother and from other relatives and friends is of great help, but the husband's attitude toward the expecting mother is of utmost importance and it may affect the future wife–husband and mother–child interaction. When a young woman patient of mine became pregnant, her husband (who probably needed psychological help more than she), angrily said, "What have you done to me!"

Labor and childbirth usually are a crisis experience, and a surgical delivery, cesarean childbirth, is a dramatic event that women abhor. A woman's physical and emotional discomforts could affect her future affectionate or resentful attitude toward the offspring.

Many women experience a short or prolonged period of depression after childbirth. The length and the severity of depression depends on the woman's personality makeup as well as on how different was the pregnancy and delivery. The postpartum depressions are more frequent in cases of absence of emotional support during pregnancy (Sawin, Hawkins, Walker, & Penticuff, 1980) and it can be reduced to a minimum by an affectionate and understanding attitude on the part of those around her, especially her husband.

Childbirth brings sudden physiological changes in a woman's life. Her own organism, which is heavily taxed in pregnancy and labor, undergoes hormonal changes, and her psychological situation presents her with new tasks and obligations. The woman's entire way of life undergoes radical changes for the newborn infant requires 24 hours of attention and care.

The mother's attitude to the newborn is influenced by several factors, among them the mother's personality makeup, the father's attitude, and the looks and behavior of the infant.

According to Field and Widmayer (1982) the mothering process has its share of disturbances and aberrations. An accumulating literature on early interaction disturbances and child neglect and abuse, for example, have both highlighted mothering as an important subject for study and implicated mothering disturbances as a source of developmental problems. Until recently the mother or father was implicated or blamed for everything from abuse to nervous tics. Increasingly the literature is suggesting that the disturbance lies in the relationship with each partner, the child and the parent, contributing to the problem.

Although all children and parents on occasion experience disturbed interactions, there are some who experience them fairly frequently. Disturbed interactions between mothers and children often appear as early as early infancy. Many of those reported are characterized by a hyperactive, controlling, or anxious mother and an unresponsive infant or a hypoactive, passive, or depressed mother and an unresponsive infant. It is not clear in many of the reports whether the infant is initially unresponsive and the mother's hyperactivity or hypoactivity is her response to the infant's unresponsiveness or whether the infant's unresponsiveness is a response to the over- or understimulating behaviors of the mother. Nonetheless the interaction is characterized by high levels of maternal stimulation and control (e.g., never letting the infant get a word in edgewise, not respecting his/her need to take breaks from the conversation, and escalating the level of stimulation as the infant gaze-averts, squirms, and fusses) or low levels of maternal stimulation and passivity (e.g., failing to provide stimulation for the infant and not responding to the infant's behavior).

The picture that emerges from these analyses of different types of interactions (feeding, face-to-face, and floor play) at different stages during the first two years of life among preterm infants and their parents is a vicious cycle of the infant being relatively inactive and unresponsive and the parent trying to engage the infant by being more and more active or stimulating, which in turn leads to more inactivity and unresponsivity on the part of the infant. Although the parent's activity appears to be directed at encouraging more activity or responsivity of the infant, that strategy is counterproductive inasmuch as it leads to less, instead of more, infant responsivity.

Although most research literature stressed the impact of parental behavior on the children, in recent years researchers have paid an increasing attention to the impact of the infants on the parents (Lipsitt, 1980). Quite often the mother's behavior becomes infantilized as if she is trying to imitate the infant. The speech patterns undergo changes and become baby talk, and face-to-face interaction endeavors to please the infant and to elicit coos and smiles.

A lot depends on the infant. Mothers' behavior greatly depends on the infants' looks, temperament, intelligence, and so on.

In many instances the mothers' attitude is related to the child's looks, gender, agility, and moods. As the child grows and attends nursery school and kindergarten, some mothers encourage and some discourage the child's growing independence. Insecure mothers tend to hold on to their children and to overcontrol their behavior (Mahler, Pine, & Bergman, 1970; Spitz, 1965). A patient of mine, Mrs. S. did not allow her 5-year-old son to attempt to dress himself and resented whatever the child dared to do without her approval and close supervision. Mothers who respect children's individuality and growing need for independence greatly contribute to their wholesome development. Those who during middle childhood pay attention to the children's intellectual and emotional needs, who show interest in their children's interaction with peers and teachers, who occasionally help them in school work and guide their extracurricular activities, are fostering children's intellectual and personality development.

Adolescence is usually a difficult time in the mother–child relationship. Most adolescents are more involved with their peer group than with their parents. The identification with the peer group enables them to attain a higher level of personality development (Wolman, 1982), but many a mother finds it difficult to accept the inevitable lessening of the bond between her and her growing children. Most adolescent boys and girls expect to be treated as adults and resent maternal care that they perceive as an obsolete and insulting infringement of their freedom and rebel against their mothers. Some authors, notably Lefrançois (1973), believe that the rebellion is not just adolescents versus mothers. The conflict has several aspects, usually impatience with oneself, the struggle for independence versus love and loyalty to the parent, and the conflicting loyalty to one's peers versus one's loyalty to the parents. In any case, adolescence is a difficult period not only for adolescent boys and girls, but also for their mothers and fathers.

11.1. Infants' Attachment to Mothers

It is apparent that the higher biological species need a longer period of maternal nurturance and protection than the lower ones. A "newborn" fish can swim, but a newborn bird needs some time and care before it can strike on its own, and a human newborn has little chance to survive without adequate care and protection. The dependence on oneself and on one's own power is the prime factor in adults—mature individuals *first* count on themselves and *then* on their friends, relatives, and others. Children first count on others, on assisting and protecting parents or parental substitutes. Children's security depends primarily on acceptance by others.

Children must receive an adequate amount of protection in order to function freely. A child has the right to be a child, and as such he deserves all the parental protection and acceptance he needs to give him the feeling of security. The very presence of strong and friendly parents or parental substitutes considerably contributes to the child's wholesome development.

Bowlby (1969, 1973, 1980) combined psychoanalytic theory with Piaget's system, ethology, and psychobiology. The infant's attachment to the mother is biologically determined and has a fundamental survival value. Human infants have an innate drive for physical proximity with the nourishing and protecting adult, and this drive is genetically transmitted into all human beings. In a tired, scared, ill, or wounded infant the search for physical proximity is heightened.

Sroufe and Waters (1977) noticed that the infants' secure relationship with the mother significantly contributes to a wholesome personality development and the future establishment of an autonomous self and self-assuredness in the peer group.

Infants over 7 months of age and especially in the second year of life demonstrate long lasting, severe distress when they are separated from their mothers (Joffe & Vaughn, 1982).

Unwanted, rejected, unloved infants in foundling homes have a high mortality rate even when they have received adequate food and medical care (Spitz, 1965; Weiniger, 1972). The decline of paternal authority is one of the most significant features of contemporary family and, as mentioned above, more and more families have two providers. The historical role of the father as the sole provider is coming to an end and with it women's dependence on their husbands.

Many a man, although wishing to have children, reacts with anxiety and psychosomatic symptoms to his wife's pregnancy. Many develop psychosomatic symptoms during their wives' pregnancy, and the symptoms somehow resemble their pregnant wives' symptoms. Shereshefsky and Yarrow (1973) maintain that almost two-thirds of men react in the above manner. On the other hand, some men react favorably to pregnancy as if it were an evidence of their masculine prowess and power. Many men also derive a great deal of satisfaction from their paternal role as protectors of the nurturing wife and the helpless infant. Some are proud of their new role and contribute to an atmosphere of warmth and security in their home.

According to Biller,

> Many fathers have masculine interests and are masculine in their peer and work relationships but are very ineffectual in their interactions with their wives and children. The stereotype of the hard-working father whose primary activity at home is lying on the couch, watching television, or sleeping is an all-too-accurate description of many fathers. If the boy's father is not consistently involved in family functioning, it is much more difficult for his son to learn to be appropriately assertive, active, independent, and competent.
>
> The father's affectionate, encouraging, and attentive behavior toward his child can be seen as aspects of paternal nurturance. There is much evidence that a warm, affectionate father–son relationship can strengthen the boy's masculine development. (1982, pp. 704 ff.)

Studying kindergarten boys, Biller found that perceived father-nurturance was related to a fantasy game measure of sex-role orientation. Other researchers also have found evidence suggesting that paternal nurturance is related to older boys' masculinity.

When the father plays a significant part in setting limits, the boy's attachment to his father seems to be facilitated *only* if there is an already established, affectionate, father–son relationship. If the father is not nurturant and is punitive the boy is likely to display a low level of father-imitation. Bandura and Walters (1959) found that adolescent boys who had highly punitive but generally nonnurturant and nonrewarding fathers exhibited relatively low father-preference and little perception of themselves as acting and thinking in the same way as their fathers.

In Biller's (1977) study with kindergarten boys, the overall amount of perceived father-influence was much more important than the perception of the fathers as dominant in a particular area of family or parent–child functioning.

There is ample evidence that well adjusted and successful individuals come from homes where the fathers were much involved and took an active part in the child rearing and the intraparental relationship was congenial and affectionate (Biller, 1977, 1982; J. Block, 1971). Maternal dominance is associated with mental disorders of children, especially boys. In a longitudinal study by J. Block, von Der Lippe, and Block (1973), the well adjusted females were brought up by rational parents who related well to one another and were involved in child rearing.

Paternal deprivation can adversely affect child's personality development. The longer the father's absence and the younger the child, the more severe was the ensuing pathology especially in male children (Trunnell, 1968). Many alcoholics, drug addicts, and antisocial individuals have experienced frequent and prolonged periods of father's absence (Rosenberg, 1969). Divorce seems to have an adverse impact on mental health of children of both sexes (Wallerstein & Kelly, 1980).

12. Patterns of Interaction

One can present all human interactions in four dimensions. One hostile (*H*) and three friendly, namely, instrumental (*I*), mutual (*M*), and vectorial (*V*). These four types are not always separate and discrete patterns and often human interactions are a combination or even confusion of the above four attitudes.

Most probably, hostile attitudes are phylogenetically older than any other. Each individual comes in physical contact with a great many other individuals. Each individual may develop *N-1*, one-to-one social relationship within a population of *N* members, an innumerable number of relations with more than one partner.

Each individual, however, participates in a limited number of associations. In a society based on freedom of association, individuals may choose a certain number of groups and organizations to which to belong. They may increase their social participation by marriage, by a change of job, by moving into a new neighborhood, or by making new friends. They may relinquish their former associations, forget schoolmates, renounce religious or political affiliations, resign from their jobs, divorce, and sever relationships with parents and other family members.

The motives for interindividual relations can be friendly, or hostile, or mixed. Traditionally, friendliness is equated with social behavior and hostility with antisocial behavior. Later, I shall explain that both types of attitudes and action, such as cooperation and competition, love and hate, friendliness and hostility, and alliance and war are *social* processes. Let us start, however, from social relations based on cooperation.

A classification of social relations, based on *motivation* of the participants in voluntary face-to-face relationships, is proposed here. One may divide social relations according to the aims of the participants, depending on whether their main purpose is the satisfaction of their own needs (instrumental), or their partners' (vectorial), or both (mutual or mutual acceptance). Several experimental and observational studies have been reported elsewhere.

People frequently join a group in order to have their own needs satisfied; they have in mind to take and not to give. In such a case the individual considers the other group members as tools or instruments. The individual joins the group only for his or her own benefit and pursues only his or her own objectives. The person joins the group because without it he or she could not satisfy his or her needs or would encounter considerable difficulties. Whenever the particular relationship or the particular group ceases to satisfy those needs, the individual will leave it.

This kind of a group, called *instrumental,* represents the usual business relationship. When a person looks for a job, he or she enters an instrumental social relationship and the objective is to *receive* a salary. The employer's attitude is instrumental also, for the only thing the employer wants is to find someone to *help* in his or her trade. When a student registers for a course, it is an instrumental arrangement; he or she wants to receive knowledge or a degree or both.

Apparently people form instrumental groups because otherwise their needs could not be satisfied. Sociability in human beings starts out of weakness and the instrumental attitude bears witness to that. A new organism starts life in a dependence upon the organism that gave life; the intrauterine life is a parasitic process of taking without giving anything in return. This parasitic, taking attitude continues in infancy; the infant is a taker and parents or parental substitutes are the givers. The infant is too weak to give; he or she must receive all the necessary supplies or will not survive. Also, a drowning person who calls for help is instrumental.

Instrumentalism does not exclude friendliness: one likes his or her car or toys. It is a selfish kind of friendliness, but it is friendliness. No one would sacrifice his or her life for a toy, but usually we like to preserve them.

During the first two years, the child learns to love others. Certain persons become the symbols of satisfaction, for they are always the object that provides the means of satisfaction. The first conditioning that the child undergoes is that persons, who fairly consistently have been the objects that have provided the infant with the means of satisfying its needs, now become satisfying objects in themselves.

The maturation and learning processes are well illustrated by the growth of the infant's power or ability to satisfy his or her own needs. The infant becomes capable of such things as holding balance, walking, grasping and holding things, and eating without assistance.

The first social contacts of the infant are the supporting and protecting adults. As soon as the infant meets other children, the situation changes. Adults were the givers, he or she was the taker; but peers are also takers. To become a giver, one has to be assured about his or her possessions. The child must feel self confident to be ready to face other children.

The readiness for social relations with peers is obviously a product of the child's maturation and learning. Yet the support the child received from adults is of importance for that readiness.

The more help, the more love and affection the child has received, the more he or she is sure of the forthcoming help. The more the child feels secure and protected, the sooner he or she will develop the feeling of self-confidence. In terms of the power and acceptance theory, the friendly and supportive attitude of parents gives the child an increasing feeling of his or her own power and enables him or her to enter the higher developmental stage of a give-and-take relationship. A very anxious, insecure child will be afraid of other children and have difficulties in relating to them on a give-and-take basis.

The mutual or mutual acceptance relationship develops gradually. In the nursery school or kindergarten the child already is presented with opposition to his or her instrumentalism. When children try to monopolize the games, books, and toys, the way out is to teach them to share, to take turns, and to trade. The adult society, teachers and parents, cannot tolerate a war of all against all. They suggest a give-and-take relationship. The child is *taught* to share, to take turns, and to trade toy for toy. The progress toward a higher developmental stage is a product of learning, but no one can learn unless he or she is ready for it. Gesell's structure function principle permits us to see the child's growth as a product of both maturation and learning. Freud's developmental stages (Fenichel, 1945, chaps. 4,5,6) also are a combination of inherited potentialities (of going through stages such as the oral and anal) with environmental influences.

Forced giving, trading, or sharing is still instrumentalism, although it already is a step forward. Initially, infants are not too willing to give; they are afraid to part with their possessions and fear they will not get them back. They must become "stronger" and more sure of their strength or of support by adults to be ready to part with their possessions for a short while. It is not only their power, but their belief in this power (or the power of and acceptance by their supporters) that matters. Children can be well developed physically and have high IQs and yet feel insecure and afraid of other children. As long as children feel weak or rejected by parental figures, they may find it difficult to enter any give-and-take relationship. The less secure any child is, the more guarding and hostile (fight or flight) will be his or her reactions to other children.

Several factors help the child to arrive at the mutual level of a voluntary give-and-take relationship. The first is the child's *own growth* and *learning* which lead toward an increasing mastery of the child's own body and acquisition of skills. Success is a good therapist; it helps to build up one's self-confidence.

The second factor is the child's undisturbed *instrumental* relationship with parental figures and other relevant adults. Several workers have observed the importance of parental approval for the development of the child's self-confidence (Adler, Sullivan, Horney). Parental acceptance and approval is the very foundation for the child's feeling of security, and the more the child is sure of continuous parental support, the more courage he or she will have in forming social relations with peers on a give-and-take basis.

The third factor is the *interaction* with peers, the rewarding experience of sharing, trading, taking turns, and helping each other. Children who are rejected by their peers and assaulted or ridiculed, for whatever reasons, may regress into a defensive guarding attitude of withdrawal and hostility. The simple fact of being among children does not necessarily encourage social development. Children may reject, hurt, and humiliate the shy schizophrenic child. The misfortunes in group living may set the development back and force more withdrawal and more world-destructive, revengeful fantasies.

Under favorable conditions the child gradually will develop and learn consideration for other children. The instrumental, exploitative type of friendship will change into a relationship based on mutual understanding. A study of friendship relationships conducted on 1,086 children and adolescents has shown that in childhood the main reasons for friendship are instrumental. A dear friend is chosen during childhood for objective rather than subjective reasons; he or she is smart, strong, quiet, clean, well ordered. Many stress benefits of friendship: He or she helps me with my lessons, tells jokes, gives me gifts, etc. The friendship is practically devoid of emotional content and exhibits little readiness for self-sacrifice.

In adolescent years the emphasis shifts to personality traits; faithfulness, loyalty, and willingness for self-sacrifice are stressed by both partners. A friend is not chosen for the benefit one derives from him. New criteria are added, among them concern for the individual, understanding of his weaknesses and faults, sympathy, and a desire to help the suffering.

This is the beginning of the mutual or mutual acceptance relationship. Each individual is willing to give; he or she gives willingly and the emotion experienced can be called friendship, consideration, or love. The individual is willing to renounce some of his or her benefits for the sake of the partner, willing to protect that partner, to make him or her happy. It is the beginning of a voluntary giving. In fact, the adolescent looks for someone to be friends with, to help, to protect, to give love to. This love can be sexual or nonsexual, or, in psychoanalytic terms, aim-inhibited.

But the loving adolescent insists on mutuality. In an answer to a questionnaire, "How is your friendship expressed?," the most frequent answers were the following: mutually reveal secrets, exchange visits, partners in trouble, mutual help, and faithfulness. Each partner is willing to give and expects the other partner to feel the same way.

In sexual relations mutuality achieves its peak in intercourse. Each partner desires to make the other partner happy and expects that the same is the desire of the other partner. Successful marriage is based on mutuality; each marital partner is determined to do his or her best for the well-being of his or her partner and expects the same from the other party.

In mutual relations the desire to give, to be friendly, to accept the other person comes to the fore. This relationship is based on the fact that *both parties have the same desire to give*. The instrumental relationship also may entail some giving; the employee who looks for a job to earn a living must *give* his or her work. But this is not the objective, and my division of social relations is based on the objectives of their participants.

In a mutual relationship, the *aim* is to give and to receive. Hence there is *love* in them, love being defined as willingness to be of help. In instrumental relationships there is the desire to receive love, but not to give it. In mutual relations there is the desire to give and to receive.

When one feels weak, he or she is inclined to seek help; he or she wants to get support to become stronger and to increase his or her chances for survival. Poor men beg. Hungry wolves attack. Children of depression brought up in deprivation tend to be acquisitive and greedy. All these types of behavior can be hostile or not, but all of them are acquisitive.

When one feels rich and strong, he or she is inclined to give away. Rich and secure individuals tend to be generous. Overflow makes one feel like giving away; the cow needs to give away milk. Self-confident individuals are prone to be considerate.

Obviously, it takes both development and learning to become capable of self-sacrifice, to give away without asking anything in return. A little child is selfish, instrumental, willing to take. This is so because the child is weak and needs support. As he or she grows and becomes stronger, the child becomes more and more capable of sharing and mutual relations.

It seems rather doubtful whether this development would take place without learning by conditioning. Life usually offers a great many opportunities to learn, and mutuality is reinforced. It seems even more difficult to answer the question of whether the ability to give without asking anything in return, the willingness to be of service to others, the charitable, unselfish, idealistic attitude called vectorialism could ever develop without learning. One obviously has to be strong enough, or rather feel strong enough, to be able to act that way, but it seems that without learning one never may become vectorial.

Several studies on social development in Israel and comparisons of Israeli youth and youth elsewhere have pointed to the sociocultural influences that help adolescents to develop the vectorial attitude of self-sacrifice for fellow men, for the homeland, faith, or social ideals. Vectorialism is an outgrowth of mutualism; it is the same willingness to give, but without asking for any compensation or reciprocation. It is the lavish willingness to give love, to be friendly with the world, to help the poor and suffering.

Parenthood is the prototype of vectorialism. Parents create life, protect it, and care for it regardless of their child's looks, health, IQ, disposition, and success. The weaker the child, the more they protect it. The more the infant needs their help, the more sympathy he or she elicits in them.

Little children could not make good parents; they demand that love be given to them; they are instrumental. So are childish adults—they could not be adequate parents. To be an adequate parent, one needs to be strong, friendly, willing to give, help, and take care of one's child without asking anything in return.

The sight of a helpless infant elicits in us the feeling of power and the willingness to help. Mature adults tend to protect infants, not only their own children. In well-balanced individuals the sight of sickness, misery, and despair elicits the desire to help and protect and stimulates them to vectorial attitudes and actions. To give without asking, without expecting anything in return, is the highest degree of love and the most profound principle of ethics.

No human being can be vectorial all the time. Some human beings never can develop a vectorial attitude, while others develop it frequently and to a great extent. And yet the most fatherly or motherly or self-sacrificing and saintly individuals, when exposed to a lethal danger, may slide down to instrumentalism and call desperately for help. Or, in black despair, they may sink below instrumentalism into the hateful rage of a wounded animal.

Normal human beings are capable of functioning adequately in all three types of social relations and can be instrumental in business, mutual in marriage, and vectorial in parenthood. Occasionally, one may combine some of these attitudes in a rational manner (Wolman, 1974).

13. Family Dynamics

One must view these interactional patterns as "ideal types" in Weber's definition. In real life people interact with one another in more than one way and, quite often, in a combination of several behavioral patterns. Well adjusted adults are capable of acting in a *hostile* manner against those who threaten their survival, try to hurt or incapacitate, take away their possessions, or hurt their dear ones and allies. One must be *instrumental* in all endeavors related to earning a livelihood; one takes a job or starts a business not for charitable reasons but for clearly understood selfish needs. Friendly relations with other people are a two-way street; one is willing to do everything for one's dear friend, spouse, or an ally, being sure that the other party will do the same; these are *mutual relationships*. Mature and self-confident adults are willing to *give without taking;* they are caring and dependent parents and in certain situations they are ready to sacrifice their own well-being for the sake of their country, religion, or any other idealistic cause.

Mature married adults relate to each other in a mutual manner and in a vectorial manner to their children; children relate to parents in an instrumental manner.

With the exception of heredity, brain damage, and poison, childhood experiences are the main cause of mental disturbance and maladjustment. Some parents go out of their way to protect their children against traumatic experiences. They extend undue overprotection and thereby cripple their children. Obviously, these efforts are doomed to fail for no parent can protect his children from unwholesome experiences, mishaps, and adverse influences. The widespread blaming of parents for childrens' emotional problems largely ignores the impact of urban decay, crime, public corruption, anti-educational television programs, and a great many other factors. Children are not brought up in a vacuum and the only thing parents can do is to give their children healthy foundations and endow them with inner strength which will enable them to cope with adverse life conditions.

Most American parents certainly provide food and shelter for their children. Unfortunately, they do not realize that sometimes they themselves unwittingly and unwillingly adversely affect the mental health of their offspring.

It is not true that every frustration and stress causes mental disorder, but the same amount of stress may cause severe damage to an undeveloped mental structure. In several consultations in mental hospitals I have seen autistic children whose mental structure was gravely damaged before it had a chance to develop. Assuming that the harmful circumstances represent the hammer, the child's personality is the anvil; one may expect the worst when it is a sledgehammer and the anvil is the not yet developed infantile mind (Wolman, 1970).

During World War II I had the opportunity to observe mothers and children in war zones. I saw children playing cheerfully in air-raid shelters in cities under heavy bombardment with practically no damage caused to their mentality because their mothers were self-assured, well adjusted women who gave their children a feeling of security. Little children scarcely were influenced by Hitler's atrocities, the collapse of France, and the fall of Europe. Their mothers' attitude, peace of mind, and affectionate yet self-assured demeanor protected the children's mental health despite the grave and imminent danger.

I visited shelters in areas removed from the battle zone and rarely attacked by enemy bombs. In one place, the anxiety-ridden mothers threw themselves on their children in a state of panic when a bomb hit a target miles away. Practically all the children in the areas have suffered severe emotional disturbances. Children who stayed during the blitz in London were better off than those separated from their parents and sent to safe peaceful areas in Great Britain (A. Freud & Burlingham, 1944).

Children see the world through the eyes and emotions of their parents and they take parental communication seriously. A hysterical mother who says "you are killing me" or a maladjusted father who says "I am going to commit suicide" may cause damage beyond repair to their children. What counts most is not what the parents really are but how they interact and how their interaction is perceived verbally or intuitively by their children. I had patients who were afraid to fall asleep at night, and tiptoed to their parents bedroom to see whether they were still alive after an evening of interparental hostility verbalized by "I'll kill you!"

It is not true that all parents are always responsible for mental disorder in their children, but many mental disorders in children are caused by parents who involve them in their emotional problems. A wholesome and satisfactory family life is not necessarily a perfect life; children can take a good deal of stress, with one exception—parental emotionality—but no child can carry the burden of parental problems.

I once had in treatment a high school girl who was overcontrolled by her "loving" mother. She had no life of her own, no thought of her own, no will of her own. She was, psychologically speaking, a not-yet born entity and the emotional umbilical cord hung like a chain around her neck. She was shy, withdrawn, had no friends, no life of her own. The mother boasted to me that she herself was active, independent, marvelous, and willing to do *everything* for her beloved daughter. At the peak of an emotional outburst, she asked me "What else can I do to help my child?" My answer was brief and firm: "Please stop doing everything for her." Obviously her overpossessive "love," which had a paralyzing effect on her daughter, was a product the mother's emotional needs. The woman *needed* her daughter and thrived on the symbiotic relationship.

The parent–child relationship is a two-way street. In my clinical practice I have come across couples whose intramarital relationship has deteriorated with the coming of the first child to the point where they no longer could meet each other's emotional expectations. According to Gove and Geerken (1977), the incidence of mental disorders is quite high among mothers of children below the age of 5. Most mothers of infants are exposed to practically incessant demands and often find it exceedingly difficult to cope with the new situation. Pregnancy and labor are taxing experiences and women have to face the child's demands while they need to restore their own physical and mental balance.

Brown and Harris (1978) reported the highest incidence of depression in young working class mothers who had a child under 6, and the lowest incidence with the same age women who had no children. The presence of three or more young children was a highly significant factor of depression in women at all socioeconomic levels.

Depressive symptoms are more frequent in women than in men, but some men react with impatience and irritability to the child's crying at night and the need to help their wives in child care. Mature and well adjusted adults take the temporary hardships in stride, help each other, and derive a great deal of pleasure from taking care of the infant; but in less stable and less mature couples the necessity for temporary inconvenience may lead to intramarital conflicts. In some of them the very fact of becoming a parent revives old emotional problems. They identify with the child and live vicariously through the child. Sometimes they ascribe to the child nonexisting features and worry about nonexisting problems that are related to their own personality and past experiences.

Some parents develop an infantile attitude to their children (which will be described below). They frequently are disappointed when the child's looks and/or behavior does not meet their expectancy.

Brody and Axelrod (1978) maintain that parental *need to be loved* sometimes is an apparent contradiction to what parenthood should be. Ideally, parenthood means *giving without asking anything in return.* Such an attitude brings the joy of giving associated with the feeling of power. Helping, caring, and protecting proves a certain degree of strength.

Following in the footsteps of M. Mahler's child development theories, Mahler, Pine, and Bergman (1970) studied the reaction of mothers to the loss of their infant's symbiotic dependence. Many a mother experiences the infant's growing independence in speech and locomotion as a threat to her need to be needed. Many fathers and mothers wish to prolong the child's dependence on them and, unwittingly, try to infantilize the child. They may refer to their 10-year-old son or daughter as "my baby," and tend to overcontrol and overprotect their children far beyond the necessary parental care.

For a great many years in private practice and in hospital settings I have treated several disturbed patients, some of them schizophrenic. In practically all cases schizophrenics were people who were prematurely forced to give love and attention to their parents instead of receiving it. All human children are born selfish and narcissistic. They are helpless creatures and unless they *receive* love, protection, and care, they may not survive. Sensitive and mature parents are fully aware of this division of roles. They expect love and affection from each other and they give to their children love combined with common sense. By the nature of their helplessness, children must be on the receiving end of the parent–child relationship (Peterson, Becher, Schoemaker, Luria, & Hellma, 1962).

In 40 years of psychotherapeutic practice I saw innumerable cases of people who, dissatisfied in each other, expected their children to compensate for their marital misfortune. It happens quite often that an immature man marries an immature woman and both of them expect their marital spouse to play the role of a loving and forgiving parent. Since no man can be a father to his wife and no woman can mother her husband, they turn to their child and involve him or her in an exploitative and/or seductive manner. Most often, it is the first-born child who gets the brunt of parental "love" and who is made to feel guilty for his or her failure to satisfy the parents' insatiable emotional needs. I saw families in which the most "beloved" child ended up in a mild or severe case of schizophrenia, while another child, feeling totally rejected, developed sociopathic personality (Wolman, 1965).

Not all children of overdemanding parents become schizophrenic but hardly anyone can escape some degree of emotional damage. Some of these children are confused about their age roles; they are never too clear whether to act as children of their parents or parents to their parents. Some of them, seduced sexually and/or emotionally, are confused in regard to their psychosexual identity and many become homosexual or bisexual. The most severe cases are overattached to one or both of their parents and are unable to develop any kind of adult life. I saw in my practice very young children whose personality was destroyed in its inception and who remained infantile, mute, and self-destructive. The milder cases live on the margin of their own lives, passive, overdependent, dreaming of power, and/or imagining that the world is against them.

In my studies of schizogenic families I arrived at the conclusion that the parents were not sick people but the family was sick. Not all parents of disturbed children (even schizophrenics) are mentally disturbed, but the patterns of intrafamilial interaction were morbid. I interviewed hundreds of families in which one or both parents were somewhat mildly immature and some of their children were severely disturbed. If the parents were married to more mature and better balanced partners, the mental disorder in their children might have been avoided. Instead, their turning to the child for love and affection played havoc with the child's mental health. As mentioned before, children must remain selfish until, through interaction with their peers, they gradually develop more mature social attitudes. In my book *Children without Childhood* (1970) I describe children who were prematurely forced to give more love to their parents than they ever could afford and therefore ended up in mental bankruptcy.

14. The Rejecting Parents

It is a highly controversial issue whether the so-called maternal instinct is fact or fiction, for a great many women have no desire to have children and some of them resent the children they do have. Maternal rejection could be caused by a variety of factors. In many cases, interparental strife is the main cause of hatred toward the children. Modern marriage is a highly complex sociological and psychological phenomenon and not too many people are capable of living together. The fact that they were or even are sexually attracted to one another does not guarantee a wholesome human relationship nor does it suffice for the development of mutual understanding, respect, and necessary compromise. In many cases, married couples unite at night and split at day; in some instances they stay together because no one else would agree to the barrage of abuse and insult. It may sound paradoxical, but I saw a number of patients who would not divorce despite the intense hatred they had for their spouses or perhaps because of that hatred. Sometimes marriage is a strong combination of a sadist with a masochist or of two sadists or two masochists who enjoy inflicting hurt and being hurt.

The arrival of a child who demands so much attention and care often is perceived by one or both parents as an intrusion on their "rights." Attention combined with shifting attitudes of attraction and repulsion are showered on the child. In many cases, men look for outside supplies of affection and leave all their hatred for their beloved wife. Women who have children are less fortunate and they bestow on their offspring a great part of their frustrated rage. Children are exceedingly sensitive to nonverbal communication and somehow are aware that the mother wishes to get rid of them and be free again. Many married couples stay together for their children's sake and use their offspring as a convenient battleground in subtle guerilla warfare or in overt outbursts of a missile war.

A rejected child may end up in a complete nervous breakdown but fortunately most children are made of more sturdy stuff. Many a rejected child develops the mentality of a hunted animal. It is sink or swim; either "I get them or they will get me." Extreme selfishness, cunning devices, lying, and exploiting other people's weakness become the only way the child believes he can survive. This psychopathic mentality which is so frequent in our society and practiced under the slogan "if you can get away with murder, why not?" is usually a result of extreme parental rejection. I saw several sociopathic individuals coming from broken homes in low socioeconomic classes. On the other hand, in wealthy families where the father and mother live side by side with each other, each of them wrapped up in making and spending money, they offer very little affection to their children. Children showered with money without love grow up in a world of emotional neglect and alienation and they may turn to a wayward life, with or without drugs, indiscriminate sexuality, and desperate futility. The parents of sociopathic children are not necessarily sociopaths, but the intraparental alienation or animosity often leads to a total rejection of children.

14.1. Child Abuse

Every year close to 500,000 children in the United States need protection against being abused. According to Field and Widmayer (1982), approximately 550,000 children a year suffer from parental abuse and neglect.

"Children have been whipped, beaten, starved, drowned, smashed against walls and floors, held in ice water baths, exposed to extreme outdoor temperatures, burned with hot irons and steam pipes . . . exposed to electric shock; forced to swallow pepper, soil, feces, urine, vinegar, alcohol and other odious materials; buried alive . . . bitten, knifed and shot" (Bakan, 1971, p. 4). Bakan maintains that people who abuse a child intend to kill him or her, for the reason of child abuse is the wish to be rid of the child (Bakan, 1971, p. 55).

Children physically mistreated by their parents learn to use violence to coerce others to obey them. Being forced to obey they learn that violent behavior can help them to attain their goals. The fact that their own parents, who are expected to be kind and loving, practice hurtful violence leads to the formation of a self-righteous behavior. The parents who hurt them justify their behavior and maintain that their actions are not hostile but conducted in the name of love. They tell the beaten child that beating will make him or her into a "better human being." The allegedly noble purposes of parents justify their cruelty, thus convincing the child that one is allowed to act in an otherwise reprehensible manner provided one has a sort of excuse.

The process of identification with the aggressive parent leads to the formation of a hostile, self-righteous superego. Beaten children learn that they have the right to do so as they please in order to attain whatever goals they may have. The idea that the "end justifies the means" becomes the guiding motive in their self-righteous and antisocial behavior.

14.2. The Rejecting-Accepting Parents

Some parents act in a self-contradictory way. Their attitude to the child is a strange combination of love and hate, of acceptance and rejection, of feeling sorry for themselves and for their children. They usually reject their child and make him or her feel guilty for being unloved. Many a patient of mine felt that he or she did not deserve their great "parental love." Some of them, torn by feelings of inferiority, did not believe that they had the right to live. Some of these patients vividly recalled that when they reached the bottom of despair, whether in severe illness, accident, or rejection, their mothers and sometimes their fathers turned around and showered them with affection and overprotection. The behavioral pattern was clearly indicated: one cannot win love by being a wholesome and successful person. Parental love can be gained through suffering and self-defeat; only those who reach the bottom of depression can expect great affection.

This masochistic pattern was ingrained in some of my patients, as if depression were the only way to win love.

Perhaps all this sounds depressing. I have been working with these people for the last 40 years, trying to remedy their maladjustment and improve their way of life. But the stakes are too high to be reduced to a psychoanalyst's office. What psychotherapists are doing is largely a repair job. The time has come to think about these problems in broader sociological terms and to think how to *improve marital and family relationships* in order to prevent or at least significantly reduce the number of people who suffer because of mismanagement by their parents.

15. Some Relevant Issues

As described in the present chapter, contemporary marriage and family are beset by hitherto unknown difficulties that call for a remedial psychotherapy. Contemporary marriage cannot go back to slavery or colonialism. Contemporary women would not accept the role of second-class citizens and their access to education, employment, business, and politics militates against the past. The three *K*'s (Kinder, Küche, Kirche) advocated by the Nazi barbarians are a sad reminder of reactionary systems, but not too many American women would agree to go back to the dark ages.

The evolution of the social status of women is not unanimously accepted by women and even less by men. Centuries of brainwashing have led to a pseudoscientific theories of an alleged "psychology of women" (Deutsch, 1945), disputed by de Beauvoir (1949), Wolman (1978), and others. It is not easy for men brought up on yesterday's ideas to accept the inevitable end of their domination, and contemporary male–female relationships often resemble a contest of power.

Marriage does not solve the problem; in many instances living in the same quarters and facing each other every day aggravates the issue. It is much easier to be kind, polite, and friendly on a date than in daily encounters, and a short-lived romantic affair gives less reason for disappointment than the daily chores of marital life.

Small wonder that many marriages go sour and end up in separation and divorce thus playing havoc with the child's feeling of security and often affecting his or her mental health (Wallerstein & Kelly, 1980). It is not the task of psychotherapists to save every marriage and become second-hand matchmakers. The task of psychotherapists is always the same, whether they deal with an individual or with a couple: *The task is to make further psychotherapy superfluous.* As soon as the patient is capable of using realistic judgment, is emotionally balanced, and is capable of assuming full responsibility for his or her deeds, that is, has the courage to live and the wisdom to make the best possible decision, the therapist's task is accomplished.

Quite often married people engage in "baby-wars," fighting about irrelevant issues and trying to impose their will on their spouses. Many of my patients acted in a domineering fashion in marriage as if playing the father or the mother of their spouse. Mrs. F., a mother of two infants, has given orders to her husband as if he were her third infant. Unfortunately, the husband, brought up by a domineering mother and weak father, usually obeyed with occasional flare-ups resembling childlike temper tantrums that threatened the survival of the marriage.

In some cases both marital partners tried to assume the parental role to each other, and the first task of the psychotherapy was to make them aware of their activities and the underlying unconscious motivation. Some patients unwittingly accept the subservient role, and the domineering partner may feel disappointed with the spouse who "acted like a parasitic helpless infant." The 36-year-old Mr. S. resented his wife's passive and idle life. Although he himself in a way contributed to his wife's idle existence by demanding that she "stay home and take care of him," after a few years he "felt disappointed" and demanded that his wife be gainfully employed and "stop being an emotional burden."

16. Indication for Marital and Family Therapy

The rapidly expanding field of marital and family therapy is a much needed and welcome phenomenon. On one hand, it offers a necessary remedy to a vast variety of contemporary marital and family problems. On the other, it is a product of growing awareness that people do not live in a vacuum and human behavior is a field phenomenon. Different aspects of human personality come to the fore in interaction, and behavior is greatly and often permanently influenced by one's social environment (Kohlberg, 1969; Mead, 1964; Parsons & Bales, 1955; Wolman, 1974, 1982). It therefore seems advisable to keep in mind the social environment of patients and marital and family therapy may be the best avenue for psychotherapy.

Contemporary psychopathology and psychotherapy cannot ignore the obvious fact that *in a vast majority of cases, with the exception of clear organic etiology, mutual disorders are a product of faulty interpersonal relationships.* One can compare noxious interaction to a hammer and anvil; the hammer blows on a sturdy surface may cause no harm, but the same blows on a fragile surface may cause damage beyond repair. Analogously, adverse situations may cause little or no harm to a sturdy personality structure, but the same adverse situations may play havoc with a weak personality. One may question the Freud-Abraham assumption that mental disorders are caused in early childhood (Fenichel, 1945), but there is no doubt that infants are more sensitive to harmful conditions than mature adults and no human being is ever totally immune to emotional harm. Thus every type of psychotherapy must take into consideration the patient's past history and the present relationships. As a rule one is more sensitive to one's close environment than to strangers, and a hostile attitude of one's spouse or parents hurts a lot.

It seems apparent that even individual psychotherapy is *social psychotherapy* in more than one way. It deals with a patient's childhood interactions with parents, siblings, mates, and adults; it must analyze the entire gamut of past and present relationships within the patient's close environment. In most cases, marriage and family represent the closest ties, thus every individual psychotherapy is, in fact, a family and/or marriage psychotherapy.

Parent–child relationships present an enormous challenge for psychotherapists. Therapists, as it will be described in the present volume, use a variety of methods to protect and/or remedy the mental health of parents and children, and their successful intervention may prevent widespread emotional difficulties of a generation.

17. References

Ahlstrom, W. M., & Havinghurst, R. R. *400 losers*. San Francisco: Jossey-Bass, 1971.

Bakan, D. *Slaughter of the innocents*. San Francisco: Jossey-Bass, 1971.

Bandura, A., & Walters, R. H. *Adolescent aggression: A study of the influence of child-rearing practices and family interrelationships*. New York: Ronald Press, 1959.

Beauvoir de, S. *Le deuxième sex*. Paris: Press Universitaires, 1949.

Biller, H. B. Fatherhood: Implications for child and adult development. In B. B. Wolman (Ed.), *Handbook of developmental psychology*. Englewood Cliffs, N.J.: Prentice-Hall, 1982.

Biller, H. B. Father absence and paternal deprivation. In B. B. Wolman (Ed.), *International Encyclopedia of Psychiatry, Psychology, Psychoanalysis, & Neurology* (Vol 5.). New York: Aesculapius, 1977. Pp. 4–11.

Blanck, R., & Blanck, G. *Marriage and personal development*. New York: Columbia University Press, 1968.

Block, D. Feelings that kill: The effect of the wish for infanticide in neurotic depression. *Psychoanalytic Review*, 1965, *52*, 51–61.

Block, J. *Lives through time*. Berkeley: Bancroft Books, 1971.

Block, J., von Der Lippe, A., & Block, J. H. Sex role and socialization. *Journal of Consulting and Clinical Psychology*, 1973, *41*, 321–341.

Bowen, M. Family therapy and family group therapy. In D. H. L. Olson (Ed.), *Treating relationships*. Lake Mills, La.: Graphic Press, 1976.

Bowlby, J. *Attachment-Separation* (Vol. 1). New York: Basic Books, 1969.

Bowlby, J. *Separation: Anxiety & anger* (Vol. 2). New York: Basic Books, 1973.

Bowlby, J. *Attachment and loss* (Vol 3). New York: Basic Books, 1980.

Brody, S., & Axelrad, S. *Mothers, fathers, and children*. New York: International Universities Press, 1978.

Brown, G. W., & Harris, T. *Social origins of depression: A study of psychiatric disorders in women*. New York: Free Press, 1978.

Burgess, E. W., Locke, H. J., & Thomes, M. M. *The family: From institution to companionship*. New York: American Book, 1963.

Cherlin, A. Work life and marital dissolution. In G. Levinger & O. Moles (Eds.), *Divorce and separation: Conflict, causes and consequences*. New York: Basic Books, 1979.

Darwin, C. *The origin of species and the descent of man*. New York: Modern Library, 1936.

Davids, A., & DeVault, S. Maternal anxiety during pregnancy and childbirth abnormalities. *Psychosomatic medicine*, 1962, *24*, 464–470.

Deutsch, H. *Psychology of women*. New York: Grune & Stratton, 1945.

Doherty, W. J., & Jacobson, N. S. Marriage and the family. In B. B. Wolman (Ed.), *Handbook of developmental psychology*. Englewood Cliffs, N.J.: Prentice-Hall, 1982.

Evans-Pritchard, E. E. *The position of women in primitive societies and other essays in social anthropology*. New York: Free Press, 1965.

Fenichel, O. *The psychoanalytic theory of neurosis*. New York: Norton, 1945.

Field, T. M., & Widmayer, S. M. Motherhood. In B. B. Wolman (Ed.), *Handbook of developmental psychology*. Englewood Cliffs, N.J.: Prentice-Hall, 1982.

Frazer, J. G. *The golden bough*. New York: Macmillan, 1945.

Freud, A., & Burlingham, D. *Infants without families*. New York: International Universities Press, 1944.

Freud, S. *New introductory lectures on psychoanalysis*. New York: Norton, 1932.

Freud, S. *An outline of psychoanalysis*. New York: Norton, 1938.

Freud, S. Three essays on the theory of sexuality. *Standard Edition* (Vol 3.). London: Hogarth press, 1954. (Originally published, 1905.)

Freud, S. Beyond pleasure principle. Standard Edition (Vol. 18.). London: Hogarth Press, 1957. (Originally published, 1920)

Freud, S. A child is being beaten. *Standard Edition* (Vol. 17.). London: Hogarth Press, 1961. (Originally published, 1919.)

Gadlin, H. Private lives and public order. In G. Levinger & H. Raush (Eds.), *Close relationships*. Amherst: University of Massachusetts Press, 1977.

Giovannoni, J. M., Conklin, J., & Liyama, S. *Child abuse and neglect*. Palo Alto, Calif.: R & E Research Associates, 1982.

Glick, P. C. Updating the life cycle of the family. *Journal of Marriage and the Family*, 1977, *39*, 5–13.

Glick, P. C. *The future of the American family*. Washington, D.C.: U.S. Government Printing Office, 1979.

Gottman, J. M. *Marital interaction: Experimental investigations*. New York: Academic Press, 1979.

Gove, W. R., & Geerken, M. R. The effect of children and employment on mental health of married men and women. *Social Forces*, 1977, *56*, 66–76.

Hartik, L. M. *Identification of personality characteristics and self-concept of battered wives*. Palo Alto, Calif.: R & E Research Associates, 1982.

Helfer, R. E., & Kempe, C. H. (Eds.). *The battered child*. Chicago: University of Chicago Press, 1968.

Hofeller, K. H. *Social, psychological, and situational factors in wife abuse*. Palo Alto, Calif.: R & E Research Associates, 1982.

Howells, J. G. (Ed.). *Advances in family psychiatry*. New York: International Universities Press, 1980.

Joffe, L. S., & Vaughn, B. E. Infant-mother attachment. In B. B. Wolman (Ed.), *Handbook of developmental psychology*. Englewood Cliffs, N.J.: Prentice-Hall, 1982.

Kelly, J. B. Divorce: An adult perspective. In B. B. Wolman (Ed.), *Handbook of developmental psychology*. Englewood Cliffs, N.J.: Prentice-Hall, 1982.

Kohlberg, L. Stage and sequence: The cognitive developmental approach to socialization. In D. Goslin (Ed.), *Handbook of socialization*. Chicago: Rand McNally, 1969.

Leach, M. (Ed.). *Dictionary of folklore*. New York: Funk & Wagnalls, 1949.

Lee, R. W. *The elements of Roman law*. London: Sweet & Maxwell, 1956.

Lefrançois, G. R. *Of children: An introduction to child development*. Belmont, Calif.: Wadsworth, 1973.

Levinger, G., & Moles, O. (Eds.). *Divorce and separation: Context, causes and consequences*. New York: Basic Books, 1979.

Lipsitt, L. (Ed.). *Advances in infant development*. Hillsdale, N.J.: Earlbaum, 1980.

Macklin, E. D. Review of research on nonmarital cohabitation in U.S.A. In B. I. Murstein (Ed.), *Exploring intimate life styles*. New York: Springer, 1978.

Mahler, M., Pine, F., & Bergman, A. The mother's reaction to her toddler's drive for individuation. In E. J. Anthony & T. Benedek (Eds.), *Parenthood*. Boston: Little Brown, 1970.

Mead, M. *Continuities in cultural revolution*. New Haven, Conn.: Yale University Press, 1964.

Murdock, G. *Social structure*. New York: Macmillan, 1949.

Nock, S. L. The life-cycle approach to family analysis. In B. B. Wolman (Ed.), *Handbook of developmental psychology*. Englewood Cliffs, N.J.: Prentice-Hall, 1982.

Parsons, T., & Bales, R. F. *Family, socialization and interaction process*. Glencoe: Free Press, 1955.

Peterson, D. R., Becher, W. C., Schoemaker, D. J., Luria, Z., & Hellma, L. A. Child behavior problems and parental attitudes. *Child Development*, 1962, *32*, 151–162.

Rheingold, H. L. (Ed.). *Maternal behavior in mammals*. New York: Wiley, 1963.

Rosenberg, C. M. Determinants of psychiatric illness in young people. *British Journal of Psychiatry*, 1969, *115*, 907–915.

Rosenfield, S. Sex differences in depression: Do women always have higher rates? *Journal of Health and Social Behavior*, 1980, *21*, 33–42.

Rossi, A. S. Transition to parenthood. *Journal of Marriage and the Family*, 1968, *30*, 26–39.

Sawin, D., Hawkins, R. C., Walker, L. D., & Penticuff, J. H. (Eds.). *Current perspectives on psychosocial risks during pregnancy* and early infancy. New York: Brunner/Mazel, 1980.

Schaffer, H. R. (Ed.). *Studies in mother–infant interactions*. New York: Academic Press, 1977.

Shainess, N. Pregnancy: Psychiatric aspects. In B. B. Wolman (Ed.), *International Encyclopedia of Psychiatry, Psychology, Psychoanalysis, & Neurology*, (Vol 9.). New York: Aesculapius, 1977.

Shereshefsky, P. M., & Yarrow, L. J. (Eds.). *Psychological aspects of first pregnancy and early postnatal adaptation*. New York: Raven Press, 1973.

Spitz, R. *The first year of life*. New York: International Universities Press, 1965.

Sroufe, L. A., & Waters, E. Attachment as an organizational construct. *Child Development*, 1977, *48*, 1184–1199.

Sumner, W. G. *Folkways*. Boston: Ginn, 1906.

Trunnell, T. L. The absent father's children's emotional disturbances. *Archives of General Psychiatry*, 1968, *19*, 180–188.

Wallerstein, J. S., & Kelly, J. B. *Surviving and breakup: How children and parents cope with divorce*. New York: Basic Books, 1980.

Weininger, O. Effects of parental deprivation: An overview of literature and report on some current research. *Psychological Reports*, 1972, *30*, 591–612.

Wilson, E. B. *Sociobiology, the new synthesis*. Cambridge: Harvard University Press, 1975.

Wolman, B. B. Family dynamics and schizophrenia. *Journal of Health and Human Behavior*, 1965, *6*, 147–155.

Wolman, B. B. *Children without childhood*. New York: Grune & Stratton, 1970.

Wolman, B. B. Power and acceptance as determinants of social relations. *International Journal of Group Tensions*, 1974, *4*, 151–183.

Wolman, B. B. Psychology of women. In B. B. Wolman (Ed.), *Psychological aspects of gynecology and obstetrics*. Oradell, N.J.: Med Economics, 1978.

Wolman, B. B. Interactional theory. In B. B. Wolman (Ed.), *Handbook of developmental psychology*. Englewood Cliffs, N.J.: Prentice-Hall, 1982.

Wolman, B. B. *Interactional psychotherapy*. New York: Van Nostrand-Reinhold, in press.

2

Individual and Marital Development

ENTROPY OR SYNERGY

JOSEPH W. NEWIRTH

The purpose of this chapter is twofold; first, to explore aspects of adult development in relationship to marriage and individual growth and, second, to attempt to integrate the conceptual perspectives of psychoanalytic object relations theory and a systems approach to family and marital therapy. In exploring aspects of adult development, it is important to emphasize the evolving life stages as a critical dimension in adult personality development, psychopathology, and family functioning. It is this new awareness of a developmental continuum (Carter & McGoldrick, 1980) extending from birth to death that has helped us to conceptualize family pathology, as well as individual disorders of the self, in which problems of intimacy and self-esteem regulation are the central dimensions. In looking at both professional and popular literature, it would seem that we are living in a time in which marriage and marital dissolution and failure have become a central concern of both professionals and lay people alike. On the professional level, one aspect of this crisis in family relations is our lack of models that can both describe and explain successful marital and family relations and the causes of failure in these relationships.

1. Models of Marital Functioning

In order to develop a model of individual and marital development we first will consider briefly the traditional reasons for, or the purposes of, marriage. In many ways this view is based on individual psychology in which motivation and purpose has been an important issue. In family theory, marriage typically has been considered an *a priori* given and the nature of its structure and the relationship difficulties have been the point of theoretical focus. The first major historical reason for marriage has been economic: the family and the marital pair is able to maintain a more economically productive and efficient relationship with each other as well as with the economy at large. This is an

JOSEPH W. NEWIRTH • Institute of Advanced Psychological Studies, Adelphi University, Garden City, New York 11530.

extension of the historical development of permanent societies in which there was a division of labor and a diversification of function. This perspective might be considered an anthropological one, as contrasted to a traditional psychoanalytic perspective that has seen marriage as an outgrowth of the evolution of successful channels of libidinal discharge. From this traditional psychoanalytic perspective, marriage would be understood in terms of the resolution of the Oedipus complex and the individual's ability to shift his or her sexual desires from the parent of the opposite sex to a new person; marriage would be seen almost exclusively in terms of the evolution of sexual dynamics.

In terms of our current experiences with marital difficulties, neither of these explanatory systems seems to work very well. The economic motivation for the maintenance of marriage seems to have become, among our patients, considerably less relevant and, in fact, we frequently see the dissolution and failure of marriage as a concomitant of greater career or financial success within the family unit. In addition, the increased public acceptance and expression of sexuality and the apparent decreasing sanctions on various sexual relationships seem to cast the notion of marriage as primarily a channel for sexual discharge into some doubt. In fact, many of our patients seem to report a lack of sexual interest and activity in their relationships for extended periods of time prior to a separation. The Freudian view of sexuality and the centrality of Freud's libido theory has been questioned on many grounds. The traditional anthropological and psychoanalytic understandings of marriage seem somewhat irrelevant to contemporary marital difficulties. How, then, are we to understand both these marital difficulties and what in fact would account for successful marital relationships?

A third perspective on the purposes of marriage would seem to be an extension of contemporary thinking about psychoanalytic object relations theory in which the most important psychological dimension is the definition and experience of the self in relation to an other. This evolution of self and object relationships has been the central concern of many contemporary psychoanalytic thinkers (Kernberg, 1976; Khan, 1974; Kohut, 1977, and Searles, 1979). Although, from a theoretical perspective, there is a great deal of difference among these and other object relations theorists, a similarity exists in the importance that each attributes to the individuals attempt to establish a meaningful identity in relation to the other. It is the lack of meaningfulness of the self in the world that is seen as the source of the greatest emotional stress, with both pathological and healthy behavior motivated by attempts to deal with this lack of meaningfulness, which is experienced phenomenologically, as either death, being invisible, or being fragmented into nonexistence. From this perspective one's identity or sense of self, which is dependent on a human context or another, is seen as the central psychological force in contrast to either the economic basis of the earlier anthropological view or the libidinal basis of the traditional Freudian psychoanalytic view.

Human development, from the object relations perspective, is thought of as the development of autonomous, whole self-structures with the recognition of the separate existance of independent objects. This process of development involves the process of projection and introjection in which individuals exploit their relationship with others. Although one would assume that these processes of projection and introjection are fairly regular aspects of relationships, it would seem that certain relationships encourage and facilitate these intense affective processes more than others. A good deal has been written about projection and introjection in psychotherapy and the possibility of growth and development in that interpersonal field. Marriage and the family also can be seen as a special interpersonal field in which there are those intense affective relationships that support increased projective and introjective activity. In a later section of this paper the characteristics of an interpersonal field that is supportive of increased projection and introjection will be discussed; with increased projective and introjective activity there is the possibility for individual growth and development for each member of the couple. This is not a static view of marriage. It would be assumed that one of the major purposes of the marital relationship would be to provide a field in which dissociated and fragmented aspects of the self can become projected into the other as well as introjected from the other. This notion of projection and introjection within marriage will be discussed more fully in a later section of this chapter.

The evolving object relations view of individual as well as marital development can be seen to have many parallels with the conceptual systems of family and marital relationships based on systems and communication theory. It is not in the scope of this chapter to discuss the parallels in the development of these two approaches which have both developed during the same time period. It is, however, noteworthy that there is this temporal as well as conceptual parallel and it is suspected that both theories were developed in response to the inadequacies of the theories that they have attempted to replace or restructure.

There are two fundamental dimensions to a systems-based family theory. The first is that the family is an organized, structured whole that is regulated by rules that both limit and determine the behavior of each family member. The second major dimension is the centrality of communication as an effort not only to convey information but to define each person in relation to the other. The communicational aspects of family organization has been discussed at great length by Watzlawick, Beavin, and Jackson (1967) and Haley (1976). Both volumes present methods of understanding the complexity of interpersonal communication within families in which members use both verbal and nonverbal information to control each other, define themselves in relation to each other, and emphasize issues of power and structural change in families. This communicational framework has been adapted by many family therapists. The area in which it has been most clearly used has been in the development of paradoxical (Pallazzoli, Boscolo, Cecchin, & Prata, 1978) and defiance-based (Papp, 1980) interventions and intervention strategies for family therapists. However, for the present, we are more interested in the structural aspects of family and marital relationships than in the communicational processes that maintain them. It is noteworthy that family therapists in their concepts of structure are emphasizing the arrangement of multiple and interdependent self- or identity definitions. This would seem to be similar to the ideas of object relations theorists.

Jackson (1968) in an early article discussed the structural aspects of family relationships and their self-regulatory or homeostatic dimensions. During this early period of family theory, the focus was on *how* the identified patient's behavior maintained the family structure and in essence kept the other family members functioning. Jackson cites several examples in which after the identified patient improved in treatment other members of the family developed symptomatic behavior. The notion that evolved during this early stage of family theory was that the family was a homeostatic or rule-governed system. However, later workers have suggested that some of these earlier notions of homeostasis, particularly as it involved the use of the analogy of a home thermostat, might in fact have been more limited in their view of family and marital functioning than was necessary. The problem during this early period of conceptualizing family structure was that the model of the home thermostat and the notions of homeostasis, suggested that the family tried to maintain a set of specific interactions. The family was seen as rigidly adhering to a set of rules analogous to the set temperature on a thermostat. The question of how the rules or thermostat changed or was recalibrated was difficult to address during this early period. It is in relation to this difficulty that the developmental perspective has been useful in suggesting that the family and its members move through a developmental continuum that requires sequentially new adaptations and the development of new structures within the family and each of its members. From the perspective of marital development (Madanes, 1981) some of the expected critical points in adult development are the following: courtship, early marriage, childbirth and dealing with the young, middle marriage, weaning parents from children, retirement, and old age. This set of developmental expectations and stages can be thought of as an external press on the family that interacts with the family's developing structure. Unlike the early model proposed by Jackson (1968) and his collaborators, this current model views the family as a subsystem within a larger system or developmental schema.

The contemporary view seems to be that a family is pathological to the degree that the family seems to inhibit or prohibit the evolution of new structures; this has been referred to as a state of morphostasis (Olson, Sprenkle, & Russell, 1979). In relation to this concept of extreme stability or impaired development, the more creative or functional family is seen as one in which new structures, new behaviors, and new roles for the family members can develop. A family process that allows for this evolutionary growth has been thought of as one that is much more typical of a healthy family structure in that it is able to meet the demands of the various life stages through a progressive structure building process. From a notion of a homeostatic or self-contained and rule-governed structural systems, family and marital theory has moved to the point of defining one aspect of pathology as being the inability to change structure to articulate itself in relation to the growing demand of progressive life stages. One element of marital or family health can be defined as the ability to change structures and to develop new roles or self-definitions in relation to the other members of the family group. In contrast to this, marital pairs who are unable to change and develop in relation to the demands or press of life-stage development can be thought of as moving toward a state of entropy.

In the early thinking about family structure homeostasis was seen as providing a potentially steady state that could be maintained; however, with the inclusion of the press from the independent temperal gradiant of the evolving life stages, a steady state appears difficult to maintain and instead we see a deteriorating, decomposing, and dying structure implied in the concept of entropy. It is here that we often see the traditional forms of marital pathology as well as family pathology function as an attempt to avoid the deterioration and dissolution of the marriage implied by the notion of entropy. In contrast to this, there is a marital and family structure in which the members are able to utilize each other in the development both of new family structures and in new aspects of their own relationship with each other and with the outside world. In talking about this second kind of family, it would seem consistent with the notion of entropy to view them as being engaged in synergistic relationships.

Olson, Sprenkle, and Russell (1979) discuss this structural aspect of marital and family theory as involving the dimension of cohesion that they see as representing the emotional bonding that the members of the family group have with one another and the degree of individual autonomy a person experiences in a family system. From their view the state we are describing as one of entropy is a function of extremely high level of family cohesion, or enmeshment, that is a reflection of the lack of differentiation and individuation among family members. In their survey of the literature they found that this high degree of cohesion was reflected in the primary goal of 87% of family therapists which was to improve the autonomy and individuation of family members. Again, pathology can be seen as an attempt within this family structure to limit this self-differentiation of the members by instituting pathological structures that then function as a control apparatus that leads to the eventual entropy of the system.

Systems-based family and marital theory delineate various structural aspects of a family. This is a way to indicate that although not physically apparent the relationships among the family members are organized, limited, and regulated by a set of interconnected rules. Similarly, in object relations theory, the conceptual development has been toward concepts that describe the patterns of relationship that regulate one individual's behavior in relation to another. Both theories are attempting to deal with the basic notions of organized relatedness and progressive differentiation and growth that are inherent in living systems as opposed to concepts that are drive-related and view behavior from a tension reduction or reinforcement model. Perhaps because of these basic concerns, family and object relations theories have adopted and used the concept of *boundary* in their conceptual schemas. The concept of boundary can be very useful because it is a spatial and therefore a relational construct and also suggests the possibility of exchange between both sides of the boundary.

In talking about the structural elements of marital or family system, it is useful to think in terms of boundaries; the differentiation both within the family and within the members of the family can be seen in terms of the kinds of boundaries that exist. In a couple, there are three parallel boundary systems that can be described. There are the individual internal boundaries of each member of the family, which frequently have been discussed in terms of the internal differentiation and integration of the individual self-structure. This has been primarily the realm in which object relations theorists have been interested. The second set of boundaries is that within the family but between family members. Here issues of rigidity, lack of role flexibility, lack of role differentiation, enmeshment, and generational boundaries tend to be concepts that reflect the family's internal boundaries. The third set of boundaries are the ones between the family and the outside community. Here we see issues that are frequently central in the precipitating events in a family or marital crisis as when there is an intrusion of the larger community on the functioning of the family system. This might be either a result of changes in the family's relationship with the larger community or in terms of the evolving life stages of the family and its members that result in changing community and social expectations that these developmental tasks bring to bear on the family.

In attempting to understand individual, adult development and its relationship to marital development, it is important to recognize these three concurrent systems of boundaries or organization. The individual level, the family or marital level, and the social or larger developmental context in which people live, are all equally important perspectives. One of the questions that this chapter wishes to raise and possibly begin to answer is how these levels are related to each other, particularly in relation to the dissolution of marriage and the state of entropy that so frequently represents current marital relationships. Scheflen (1978) discusses a patient's smile during the course of a family therapy session and finds that it can be viewed from individual, communicational, and structural perspectives. It is clear that none of these perspectives is in fact more valid than the other but each represents a different mode of understanding and explanation that a therapist in working with the family might attempt to use. Scheflen points out how these various modes of explanation can reflect both a therapist's bias and more conscious therapeutic goals. It would seem that one important suggestion would be to use these different levels of organization and explanation more consciously and therapeutically to achieve one's therapy goals and to avoid the inherent bias in the use of one explanatory system.

The next section will discuss a clinical example of marital entropy to illustrate the relationship between the individual, marital, and social developmental levels of organization that would need to be accounted for. The last section of the chapter will attempt to integrate object relations theory and family theory in terms of marital entropy and synergistic relations.

Case Study. The following case history represents an example of marital pathology that illustrates the interaction of the organizational levels of the individual, the couple, and the social developmental context. The couple entered treatment at a point when the marriage was about to end. The relationship had deteriorated to a state of entropy in which there was little conversation, joint activity, shared concern, or sexuality and the current interactions involved the minimum exchange necessary for the maintenance of the family as a social-economic unit in the community. The initial contact was made by Mr. E., who said that he was uncertain whether he had an individual or marital problem. During our first interview, Mr. E. said that he had been very unhappy with his marriage for the past three years and that he had become more distant, less involved, and sexually unattached to his wife. He described an extremely dreary and distant relationship in which the major nonfinancial interactions involved either his wife's complaining about his not taking more interest in their home and family or his resentments about her unwillingness to do new things or participate in his few athletic interests. He presented his assessment of the current marital situation very thoroughly and in a well thought out, dispassionate, and affectless way. Mr. E., who was in his mid to late thirties, was a successful attorney. He said that coming for this consultation was the result of his inability to understand clearly what had happened to his marriage and that he wanted to decide in the immediate future whether he would be divorced.

The aspect of the marriage that made Mr. E. feel most hopeless was his feeling that his wife, Mrs. E., was becoming more and more like her mother. The issue of Mrs. E.'s mother played an important part in the family dynamics. First, Mr. E. was concerned that his wife would become like his mother-in-law: fat, unattractive, cynical, angry, bossy, and contemptuous toward him. As the treatment evolved, it seemed that Mr. E.'s view of his mother-in-law was confirmed by his wife who felt rather guilty toward her mother. Mrs. E. felt compelled to compensate her mother for having had what appeared to be a rather unhappy and impoverished life. It was Mrs. E.'s attempts to give to her mother over the years that represented the major source of conflict in this couple who both tended to avoid direct interpersonal conflict and yet had been able to provide support for each other in each of their developing professional careers.

The E.'s had been married for 15 years; they had met during the end of college and married after graduation while Mr. E. was in law school and Mrs. E. was working. After Mr. E. graduated from law school, he encouraged and supported Mrs. E.'s desire to go to medical school and to pursue a residency. During these early years of marriage, the E.'s had two children; they both seemed to share both the responsibilities and the emotional aspects of parenthood with little difficulty. They came from similar socioeconomic and religious backgrounds. In many ways both Mr. and Mrs. E. found the deterioration of their relationship and the resultant entropy perplexing. From their perspective, they had managed to achieve their earlier dreams but during this subsequent period of their life found that everything seemed hollow, lifeless, and loveless.

In speaking with Mr. E., it seemed that the issue to be addressed clearly involved both a failure in their marital development and a failure of individual development. I suggested that he tell his wife about our meeting and that we might begin to meet together for marital therapy.

The joint marital interviews focused on three issues; Mrs. E.'s surprise and despondency with regard to the failure in their marriage; the time that Mrs. E. was occupied with her parents and their place in the marital relationship; and Mr. E.'s isolation and lack of attention and affection for Mrs. E. Mrs. E. did not seem to be aware of their marital difficulties, even though months earlier after a vacation, Mr. E. had made it clear that he was extremely unhappy with their relationship. Mrs. E. felt that her husband's unhappiness did not have to do with their relationship, but rather with dissatisfactions arising from work. Shortly after discussing this, she said that she had felt sorry about her own career and wondered whether she and her marriage would be better off if she stayed home and did not work. They each focused most of their attention and energy on work issues and each thought the other was unhappy with his or her career. Most of the discussion about work and career had a somber, depressed, burdened tone, as if both were frightened of a strict and critical boss. This was striking because each had a practice that objectively was fairly successful. This suggested that the relationship had been arrested at the stage of early marriage in which the couple is coming to terms with the adult world of work.

Neither Mr. or Mrs. E. had been able to acknowledge the pleasure and success that they received from their respective careers. Their relationship had been well adapted to the earlier period of their personal and career development when each had experienced difficulties and had been able to turn to the other for both emotional and financial support. In many ways, their career-focused relationship had become stuck at an earlier period of career and individual development. This difficulty reflected both a pathological development of a formerly constructive stage in their marriage and difficulties that both Mr. & Mrs. E. had with the integration of playful and exhibitionistic aspects of their identities.

The difficulties that both reported in relationship to Mrs. E.'s mother involved lengthy visits from Mrs. E.'s parents and her guilt toward her mother. Mrs. E.'s mother was an angry, bitter, cynical person who demanded a great deal of attention from her daughter and who seemed to use her own severely emotionally disturbed husband as a cross to be carried. Mrs. E. acted as if she had to compensate her mother for this suffering and also seemed to be unable to set limits or express resentment at her mother's demandingness. It seemed as if Mrs. E. functioned as the successful son that her mother did not have and that being this would compensate her for her inadequate husband. Mrs. E.'s identification with her mother's idealized masculine self was a critical aspect both of her own development and of her marital development. Mr. E. also was identified with the idealized masculine self and strivings of his parents and focused most of his concerns on his developing and successful career. It was after both Mr. and Mrs. E. had achieved success in the world of work that their idealized masculine self structures were oriented toward, that the marriage became barren and moved into a state of entropy. During the period that Mr. & Mrs. E. had felt good in their relationship each was able to see the other actualizing and developing a significant self-structure involving achievement and masculine identity. They were, however, unable to differentiate beyond this position or role of successful adolescent son, the one who achieves for the parent, into roles that emphasized playfulness, sexuality, and differences between man and woman rather than similarity.

From a structural framework, Mr. & Mrs. E. had developed a symmetrical relationship (Watzlawick *et al.*, 1967). That is one in which similarity as opposed to difference was emphasized, in which there was an emphasis on competition, and in which relationships outside of the marital dyad were minimized because any new relationships or achievements would introduce complimentary components into the relationship and threaten its symmetrical structure.

One focus of the treatment was on the lack of complimentarity of roles, which also introduced greater differentiation and individuation. In terms of this shift there was an emphasis on the development of more sensual, sexual, and enjoyable aspects of Mr. & Mrs. E. and an attempt to bring this into the marital relationship. Mr. E. had a great deal of difficulty in developing aspects of himself that were not primarily related to career achievements and to the hypermasculine idealized self, and Mrs. E. had been very reluctant to express her interest and desire in more affectional and sensual experiences for fear of disturbing Mr. E.

In conceptualizing the structural and dynamic considerations in this marital pair from the three organizational levels or the three types of boundaries discussed earlier we would start with the change in their position with regard to the social-developmental context. Here, the change in their relationship is based on the expectations that accompanied the change in their life stage. Mr. & Mrs. E.'s relationship was well suited to the period of career development and the early stages of their professional careers. As each achieved success in his or her career, there was more social pressure or force directed at becoming more involved in recreational and social pursuits, both as a couple and with their individual peer groups. There was more freedom to be away from home and less need to provide a protected haven from a dangerous and fear inducing external world. Because of this change in the social expectations that accompanied the change in their life stage, the boundary structure between the social context and the family became more opened. As a result of this, the prolonged visits from Mrs. E.'s bitter, demanding, and unhappy parents became more disturbing because Mr. and Mrs. E. no longer needed confirmation of a view of the world as a frightening, unrewarding, and dangerous place. During the earlier stage of their marital development, the boundary between the family and the social context was rigid and tightly drawn so that the couple supported each other in their fearful struggle with the world. As they each achieved success in the world, they no longer needed this rigid boundary and became less able to assimilate the essentially paranoid view espoused by Mrs. E.'s mother. However, rather than being able to develop a new structure in this sphere, each became more despondent and overtly and covertly critical of the other.

The second set of boundaries, that between family members, also demonstrates critical problems related to the development of entropy within this couple. Here we see not the emphasis on the rigid boundaries between the couple and the external world but fairly porous boundaries resulting in a symbiotic or merged relationship between the couple with little opportunity for the development of separate interests or activities. We see a pattern of enmeshment with the separation modulated only by career interests. In this couple the communicational structure is one of symmetry in which there is an emphasis on equality, similarity, and competition. Again, this symmetrical and symbiotic or enmeshed internal structure of the family was fairly adaptive during the earlier phase of the couple's development. With the change in their positions, both in terms of individual and marital development, however, this pattern became pathologically symbiotic with the symmetrical aspects becoming more limiting and internally destructive. In terms of the couple's internal individual self-boundaries, these are well articulated idealized masculine self-structures, in which both Mr. and Mrs. E. organized their individual lives in the area of achievement and minimized those other aspects of the self that are associated with nurturance, play and admiration. Using Kohut's (1971) notions of the development of the self, both Mr. and Mrs. E.'s self-structures were organized around the idealized parent images and were arrested in the development of their exhibitionistic self with its complementary mirroring self-object. At the point of beginning treatment this couple had rigidly isolated themselves from their peer groups and the community at large and had tried to maintain themselves rigidly in a developmental time frame that had been appropriate during their early years of marriage. Between themselves, as a couple, the symbiotic and symmetrical pattern had brought them to a state of entropy in which the redundancy and lack of differentiation led to their experience of barren, lifeless inactivity. As individuals they had experienced a minimal development of their grandiose exhibitionistic selves (Kohut, 1971). Both Mr. & Mrs. E. had introjected the masculine-achievement oriented components of their parents desires and fantasies.

The treatment followed this structural and dynamic assessment. We attempted to expand or reframe the couple's awareness of their crisis into an appropriate developmental framework. The symmetrical pattern was focused on both in terms of the inherent competitiveness and the need for a more complementary and differentiated experience. The individual difficulties, the absence of a mirroring as opposed to idealized parental self-experience, was focused on by suggestions and exercises that led to their experiences of admiration and taking pleasure in themselves as well as each other. The treatment itself was considerably more complex than this schematic description would suggest, however, and it is important to emphasize that it was organized concurrently around these three systems of parallel boundaries.

2. Individual and Marital Development

The view of individual and marital development presented here is that there is an independent developmental continuum that requires the individual, couple, and family continuously to develop new structures and modes of relatedness. From this view, structures and modes of relatedness that are constructive and healthy at one point along this temperal gradiant become destructive and pathological and result in states of entropy if they are maintained beyond their social-developmental context. In our use of the term *social-developmental context* we wish to emphasize that each of these abstract positions on the temperal gradiant have specific expectations and consequences in terms of the individual's, couple's, and family's relationship to the social community. The importance of these psychological intrusions into the family system are as important as the physical intrusions into the family space that can occur as members of the family evoke physical responses from the community at large. Given the importance of the social-developmental context we would like to focus on the other two boundary systems, that between the members of the couple or family, the intrafamilial boundary structures, and its relationship to the intraindividual boundary structures or the individual's self-structures.

Before continuing with this discussion, I would like to expand briefly on an aspect of the earlier discussion, that is the psychological purpose of marriage from an object relations perspective. It is obvious that one of the great events of evolution was the development of the human family, because, as we can see in terms of the history of literature and art, it has been the ground, the laboratory, and the crucible for human development. It is within the social structure of the family, which has been referred to as a group with a history (Haley, 1961), that people are able to have their needs satisfied, hammer out and develop their individual identities, and have a field in which they can actualize the best and the worst that they potentially are. It is these efforts of expression, experience, and ultimately self-organization that move the individual from a disorganized set of experiences to an individual who can relate to and take responsibility for themselves and their immediate world. It is these processes within the family that lead to the development of a self that is intimately connected to another and a particular socio-historical purpose. Thus, the family is both the stage on which identity is developed and a unit of the larger social community. In focusing on the marital couple, we see a somewhat simplified version of the process of identity formation and growth in adulthood.

In an earlier section it was suggested that the marital relationship was one of those special interpersonal fields that facilitate individual development through an activation and encouragement of projective and introjective processes. This idea of a special interpersonal field can be understood as a function of the interaction between the three systems of boundaries, each of which are a necessary aspect of the establishment of a marital relationship.

The notion of marital entropy or the deterioration and deadening of a marital system was illustrated in the discussion of the case of Mr. and Mrs. E. This was a family that had a high degree of enmeshment and was organized symmetrically. It was our understanding that this organization of the couple had served an important adaptive purpose during the earlier part of their relationship and became dysfunctional as they progressed through the social-developmental continuum. In working with them as a couple, using a family treatment format, this marital crisis was resolved allowing for a continuation of their development. However, it would be helpful for our understanding of human development to look more closely at the relationships between the individuals involved and their marital relationship.

Enmeshment or high degrees of cohesion are ways of structurally describing individuals who are extremely dependent; have poor boundaries; have few independent friends, interests, and recreational pursuits; and who become confusingly muddy about space, time, and decision making. From an object relations perspective each member of the couple becomes easily merged, has not developed a firm sense of self, has poor self-object constancy and, therefore, has developed a symbiotic form of relatedness. It is important for us to note that from the object relations perspective being symbiotically related is not in and of itself pathological, but rather reflects a particular developmental position and mode of relatedness in which projective identification and introjection dominate as ways of organizing experience and being in the world. In several of his papers Searles (1979) discusses both healthy and pathological symbiosis and the way in which psychological growth and autonomy develops out of the related processes of introjection (or identification) and projection. Searles's conceptual framework will be used to discuss the dynamics of marital and individual development.

In a marital relationship in which the couple has moved into a state of entropy (Mr. and Mrs. E., for example), it would be conceived of as one of pathological symbiosis. Each member becomes a part of a whole person occupying a relatively fixed role and their affective tone is constricted, incomplete, and unfulfilled. The constriction frequently is related to both unconscious hatred and rage that are associated with these identifications, as well as with grief, and the unmourned aspects of the parents' lost possibilities. For a couple like the E.'s, their attempt to fulfill the parental wish, to actualize the parents' idealized successful male self, was an attempt to bring new life to their parents and to save their parents from the perceived hopeless and helpless living death that they perceived their parents to have. Just as an acting-out adolescent is attempting to rescue or save his or her parents, so in this situation, through the exclusive development of the introjected idealized self-object, the couple is attempting to save the parents of their childhood. The pathological elements in the symbiotic relationship arises out of the couple's inability to appreciate and enjoy their achievements in their present reality, that is, to maintain their self-development and still belong to their childhood parents. This leads to fear of the other's envy and hostility, which can be manifested in self-derogation or in critical attacks on the spouse.

If this self-development has not been integrated into a realistic identity or self-structure, it can be lost or stolen at any time; it is part of the uncontrollable world of the not me. The affective exhaustion that is a concomitant of the state of entropy arises out of the need to control one's hostility toward the other and from the feelings of loss for this early symbiotic and hopeful fusion with the parents that does not materialize. It is not uncommon during this marital organization for each member of the marital pair to feel distrustful and accusatory toward the other because of the predominance of projective identifications in which the spouse becomes the container for the other's hostile and destructive feelings. Entropy, or a pathologically symbiotic relationship, arises both from the couple's inability to integrate the successful actualization of the internal idealized self-object into a new personal and marital identity and from their inability to mourn the loss and to acknowledge they cannot rescue or save the parents of their childhood.

In an earlier section of this chapter it was suggested that the family and marital relationship are among several special interpersonal fields that regularly allow for the continued evolution and development of the self. The constructive or healthy aspect of the symbiotic relationship which is inherent in marriage encourages and facilitates the isolation of the marital couple from the social-developmental context of the wider society. This boundary between the couple and the wider social field facilitates the processes associated with increased affective relatedness as well as the processes of projection and introjection (or identification) which then can lead to the development and growth of the individual. Our understanding of these processes of projection and introjection is still in a rudimentary phase, with some authors (Kernberg, 1976; Klein, 1975) emphasizing projection and projective identification while others (Kohut, 1977; Searles, 1979) emphasize processes of introjection and identification. It is not within the scope of the present chapter to discuss the similarities and dissimilarities between those complementary processes of projection and introjection.

Searles (1979), Kohut (1977), and Winnicott (1975) seem to emphasize processes associated with introjection, or identification, or holding as significant aspects of the development of the self-structure. This notion seems to involve the psychological importance and developmental necessity of the self-object's, that is, the important other's, empathic identification and imaginative elaboration of the love objects, self, activity, and affective existence. It is within this process of affective identification that the other's life takes shape within the spouse's, or parent's, or therapist's inner experiential world. It is through this process of empathic identification or holding or mirroring that the self develops within the loving or hating self-object. The direction of this developmental process is independent of the process itself. This can be either a process of entropy or synergy, but in either case, requires minimally two participants. The marital field is one of those interpersonal areas in which the potential for matural identification exists and within which there can be, through this process of identification, further elaboration of the self.

Interestingly, this idea of the progressive development of the self within marriage was foreshadowed in Jung's (1971) work on the functioning of archetypes. He suggested that the limitations in the development of one's gender identity can be overcome through later development during adulthood, where one can identify with the opposite gender components and become more like one's spouse. As a result of these complex processes of identification, each spouse then can develop aspects of his or her self that had been unavailable to them in their earlier lives. These processes of matural projection and identification, which are among the important psychological dimensions of marriage, can result in either progressive, synergistic development or states of entropy that both mark and initiate much marital and family pathology.

The concept of identification and introjection has been used in this discussion both to represent a process of internalizing aspects of another and as a noun to represent an individual's conscious or unconscious self-structure. In terms of its use as a structural construct, it has become increasingly essential to discussions of object relations theory and self-psychology. In its most essential form it is not merely a representation or verbal description of a belief system (i.e., I am a man), but rather a schema that organizes one's perceptions of self and the world, one's actions within the world, and the evocative potential for inducing complimentary behavior in the other. This internal construct, that is the introjects, is at the heart of processes of projection and introjection. This has been conceived of as an internal fantasy that organizes the individual's behavior affects and perceptions. The value of conceptualizing this process as a fantasy is that it implies an active organizational force that takes into account other people, time, and space in the patterns of relationship. It has been our experience that just as individual identity can be understood through the articulation of a cure fantasy system marital relationships can be understood in terms of a joint, conscious, or unconscious fantasy that can be articulated. This fantasy, or marital identity, always has deteriorated in couples who are in a state of entropy. In contrast to this is the rich and frequently verbalized fantasy of their marital identity in couples who have a synergistic relationship. It is the ability to participate affectively in this joint identity formation while at the same time being able to affirm the other through processes of identification and idealization that leads to the synergistic and creative potentials of marital relationships.

3. Summary and Conclusions

It has been the intent of this chapter to suggest the mutual benefit and, hopefully, the synergistic potential, of combining psychoanalytic object relations theory with the structural theory of marital and family therapy. In the course of this process, the conceptual movement has been away from the experiential realities of life and into abstract theoretical language. As a way of bridging the dissonance between experience and abstraction we would like to reemphasize the notion of identity (Kernberg, 1976) as a concept that expresses the phenomenological and theoretical realities of the self-structure. This concept represents both a conscious and unconscious view of the individual in relation to his or her social-developmental context; it represents the person acting (Shafer, 1976) as opposed to being driven within his or her social-developmental context. In terms of marital as opposed to individual identity, there is a parallel process that might be referred to as a family identity, which captures similar dimensions of both the couple and the family being identified by and acting within its social-developmental context. This phenomenological experience of having a conscious or recognizable marital or family identity seems to be a requirement for a creative, synergistic relationship. It represents in awareness the structures that are being created out of the introjective and projective processes within the affective relationship of the marital dyad. Where this identity is nonexistent it is an indication of a state of entropy, and where it reflects hatred and the projection of hostility it is most likely to reflect a destructive and socially acting-out family relationship. To reemphasize the initial concept, this chapter proposes that one of the primary functions of marriage is the development of an affective field within which individuals can develop creative self-structures and joint marital identities, with which they can creatively adapt to and enjoy the full potential of their developing life stages and contribute to the evolving social community within which they find themselves. Psychological health can be defined as the ability to have a developing, articulated, individual, marital, and group identity.

4. References

Carter, E. A., & McGoldrick, M. (Eds.). *The family life cycle.* New York: Gardiner Press, 1980.

Haley, J. Family experiments: A new type of experimentation. *Family Process,* 1961, *1,* 265–293.

Haley, J. *Problem solving therapy.* San Francisco: Jossey-Bass, 1976.

Jackson, D. D. The question of family homeostasis. In D. D. Jackson (Ed.), *Communication, Family and Marriage.* Palo Alto, Calif.: Science and Behavior Books, 1968.

Jung, C. C. The mother archetype. In C. C. Jung, *Four archetypes.* Princeton, N.J.: Princeton University Press, 1971.

Kernberg, O. *Object relations theory and clinical psychoanalysis.* New York: Jason Aronson, 1976.

Khan, M. M. *The privacy of the self.* New York: International Universities Press, 1974.

Klein, M. *Envy and gratitude and other works.* New York: Delacourte Press/Seymour Lawrence, 1975.

Kohut, H. *The analysis of the self.* New York: International Universities Press, 1971.

Kohut, H. *The restoration of the self.* New York: International Universities Press, 1977.

Madanes, C. *Strategic family therapy.* San Francisco: Jossey-Bass, 1981.

Olson, D. H., Sprenkle, D. H., & Russell, C. Circumplex model of marital and family systems, *Family Process,* 1979, *18,* 3–28.

Pallazzoli, M. S., Boscolo, L., Cecchin, G., & Prata, G. *Paradox and counterparadox.* New York: Jason Aronson, 1978.

Papp, P. The Greek chorus and other techniques of family therapy. *Family Process,* 1980, *19,* 45–58.

Schafer, R. *A New Language for Psychoanalysis.* New Haven: Yale University Press, 1976.

Scheflen, A. E. Susan smiled: An explanation in family therapy, *Family Process, 17,* 1978, 59–68.

Searles, H. *Countertransference and related topics* New York: International Universities Press, 1979.

Watzlawick, P., Beavin, J. H., & Jackson, D. P. *Pragmatics of human communication.* New York: Norton, 1967.

Winnicott, D. W. *Through pediatrics to psychoanalysis.* New York: Basic Books, 1975.

3

Marriage

AN UNEQUAL PARTNERSHIP

JANICE M. STEIL

1. The Myth of Equality

Two decades ago, Blood and Wolfe (1960), in a singularly influential study of 731 urban and suburban wives and 178 farm wives, concluded that "the average Detroit marriage is properly labeled equalitarian" (p. 23). Further, they asserted, "the American family has changed its authority pattern from one of patriarchal male dominance to one of equalitarian sharing" (p. 47). It is the contention of this chapter that the assertion of equality as the normative condition in American marriage relationships not only was unwarranted at the time but continues as an unwarranted assertion in the eighties. Neither Blood and Wolfe's own data nor that from subsequent investigations supports the conclusion of equality.

Blood and Wolfe's study was a major attempt to assess the social structure of families on the basis of the power positions of husbands and wives (as measured by decision-making patterns) and the division of labor (as measured by performance of domestic tasks). Contrary to subsequent investigators who have tended to use task allocation and performance as one indicator of relative power and status, Blood and Wolfe viewed the division of labor as separate from, though not unrelated to, their measure of family power. Their conclusions regarding equality in the power structure are based on the wives reporting of "who usually makes the final decision about" eight areas of family life (p. 20). The eight decision areas purportedly were selected to meet the criteria of importance, universality, and representativeness of masculine versus feminine spheres. The inclusion of the last criterion reflects a separate but equal ideology that is in itself questionable. Scores were assigned on the basis of responses that ranged from "husband always" to "wife always" (makes the final decision) for each area and were summed on an equal weighted basis. Blood and Wolfe's measure has been widely used in subsequent studies and widely criticized by a number of investigators (Cromwell & Olson, 1975;

JANICE M. STEIL • Institute of Advanced Psychological Studies, Adelphi University, Garden City, New York 11530.

Gillespie, 1971; McDonald, 1980; Safilios-Rothschild, 1969, 1970; Sprey, 1972, 1975; Turk & Bell, 1972). For our purposes, then, we will note only the most relevant issues.

We begin at the outset by questioning whether the authors met their own criterion of each decision being of equal importance in terms of its impact on family life. Decision areas ranged from who makes the final decision regarding what jobs the husband should take to who decides how much money the family can afford to spend per week on food. There is no indication that either Blood and Wolfe or subsequent investigators made any attempt to obtain independent ratings of the relative importance of these areas. Common sense, however, suggests not only that husband's job has a greater impact on family life (certainly in terms of geographic location, standard of living, and time available to spend with family members) but also that the latter area may in fact be determined by the former (husband's job). The failure to achieve equality of importance in the decision-making areas clearly challenges both the appropriateness of equal weighting and, consequently, the validity of the final score as a measure of marital power. With this caveat in mind, we note that 90% of Blood and Wolfe's respondents reported that husbands always make the final decision regarding husband's job and 41% reported that wives always make the final decision regarding food. Food is, in fact, the area in which wives reportedly have the most decision-making power. If these areas are not in fact of equal importance, the equal weighting procedure skews the final scores in the direction of inflating wives' overall influence on the basis of greater say in less important areas. The two of the eight areas that, on face value, seem to be most equal in importance are who makes the final decision regarding what job the husband should take and who makes the final decision regarding whether or not the wife should go to work or quit work. In fact, although 90% of the husbands are reported to have the final say regarding their own job, only 39% of the wives are reported as having the final say regarding whether they should or should not work. On the other end of the spectrum, only 1% of wives reportedly have the final say regarding husband's job but 26% of husbands are reported as having the final say regarding whether or not their wife should work. Husbands are more than twice as likely to have the final say regarding their wife's working (26%) than they are regarding the food budget (10%). This suggests the validity of Safilios-Rothschild's (1969, 1970) point that decision making in specific areas may be more a reflection of its relative unimportance than a measure of power. Despite this biasing which we have suggested inflates the wife's power score by according equal weight to her final say in less important and relegated decisions, Blood and Wolfe still found the overall mean scores to reflect husband dominance.

The authors then categorized the families into four groups on the basis of their self-reported decision-making patterns. These were husband dominant; wife dominant; and, following Herbst (1952), syncratic (where most of the decisions are made jointly by husband and wife); and autonomic (where approximately equal numbers of decisions are made separately by each spouse). Even in combining the syncratic and autonomic categories, and admittedly including couples in which the mean scores reflected some degree of husband dominance, Blood and Wolfe found less than half the families could be categorized as egalitarian. In addition, with regard to task allocation, which currently is viewed as one indicator of spouse's relative power and status, Blood and Wolfe found that the predominant picture revealed specialized task performance along traditional sex lines. The median family had a completely stereotyped allocation of five of seven tasks, leaving only two for even marginal variation.

Blood and Wolfe's study of family decision making remains one of the most influential attempts at investigating the power structure of American marriages and is the paramount example of one of the three domains identified by Olson and Cromwell (1975) as the focus of almost all studies of family power. The three domains generally delineated are: bases of family power, family power processes, and family power outcomes. Studies in the area of family power outcomes (including Blood and Wolfe) frequently investigate issues involving who makes decisions and who wins, and have been the subject of more research than the other two combined.

More than a decade after Blood and Wolfe's study, Centers, Raven, and Rodriques (1971) replicated it with a sample of 776 husbands and wives in the Los Angeles area. Using the same instrument, they found close agreement in the reports of husbands and wives, and a similar distribution of decision-making types. Also consistent with the findings of Blood and Wolfe, husbands' mean power continued to be somewhat greater than wives. Centers *et al.* demonstrated the dramatic effect that investigators' choice of decision areas can have on the overall findings. A series of decisions normally perceived as predominantly feminine (e.g., how to decorate or furnish the house or what the family will have for dinner) were added to the original Blood and Wolfe items. Overall scores computed on the basis of the original eight items were compared with scores based on the supplemented measure with the result that family decision-making types changed from 34% husband dominated to only 9% husband dominated, and from 29% autonomic to 68% autonomic. If one were to accept decisions regarding the dinner menu as valid indicators of power the proportion of alleged egalitarian marriages would soar.

A study by C. L. Johnson (1975) of authority and power on Japanese–American marriages further illustrates the limitations of restricting studies of power to measures of decision making. C. L. Johnson found little agreement between the response to a Blood and Wolfe summated decision-making score and data obtained from open-ended discussions. The decision-making data would have suggested an egalitarian structure for a majority of the Japanese–American marriages in the sample. Yet most of the wives clearly placed themselves in a subordinate position. Thus, the author concluded that while the Japanese-American wives played active roles in decision making, especially in regard to child care, they did so by right of relegation of power from their husbands.

In addition to the Blood and Wolfe summated score, other more direct measures have also been used. Heer (1962) asked, "When there's a really important decision on which you two are likely to disagree, who usually wins out?" In families where the wife is unemployed over 50% of both middle-class husbands and wives reported that the husband had more influence. Responses of working-class families and families of employed wives were less likely to report husband dominance.

Turk and Bell (1972) asked a sample of 336 Canadian households, "who is the real boss in your family?" Seventy-six% of wives responded that the husband was the boss compared to only 13% who responded that power was shared equally. Scanzoni (1972) asked respondents to list "the four things that you and your spouse have disagreed upon most often." For each of the listed areas, respondants were then asked, "when you disagree about ______, who usually gets his way?" Responses indicated a clear pattern of male dominance, with a greater percentage of husbands than wives reportedly getting their way in each of the four conflict areas.

Studies in the domain of the bases of family power have been the second most influential (Olson & Cromwell, 1975a). These studies evolved from the early work of French and Raven (1959) and, subsequently, Raven and Kruglanski (1970) and Raven (1974), who distinguished six sources of power (reward, coercive, legitimate, expert, referent, and informational) and conceptualized the differential impact of each on the direction and quality of interpersonal relationships. P. Johnson (1976, 1978) reports that access to specific power bases is sex-linked. Both males and females perceive reward, coercive, legitimate, expert, and informational power as more associated with men and referent, helplessness, and indirect information as more associated with women. P. Johnson conceptualized the bases of power along three dimensions: direct–indirect, concrete–personal, and competent–helpless. Women, it was asserted, have less access in reality and expectations to concrete resources (e.g., money, knowledge, physical strength) and competence, leaving them with indirect (i.e., manipulative), personal, and helpless modes of influence. Although each of these may be effective in the short run, P. Johnson suggests that in the long run each is likely to have negative consequences, particularly in fostering or maintaining subordinated positions, dependency, and lowered self-esteem. In an investigation of marital couples Raven, Centers, and Rodriques (1975) found that expert and referent power were considered the most likely bases of influence in marriage; legitimate power was next; and coercive power was reportedly the least likely basis of influence. Anticipating P. Johnson's subsequent work, they found that wives were more likely to attribute expert power to their spouses than were husbands (37% vs. 20%). For husbands, referent power was highlighted as the most important basis of power for their wives. A more recent study of power strategies in intimate relationships (Falbo & Peplau, 1980) found that men were more likely to report using bilateral and direct strategies whereas women were more likely to report using unilateral and indirect strategies. These differences, the authors suggested, were reflective of gender differences in power in general and a pattern of male dominance in intimate relationships. Because they expect compliance, the authors assert, men are more likely to use bilateral and direct strategies in their influence attempts. Conversely, because women anticipate noncompliance they are more likely than men to report the use of unilateral strategies that do not require the partner's cooperation.

The third domain, processes of power, has rarely been the focus of empirical investigation (Olson & Cromwell, 1975a). Those studies that have been done generally have employed observational methods to study interaction variables such as assertiveness and control. An example of this type is the study by Cromwell, Klein, and Weiting (1975) which used two observational methods (SIMFAM and Kenkel) to measure each of three traits: assertiveness, control, and sociability. The measure of assertiveness was computed to reflect all power statements or attempts at influence by an individual. The control measure was computed to reflect only those power statements that were successful. Despite a general tendency for observational methods to reflect less husband dominance than self-report measures (Turk & Bell, 1972), the study showed reasonably balanced assertiveness by the Kenkel method and father domination using the SIMFAM method. For control, seemingly the most relevant measure, the scores were consistent across methods indicating a slight tendency for fathers to exercise more control than mothers.

Perhaps because of the pervasive theoretical and methodological dissatisfaction with most attempts to assess marital power, the prevalence of these types of studies seem to have decreased. Studies using other indications of marital influence are no more likely to support an equalitarian view, however.

2. The Dual Career Couple

In the last decade, there has been a surge of interest in studying the dual career family, defined as "one in which both heads of households pursue careers (as compared to jobs) and at the same time maintain a family life together'' (Rapaport & Rapaport, 1971, p. 519). The dual career family is perceived as the most egalitarian of marriages and the harbinger of future family patterns. Even among such couples, however, there is a consistent pattern of inequality in both the domestic and occupational spheres. It has been shown, for example, that only husbands' occupational characteristics and prestige affect families' occupational migrational probability. Neither wives' occupational prestige, income, nor opportunities for employment in their field elsewhere in the country affects the migration of dual career couples (Duncan & Perrucci, 1976). Further, ''when employment pressures require, the wife's career is more likely to be considered as secondary, her job is more likely to be part-time or non-tenure track, and her pay and level are likely to be less than her husband's'' (Bryson & Bryson, 1980, p. 257). In the domestic sphere, household management and work are not evenly shared (Lopata, Barnewolt, & Norr, 1980). Wives are more likely than their husbands to have to curtail career involvements in favor of family demands and both partners seem to accept as inevitable that women have to bear the main brunt of child care and domestic organization (Rapaport & Rapaport, 1976). Further, as Rapaport and Rapaport observe, tension lines often develop. In their sample, ''the main tension lines for men were in the area of how much responsibility (as distinct from participation) to take in the home, and how much occupational achievement to *tolerate* (emphasis added) in their wives'' (1976, p. 312). Despite an essentially supportive orientation, both partners seem to endorse some level of male dominance. Thus, Rapaport and Rapaport report ''Mr. O encourages his wife to pursue her career . . . but the amount of her income relative to his is a point of some tension between them. . . . With the X's the central issue is authority . . . he did not wish actually to have her in authority over the job on which he himself was working'' (1969, pp. 16–17). Wives, it seems, collude in this process (Poloma & Garland, 1971). A tactic sometimes observed in wives for dealing with the identity tension points is for her to de-emphasize her career position while in the home context by presenting it as a series of accidents or improvisations (Rapaport & Rapaport, 1969, p. 18). Thus, it seems that dual career couples are not egalitarian. As Bryson and Bryson concluded, ''They tend to divide household responsibilities along sex-stereotypic lines and to place differential values on their careers. It also seems clear that the pressures for such differentiation falls disproportionately upon the wife'' (1980, p. 256).

3. Factors Associated with Husband Dominance

Family size, social class, ethnicity, husband's income, and wife's employment status consistently have been associated with the extent of the husband's dominance. Black husbands have less power than white husbands (Blood & Wolfe, 1960). Centers *et al.* (1971) found Oriental husbands to have more influence than whites and found black husbands to have the least. Scanzoni and Szinovacy (1980) suggest that black couples may be more sex role egalitarian than whites. Working-class husbands have less power than middle-class husbands (Heer, 1958, 1962). White middle-class housewives may well have less power in their marital relationships than any group. Further, the better educated and more successful their husband, the less power wives are likely to have (Blood & Wolfe, 1960; Ericksen, Yancey, & Ericksen, 1979; Heer,1958, 1962; Hoffman, 1960). This finding seems in some senses counterintuitive since one may associate higher levels of education and social class with more egalitarian ideologies. As Goode (1963/1970) points out, however, "lower class men concede fewer rights ideologically than their women in fact obtain; and the more educated men are likely to concede more rights ideologically than they, in fact, grant" (1970, p. 21). It may well be a two-way street. Housewives are more likely than employed women to endorse traditional sex-role ideologies (Beckman & Houser, 1979; Hoffman, 1960; Mason & Bumpass, 1975) and it also has been reported that the higher a husband's income, the more likely his wife is to endorse the legitimacy of his power on the basis of traditional male authority (Scanzoni, 1972). A wife's employment is negatively associated with family size and husband's income and occupation level. Employed wives are consistently shown to be less likely to endorse traditional ideologies, to have more say in decision making, and to enjoy a somewhat more egalitarian division of family roles than nonemployed wives (Beckman & Houser, 1979; Blood & Hamblin, 1958; Blood & Wolfe, 1960; Crosby, 1982; Heer, 1962; Hoffman, 1960; Mason & Bumpass, 1975; Radloff, 1975). Among wives who are employed, most studies report that influence and task sharing tend to be greater for those who work full time.

Studies that ask who has the prime *responsibility* for domestic tasks, however, show no difference (Lopata *et al.*, 1980). Number of years worked (Blood & Wolfe, 1960) and continuity and pattern of employment also may be associated with an increase in the wife's influence but not with increased sharing of child-care responsibilities (Weingartern, 1976). Finally, Centers *et al.* (1971) and Scanzoni and Szinovacy (1980) note that the husband's influence is greatest in first marriages and is least when both partners have remarried. Thus, it seems clear that the wife's marital influence is greater when there are no or few young children, when her husband's income is less, and when she pursues a full-time career. Yet as Ericksen *et al.* point out, the definitions are loose and the sharing is at best relative. Husbands do not have to do exactly half the housework or child care, nor do wives have to work as many hours in paid employment for the tasks to be called shared. "Even when the wife is well educated and working, and the husband is not successful, she tends to do more around the house than he does, and were our measurement of role sharing strict enough to only include absolutely equal patterns, we would lose all our cases" (1978, p. 311).

4. Inequality and Mental Health

We would like to address the issue of the relationship between the pattern of inequality in marital relationships and spouses' physical and emotional well-being. It seems, however, that surprisingly few studies have attempted such an assessment. Some attempts were made to examine the relationship between marital power (as measured by decision-making and influence patterns) and marital satisfaction and emotional well-being (as measured by wives' satisfaction with levels of companionship and help with problem solving). Most of these studies found increased satisfaction in the more "egalitarian" marriages (Blood & Wolfe, 1960; Corrales, 1975; Rainwater, 1965). Corrales's findings were ambiguous though they did suggest that behavior that is more conducive to building self-and other esteem seems to be more effectively communicated in an egalitarian interaction structure. Bahr and Rollins (1971) found egalitarians to be more adaptive in meeting simulated crisis situations. We are aware of no studies, however, that directly assessed the relationship between varying authority patterns within marriage and specific indicators of physical and/or mental health. The question, then, must be addressed indirectly and from the perspective of marital roles as reflective of societal gender roles.

Broverman, Vogel, Broverman, Clarkson, and Rosenkrantz (1972) demonstrated that pervasive differences exist in societal conceptions of the characteristics associated with masculinity and femininity and that these differences reflect inequality. Masculine-associated traits are more positively viewed and valued, and behavioral attributes indicative of an ideal health pattern are more often considered by clinicians as healthy for men than for women. Chessler (1972) and Cloward and Piven (1979) argue that patterns of mental illness are societally determined and influenced primarily by patterns of gender role socialization. This view is supported by epidemiological data showing differential distributions of males and females in specific types of mental disorders and a greater incidence, overall, of mental illness in females. A relationship between marital status and mental health also exists with a greater incidence of mental illness among the unmarried as compared to the married. Contrary to the overall pattern, however, unmarried males fare less well than unmarried females. Among the married, women have higher incidences of mental illness than men.

It has been asserted that the greater incidence of mental illness in women is due neither to greater biological vulnerability nor to differential patterns of help-seeking behavior (Gove, 1972; Weissman & Klerman, 1977) but rather to characteristics of the female role, particularly the married woman's role as housewife. Bernard (1972) reviewed the incidences of poor mental and emotional health among housewives (all of whom were presumed to be married) and working women, (three-fifths of whom also were married). In 11 of 12 symptoms of psychological distress, the working women were found to be overwhelmingly better off than the housewives. Bernard concluded that the major reason for this was the status denigration that marriage brings to housewives.

Gove (1972) suggests that the absence of employment compounds the situation for housewives by depriving them of alternate sources of gratification when the housewife role is unsatisfying. This position suggests that if marriage fails to bring satisfaction the employed worker can turn to an alternate source of satisfaction, the job, whereas the housewife cannot. By extension, then, marital satisfaction should be a greater determinant of both global satisfaction and health for housewives than for husbands or employed wives. Measures of marital satisfaction have, in fact, been found to be strongly related to various indices of physical, but especially mental, health. Consistent with Gove's (1972) hypothesis, these measures seem more strongly related for women than for men, but the data were not analyzed to compare the relationship for wives who were employed as compared to those who were not (Renne, 1970). Women have been found to be more dissatisfied with their marriages than men (Renne, 1970), though not always according to Glenn (1975), who also found a stronger relationship between measures of marital happiness and global happiness for women than for men. Again, however, the data were not analyzed for differences between employed as compared to unemployed wives. Two studies explicitly examined the relationship between roles and mental illness among the married (Gove & Geerken, 1977; Radloff, 1975). In both, unemployed housewives fared the worst, employed husbands the best, and employed wives consistently scored somewhere in between. Unemployed housewives were most likely to report that they felt confronted by incessant demands, that they more frequently desired to be alone, and more frequently felt lonely. Housewives also reported the highest prevalence of 14 general psychiatric symptoms and experienced the highest incidences of depression. Yet, as Radloff (1975) points out, the dual role hypothesis can explain the poor position of housewives as compared to employed wives but not the difference between employed wives and employed husbands. The role of housewife seems to be only part of the explanation. Radloff reports further, "neither working nor happiness with jobs and/or marriage makes married women as healthy as comparable married men" (1975, p. 259). Anticipating the position we are about to assert, Radloff suggested that on the basis of her findings, at least for incidences of depression, one must consider its relationship to feelings of powerlessness and learned helplessness (Seligman & Garber, 1980).

Because the incidences of mental illness are fewer for married women than for the unmarried, it cannot be said that marriage, per se, is detrimental to women's health. Yet, married women clearly do not fare as well as married men and, among married women, unemployed housewives do not fare as well as the employed. The pattern, we suggest, mirrors the societal and marital pattern of inequality. From this perspective, responses to Gove and Geerken's (1977) measure of incessant demands may reflect feelings of powerlessness, just as the desire to be alone may reflect a wish to escape that which feels both controlling and uncontrollable. The evidence may be inconclusive and our position, therefore, must be circumspect. We hypothesize, however, that emotional well-being and mental health may be associated less with marriage than it is with the extent to which the relationship reflects, or is a measure of, relative equality of status and power between the partners. This hypothesis remains to be tested. Existing data, however, clearly do not refute it.

5. From Equity to Equality

> Marriage exists when two or more persons share expressive and economic interdependencies.
>
> —Scanzoni, 1972, p. 54

> Status must be defined by its relations of obligations and rights with respect to other positions.
>
> —Goode, 1963/1970, p. 54

Deutsch (1975) identifies equity, equality, and need as distinct principles on which to base the distribution of the conditions and goods that affect individual well-being. Well-being is broadly defined to include its psychological, physiological, economic, and social aspects. Each principle, he asserts, represents a distinct value system and has differential implications for the course of human interaction. The equity principle is associated with the goal of economic productivity and distributes outcomes on the basis of valued contributions. Equity, according to Deutsch, undermines the basis of mutual and self-respect by signifying that the different participants in a relationship do not have the same value. When equity is the basis of distribution, people come to be regarded primarily in terms of their economic utility. The principle of equality, by contrast, is associated with the goal of fostering and maintaining enjoyable social relations. It supports the basis of mutual respect that underlies enjoyable relationships and does not evoke the deleterious emotions that undermine them.

Contrary to expectation and myth, contemporary marriage relationships seem to be based primarily on principles of equity rather than equality with the consequent ramifications elucidated by Deutsch. This equity orientation reflects the institution's historically economic roots and a societal ideology that values the economic over the expressive. As a consequence, traditional gender roles are not separate but equal, but separate and unequal. By extension, then, the achievement of equality in marital relationships requires either a societal reordering of its values or the elimination of gender-based role specialization and the emergence of equal rights and equal duties for each partner in both the instrumental and the expressive domains.

Scanzoni (1972) suggests a continuum of married female statuses in relation to husbands. This continuum extends from wife as property to wife as equal partner, with wife as complement and wife as junior partner as intermediary steps. Wife as property is characterized by high rights and duties for the husband in the instrumental domain and high rights and low duties in the expressive domain. The wife's role, by contrast, is high on duties in both the expressive and instrumental domains and low on rights in both. In the wife as compliment category, the husband remains the dominant figure. The needs and interests of the husband and his occupation, as well as the needs and interests of the children, are more important for the wife than are her own. She has fewer instrumental rights and more such duties than her husband. On the other end of the continuum, equality is characterized by equal rights and duties by both husband and wife in both domains. Equality of rights and duties in both domains, however, cannot be achieved in a system that prescribes differential responsibilities and entitlements for each on the basis of sex. Consequently, role specialization, as currently prescribed, must be replaced by role interchangeability and free choice. Yet, how is this to be achieved in a society that socializes its women to be expressive but not instrumental and its men to be instrumental and not expressive? Family structures both reflect and perpetuate societal norms and values. If equality is to be achieved, change must take place not only within marital relationships but within the society as a whole. Such change will not occur, we assert, until stereotypic gender roles are perceived not only as separate and unequal; but unequal and unjust. Yet, traditional ideologies lower women's instrumental aspirations and the absence of instrumentally achieving women as the comparison norm serves to limit the awareness of a discrepancy between what is and what should be.

An extensive literature suggests that for women to perceive their position as unjust they must be aware that other possibilities exist, must want such possibilities for themselves, must believe that they are entitled to them, and must lack a sense of personal responsibility for not having them (see Crosby, 1976, 1982, for reviews). Women support husband dominance because they believe both in the appropriateness and importance of the male role as bread winner and in the importance and appropriateness of women's role as nurturer (both to their husbands and to their children) (Sanders & Steil, 1983). This belief is both ideologically and pragmatically determined. Yet, it has important consequences for women's perceptions of their possibilities, their responsibilities, their wants, and their entitlements (Weinglass & Steil, 1981). If women are to achieve equality, they must perceive it as their *entitlement* and be willing to assume the concordant responsibilities. This involves assuming equal responsibility in the instrumental sphere and accepting only equal responsibility in the expressive. We do not underestimate the psychological and practical difficulties of such a reorientation, and it is not our intent to ignore the importance of partner (Bailyn, 1970; Houseknecht & Macke, 1981; Rapaport & Rapaport 1976) and societal support. Nor do we suggest that women are to blame for the unequal position they hold. Yet, as women disproportionately bear the costs (as our review suggests), so they also must assume the initiative disproportionately. Although the process of reorientation may be difficult, recent investigations suggest that the achievement of equality may have particular benefits for women.

In a review of the literature on sex roles and mental health, Gilbert (1981) concludes that androgynous individuals (those who possess high degrees of masculine instrumental attributes *and* of feminine expressive attributes) typically have an advantage over feminine individuals (those who possess high degrees of expressive but low degrees of instrumental attributes). Androgynous individuals of both sexes only sometimes have an advantage over masculine individuals on measures of social competency, self-esteem, and personal adjustment. They typically, however, have an advantage over feminine individuals. Although the move toward equality may be facilitated by highlighting the benefits that will accrue to men as well as to women (Pleck, 1976), males, overall, "are not about to upset the status quo that provides them with such a favorable position" (Scanzoni, 1972). The reorientation is likely to lead to an increase in the number of women who remain unmarried, and will, in the short term, produce increased stress among the married. As equality is achieved, however, there should be obvious improvements for all.

6. References

Bahr, S. J., & Rollins, B. C. Crisis and conjugal power. *Journal of Marriage and the Family*, 1971, *33*, 360–367.

Bailyn, L. Career and family orientations of husbands and wives in relation to marital happiness. *Human Relations*, 1970, *23*, 97–113.

Beckman, L. J., & Houser, B. B. The more you have, the more you do: the relationship between wife's employment, sex-role attitutes, and household behavior. *Psychology of Women Quarterly*, Winter 1979, *4* (2), 160–174.

Bernard, J. *The future of marriage*. New York: World, 1972.

Blood, R. O. & Hamblin, R. L. The effect of the wife's employment on the family power structure. *Social Forces*, 36, May 1958, 347–352.

Blood, R. O., & Wolfe, D. M. *Husbands and wives*. Glencoe, Ill.: The Free Press, 1960.

Broverman, I. K., Vogel, S. R., Broverman, D. N., Clarkson, F. E., & Rosenkrantz, P. S. Sex-role stereotypes: A current appraisal. *Journal of Social Issues*, 1972, *28*(2), 59–78.

Bryson, J., & Bryson, R. Salary and job performance differences in dual career couples. In F. Pepitone-Rockwell (Ed.), *Dual career couples*, Beverly Hills: Sage, 1980.

Centers, R., Raven, B., & Rodriques, A. Conjugal power structure: a re-examination. *American Sociological Review*, 1971, *36*, 264–278.

Chessler, P. *Women and madness*. New York: Doubleday, 1972.

Cloward, R. A., & Piven, F. Hidden protest: The channeling of female innovation and resistance. *Signs*, *4*(41), 1979.

Corrales, R. G. Power and satisfaction in early marriage. In R. Cromwell & D. Olson (Eds.), *Power in families*. New York: Wiley, 1975.

Cromwell, R., & Olson, D. *Power in families*. New York: Wiley, 1975.

Cromwell, R., Klein, D., & Weiting, S. Family power: A multitrait-multimethod analysis. In R. Cromwell & D. Olson (Eds.), *Power in families*. New York: Wiley, 1975.

Crosby, F. A model of egoistical relative deprivation. *Psychological Review*, 1976, *83*, 85–113.

Crosby, F. *Relative deprivation and working women*. New York: Oxford University Press, 1982.

Deutsch, M. Equity, equality and need: What determines which value will be used as the basis of distributive justice? In M. J. Lerner (Ed.), *The Journal of Social Issues*, 1975, *31*(3), 137–150.

Duncan, R. P., & Perrucci, C. C. Dual occupation families and migration. *American Sociological Review*, 1976, *41*, 252–261.

Ericksen, J. A., Yancey, W. L., & Ericksen, E. P. The division of family roles. *Journal of Marriage and the Family*, 1979, *41*, 301–313.

Falbo, J., & Peplau, L. A. Power strategies in intimate relationships. *Journal of Personality and Social Psychology*, 1980, *38*, 618–628.

French, J. R., & Raven, B. The bases of social power. In D. Cartwright (Ed.), *Studies in social power*. Ann Arbor, Mich.: Institute for Social Research, 1959.

Gilbert, L. A. Toward mental health: The benefits of psychological androgyny, *Professional Psychology*, 1981, *12*(1), 29–38.

Gillespie, D. L. Who has the power? The marital struggle. *Journal of Marriage and the Family,* 1971, *33,* 445–458.
Glenn, N. D. The contribution of marriage to the psychological well being of males and females. *Journal of Marriage and the Family,* 1975, *37,* 594–601.
Goode, W. J. *World Revolution and Family Patterns.* New York: The Free Press, 1970. (Originally published, 1963)
Gove, W. R. The relationship between sex roles, marital status and mental illness. *Social Forces,* 1972, *51,* 34–45.
Gove, W. R., & Geerken, M. R. The effect of children and employment on the mental health of married men and women. *Social Forces,* 1977, *56,* 66–76.
Heer, D. M. Dominance and the working wife. *Social Forces,* 1958, *36,* 341–347.
Heer, D. M. Husband and wife perceptions of family power structure. *Marriage and Family Living,* 1962, *24,* 65–67.
Heer, D. M. The measurement and bases of family power: An overview. *Marriage and Family Living,* 1963, *25,* 133–139.
Herbst, P. G. The measurement of family relationships. *Human Relations,* 1952, *5,* 3–35.
Hoffman, L. W. Effects of the employment of mothers on parental power relations and the division of household tasks. *Marriage and Family Living,* 1960, *22,* 27–35.
Houseknecht, S. K., & Macke, A. S. Combining marriage and career: The marital adjustment of professional women. *Journal of Marriage and the Family,* 1981, *43,* 651–661.
Johnson, C. L. Authority and power in Japanese–American marriage. In R. Cromwell & D. Olsen, 1975 (Eds.), *Power in Families,* New York: Wiley, 1975.
Johnson, P. Women and power: Toward a theory of effectiveness. *Journal of Social Issues,* 1976, *32*(3), 99–110.
Johnson, P. Women and interpersonal power. In I. Frieze, *Women and Sex Roles.* New York: W. W. Norton, 1978.
Lopata, H., Barnewolt, D., & Norr, K. Spouses contributions to each other's roles. In Pepitone-Rockwell F. (Ed.), *Dual career couples.* Beverly Hills: Sage, 1980.
Mason, K. O., & Bumpass, L. L. Women's sex role ideology, 1970. *American Journal of Sociology,* 1975, *80,* 1212–1219.
McDonald, G. W. Family power: the assessment of a decade of theory and research, 1970–1979. *Journal of Marriage and the Family,* 1980, *42,* 841–854.
Olson, D. H., & Cromwell, R. E. Methodological issues in family power. In Cromwell, R., & Olson, D., *Power in Families.* New York. Wiley, 1975a.
Olson, D. H., & Cromwell, R. E. Power in families. In Cromwell, R., and Olson, D., *Power in Families.* New York: Wiley, 1975b.
Paloma, M. M., & Garland, T. N. The married professional woman: A study in tolerance of domestication. *Journal of Marriage and the Family,* 1971, *33,* 146–154.
Pleck, J. The male sex role: Definitions, problems, and sources of change. *Journal of Social Issues,* 1976, *32,* 155–164.
Radloff, L. Sex differences in depression: The effects of occupation and marital status. *Sex Roles,* 1975, *1*(3), 249–265.
Rainwater, L. *Family design.* Chicago: Aldine, 1965.
Rapaport, R., & Rapaport, R. The Dual Career family. *Human Relations,* 1969, vol. *22,* no.(1), 3–30.
Rapaport, R., & Rapaport, R. N. Further considerations on the dual career family. *Human Relations,* 1971, *24*(6), 519–533.
Rapaport, R., & Rapaport, R. *Dual-career families re-examined.* New York: Harper & Row, 1976.
Raven, B. The comparative analysis of power and power preference. In J. T. Tedeschi (Ed.), *Perspectives on social power,* Chicago: Aldine, 1974.
Raven, B., Centers, R., & Rodriques, A. The bases of conjugal power. In R. Cromwell & D. Olson (Eds.), *Power in families,* New York: Wiley, 1975.
Raven, B., & Kruglanski, A. Conflict and power. In P. Swingle (Ed.), *The structure of conflict.* New York: Academic Press, 1970.
Renne, K. Correlates of dissatisfaction in marriage. *Journal of Marriage and the Family,* 1970, *32,* 54–67.
Safilios-Rothschild, C. Family sociology or wives family sociology? A cross cultural examination of decision making. *Journal of Marriage and the Family,* 1969, *31*(2), 290–301.

Safilios-Rothschild, C. The study of family power structure: A review 1960–1969. *Journal of Marriage and the Family,* 1970, *32,* 539–552.

Safilios-Rothschild, C. A macro and micro examination of family power and love: An exchange model. *Journal of Marriage and the Family,* 1976, *38,* 355–362.

Sanders, A., & Steil, J. *Women, marital status and careers: Paradoxes and parallexes.* Paper presented at the meetings of the Eastern Psychological Association, April 1983, Philadelphia.

Scanzoni, J. *Sexual bargaining: Power politics in the American marriage.* Englewood Cliffs, N.J.: Prentice-Hall, 1972.

Scanzoni, J., & Fox, G. L. Sex roles, family and society: The seventies and beyond. *Journal of Marriage and the Family,* 1980, *42,* 743–756.

Scanzoni, J., & Szinovacy, M. *Family decision-making: A developmental sex role model.* Beverly Hills: Sage, 1980.

Seligman, M., & Garber, J. *Human helplessness: Theory and applications.* New York: Academic Press, 1980.

Sprey, J. Family power structure: A critical comment. *Journal of Marriage and the Family,* 1972, *34,* 235–238.

Sprey, J. Family power and process: Toward a conceptual integration. In R. Cromwell & D. Olson (Eds.), *Power in families.* New York: Wiley, 1975.

Turk, J. L., & Bell, N. W. Measuring power in families. *Journal of Marriage and the Family,* 1972, *34,* 215–223.

Weingarten, K. The employment pattern of professional couples and their distribution of involvement in the family. *Psychology of Women Quarterly,* Fall 1978, *3*(1), 43–52.

Weinglass, J., & Steil, J. *When is unequal unfair: The role of ideology.* Paper presented at the meetings of the American Psychological Association, Los Angeles, August 1981. (ERIC document Reproduction Service No. ED 2185330)

Weissman, M., & Klerman, G. L. Sex differences and the epidemiology of depression. *Archives of General Psychiatry,* 1977, *34,* 98–111.

4

Human Systems and Communication Theory

LYNN SEGAL AND JANET BEAVIN BAVELAS

For the past 30 years family therapists repeatedly have referred to "systems theory" as a means of explaining and legitimizing the treatment of the whole family. As a consequence of this repeated pairing (in schools, books, and seminars), most mental health professionals have come to assume that "family treatment" and "systems work" are synonymous or interchangeable sets of ideas. But is this really the case? As Bowen (1976) writes,

> In the past decade, the term [systems] has become popularized and overused to the point of being meaningless. . . . It is grossly inaccurate to consider family systems theory as synonymous with general systems, although it is accurate to think of family systems theory as somehow fitting into the broad framework of general systems theory. (p. 62)

Agreeing with Bowen and not wishing to compound this state of confusion, we have attempted to organize this chapter along slightly different lines than those usually found in the literature, which begin by simply defining basic concepts and illustrating how they apply to family functioning. In Section 1, important issues and events that served to make up the historical and philosophical context of family systems theory will be described and discussed. In Section 2, basic concepts from General System Theory will be defined and their application to the family illustrated. Section 3 introduces some basic axioms of human communication theory and the particular communicational pathologies they imply. Finally, in Section 4, some critical, even controversial, issues in current practice will be explored.

1. Background

Family therapy as a treatment modality is now in its fourth decade, and working with two or more family members is so commonplace that it is easy to assume that family treatment was always a viable idea in the history of psychiatry and psychotherapy. But

LYNN SEGAL • Mental Research Institute, 555 Middlefield Road, Palo Alto, California 94301. JANET BEAVIN BAVELAS • Department of Psychology, University of Victoria, Victoria, British Columbia, Canada V8W 2Y2.

this was far from the case. In the early 1950s, psychoanalysis was the established mode of treatment, and its theoretical assumptions actually proscribed therapist contact with family members. As Bowen notes, "Some hospitals had a therapist to deal with the carefully protected intrapsychic process, another psychiatrist to handle reality matters and administrative procedures, and a social worker to talk to relatives" (1975, p. 368).

However, as Guerin (1976, p. 3) suggests, whenever "any ideology becomes established, professional outsiders—'change merchants'—in the field become impatient with its limitations," and begin experimenting with new ideas. Given the sanctions against the therapist's contact with family members (i.e., contaminating the transference), there were two major conditions that legitimized treating the whole family. First, family treatment was called research. Second, this "research" was done on clinical problems that did not respond well to the established psychotherapies of that time (e.g., the problems of delinquency and schizophrenia).

One such research program of particular importance was the Bateson Project, funded by the Rockefeller Foundation to study communication. Gregory Bateson had been a participant in the Josiah Macy conferences, begun during the 1940s, which were interdisciplinary meetings concerned with information, feedback, and systems theory.

In 1951, with Jurgen Ruesch, Bateson wrote *Communication: The Social Matrix of Psychiatry*. Their purpose was explicit—to present "the broader aspects of communication, to conceptualize interpersonal and psychotherapeutic events by considering the individual within the framework of a social situation" (Ruesch, 1951, p. 3). One might speculate that the Bateson Project was an attempt to test empirically many of the ideas and hypotheses set down in the 1951 volume. A group now well known in the field of family therapy, including Don Jackson, John Weakland, and Jay Haley, studied a variety of communicational phenomena—humor, the nature of metaphor, popular film, ventriloquism, animal behavior, training guide dogs for the blind, and the nature of play. The Bateson Project is most noted for its 1956 paper (Bateson *et al.*) "Toward a Theory of Schizophrenia," a seminal work primarily identified with the "double-bind" theory of schizophrenia. Of even greater importance, however, are its more general implications for viewing disturbed behavior as disturbed *communicative* behavior that is maintained and structured by interaction with others in a social context. Jackson (1965) summarized this new viewpoint as follows: "Thus symptoms, defenses, character structure, and personality can be seen as terms describing an individual's typical interactions which occur in response to a particular interpersonal context" (p. 1).

It is worth noting that the three most important words in Jackson's statement are "can be seen," for they imply that there is a whole new way of conceptualizing disturbed behavior (psychopathology) and therefore a whole new way of treating it. This is not simply an additional theory about the nature of human behavior but, as Wilder (1976) suggests, a paradigmatic leap in conceptualization à la Kuhn, to what might be called a new epistemology, that is, a new way of thinking about what we can know. Most psychological and behavioral models reflect the traditional epistemology of physics, based on energy and the first law of thermodynamics (the transformation of energy). This new epistemology was based on the concept of information, on circular rather than linear causality, on pattern, stochastic process, entropy, and—in a sense—the second law of thermodynamics. From this perspective it is not the material structure that defines an object but its organization as defined by the patterns of interaction among its parts. So it is not the nature of the components that are important, but their interrelations.

In 1967, Watzlawick, Beavin, and Jackson delineated the implications this shift in thinking held in store for psychotherapists:

> Failure to realize the intricacies of the relationships between an event and the matrix in which it takes place, between an organism and its environment, either confronts the observer with something "mysterious" or induces him to attribute to his object of study certain properties the object may not possess. Compared with the wide acceptance of this fact in biology, the behavioral sciences seem still to base themselves to a large extent on a monadic view of the individual and on the time-honored method of isolating variables. This becomes particularly obvious when the object of study is disturbed behavior. If a person exhibiting disturbed behavior (psychopathology) is studied in isolation, then the inquiry must be concerned with the *nature* of the condition and, in a wider sense, with the *nature* of the human mind. If the limits of the inquiry are extended to include the effects of this behavior on others, their reactions to it, and the context in which all of this takes place, the focus shifts from the artificially isolated monad to the *relationship* between the parts of a wider system. The observer of human behavior then turns from an inferential study of the mind to the study of the observable manifestations of relationship.
>
> *The vehicle of these manifestations is communication*. (p. 21)

Summarizing what has been developed so far, first, and most important, all individual behavior can be understood as a part of something larger, that is, interpersonal behavior, from which individual behavior derives its meaning and motives. Although there are differences among the various theories of family therapy, almost all agree that the individual is best understood as part of a larger social context, usually defined as the family. This basic assumption is the fundamental argument legitimizing most family treatment. Second, if one is studying interaction, the focus of study shifts from what goes on inside a person to what takes place between people, the study of relationships. Third, the study of relationships is the study of interpersonal communication. Fourth, studying the patterns of communication in a family has many similarities to the kind of study conducted by general system theorists, who seek to discover isomorphic relationships between various and, at times, seemingly dissimilar systems.

Buckley's (1968) collection, from which much of the following is drawn, is a thorough sourcebook on the origins and diversity of modern systems work; in his Foreword, Rapoport defines a system as

> a whole which functions as a whole by virtue of the interdependence of its parts . . . , and the method which aims at discovering how this is brought about in the widest variety of systems has been called General System Theory. General System Theory seeks to classify systems by the way their components are *organized* (interrelated) and to derive the "laws," or typical patterns of behavior, for the different classes of systems singled out by the taxonomy. (Rapoport, 1968, p. xvii)

In one sense the formal study of systems, as stated in Rapoport's definition, is not new. Classical science had been studying systems for centuries, but in another sense it is very new. The study of "wholes" in this manner represented a step forward for the biological and social sciences whose progress was previously hampered by the fact that the scientific method was essentially defined by the physical sciences. Classical or Newtonian science studied physical systems that were seen as conglomerates of parts rather than as functional wholes. The systems studied by classical science could be understood by taking them apart and analyzing the pieces, then adding such knowledge together to generate a model of the whole. As Deutsch (1968) explains:

> The classical concept or model of mechanism implied the notion of a whole which was completely equal to the sum of its parts; which could be run in reverse; and which would behave in exactly identical fashion no matter how often those parts were disassembled and put together again, and irrespective of the sequence in which the disassembling or reassembling would take place. It implied consequently the notion that the parts were never significantly modified by each other, nor by their own past, and that each part once placed into its appropriate position, with its appropriate momentum, would stay exactly there and continue to fulfill its completely and uniquely determined function. (p. 388)

There is no doubt that this form of science—controlled experiment, isolation of variables, mathematical analysis of simple relationships, such as, two-variable relationships—was highly successful. Mathematical physics, the queen of the hard sciences, had been immensely successful in studying a large number of divergent phenomena, including electricity, light, magnetism, heat, sound, and mechanics, the study of moving bodies. As Rapoport (1968) suggests, this success was directly attributable to the *analytic method* of investigation described above. There was a clear relationship between what mathematical physics studied and its success: It studied those phenomena that yielded to its methodology.

This state of affairs created problems for the other two branches of sciences, the biological and social sciences. Oversimplified, the dilemma was as follows: The analytic method of physics was seen by the scientific community as the pinnacle of the scientific method, yet was unsuited to the subject matter at hand. As Bertalanffy (1968) stated, "Up to recent times the field of science as a nomothetic endeavor, i.e., trying to establish an explanatory and predictive system of laws was practically identical with theoretical physics" (p. 12). Unfortunately, the subject matter that most interested biological and social scientists did not reveal its secrets via the analytic methods of physics.

Biological and social scientists studied phenomena that were immensely complex. In some cases one could not even begin to account for all the variables, much less attempt to organize them into a mathematical equation. Conversely, the physicist's explanation of events *is* a mathematical one, usually in the form of equations (differential equations) consisting of two variables. When one moves into three variables, the formalism of mathematics is already in trouble. (Now, with the aid of computers, mathematicians can make approximations for three-variable equations.) So physicists essentially took the position that "their" scientific method might apply to biological and social systems, but mathematics was not yet sufficiently developed to aid scientists in writing such complicated equations. One might say this amounted to relegating the "scientific study" of biological and social phenomena to the distant future.

Other groups of scientists, known as vitalists, took a rather different position regarding the study of living processes. They claimed that there were entirely different sets of laws governing the behavior of living processes, and it was not simply a matter of being able to write differential equations for complex phenomena. Vitalists argued that living matter, and particularly human beings, show purpose and intention. Their behavior is goal-directed. This implies there is causality that pulls from the future as well as the more commonly held idea of causality (determinism) that pushes from the past. Known initially as teleology, these ideas come directly from Aristotelian philosophy, which posited final causes as a way of explaining the motion of moving objects. Aristotle suggested that there is a natural resting place for objects, and if disturbed they seek to return to this place. For example, the natural resting place of rocks is the earth; thus they always fall to the ground. The natural resting place of smoke is the heavens and that is why smoke rises. A bird flies in order to return to its nest in the tree.

Mathematical physics rejected teleological explanation. It is important to note, as does Rapoport (1968), that they did not do this solely by philosophical edict. Rather, they were in fact capable of writing strictly deterministic equations that were sufficient to predict future events. But human beings, alone or in groups, do act with purpose, conscious or not, and this posed problems for classical science. Ludwig von Bertalanffy, one of the architects of General System Theory, writes,

> In the biological, behavioral and sociological fields, there exist predominant problems which were neglected in classical science or rather which did not enter into its considerations. If we look at a living organism, we observe an amazing order, maintenance in continuous change, regulation and apparent teleology. Similarly, in human behavior goal-seeking and purposiveness cannot be overlooked, even if we accept a strictly behavioristic standpoint. However, concepts like organization, directiveness, teleology, etc., just do not appear in the classic system of science. As a matter of fact, in the so-called mechanistic world view based upon classical physics, they were considered illusory or metaphysical. This means, to the biologist for example, that just the specific problems of living nature appeared to lie beyond the legitimate field of science. (1968, p. 12)

Obviously, biological and social scientists did not simply give up their studies because their methodology did not conform to the scientific methods of physics. The problem was circumvented by utilizing concepts that were outside the realm of concepts used in the physical sciences: adaptation, behavior, organism, etc. The single most important feature of these concepts is their attempt to represent ''irreducible wholes in place of physically measurable variables'' (Rapoport, 1968, p. xvii). So we have come full circle returning to our definition of a system—a whole that functions as a whole by virtue of the interdependence of its parts.

Given this brief historical and theoretical overview of General System Theory and some of its early links to family therapy (e.g., the Bateson Project), let us now turn to a more formal examination of key concepts derived from General System Theory and how they are exemplified in family interaction.

2. Systems Concepts Applied to the Family

In recent years, we have all learned ''systems thinking,'' whether we knew it or not, simply by becoming more aware of the physical environment and threats to its ecology. For ecology[1] is a systems concept, encapsulating the interrelatedness of different forms of life that create and share a common environment. In any particular place, people, animals, plants, birds, air, and soil all form an ecological system, affecting each other so intimately that it would be foolish to consider them separately, as if they occupied separate houses.

Similarly, many psychiatrists and psychotherapists, whose professional interest was the individual person, began to ask whether it might be useful to consider the individual as existing in a special kind of ecological system, namely, his or her family. Thus, the beginnings of a systems approach to the family were extremely simple in that professionals began to look past and around the patient and to ''see'' for the first time his or her family. However, just as when a camera changes focus the new scene is blurred and often unrecognizable, one does not necessarily know *how* to see the new phenomenon. A new focus, a new language, a new kind of thinking was needed. Imagine the excitement as the

[1]Literally, ''the study of the house,'' meaning the study of the pattern of relationships between organisms and their environments sharing a common ''house.''

infant "systems theory" began to speak a language that family theorists urgently needed in order to understand and convey what they were seeing by expanding their focus from the individual to the family.

Thus, for those of us interested in the family, a systems approach is an essential conceptual tool. Learning to use it teaches us how to see the family as something quite different than an aggregation of individual identities, psyches, or roles. The systems approach to the family has also, in our opinion, made a contribution to General System Theory by expanding its referents and to the social sciences by introducing a new way of thinking about social interaction, one that is extremely unlikely to have emerged from the study of groups of strangers, whose systemic aspects are ephemeral at best.

2.1. Basic Terms and Concepts[2]

A system is "a set of objects together with relationships between the objects and their attributes" (Hall & Fagan, 1956, p. 18). When the "objects" happen to be people in relationships with other people, one of the most important attributes they have is their communicative behaviors (see Section 3, below). Thus, a family system is a special set of people with relationships among them; these relationships are established, maintained, and evidenced by their *communication* with each other. Any system is essentially a set of relationships; in a family system, those relationships are tangible in the form of their observable communication. In general, any human interactional system can be defined as "persons-communicating-with-other-persons." Note that even this simplest definition of a system has the effect of putting the "objects" in the background and bringing their relationships to the foreground. A family system is not a list of family members; it is a description of the relationships between and among family members. Moreover, as will be seen below, insofar as family relationships endure, they form *patterns over time*, and it is this patterning over time that is the essence of a family system.

These relationships and patterns make a family system, like any other system, *whole, not summative*. That is, it is a unit of analysis that cannot be reduced further. A non-systems approach to the family would be to enumerate and study each individual family member as an individual personality, with the plan of "adding these up" to form the family. This strategy of reduction to smaller units is almost irresistible, especially when, as in this case, the smaller unit is an individual person—the "natural" unit of psychology and indeed of our intuitive perception. Unfortunately, no advocate of reductionism has ever made it clear precisely how the parts are going to be put together in that great summation of the future. How will a family be understood by the understanding of its individual members? The systems view says it will not be, any more than a square can be understood or even seen by studying separately four unassembled lines. The essence of a system is its complexity, its relationships, the ways in which the subparts are connected. Systems theory says we must start with this, rather than hoping it will somehow all fall together at the end. We focus on the whole, and see parts only in the context of that whole, rather than collecting parts and hoping someday they will add up to the whole. These are the complementary principles of *wholeness* and *nonsummativity*.

If these principles make sense, they raise a vexing question: What size is the whole? How much must be included? If we reject reductionism, must we take in nothing less than

[2]Much of the following is adapted from Watzlawick, Beavin, and Jackson (1967, Chapters 4 and 5) where more details and further examples can be found.

everything? That is, having defined "system" in the abstract, it is now necessary to define any particular system concretely and finitely. If a family were a *closed system,* this would be easy, because the system would be entirely defined by its members. Closed systems are those that exist as isolated units, like a mixture of chemicals in a container. For a family to be an interpersonally closed system would mean that it had no outside communication and therefore no relationships with other possible components. They would be the only persons communicating with each other, so their system boundary could be drawn easily and it would be a boundary over which nothing passed. Obviously, no families (nor any living systems) are so isolated. Their boundaries are open to many interactions with other persons; individual members may form strong relationships with nonmemebers; and a particular family exists in the context of a larger, extended family. An *open system* has precisely this annoying multiplicity of inclusion and exclusion, so that defining it is trickier, but more interesting. A useful principle for this purpose is that of *hierarchical relationships,* in which an *environment* subsumes a system, which in turn contains several *subsystems.* For example, the extended family may be an "environment" containing several nuclear family systems. Each of the latter may contain significant subsystems of, say, spouses, of children, or of cross-generational coalitions. It may be useful for some therapeutic purposes to focus only on the main system; or on the subsystems that make it up; or, expanding, to fit the system into its next-level environment. Being given such sliding concepts is not the same as being given license to define a particular system as "any or all of the above." Instead, it sets a homework problem: For this family, define the system relevant for therapy; define its subsystems and also its environment(s). The criterion will be the influences exchanged. The eldest child, now living away from home, may still have a substantial reciprocal influence with the family; or the communication may be so attenuated that this is in fact an environment–system relationship for purposes of studying this family.

All of the above terms and concepts are focused on the first issue of *what* a system is (and is not). But a system is not simply a new unit of analysis, a container with more pieces in it than the traditional, monadic unit. (Indeed, it would be foolish to imply that no one ever thought of individuals as living in families until systems theory came along.) The systems approach is also a commitment to look at *how* these parts are connected, and this is a commitment to process as well as structure. In some cases, this process may define the system entirely:

> The open system may attain a time-independent state *independent of initial conditions* and *determined only by the system parameters.* (von Bertalanffy, 1968, p. 18; italics added)

In other words, the system may be describable solely in terms of its present process: how it works now. The broad term for this principle is *equifinality,* which rejects the "genetic fallacy" (Langer, 1942) that initial causes dictate outcomes. Equifinality is the proposition that, in open systems, the process determines the outcome—many beginnings can lead to the same outcome, and the same beginning can lead to quite different outcomes—because *the process can override the initial conditions and become the sole causal factor.*

This is a radical scientific statement. Logical scientific thought has for centuries defined cause–effect relations in one direction: *A* leads to *B,* in a linear temporal sequence. To someone who thinks of the natural order of events as a trail of footprints walking in one direction this must seem a pirouette into chaos. It is impossible that *B* also affects *A,* which affects *B,* and so on, impossible because we have been deeply taught to equate order with a one-way sequence in time. Since this is also our intuitive perception of "the march of time," it is not surprising that traditional psychological thought also has been that the "why" of the present is always to be sought in the past—parents cause children's behavior, childhood causes adult personality, and so forth. What is the alternative?

Unravelling an alternative requires first an insight into the distortion of time that the usual kind of psychological thinking represents. Take the proposition that parental behavior reinforces a child's behavior; for example, that some parents inadvertently reward their child's disruptive behavior by giving it their attention and concern, so the child's behavior continues because it is attention-getting. This very reasonable statement has, on close examination, imposed the following temporal distortions. Many different parental behaviors, widely separated in time, have been cut out of their natural context and put in the observer's category, called "rewarding behavior." Similarly, many of the child's actions have been taken out of their place in the flow of time and frozen into another behavior category, "disruptive behavior." Then these categories are put in a fixed temporal order and one is said to "cause" the other. Oddly, in this particular example, it is the category that comes "afterward" (the reward) that is said to cause the category that has been placed "before." Common sense would demand at least that the category of the child's disruptive behavior, if placed "first," must be said to cause the rewarding behavior. By now the reader will be thinking that it is obvious *both* are causes. The child's behavior leads to the parents' and the parents' behavior leads to the child's, in a circular fashion. And this is the systems view. The events are connected not by an arrow but by a circle. The arrow and the circle and the events they connect are abstractions from the flow of events over the time period under study. Neither is the "real" or "accurate" or "true," much less the only scientific way, of representing that ultimate abstraction, time itself.

In brief, a systems process approach is again a useful exercise: What circles are happening in this family? Are there behaviors that lead to other behaviors that lead back to themselves? For example, in O'Neill's *Long Day's Journey into Night,* the family members watch the mother closely, which makes her visibly nervous, which makes them watch her closely . . . until the circle winds into a spiral leading to the return of her addiction, which they all fear. The above description also could have begun: the mother is visibly nervous, which makes them watch her closely, etc. Our addiction, as analysts of human behavior, is to "beginnings" and "causes"; we cannot help thinking that it *must* start somewhere. And well it may, but it may not matter any more where it started—which is the principle of equifinality.[3]

A family system may operate by any of a variety of particular equifinal processes, and, as in the definition of the system, it is the observer/analyst's task to identify the particular process operating and relevant in a particular case. Two general kinds of process, negative and positive feedback, are the most well known. Open systems, in which input is possible, are likely to deal with that input by a *feedback* process. This much misused term is actually a description not of an individual action but of an entire system's sequential function. For example, *negative feedback*[4] is the organization of the system to maintain stability (homeostasis) and to prevent change. Suppose the child, at about age 18, begins to leave the family, which would be a major change in the system. Some families might react to the child's initial moves by strong countermeasures: dissuading the child, becoming helpless and needing care from him or her, or even labeling the effort to

[3]See Sluzki (1981) for a clinical discussion and illustration of this point.

[4]The principle by which a thermostat or any homeostatic system operates.

leave as deviant and "rescuing" the child from such an action. In some cases, where the child has not left home successfully by his or her mid-twenties (e.g., Haley, 1980), then it may be even more apparent that everyone, including the child, is contributing the essential elements of a negative feedback system. The parents may urge the child to go out on his or her own; the child does so, but things somehow go awry, and the child must be rescued and brought home again. The essential process is as follows: A change begins, is detected by the system, which counteracts the change, and the system restores homeostasis. In the end, nothing changes, because negative (change-negating) feedback is operating. It does not matter who takes which roles, whether the child tries to leave or stay or whether the parents try to push or pull, at any particular time. The system rule is to prevent this change, and a process of negative feedback characteristic of the family as a whole will maintain the status quo over time (cf. Jackson, 1959).

A *positive feedback* process, on the other hand, will increase change over time. It may be, for example, that the parents' and the child's reaction to his or her forays into the outside world is to encourage and increase these; independence is engendered by all. This eventually will change the system so much that a member (the child) leaves and the system is now reconstituted.

Two important points about positive and negative feedback: First, they do *not* correspond to positive and negative reinforcement, because the latter refer to single acts by individuals, not to a systemic process. Furthermore, either of these acts of reinforcement may be part of either feedback cycle. For example, parents may negatively reinforce (by punishing or withdrawing reward for) the child's independence or they may positively reinforce (reward or withdraw punishment for) dependence. Either would be part of and maintain a negative feedback system for the entire family.

Second, there is nothing inherently good or bad about either feedback system in a family; this depends on what the family wants and what works for its members at various stages in family life. When the child is too young, a system that pushes him out of the family by positive feedback is likely to be harmful; by late adolescence, such a feedback cycle is considered desirable in many cultures. Similarly, in the parental subsystem, a positive feedback cycle between husband and wife could mean escalating competition in a "tit-for-tat" that quickly drives them apart; or it could take the form of increasing growth and autonomy, desired by both as their family grows up. In other words, these feedback processes are mechanisms, not values or outcomes. They are part of a language for describing *how* a family system operates.

In this section, we have defined a family system, some of its important properties, and some of the processes by which it may operate. Taken together, these offer a different way to look at individuals within their family context, one that in our experience always has repaid the effort of using the concepts and applying them in particular cases.

3. Communication Assumptions Behind a Systems Approach

Just as cybernetics is associated with information processing, so the systems approach to the family is associated with interpersonal communication theory. As noted above, a basic definition of a family system, or any interpersonal system, is persons-communicating-with-other-persons. How else could they have relationships with each other? So, while the communication "axioms" to be given in this section may not be the only or necessary ones, some set of assumptions like them are required for further definition and observation of the family as a system.

Closed systems operate by energy exchange, but open systems—and especially those of interest to modern systems theorists—exchange *information* in addition to or instead of physical energy. Most of our relations with others in society are based on and regulated by our communication with them. Instead of using formal memos, television ads, and computers, families typically communicate face-to-face, by phone, and by notes or letters. Whatever the medium, we will reassert below that (1) it is impossible *not* to communicate, at least in the presence of another person; (2) all communication defines, maintains, or changes the nature of the *relationship* between communicants; and (3) the communicants (and observers) often *punctuate* their communication in such ways as to produce quite different interpretations of the same events.[5]

First, in the presence of a potential receiver, "one cannot not communicate," which is to say that all behavior is communicative, or that any behavior may be seen (by self or other) as communicative or at least as informative. For example, standing in front of one's spouse in long silence after a question has been asked may be interpreted as "I don't want to answer," "I didn't hear you," or "the discussion is over." Doing nothing but ignoring the other person (even in stranger-relationships) probably conveys the message "I don't wish to communicate with you." In brief, we are all communicating all of the time. This may be seen as delightful or as a trap, but it is our firm assumption. It is, however, then crucial to go on to make a distinction between *communicative* and *informative* events. An event is informative if, even by inference, it changes one's state of knowledge, reduces uncertainty, or changes the probability of any proposition. Thus, a cloudy sky is informative regarding the probability of rain (although the sky does not communicate with us). A useful, traditional definition of communication is "the intentional use of a shared code (e.g., language) to convey information." Note the key addition here is the notion of *intention,* a highly inferential concept most of us would rather avoid. However, if we insist on saying that all behavior is communication, then we also have said that all behavior was intended to convey something, and the door is open to arguments (among professionals and laypersons alike) about what was intended, whether this was conscious or unconscious, and who is to say what and whether. This is especially problematic when we include nonverbal communication, which does not have a code as clearly shared as verbal language (cf. Wiener, Devoe, Rubinow, & Geller, 1972).

One way to solve this problem is to abandon a monolithic definition of communication for one that identifies these sources of discrepancy. On the one hand, there can be *sender* communication—the sender intended to encode a given message and to send it to the receiver(s), for example, "I hate you." It may be that this message was not heard, or was reinterpreted ("She's crazy, she doesn't mean it"), but the sender communicated, or attempted to send this information. On the other hand, there can be communication from the viewpoint of the *receiver*—the receiver decoded a message from someone's behavior and believes this to be a message; your silence means you agree. Whether or not the sender intended to send this or any other message, the receiver got one, because he or she extracted information from the other's behavior (e.g., by attribution of intention). Obviously, when sender and receiver agree about the message sent and received, we have a third kind of communication, a *mutual* communicative act. Thus, the principle that "all behavior is communication" breaks down into all behavior being sender, receiver, or mutual communication. The important reason for including sender and receiver commu-

[5]These axioms have been adapted and somewhat modified from Watzlawick, Beavin, and Jackson (1967, Chapters 2 and 3), where a fuller statement and both normal and pathological examples can be found.

nication is that, although they are not mutual, they do affect behavior and relationships profoundly. The reader easily can imagine any number of other examples where problems can arise because of these two kinds of communication, where message sent does not equal message received.

Thus, we have set a stage on which every behavior is in some sense communicative, to the sender, to the receiver, or to both. What is being communicated, that is, what is the information being sent? Obviously, a great deal of the time, including in families, it is the exchange of facts, opinion, perceptions, wishes, and the whole gamut of information about the world, including ourselves. People talk about what they talk about; their communication is in one sense "about" the content of their messages. To this we add another dimension, and dogmatically again: All communication conveys not only *content* but also information about the *relationship* between the participants. For example, the imperative "Take out the garbage" not only conveys what the sender wants done (this is the content aspect), but also conveys a certain relationship between sender and receiver, that is, one in which this order can be given.

Usually, the relationship aspect of communication must be inferred. People do sometimes talk to each other about the nature of their relationship ("I'm going to be in charge," or "We'll act as equals," or "I'm dependent on you"). But whether or not such explicit relationship definition is going on from time to time, we propose that it is always happening implicitly whenever people communicate (which is whenever they behave in each other's presence). Couples argue over trivial matters, both knowing that the point at issue is the relationship, not whether one of them came home late or not. An offer of a ride, a decision to stay for dinner, a longish silence, and other equally trivial content events can signal the beginning of a more intimate relationship. Most of us are especially aware of the relationship implications of communication content when we begin, end, or change a relationship. But even in established relationships such as in some families, the everyday communication continues to carry information that the relationship continues "as usual."

The assumption that there always is this implicit aspect to every message is an important one, for we have defined family systems principally at this (relationship) level; for our purposes, it is less important where the child goes to college than how this decision is made and by whom. A critic of this position could say that such inferences cannot be proven except by intuition; who can say whether they affect behavior? Even more, the relationship inference could be a figment of the experts' imaginations, never or only randomly made by participants. In an initial effort to test this issue, Chovil (1980) examined whether laypersons could systematically encode and decode relationship using communication content. One group of subjects were asked to write "scripts" depicting brief dialogues between dyads with certain (varied) relationship characteristics (e.g., competitive, informal, and intellectual). Another group of subjects were given only the scripts and asked to say what kind of relationship was there. Note that, in the scripts, no one talked about the relationship; they talked about wallpaper, school courses, and jobs. Yet the second group of subjects usually guessed the kind of relationship with high accuracy. It appears that we do have some consensus about how content leads to relationship inferences, which implies that this is a "real" and operative part of interpersonal communication.

So far, in this and the previous section, communication between members of a family system has been viewed from "on high," that is, as if by someone totally uninvolved and committed to a systems, rather than a monadic, viewpoint. Our thesis is that this is a very useful way to look at communicative behavior, as an unpunctuated stream of mutually causal events. However, it is not the way that people (including experts) usually look at their own or others' behavior. Everyone from the family members quarreling about blame to the expert who proposes a "schizophrenogenic mother" has *punctuated* the sequence of communicational events, so that some are now seen as coming first and especially as causing other events. It is one thing for us to say this is a less useful way to look at communication than, say, as an equifinal process. But it would be quite another to ignore that people do this most of the time, often leading to distortions of the communication and problems in the system. Even among children, "who started it" is crucial, as it is for adult quarrels. Some punctuations can function quite beneficially, if accepted by all; for example, a shared belief that one partner always initiates and the other agrees and supports (even though an observer might see a lot of initiation and negotiation in that agreement and support).

The punctuation of the sequence of events probably satisfies the above-mentioned "addiction" to beginnings and causes. It is hard to accept that, in an ongoing system, we always come in in the middle—that every sequence should begin and end with an ellipsis rather than being cut by us into linear segments of clear cause and effect. We should not avoid punctuation any more than we should avoid communicating or defining relationships—we cannot. But we can be aware that many "communication problems," and many other problems, such as identifying one person as the "patient" in the family, are the result of such punctuation, so that the present punctuation should be examined and, perhaps, changed.

4. Current Issues Affecting Practice

Thus far, we have emphasized the continuity of development of systems thinking and the interrelatedness of its main principles. Unfortunately, there is a tendency to think of systems theory, including a systems approach to the family, as a kind of "central dogma," capable of taking only certain inevitable directions, which are embraced with unanimity. In this last section, we will try to dispel this belief by examining some of the critical, unresolved issues about the relationship of theory to the practice of family therapy. Like any healthy new field, family systems theory is still developing. Development means divergence, and we would like to show how the same premises can lead to different conclusions about practice, leaving us with many important issues to debate. Given the complexity of this subject, our examination can be neither complete nor thorough, for such an undertaking would easily fill a separate book.[6] Rather we have selected some of the many differences among the schools of family therapy, differences that derive from what seems to be a common theoretical orientation: understanding the family as a system exhibiting organization and behavioral patterns that are common to all open systems.

We will discuss three such issues: *who is seen* during the interview; what is the *aim or purpose* of therapy (the therapist's goal in its most general sense); and what is *the nature of the problem*. It will become obvious that these are interdependent questions, based on similar issues. But for purposes of examination and discussion, we are forced to treat them as if they could be understood separately. In this sense, their relationship with

[6]A good further discussion can be found in Tolson and Reid (1981).

each other might be described as a circle. So the order in which they are taken up is in fact arbitrary.

4.1. Who Is to be Seen

Many family therapists believe that the entire nuclear family (and in some cases also the extended family) should attend each treatment interview. Aside from historical precedent, this principle of practice rests upon the basic assumption that the family system is the *unit* of treatment and is best diagnosed and treated as a complete "whole." Supporting theoretical arguments are as follows: (1) The family as a "whole" entity cannot be understood in an additive, piecemeal fashion, that is, by interviewing individual family members, assessing each person separately, and adding them up to derive a picture of the family unit. (2) Having the entire family attend the interview affords the therapist direct observation of the system, that is, direct observation of family rules that for the most part are beyond the conscious awareness of the family members. (Not that they are "unconscious," i.e., repressed. Rather, they are analogous to the grammatical rules observed by a linguist but unknown to the native speaker who follows them systematically.) (3) The process of diagnosing the family rules is also a means of directly intervening in the system, since to describe and define a pattern of interaction also may block its reoccurrence. (4) Direct observation of the identified patient in the social context of his or her family affords a deeper and more direct understanding of the presenting complaint.

Conversely, there is another set of arguments based upon systems-communication theory that makes a good case for *not* necessarily seeing the entire family. First, one of the most fundamental assumptions in communication theory is that behavior, seen as communication, is defined and structured by the social context in which it takes place. Using this premise, one can argue that the family behavior one observes in the context of a psychiatric interview is just that: the family's "public face," so to speak, with a psychotherapist, in his office. Rather than being representative of the system in a way that transcends context, the family's behavior is highly determined by the context. Even if the therapist conducts a home interview the same argument would apply. One cannot escape social context.

Second, seeing the entire family has its drawbacks. The therapist may spend what precious clinical time is available playing referee to repetitious marital or child–parent fights whose content changes while the basic interactional pattern remains the same, offering no new information for treatment. Dealing with a family group is more difficult than dealing with one or two people in an interview, especially when some of them do not wish to be present, or the family aligns against the therapist. Is this expenditure of time and effort worth its potential benefits?

Third, since the context in which communication takes place defines its meaning, having the entire family present at an interview can inhibit data collection and constrict the therapist's maneuverability, particularly in the area of interventions. For instance, suppose the therapist correctly makes a simple but important observation about the interaction between a parent and child, namely, the more the parent presses for some behavioral change, the more the child resists such a change. The therapist may assume that if the parent could be convinced to "back off," that is, refrain from pushing verbally, the child might respond in a positive manner. However, if the parent is told to do this in front of the child, in a context of discussing the child's misbehavior, the intended change is, in one sense, redefined by the context as "silent nagging." That is, since the child has heard the therapist tell the parent to back off as a means of getting the child to behave better, the meaning of the parent's silence simply becomes another form of pushing. Conversely, if the child is not present during such an instruction and the parent is told to do this without explaining it to the child, then the meaning of the parent's new communication (silence) is quite different. From the child's perspective, the parent has "backed off."

4.2. Treating Problems versus Treating Families

At first glance this distinction might be somewhat puzzling. Surely, family therapists treat both problems and families. This is true. However, there is an important distinction between what is considered the primary focus of treatment: the problem or the family.

Those therapists who operate from a model of "normality" or some ideal of family organization and functioning usually think of their work as treating families. They will tend to see other aspects of family functioning, in addition to the presenting complaint, as dysfunctional or pathological and take corrective action for them as well. Many therapists of this persuasion assume that the presenting complaint is a symptom of more fundamental family problems, which even may be beyond the conscious awareness of the family members.

Then there are those family therapists who refrain from using a normal or ideal model by which to judge family functioning, who operate from a problem-solving model. Following the maxim that the system is its own best explanation, they seek to discover which patterns of interaction within the family perpetuate the presenting complaints and to plan their interventions accordingly. Rather than automatically assuming that the family is the system to be treated, they view the problem and the ways in which the identified patient and others attempt to cope with or solve the problem as an interacting system, one that exhibits the same principles outlined in systems theory: interaction, circular casuality, feedback, and homeostasis.

4.3. The Nature of the Problem

Probably the most controversial issue among family practitioners (and for that matter, all psychotherapists) centers on what is defined as the "problem" and therefore what assumptions are made regarding "why" the problem persists. Traditionally, the presenting complaints of psychotherapy patients have been viewed as "symptoms" of something else called the *real* problem, which was viewed as the cause of the symptoms. In this view, there is the usual linear relationship between the underlying cause (the problem) and the symptom. Throughout history there has been a wide variety of interpretations and assumptions regarding the causal sources of "deviant behavior": planetary interaction, deities and devils, heredity, biology, economics, individual psychology or intrapsychic make-up, and, new on the list, family interaction. It has become "the real problem."

However, family interaction does not represent a single unified theory about the nature and causes of human problems. There is a wide range of views regarding what is a problem and how it might be causally related to the family system. First, family therapists differ as to whether or not the presenting complaint is defined as the problem, in and of itself, or a sign of something deeper, which implicitly if not explicitly redefines the presenting complaint as a symptom—a symptom of a family organization that is then defined as the problem. Second, practitioners differ on just what type of causal relationship does exist between the presenting complaint and family interaction. These differences might be described as a set of positions along a continuum.

On one end of the continuum are those therapists who assume the presenting complaint is symptomatic of family dysfunction and that it serves the purpose of solving a deeper problem in the family, one that the members are not ready or able to deal with on a conscious level. This position is analogous to the relationship between defenses, symptoms, and problems found in the traditional psychodynamic theory of the individual. On the other end of the continuum are those therapists who assume the presenting complaint *is* the problem and it is ''unwittingly'' being perpetuated by the interaction with significant others, including family members, who are seen as making a logical error in the way they go about attempting to cope or to solve the problem.

In between these two extremes there are those therapists who view the presenting complaint, such as Johnny's delinquency or Mary's anorexia, as the problem rather than the symptom, but assume that it is causally related to the more general structure or organization of the entire family unit. Another school of family therapists would take a similar position regarding Johnny or Mary's problem, but also would include the additional theoretical concept of family life cycle. Observing that all families undergo specific stages of development over time, they might assume that the identified patient's problem is a sign that the family is stuck in one of its developmental stages.

Based upon these different views of problems and their causes one finds corresponding treatment principles: who is seen, how the interview is conducted, what information is gathered, how it is processed, and what interventions are formulated and implemented. Our main point is simply that these highly diverse schools of treatment share a *common* theoretical perspective, systems and communication theory, as the basis for their divergent assumptions and practices, although this is not always easy to discern from the literature.

5. Summary

Throughout this chapter we have attempted to illustrate that ''systems work'' represents a new way of thinking about the world. Arising in reaction to the constraints of classical science, in just 40 years systems thinking has grown and prospered, becoming a legitimate science in its own right. One of its many applications is in the field of family treatment. As suggested in our discussion of some of the current issues in the family treatment field, working from a systems perspective does not mean that practitioners and theorists have discovered a single, unified way of understanding the family and its problems. There has always been a wide divergence of views, hypotheses, models, and methods, all of which, to some degree, are legitimized by reference to the more general systems model. We believe this is a desirable state of affairs. In our opinion no one has yet cornered the true understanding of human behavior, and the data of most psychotherapy outcome studies suggest we have a long way to go to help people solve their problems in living.

6. References

Bateson, G., Jackson, D. D., Haley, J., & Weakland, J. H. Toward a theory of schizophrenia. *Behavioral Science*, 1956, *1*, 251–264.

Bertalanffy, L. von. General system theory—A critical review. In W. Buckley (Ed.), *Modern systems research for the behavioral scientist.* Chicago: Aldine, 1968.

Bowen, M. Family therapy after twenty years. In D. X. Freedman & J. E. Dyrud (Eds.), *American handbook of psychiatry* (2nd ed.) (vol. 5). *Treatment* New York: Basic Books, 1975.

Bowen, M. Theory in the practice of psychotherapy. In P. J. Guerin, Jr. (Ed.), *Family therapy: Theory and practice.* New York: Garner Press, 1976.

Buckley, W. (Ed.). *Modern systems research for the behavioral scientist.* Chicago: Aldine, 1968.

Chovil, N. A test of encoding and decoding relationship messages. Unpublished honours thesis, University of Victoria, B.C., Canada, 1980.

Deutsch, K. W. Toward a cybernetic model of man and society. In W. Buckley (Ed.), *Modern systems research for the behavioral scientist.* Chicago: Aldine, 1968.

Guerin, P. J., Jr. Family therapy: The first twenty-five years. In P. J. Guerin, Jr. (Ed.), *Family therapy: Theory and practice.* New York: Gardner Press, 1976.

Haley, J. *Leaving home: The therapy of disturbed young people.* New York: McGraw-Hill, 1980.

Hall, A. D., & Fagen, R. E. Definition of system. *General Systems Yearbook,* 1956, *1,* 18–28.

Jackson, D. D. Family interaction, family homeostasis, and some implications for conjoint family psychotherapy. In J. Masserman (Ed.), *Individual and familial dynamics.* New York: Grune & Stratton, 1959.

Jackson, D. D. The study of the family. *Family Process,* 1965, *4,* 1–20.

Langer, S. K. *Philosophy in a new key.* Cambridge: Harvard University Press, 1942.

Rapoport, A. Foreword. In W. Buckley (Ed.), *Modern systems research for the behavioral scientist.* Chicago: Aldine, 1968.

Ruesch, J., & Bateson, G. *Communication: The social matrix of psychiatry.* New York: Norton, 1951.

Sluzki, C. E. Process of symptom production and patterns of symptom maintenance. *Journal of Marital and Family Therapy,* 1981, *7,* 273–280.

Tolson, E. R., & Reid, W. J. *Models of family therapy.* New York: Columbia University Press, 1981.

Watzlawick, P., Beavin, J., & Jackson, D. D. *Pragmatics of human communication: A study of interactional patterns, pathologies, and paradoxes.* New York: Norton, 1967.

Wiener, M., Devoe, S., Rubinow, S., & Geller, J. Nonverbal behavior and nonverbal communication. *Psychological Review,* 1972, *79,* 185–214.

Wilder, C. The Palo Alto Group: Difficulties and directions of the interactional view for human communication research. *Human Communication Research,* 1976, *5,* 171–186.

5

Historical Roots of Contemporary Family Therapy

IRENE GOLDENBERG AND HERBERT GOLDENBERG

> But before I treat a patient like yourself I need to know a great deal more about him than the patient himself can always tell me. Indeed, it is often the case that my patients are only pieces of a total situation which I have to explore. The single patient who is ill by himself, is rather the exception.
>
> —T. S. Eliot, *The Cocktail Party*, 1949

Can the precise moment of an event, such as the beginning of a scientific discipline or profession, be pinpointed with any degree of accuracy? In the case of the family therapy movement, as in similar situations, probably not. As Mueller (1979) points out, as one attempts to decide which of several persons or which one of several dates seems most appropriate to mark a "beginning," it becomes apparent that what we gain from such an exercise is found less in understanding "when, where, and who" and more in an appreciation of "what" was begun. Whether in art or literature, in research or professional practice, the traditional inward looking view of Western man began to be viewed as too constricting without a view of the social context in which that person functioned. Typically, that context involved interaction within the family structure. In order to change the maladaptive, problematic, or dysfunctional behavior, some clinicians began to recognize it would be necessary to alter the context in which that behavior occurred. Without necessarily stating it as such—or perhaps without themselves even realizing it—they had adopted a family therapy orientation to therapeutic intervention.

1. Setting the Stage: Developing an Outlook beyond the Individual

The decade following the end of World War II frequently is cited as the period when researchers and practitioners alike began to study the family's role in the creation and

IRENE GOLDENBERG • Department of Psychiatry, University of California at Los Angeles, School of Medicine, Los Angeles, California 90024. **HERBERT GOLDENBERG** • Department of Psychology, California State University, Los Angeles, California 90032.

maintenance of psychological disturbance in one or more of its members. Clearly, the sudden reuniting of families after the war brought with it inevitable stresses and strains. Delayed marriages, hasty marriages, the baby boom, and a greater acceptance of divorce resulted in many cases in a bewildering array of pressures within the family. At the same time outside pressures—new educational experiences, new jobs, the A-bomb, mortgages, etc.—impinged further on family equilibrium. Not surprisingly, people caught up in these situations sought professional help from mental health specialists who themselves had gained recent respectability as a result of wartime experiences. As it became more and more acceptable for people from whatever social or educational background to seek psychological aid, more people availed themselves of the opportunity to get help with problems involving marital discord, separation and divorce, emotional breakdown within the family, delinquency, problems with in-laws, and so forth.

Although most practitioners continued to offer individual treatment, a small number were beginning to inquire about family relationships, transactions between family members that needed amelioration if individual well-being was ever to be achieved. Goldenberg and Goldenberg (1980) cite five seemingly independent scientific and clinical developments that coalesced in the late 1940s and early 1950s into what we now know to be the family therapy movement. These include: (1) the extension of psychoanalytic treatment to a full range of emotional problems, eventually including work with whole families; (2) the introduction of general systems theory, with its emphasis on exploring relationships between parts that make up an interrelated whole; (3) the investigation of the family's role in the development of schizophrenia in one of its members; (4) the evolvement of the fields of child guidance and marital counseling; and (5) the increased interest in new clinical techniques such as group therapy and milieu therapy.

1.1. The Psychoanalytic Connection

As early as 1909, in a trailblazing paper analyzing a phobia in a 5-year-old boy, Freud (1955) recognized the family's effect on an individual's character formation and symptomatic behavior. A year earlier, Freud had been consulted by the father of "Little Hans" because the boy had developed a severe phobia in regard to horses. Hans refused to go out into the street for fear that a horse might bite him. Believing the child to be unconsciously equating the horse with his father, Freud speculated that the boy feared castration, ostensibly by the horse, but unconsciously by his father. Freud hypothesized further that Hans was displacing anxiety associated with his Oedipus Complex. Learning that Hans had witnessed a horse falling down in the street, Freud theorized that Hans unconsciously associated the scene with his father, since he wanted his father to be hurt. By substituting the fear of his father into a phobia about being bitten by the horse, Hans was able to displace his fear onto a substitute object—the psychoanalytic prototype of what occurs in the development of a phobia.

Although Bloch and LaPerriere (1973) cite the case of Little Hans as the first recorded example of child analysis and family therapy, the fact is that Freud chose not to work with either the child or the entire family. Instead, he encouraged Hans's father, a physician, to treat his son under Freud's supervision. (Here Freud anticipated the current family therapist's use of family members as change agents.) While Hans ultimately was relieved of his phobic symptoms, the pattern of individually focused clinical intervention was maintained. As Bowen (1978) has noted, the longtime insistence by psychoanalysts that their treatment not be "contaminated" by contact with the patient's relatives had a retarding effect on the early growth of the family therapy movement.

Alfred Adler, often credited with being a founder of the child guidance movement, also recognized the family's role in the personality development of individual family members. To Adler, both the individual's conscious personal and social goals and that person's subsequent goal-directed behavior were best understood by understanding the environment or social context in which that behavior emerged and took place. Such factors as the family constellation, position and role in the family, sibling rivalries, and so forth, all point to Adler's awareness of the key part that early family experiences play in adult behavior. Although, like Freud, Adler did not work therapeutically with an entire family, some clinicians (e.g., Christensen, 1971) believe Adler's thinking had a positive influence on the modern view of families as a social system. Adler's emphasis on the relationship between siblings, and not only the mother–child interaction, helped turn attention to other family members.

Finally, Harry Stack Sullivan, trained in psychoanalysis but also influenced by some of the early sociologists and social psychologists, emphasized the role of interpersonal relationships in personality development. From the late 1920s until his untimely death in 1949, Sullivan stressed the importance of communication and other social interactions that occur throughout life; to Sullivan, human beings are essentially products of their social interactions. To fully understand a person, he argued, one must investigate "the relatively enduring pattern of recurrent interpersonal situations which characterize a human life" (Sullivan, 1953, pp. 110–111). Sullivan's therapeutic innovations were particularly directed at schizophrenia. His approach to treating this disorder, along with his disciple, Frieda Fromm-Reichmann, attracted psychiatrists such as Murray Bowen and Don Jackson, both of whom were to become outstanding leaders in the emerging field of family therapy. Sullivan stressed the repetitive nature of interactions, foreshadowing the importance of roles in understanding family transactional patterns.

1.2. General Systems Theory

Beginning in the 1940s, Ludwig von Bertalanffy, a biologist, offered a comprehensive theoretical model that was to provide a framework for viewing seemingly unrelated phenomena and understanding how they represent interrelated components of a larger system. According to his conceptualizations (Bertalanffy, 1968) a system is made up of interconnected and interdependent parts that together make up an entity. To fully comprehend how something works, he contended, we must first study the transactional process taking place between the component parts of the system, and not merely add up what each part contributes.

Systems thinking offered a new paradigm, a shift beyond the classical linear thinking of the past. Such concepts as open and closed systems were introduced; the former have permeable boundaries, allowing freer interaction between subsystems, and thus are likely to function in an orderly manner, while the latter, with impermeable boundaries, are prone to disorder or entropy. Living systems are a special subset of open systems (Miller, 1978). Since systems have wholeness, with the totality greater than the sum of its parts, one cannot understand any separate part without understanding its connection to the other parts. (The implications of this last statement soon were seen as particularly relevant to family research.) To gain insight into a system, one must observe the relationship between the parts—*what* is happening between them—rather than focus on each part separately or search for *why* whatever is happening really is taking place. This last point—to pay attention to what transpires in the present—would become particularly germane to the later practice of family therapy.

2. The 1950s: I. Schizophrenia Research

At least four major research groups, along with a number of individual theorists, researchers, and practitioners, launched programs in the early 1950s, primarily investigating what role the family played in the etiology of schizophrenia in one of its members. Working independently at first, they did not really become aware of each other's research endeavors until late in the decade—1957—when a number of schizophrenic-family researchers met together for the first time at a national convention of the American Orthopsychiatric Association.

2.1. Bateson and the Palo Alto Group

An anthropologist by training and experience, Gregory Bateson had been attracted to the ideas of Norbert Weiner, the eminent cyberneticist, immediately after World War II. They participated together in a series of conferences sponsored by the Macy Foundation and a number of seminal ideas in systems and communication theory arose (Stanton, 1981). Bateson soon joined the Langley Porter Neuropsychiatric Institute in San Francisco as a research associate and, in 1952, in connection with the Palo Alto VA Hospital, he was awarded a grant to study patterns and paradoxes of communication in animals as well as humans. Soon he was joined by Jay Haley, then a graduate student studying communication, and John Weakland, a former chemical engineer with training in cultural anthropology; soon Don Jackson, a psychiatrist experienced in working with schizophrenics and their families, signed on as consultant to the research project. From this project, in which the ideas of cybernetics and schizophrenic-family communications patterns became interrelated, emerged the breakthrough double-bind theory of schizophrenia (Bateson, Jackson, Haley, & Weakland, 1956).

According to this theory, a double-bind situation is one in which a person receives contradictory messages from the same individual; he or she is called upon to make some response, but is doomed to failure whatever he or she chooses. As Haley (1976a) was later to put it, schizophrenia was conceptualized as resulting from children caught in paradoxical situations by a parent who "is driven not only to punish the children's demand for love, but also to punish any indication which the child may give that he knows that he is not loved" (p. 67).

Although remaining on as a consultant to the Bateson project, Jackson, the clinician, set up the Mental Research Institute in 1959 to more closely study family intervention strategies for treating schizophrenics. In that same year, Virginia Satir, a social worker at the Chicago Psychiatric Institute, sought out Jackson—she had been advised to do so by Murray Bowen (Guerin, 1976)—and quickly became a key figure in the emerging family therapy movement.

2.2. Lidz and Pathological Families

Initially unaware of the work of Bateson's group, Theodore Lidz and his associates (Stephen Fleck, Alice Cornelison, and Dorothy Terry) at Yale adopted a psychoanalytic position in studying a small group of young hospitalized schizophrenics and their families. They viewed schizophrenia as a ''deficiency disease'' resulting from the family's failure to provide the essentials for integrated personality development. More specifically, they pointed to the parents' (usually the mother's) own arrested development as leading to the inability to meet the child's nurturance needs. As a result, the child experiences profound insecurity and is unable, as an adult, to achieve any sense of autonomy or clear role differentiation. Lidz argued that it was the psychodynamics of each of the parents that causes the pathological family system primarily responsible for the development of schizophrenic behavior in their child.

In particular, Lidz and his associates (Lidz, Cornelison, Fleck, & Terry, 1957) described two patterns of chronic marital discord characteristic of families of schizophrenics. In one (labeled ''marital schism'') there is disharmony, the undermining of one another, and frequent threats of divorce. In the other (''marital skew'') serious psychological disturbance in one parent dominates the household, and mutually destructive patterns exist, although the family pretends the home situation is normal. Their research indicated that marital schism often preceded schizophrenia in a daughter and marital skew was often an antecedent of schizophrenia in a son.

2.3. Bowen and Family Systems

Psychoanalytic in his early orientation, Murray Bowen began his research on schizophrenia and the family in the early 1950s by zeroing in on the mother–child symbiotic relationship. By the time he moved to the National Institute of Mental Health near Washington, D.C., in the mid-1950s, Bowen started hospitalizing the entire family for six months or more in order to study their stereotyped role designations and restrictive interactive patterns. Although the project initially provided separate therapists for each family member, families soon were seen together and progress was correspondingly more rapid. In a short while individual psychotherapy was discontinued and all new families were seen together as a group (Bowen, 1960). Seen from today's perspective as the ''Camelot of family research'' (Guerin, 1976, p. 9), the highly innovative project failed to win NIMH administrative support, and by 1956 Bowen moved to nearby Georgetown University. However, the sudden death of his sponsor there resulted in Bowen failing to move his staff and the project to the new setting, so that the promising research was terminated. Nonetheless, Bowen continued at Georgetown, training family therapists, carrying out research, and formulating a set of theories of family development and family therapy.

Bowen pointed out the emotional distance between the parents of schizophrenics. Terming the situation ''emotional divorce,'' he described the relationships as first vacillating between overcloseness and overdistance before eventually becoming fixed at an emotional distance. He observed that typically their single area of joint activity was the rearing of children, particularly those who seemed helpless, needy, and psychologically disturbed. Bowen proposed the intriguing notion—it later came to be known as his three generation hypothesis—that schizophrenia is a process spanning at least three generations. According to his formulations, one, or more likely, both parents of a schizophrenic are troubled, immature persons who have themselves experienced serious emotional conflicts with their own parents and now are subjecting one of their offspring to similar conflict situations. Bowen first reported on his work at the 1957 Ortho meetings and has remained perhaps the leading theoretician in the family therapy movement.

2.4. Wynne and Pseudomutuality

Succeeding Bowen at the family section at NIMH, Lyman Wynne and his associates (Margaret Singer, Christopher Beels, Irving Ryckoff, Juliana Day, and Stanley Hirsch) were interested particularly in how individual identities are formed within a family. Having been trained in social psychology as well as psychiatry, Wynne was particularly intrigued by the parallel (and sometimes conflicting) needs of a child to develop a sense of personal identity and at the same time develop intimate relationships with others within the family. Through the study of the family organization of schizophrenics, the Wynne group observed that the members often related to one another by pseudomutuality (Wynne, Ryckoff, Day, & Hirsch, 1958). By this they meant that family members made a determined attempt to maintain the appearance of an open relationship where there was mutual understanding, but in fact maintained great distance between one another. What they do have in common, observed Wynne, was a series of shared maneuvers designed to defend against pervasive feelings of meaninglessness and emptiness among all family members.

The schizophrenic fails to develop a clear self-identity largely because of the blurred, ambiguous, and confused communication patterns within the family. To be a member of a pseudomutual family is to become disoriented and lose one's boundaries. As a consequence, according to these investigations, the role structure within the family becomes rigidified, the schizophrenic remains dependent on his or her assigned place, and finally is caught up in the family pathology and cannot escape. Involvement within one's family becomes all-encompassing, so that the schizophrenic, with a poor sense of self, ultimately fears outside relationships, preferring the familiar enclosed and safe family boundaries. Wynne's focus on family role relationships led to further research with families of schizophrenics, an area where he continues to be productive in his present post at the University of Rochester Medical School.

3. The 1950s: II. Treating Troubled Families

Beyond these four major groups, led by Bateson, Lidz, Bowen, and Wynne, several key individuals in the 1950s deserve inclusion as being among the founders of family therapy. Christian Midelfort (1957), a staff psychiatrist in a small Wisconsin community hospital, delivered a paper to the 1952 American Psychiatric Association convention on his experiences working with relatives of psychiatric patients who were hospitalized or receiving outpatient treatment. Unfortunately, Midelfort's pioneering efforts are all but forgotten by most present-day family therapists, since his geographic isolation kept him from the mainstream of activity and exchange of ideas and techniques taking place late in the decade. Similarly, Laing and Esterton (1970) in England reported on 11 schizophrenics, focusing on the destructive role played by their family's transactional patterns; here, too, however, while he produced a popular idea particularly appealing to those who designated themselves as radical therapists, Laing's geographic remoteness and iconoclastic views of treatment prevented an intimate role in the burgeoning American family therapy.

Three pioneers—John Bell, Nathan Ackerman, and Carl Whitaker—do stand out as highly influential. Bell (1961), a psychologist, and Ackerman (1958), a child psychiatrist, independently produced the founding documents for the new profession. In a frequently told story, Bell, while visiting the Tavistock Clinic in London in 1951, was told that John

Bowlby, a British psychiatrist, was experimenting with having entire families come to see him. Mistakenly believing Bowlby was treating the entire family—he actually had seen the family members individually and only occasionally together—Bell began treating whole families together once back in the United States. His groundbreaking monograph, which unfortunately for him was not published until 1961, detailed some of the first known experiences in family therapy.

Ackerman, trained in psychoanalysis, saw the family as a system of interacting personalities. His approach to treatment involved simultaneous intervention at several levels: the internal personality organization of each member, the dynamics of family role adaptation, the behavior of the family as an ongoing social system. In one sense, Ackerman represents a bridge between psychoanalysis, and its concern with uncovering and working through individual unresolved intrapsychic conflicts, and systems theory, with its view of the family as made up of interacting units caught up in recurring, predictable transactional patterns. As Ackerman saw it, an individual's symptoms, in family terms, was a unit of interpersonal behavior reflected in a constellation of shared family conflict, anxiety, and defense. He focused particularly on a family's "interlocking pathologies," the various disabilities within the family that are dependent on each other for expression and control. Working primarily with nonschizophrenic families (unlike most of his colleagues during the 1950s), he founded the Family Institute in New York City to provide clinical services as well as train future family therapists.

Carl Whitaker, a psychiatrist, had worked at Oak Ridge, Tennessee, during World War II, and began at that time occasionally to include other family members in his therapy sessions with his patients. Moving on to Emory University in Atlanta, where for a brief period he worked with schizophrenics and their families, he then turned his attention to working with couples together (Whitaker, 1958). Claiming to be atheoretical in outlook, Whitaker increasingly attempted a number of innovative techniques (e.g., cotherapy, the inclusion of intergenerational members) stemming largely from an experiential viewpoint. That is, he emphasized the therapist's use of self to make an impact and help the family achieve a more caring, more intimate set of relationships among its members. Difficult to classify because of his irreverent style, Whitaker nevertheless was a key figure by the late 1950s, having gained further recognition for including extended family members in the family therapy process.

4. The 1960s: The Rush to Practice

By the early 1960s, many therapists, trained to work with individuals, were beginning to take notice of family therapy. Attention began to be paid not only to the introduction of another new therapeutic technique—there were many new approaches being proposed during that period—but also to the paradigmatic shift in thinking this approach required. As Haley (1971) later noted, adopting the family therapy perspective meant no longer seeing symptoms or problematic behavior emanating from a single "sick" individual. Instead, dysfunctional behavior was to be viewed as the product of a dysfunctional relationship. The symptom bearer—the "identified patient"—was merely expressing the family's disequilibrium. As Satir (1967) put it, that person's symptoms were a message that he or she is distorting self-growth in order to try to alleviate "family pain." The goal of treatment, then, was to change the family's interaction patterns. Put another way, the family therapist's message was that treatment goals needed to shift from changing the person to changing the sequences of behavior between persons.

In 1962, Ackerman in New York and Jackson in Palo Alto together founded the first, and still the most influential, journal in the field, *Family Process,* with Jay Haley as its first editor. From the start, the journal was a unifying influence, bringing various family therapists in closer touch with what each was doing in research and practice. A number of national conferences (e.g., Boszormenyi-Nagy & Framo, 1965; Zuk & Boszormenyi-Nagy, 1967) followed and family therapy was becoming a recognized part of most psychiatric and psychological annual meetings. As Bowen (1976) later recalled, many of these conferences were characterized by the presentation by dozens of new therapists eager to describe clinical intervention techniques now involving entire families. This rush to practice before adequate research underpinnings or any comprehensive conceptual formulations were available characterized the 1960s. In what Bowen (1976) refers to as "therapeutic evangelism," a multitude of therapeutic methods and procedures were introduced. In their therapeutic zeal, oblivious to theory, many therapists simply grafted some familiar concepts of individual psychotherapy, and especially psychoanalysis, onto understanding and dealing with family dilemmas.

Perhaps the one noteworthy exception to practice over theory and research among family therapists during this period was the effort by Salvador Minuchin and his associates (Minuchin, Montalvo, Guerney, Rosman, & Schumer, 1967) to study the structure of urban slum families and develop innovative clinical techniques for successful therapeutic intervention. Supported by a federal grant, at a time of exciting social change and experimentation taking place in the United States, Minuchin's group set out to study the communication patterns and interaction patterns among 12 low socioeconomic families with delinquent children. Were there special ways of conceptualizing the problems of these poor, unstable, disorganized families? Did family therapy offer any practical solutions to the urgent day-to-day survival problems generated by their dire circumstances?

Of the 12 families studied, Minuchin found that more than three-fourths had no fathers or stable father-figures, forcing the mother to head the single-parent family. Typically, verbal communication was sparse. In those families with the father present, he was considered a peripheral member and rarely spoke with his wife. Similarly, the children communicated little with each other, although each child might talk to the mother. Minuchin and his associates distinguished two types of family interaction patterns: enmeshed (intertwined and overinvolved in each other's lives) and disengaged (isolated and unrelated to one another, in which parents abdicated authority). The extremes of each position (or continued alteration between the two) seemed to characterize relationships within these families. If the mother was available for nurturant needs, she tended to become anxious when called on to provide guidance or exercise control. Thirty weekly family therapy sessions, aimed at action rather than insight, and at integrating feelings and behavior rather than merely expressing feelings, resulted in improved structural changes in seven of the families. In general, they tended to be better able to explore alternate ways of coping with family stress and to interact without going to either extreme of enmeshment or disengagement. A greater range of emotional expression developed. Parents accepted their roles more readily, and they showed improved guidance and control over their children.

Minuchin's work with impoverished, multiproblem families at the Wiltwyck School in New York as well as in the project reported above led him into developing his theories on the importance of understanding the family structure and process as well as developing more concrete, here and now therapeutic techniques for reaching the entire family that did not require a high level of verbal sophistication. In 1965 he became director of the

Philadelphia Child Guidance Clinic, working primarily with working-class families. Soon he invited Jay Haley from Palo Alto to join him and together with others developed in more detail the structural approach to understanding and treating families of various socioeconomic strata (Minuchin, 1974).

As the 1960s grew to a close, interest and enthusiasm for family therapy was widespread, and numerous well attended regional meetings and workshops were taking place, not only in the United States, but in Canada, England, Israel, Italy, Australia, West Germany, and elsewhere. Satir's 1967 book, *Conjoint Family Therapy,* did much to popularize the approach, and Haley and Hoffman (1967) offered *Techniques of Family Therapy* in which a number of leading practitioners (e.g., Satir, Jackson, Whitaker) presented verbatim transcripts of their family therapy interviews and then answered questions about their theoretical positions and intervention procedures. Freestanding family therapy institutes (e.g., Chicago Family Institute) or those connected with hospitals (e.g., Family Studies Section of Bronx State Hospital, affiliated with the Albert Einstein College of Medicine) were established in major cities. In 1967, Mara Palazzoli-Selvini, initially influenced by the work of Wynne and his associates on communication patterns within families with a schizophrenic member, established the Institute for Family Study in Milan, Italy, later to become an influential force in family therapy, which employed paradoxical techniques, particularly with anoretic children (Palazzoli-Selvini, 1970).

5. The 1970s: Innovation and Self-Examination

Technique continued to outdistance theory into the 1970s, as various innovative practitioners developed and demonstrated a number of worthwhile methods for working with families on videotape and in front of students and colleagues worldwide. These methods included: treating several families simultaneously as in multiple family therapy (Laqueur, 1976); visiting families occasionally or regularly for therapy sessions at home (Speck, 1964); bringing families together for an intensive, crisis-focused two days of continuing interaction with a team of mental health professionals, as in multiple impact therapy (MacGregor, Ritchie, Serrano, & Schuster, 1964); working in the home with a family group, including the extended family members, friends, neighbors, employers, and so on, as in network therapy (Speck & Attneave, 1973); utilizing behavior modification principles for changing family interactive patterns (LeBow, 1972); brief therapy focusing on specific problem resolution (Weakland, Fisch, Watzlawick, & Bodin, 1974); outpatient family crisis intervention in place of hospitalizing a disturbed, scapegoated member (Langsley, Pittman, Machotka, & Flomenhaft, 1968); and many more. Videotaping family therapy sessions for immediate playback to family members (Alger, 1976) and using a family sculpturing and choreography technique, showing physically and visually through poses how each person sees each other rather than using words to do so (Papp, 1976), seem to be especially promising new ideas for diagnosing and changing dysfunctional family patterns.

At the same time, some efforts at conceptualizing what was transpiring in the still relatively new field of family therapy were bearing fruit. The Group for the Advancement of Psychiatry (1970) survey of a broad sample of family therapists found the majority to be young, dissatisfied with the results of individual treatment, and looking for a more efficient method of therapeutic intervention. When asked to indicate their primary and secondary goals from among eight classes of possible goals, over 90% of the 290 respondents listed "improved communication" within the family as their primary goal; not a single respondent said it was rarely or never a goal. However, improvement in individual task performance or individual symptomatic improvement was more likely to be a secondary goal. This indicates that these goals had by no means been abandoned, but that change in only part of a family was given less emphasis than such family-wide change as improved communication. These therapists ranked the following as most influential: Satir, Ackerman, Jackson, Haley, Bowen, Wynne, Bateson, Bell, and Boszormenyi-Nagy.

No single approach to family therapy had yet gained ascendance, although the systems-based ideology appeared to be attracting more and more adherents over the psychoanalytic perspective, particularly after Ackerman's death in 1971. Although it was still too soon to say that various viewpoints had hardened into "schools," several clusters, each with a unique viewpoint, were appearing. Goldenberg and Goldenberg (1980) have classified these as: psychodynamic (Ackerman, Bowen, Framo, Borzormenyi-Nagy, and Whitaker); communications and the "strategic" approach (Jackson, Haley, Satir, Watzlawick, Erickson, Zuk, Hoffman, and Palazzoli-Selvini); "structural" (Minuchin, Kantor, Stanton, Aponte, Montalvo); and behavioral (Stuart, Liberman, Patterson, and Jacobson).

Two parallel developments must take place before any set of therapeutic procedures can gain scientific respectability: (1) There must exist some cogent body of theory operationally stated and put into a form where its hypotheses can be tested, and (2) the effectiveness of the approach must be systematically researched and established. A number of attempts at theory building took place during the seventies, as several master family therapists presented the theoretical underpinnings of their particular methods. Minuchin's (1974) exposition of the structural theory, Bell's (1975) and Bowen's (1978) collection of papers outlining their social psychological and systems approaches, respectively, Watzlawick, Weakland, and Fisch's (1974) use of paradox and other strategies for achieving change, Haley's (1976) problem-focused approach and Napier and Whitaker's (1978) discussion of their experiential methods stand out particularly for their clarity of presentation and contribution to theory-building.

As for outcome research, Wells, Dilkes, and Trevelli (1972) were able to locate only 18 such studies published between 1950 and 1970. Of these, only two met their meager search criteria for adequately designed research (i.e., three or more families included and outcome measures explicity stated). Most either lacked a "no treatment" control group against which to compare changes in the experimental group undergoing family therapy, failed to use independent judges to evaluate change, or did not provide pre- and post-therapy measurements. A later survey (Wells & Dezen, 1978) was somewhat more encouraging, in that 20 adequately designed nonbehavioral family therapy projects were found. To these must be added the increased involvement of behaviorists in family therapy and their generally careful objective measures of attitude and behavior changes within a family. Gurman and Kniskern's (1978) broader survey of both marital and family therapy outcome investigations turned up 200 such adequate studies (after a search of close to 5,000 published studies). Their data indicate an overall improvement rate of two-thirds of all cases. These results are persuasive enough for them to question the value of seeing individuals separately for marital problems. In addition, their results indicated that "every study to date that has compared family therapy with other types of treatment has shown family therapy to be equal or superior" (p. 835.)

Despite these encouraging words, however, family therapy outcome research is still in its infancy. As Wells and Dezen (1978) pointed out, most family therapy approaches, in some instance led by major figures[1] in the field, "have never submitted their methods to empirical testing and, indeed, seem oblivious to such a need" (p. 266). Such systematic evaluations need to be given the highest priority in the 1980s.

6. The 1980s: The Professionalization of Family Therapy

Now into its "over-thirty" adult years, the family therapy movement is showing many signs of maturity, respectability, and prosperity. Two professional organizations now exist, the American Association for Marriage and Family Therapy (AAMFT) and the American Family Therapy Association (AFTA). The former, in existence since 1942 (when it was called the American Association of Marriage Counselors), grew enormously during the seventies—from less than 1,000 members in 1970 to over 7,500 by 1979, an increase of 777%. Its members come from a variety of related disciplines—psychologists, physicians, educators, social workers, clergymen, lawyers. The AFTA, organized in 1977, is a far smaller group of selected senior members working in the family therapy field.

Another perspective on the rapid growth of the field might be glimpsed from the number of publications that have begun within the last 20 years. In addition to *Family Process,* there are the *Journal of Marital and Family Therapy* (formerly the *Journal of Marriage and Family Counseling*), *Family Therapy, Family Coordinator, American Journal of Family Therapy, Journal of Family Therapy, International Journal of Family Therapy, Journal of Sex and Marital Therapy, Journal of Marriage and the Family, Journal of Divorce, Alternate Life Styles, Australian Journal of Family Therapy,* and others in at least half a dozen other languages.

Family therapy has become an international movement, as clinicians lecture and demonstrate techniques throughout the world, international congresses are held regularly, and professionals visit their colleagues in other countries to learn about advances and exchange ideas. Training in family therapy, now an integral part of most clinical training programs and family institutes, offering training along with clinical services, has become more prevalent, particularly in large cities. Both the AAMFT and the AFTA have become interested in setting standards for training future family therapists and a significant number of members in each group is interested in setting up committees to accredit such training programs.

No longer the radical departure it represented three decades ago, where is the field headed? What are the problems to which family clinicians in the eighties must pay attention? At least four major deficiencies still exist: (1) The field requires a broader set of theoretical conceptions (What distinguishes functional from dysfunctional families? What factor outside of the family influence interaction within the family? How does the "identified patient" get chosen? Can dysfunction be prevented?); (2) more attention needs to be paid to cultural influences on family functioning (What is the effect of ethnicity, race, subcultural identity, and bilingualism on personal and family development?); (3) family

[1]An outstanding exception is Minuchin, who studied the effect of structural therapy with cases of anorexia nervosa (Minuchin, Rosman, & Baker, 1978). Basing the evaluation on 50 adolescent anoretics seen for therapy together with their families for an average of six months, Minuchin and his associates found 86% of the cases were judged to have recovered from both the anorexia and its psychological components. These highly positive results persisted at subsequent follow-up evaluations extending over several years.

therapy programs need to be extended to new settings (outreach programs into the community, general hospitals, rehabilitation programs, and all of a community's comprehensive mental health services); and (4) family therapy theories and techniques must be evaluated more systematically (What kind of family therapy technique, by what kind of therapist, is most likely to lead to what specific result in which types of families?).

New ways of training, new populations to serve, new settings for clinical activities, new and better documented family therapy techniques—these are the challenges of the 1980s. Family therapy has gained acceptance and respectability; it dare not become complacent.

7. References

Ackerman, N. W. *The psychodynamics of family life.* New York: Basic Books, 1958.

Alger, I. Integrating immediate video playback in family therapy. In P. J. Guerin, Jr. (Ed.), *Family therapy: Theory and practice.* New York: Gardner Press, 1976.

Bateson, G., Jackson, D., Haley, J., & Weakland, J. Towards a theory of schizophrenia. *Behavioral Science,* 1956, *1,* 251–264.

Bell, J. E. *Family group therapy* (Public Health Monograph No. 64). Washington, D.C.: U.S. Government Printing Office, 1961.

Bell, J. E. *Family therapy.* New York: Jason Aronson, 1975.

Bertalanffy, L. von. *General systems theory: Foundation, development, applications.* New York: Braziller, 1968.

Bloch, D. A., & LaPerriere, K. Techniques of family therapy: A conceptual frame. In D. A. Bloch (Ed.), *Techniques of family psychotherapy: A primer.* New York: Grune & Stratton, 1973.

Boszormenyi-Nagy, I., & Framo, J. L. *Intensive family therapy: Theoretical and practical aspects.* New York: Harper & Row, 1965.

Bowen, M. A family concept of schizophrenia. In D. D. Jackson (Ed.), *The etiology of schizophrenia.* New York: Basic Books, 1960.

Bowen, M. Theory in the practice of psychotherapy. In P. J. Guerin, Jr. (Ed.), *Family therapy: Theory and practice.* New York: Gardner Press, 1976.

Bowen, M. *Family therapy in clinical practice.* New York: Jason Aronson, 1978.

Christensen, O. Family counseling: An Adlerian orientation. In G. Gazda (Ed.), *Proceedings of a symposium of family counseling and therapy.* Athens, Ga.: University of Georgia Press, 1971.

Freud, S. Analysis of a phobia in a five-year-old boy (1909). *The standard edition of the complete psychological works of Sigmund Freud* (Vol. 10). London: Hogarth Press, 1955.

Goldenberg, I., & Goldenberg, H. *Family therapy: An overview.* Monterey, Calif.: Brooks/Cole, 1980.

Group for the Advancement of Psychiatry. *The field of family therapy* (Report No. 78). New York: Author, 1970.

Guerin, P. J., Jr. Family therapy: The first twenty-five years. In P. J. Guerin, Jr. (Ed.), *Family therapy: Theory and practice.* New York: Gardner Press, 1976.

Gurman, A. S., & Kniskern, D. P. Research on marital and family therapy: Progress, perspective, and prospect. In S. L. Garfield & A. E. Bergin (Eds.), *Handbook of psychotherapy and behavior change: An empirical analysis* (2nd ed.). New York: Wiley, 1978.

Haley, J. Family therapy: A radical change. In J. Haley (Ed.), *Changing families: A family therapy reader.* New York: Grune & Stratton, 1971.

Haley, J. Development of theory: A history of a research project. In C. E. Sluzki & D. C. Ransom (Eds.), *Double bind: The foundation of a communications approach to the family.* New York: Grune & Stratton, 1976. (a)

Haley, J. *Problem-solving therapy.* San Francisco: Jossey-Bass, 1976. (b)

Haley, J., & Hoffman, L. *Techniques of family therapy.* New York: Basic Books, 1967.

Laing, R. D., & Esterton, A. *Sanity, madness and the family.* Middlesex, England: Penguin, 1970.

Langsley, D. G., Pittman, F. S., Machotka, P., & Flomenhaft, K. Family crisis therapy: Results and implications. *Family Process,* 1968, *7,* 145–158.

Laqueur, H. P. Multiple family therapy. In P. J. Guerin, Jr. (Ed.), *Family therapy: Theory and practice.* New York: Gardner Press, 1976.

LeBow, M. D. Behavior modification for the family. In G. D. Erickson & T. P. Hogan (Eds.), *Family therapy: An introduction to theory and treatment.* Monterey, Calif.: Brooks/Cole, 1972.

Lidz, T., Cornelison, A., Fleck, S., & Terry, D. The intrafamilial environment of schizophrenic patients. II. Marital schism and marital skew. *American Journal of Psychiatry,* 1957, *114,* 241–248.

MacGregor, R., Ritchie, A. N., Serrano, A. C., & Schuster, F. P. *Multiple impact therapy with families.* New York: McGraw-Hill, 1964.

Midelfort, C. F. *The family in psychotherapy.* New York: McGraw-Hill, 1957.

Miller, J. G. *Living systems.* New York: McGraw-Hill, 1978.

Minuchin, S. *Families and family therapy.* Cambridge: Harvard University Press, 1974.

Minuchin, S., Montalvo, B., Guerney, B. G., Jr., Rosman, B. L., & Schumer, F. *Families of the slums: An exploration of their structure and treatment.* New York: Basic Books, 1967.

Minuchin, S., Rosman, B. L., & Baker, L. *Psychosomatic families: Anorexia nervosa in context.* Cambridge: Harvard University Press, 1978.

Mueller, C. G. Some origins of psychology as science. In M. R. Rosenzweig & L. W. Porter (Eds.), *Annual review of psychology* (Vol. 30). Palo Alto, Calif.: Annual Reviews, 1979.

Napier, A. Y., & Whitaker, C. A. *The family crucible.* New York: Harper & Row, 1978.

Palazzoli-Selvini, M. The families of patients with anorexia nervosa. In E. J. Anthony & C. Koupernik (Eds.), *The child and his family.* New York: Wiley, 1970.

Papp, P. Family choreography. In P. J. Guerin, Jr. (Ed.), *Family therapy: Theory and practice.* New York: Gardner Press, 1976.

Satir, V. *Conjoint family therapy.* Palo Alto, Calif.: Science and Behavior Books, 1967.

Speck, R. V. Family therapy in the home. *Journal of Marriage and the Family,* 1964, *26,* 72–76.

Speck, R. V., & Attneave, C. L. *Family networks.* New York: Pantheon Books, 1973.

Stanton, M. D. Strategic approaches to family therapy. In A. S. Gurman & D. P. Kniskern (Eds.), *Handbook of family therapy.* New York: Brunner/Mazel, 1981.

Sullivan, H. S. *The interpersonal theory of psychiatry.* New York: Norton, 1953.

Watzlawick, P., Weakland, J. H., & Fisch, R. *Change: Principles of problem formation and problem resolution.* New York: Norton, 1974.

Weakland, J. H., Fisch, R., Watzlawick, P., & Bodin, A. M. Brief therapy: Focused problem resolution. *Family Process,* 1974, *13,* 141–167.

Wells, R. A., & Dezen, A. E. The results of family therapy revisited: The nonbehaviorial methods. *Family Process,* 1978, *17,* 251–274.

Wells, R. A., Dilkes, T. C., & Trivelli, N. The results of family therapy: A critical review of the literature. *Family Process,* 1972, *11,* 189–207.

Whitaker, C. A. Psychotherapy with couples. *American Journal of Psychotherapy.* 1958, *12,* 18–23.

Wynne, L. C., Ryckoff, I. M., Day, J., & Hirsch, S. I. Pseudomutuality in the family relationships of schizophrenics. *Psychiatry,* 1958, *21,* 191–206.

Zuk, G., & Boszormenyi-Nagy, I. (Eds.). *Family therapy and disturbed families.* Palo Alto, Calif.: Science and Behavior Books, 1967.

6

Research on Marital and Family Therapy

ANSWERS, ISSUES, AND RECOMMENDATIONS FOR THE FUTURE

THOMAS C. TODD AND M. DUNCAN STANTON

This chapter has been written with both clinicians and reseachers in mind. Regarding the former, we believe that it is important for the practicing clinician or clinical student to know what conclusions safely can be drawn from existing research on marital and family therapy and to know which areas are still speculative as far as research evidence is concerned. We also will raise a number of design issues in the belief that clinicians need to be sophisticated consumers of journal articles and research. Finally, we recognize that nonresearchers are often in a position to have an important influence on future research.

Researchers in marital and family therapy also should find much of substance in these pages. Those who are familiar with previous reviews already are aware that there are many controversial issues of research design and strategy; this chapter will offer our own positions and experience relative to them.

Much of this material has an admittedly subjective and personal flavor for two important reasons. First, we agree with Lebow (1981) that it is important for both researchers and reviewers of research to be explicit about their values and assumptions, since some subjectivity is inevitable. Second, we feel that the best way to illustrate certain crucial research dilemmas and inevitable trade-offs is through concrete examples, and our own research has provided us wth much rich, explicative material toward this end. The problems we have encountered should illustrate the kinds of compromises, research evolution, and unanticipated changes that are typical of *all* research, yet are rarely mentioned in print.

We should also be clear from the outset that we are not attempting yet another exhaustive, repetitious review of the research in marital and family therapy. We are in full agreement with Gurman and Kniskern (1981): "At the present time, we believe that there

THOMAS C. TODD • Harlem Valley Psychiatric Center and Philadelphia Child Guidance Clinic, Philadelphia, Pennsylvania 19104. **M. DUNCAN STANTON** • University of Pennsylvania School of Medicine and Philadelphia Child Guidance Clinic, Philadelphia, Pennsylvania 19104.

is no need or justification for further detailed reviews of the outcome literature. . . . What is needed, in our opinion, is not a re-mastication of what has already been digested, but a re-direction and re-focus toward identifying what needs to be studied in the future, and toward the identification of the clinically most relevant questions needing answers'' (p. 743). This review is offered in that spirit. Readers interested in more detailed summaries are referred to a number of major reviews, including DeWitt (1978), Gurman and Kniskern (1978a, 1978c), Jacobson (1978), Jacobson and Martin (1976), Olson, Russell, and Sprenkle (1980), Pinsof (1981), and Wells and Dezen (1978).[1]

This chapter is not intended as a review of basic research methodology in marital and family therapy. Excellent reviews of this area are already available and are listed in Gurman and Kniskern (1981, p. 745). We will begin by offering a brief summary of what research answers currently exist, followed by a detailed analysis of significant issues that remain and our own recommendations for addressing them.

1. What Is Currently Known about the Effectiveness of Marital and Family Therapy?

1.1. Is There General Consensus about What Is Known?

Before presenting a summary of research evidence, it is important to address the issue of whether there is a general consensus among the major reviews in the area. Easy generalizations are prevented by a number of areas of sharp disagreement, particularly between the more behaviorally oriented reviewers, especially Jacobson (1978; Jacobson & Weiss, 1978) and Wells and Dezen (1978a, 1978b), and the nonbehaviorists, such as Gurman and his colleagues (Gurman & Kniskern, 1978a; Gurman & Knudson, 1978; Gurman & Klein, 1980; Gurman, Knudson, & Kniskern, 1978). Two such areas of controversy prevail:

1.1.1. There Are Significant Disagreements about Basic Design Quality Issues

One of the most fundamental disagreements concerns the value of uncontrolled or otherwise weak studies in contributing to an overall body of knowledge. Gurman and Kniskern (1978c) reviewed over 200 reports of marital and family therapy research. Although they were quick to admit that many of these studies were seriously flawed, they nevertheless used the overall pattern of results to draw some general conclusions.

Jacobson (1978) disagrees completely with this reviewing strategy: ''One hundred uncontrolled investigations of a given treatment, all suggesting improvement among treatment couples, constitute 100 uninterpretable studies; even when considered together, the cumulative total of these studies fails to establish causal relationships between a given treatment and positive change'' (p. 401). Needless to say, stringent application of this principle has led Jacobson to consider only a very small number of studies that he regards as adequate on methodological grounds.

Another major design quality issue concerns the comparative merits of various

[1]A comprehensive list of review articles in family therapy research can be found in Gurman and Kniskern (1981, p. 743).

control groups or other comparative designs. Jacobson (1978) considers the wait-list control group the *sine qua non* of an adequate research design. Gurman and Kniskern (1981) have noted what they consider significant problems with this design, preferring a design strategy known as "Treatment on Demand." This issue, together with our own views on this controversy, will be discussed in detail below. For the present, it is primarily important to note that such disagreements about design can have a major impact upon the selection of research studies chosen for review, and therefore on the conclusions drawn from such reviews.

1.1.2. The Comparative Effectiveness of Behavioral Marital and Family Therapy

Controversy about design issues such as the above has led to heated disagreement about the comparative value of behavioral and nonbehavioral approaches. Jacobson (1978) contends that there is insufficient research evidence available to support claims of effectiveness of nonbehavioral marital therapy. This is particularly true of the large number of studies that rely exclusively on therapist or patient self-reports. (To be fair, it is important to mention that Jacobson's stringent standards lead him to make similarly conservative conclusions about many behavioral approaches.)

On the other hand, Gurman and Kniskern (1981), reach radically different conclusions because of other design considerations. They are especially concerned about the use of nonclinical or moderately disturbed populations in many studies of behavioral marital therapy. For this reason, they maintain that current evidence on behavioral marital therapy has documented its effectiveness only with minimally to moderately disturbed couples.

1.1.3. What Conclusions about Effectiveness Can Safely Be Drawn?

In general, our conclusions do not differ substantially from other nonbehavioral reviewers, especially Gurman and Kniskern (1978c, 1981) and Olson *et al.* (1980), and generally are consistent with those of Jacobson (1978). Since comparison of behavioral and nonbehavioral methods is so controversial, this comparison is dealt with separately in the following section.

We believe that the following general conclusions can be safely drawn from the body of research evidence that has accumulated over approximately the last decade.

1. *When the presenting complaint is a marital problem, treatment outcome is significantly better when both spouses are included.* This is one of the most striking conclusions offered by Gurman and Kniskern (1978c) and one with the most immediate clinical implications. They found an overall improvement rate of 65% for treatment involving both spouses (whether conjoint or collaborative), compared to 48% for individual therapy. Similarly, they found the deterioration rate of individual therapy (11.6%) to be almost double that for marital treatment involving both partners (5.6%). Finally, in studies comparing conjoint marital approaches with alternative treatments, the former was shown to be superior in 70% of the comparisons and inferior in only 5%. This is a strong and very important conclusion for marital therapy, but it is important not to overgeneral-

ize. For example, it may be premature to claim superiority for marital treatment when the presenting problem is an "individual" one (e.g., wife's depression).

2. *Family therapy appears to be equally or more effective than individual and other treatment approaches.* Gurman and Kniskern (1978c) examined 14 studies comparing nonbehavioral family therapy with other modalities. Family therapy emerged superior in 10 of these and equal in the remainder. Further, this trend remained irrespective of whether studies with "poor" design were included or not. In a separate analysis, these authors also estimated the overall improvement rate for cases seen in family therapy to be 73%.
3. *Marital and family therapies can cause deterioration, with approximately the same frequency as other modalities.* We agree with Gurman and Kniskern (1978b) that the question of deterioration in psychotherapy is insufficiently addressed. The apparent rates of deterioration that can be attributed to marital or family therapy (5 to 10%) are comparable to rates reported for individual and group psychotherapy. Gurman and Kniskern (1978b) have identified a set of *therapist* (as opposed to technique) factors that appear to be predictably associated with such poor marital and family therapy outcomes:

> The available evidence points to a composite picture of deterioration in marital-family therapy being facilitated by a therapist with poor relationship skills who directly attacks "loaded" issues and family members' defenses very early in treatment, fails to intervene in or interpret intrafamily confrontation in ongoing treatment, and does little to structure and guide the opening of therapy or to support family members. Such a style is even more likely to be counter therapeutic with patients who have weak ego-defenses or feel threatened by the nature or very fact of being in treatment. (p. 14)

4. *In certain specific clinical conditions, particular marital or family therapy approaches currently should be regarded as among the "treatments of choice."*

   There is significant evidence for the efficacy of certain marital or family approaches with particular presenting problems. Although there is a dearth of comparisons across modalities, these methods definitely should be considered for clinical application. Most of them probably could serve as appropriate bench marks in testing the effectiveness of new approaches.

   Below are listed a number of presenting problems and the various marital and family approaches that have yielded some degree of documented effectiveness with them. This (abbreviated) list is generally adapted from Olson *et al.* (1980):

   a. Alcoholism. Behavioral exchange contracting, conjoint couples groups
   b. Drug abuse. Structural family therapy, strategic family therapy, multiple family therapy
   c. Juvenile status offense. Functional family therapy, which uses both behavioral and strategic techniques (Barton & Alexander, 1981; Stanton, 1981; Stanton & Todd, 1980), structural family therapy
   d. Adolescent psychopathology. Conjoint interactional family therapy, Zuk's triadic approach
   e. Childhood conduct problems. Behavioral family therapy
   f. School and work phobias. Multiple family therapy, family crisis intervention
   g. Psychosomatic symptoms. Structural family therapy, strategic family therapy
   h. Adult depression. Drug therapy plus marital therapy

i. *Marital distress.* Behavioral exchange contracting
j. *Sexual dysfunction.* Behavioral marital therapy (conjoint)

5. *There is little comparative evidence that one marital or family therapy approach is superior to all others across a wide range of presenting problems.* Although there is currently a climate in which the various "schools" of family therapy claim, or subtly imply, superiority over competing schools, there is little research evidence to support such claims (Olson *et al.*, 1980). No systematic comparisons across "schools" have as yet been completed.[2] In fact, as Kniskern and Gurman (1981) have recently pointed out, many of the most influential marital and family therapy approaches, most notably the Bowenian and psychodynamic approaches, have not received even the most rudimentary empirical validation. The vast majority of the studies have come from a small number of "camps," most notably behavioral marital therapy, operant approaches to children, functional family therapy, and structural family therapy.
6. *Short-term and time-limited marital and family therapy is as effective as longer term therapy.* This conclusion seems equally valid for nonbehavioral (Gurman & Kniskern, 1981) and behavioral methods (Jacobson, 1978). Gurman and Kniskern (1982) note that marital and family therapy are often of brief duration. Two-thirds of the studies they reviewed examined therapies that lasted from 1 to 20 sessions, with a mean of approximately 9 sessions.
7. *The involvement of the father in family therapy substantially increases the likelihood of successful outcome.* Similar to the importance of inclusion of the spouse in marital therapy, inclusion of the father in therapy appears to be one of the most critical factors in success (Love, Kaswan, & Bugental, 1972; R. Shapiro & Budman, 1973). Although there is much clinical controversy about who should be included in sessions, no other general conclusions safely can be drawn at present.
8. *A wide variety of patient and family characteristics have shown little or no relation to treatment outcome.* Many patient characteristics (especially diagnosis), family interaction patterns (e.g., enmeshed, pseudomutual), family constellation variables, and demographic variables have shown unpredictable relationships to the outcome of therapy. It is noteworthy, however, that virtually all of the successful research projects to date have been based on populations identified according to the symptoms of the index patient. (See Number 4, above.) Thus far, despite the plethora of family theories and typologies, the field has yet to isolate factors of general importance.
9. *There is no empirical evidence for the superiority of the common practice of cotherapy, compared to therapy conducted by a single therapist.* Although many "no difference" statements can be made in the field of marital and family therapy, the lack of evidence for the effectiveness of cotherapy seems critically important in view of cost considerations.
10. *There is little empirical evidence to support claims of comparative effectiveness of behavioral marital or family therapy over nonbehavioral methods or vice versa.*

[2]As of this writing, the study by Winter and Kolevson (1982) comparing the approaches of Bowen, Haley, and Satir is still in progress.

There are few studies that systematically compare behavioral and nonbehavioral marital or family therapies. Indirect comparisons (which contrast the two bodies of research) are particularly difficult to evaluate due to the extreme differences between these two domains, as we will see in the next section.

1.1.4. Specific Issues in Comparing Behavioral and Nonbehavioral Approaches

Controversy between behavioral researchers and reviewers and their nonbehavioral counterparts has consumed much space in the literature on marital and family therapy research. Generally it seems that these exchanges have generated more heat than light, leaving the opposing camps as far apart as ever and with few "converts" crossing over to the opposite side. It would be foolhardy to attempt to recapitulate these discussions; the interested reader is invited to delve into the series of articles, replies, and rejoinders that have been published (Gurman & Kniskern, 1978a, 1978d; Gurman & Knudson, 1978; Gurman, Knudson, & Kniskern, 1978; Jacobson & Weiss, 1978; Wells & Dezen, 1978a, 1978b).

We do, however, believe that these exchanges have highlighted certain core assumptions and world views that differentiate the two approaches and that it is worthwhile to underscore some of them, with their (inevitable) consequences. As Colapinto (1979) has astutely observed, this controversy is a conflict between alternative epistemologies. One would therefore be misguided to believe that empirical evidence ever will resolve the argument. These different epistemologies lead to major differences in the definition of critical concepts such as "problems," "causes," "solutions," and "therapeutic goals." As such, it is inevitable that "success" in one framework may be labeled as the "problem" in another, as Colapinto illustrates with pointed examples. Of course, we ourselves are prisoners of our own epistemology as much as anyone else, so we can only hope to show how our own epistemology leads us to positions that are consistent or inconsistent with either the behavioral or nonbehavioral position.

We clearly owe a major debt to Gurman and Kniskern as far as research in marital and family therapy is concerned and share many of their views on research design and strategy. On the other hand, we do differ from them in our view of treatment, which leads us to major differences in research priorities.

Gurman and Kniskern (1978c) have described their framework as a "psychodynamic-systems" perspective, although Colapinto (1979, p. 438) has criticized their position as a subordination of systems concepts within a basically psychodynamic approach. Clearly, our major difference with their view is their emphasis on psychodynamics and history. We place much less emphasis on intrapsychic factors within the family and on similar factors for the therapist. Instead, it will come as no surprise to those familiar with the structural/strategic framework to learn that our emphasis is upon present interaction and the operations of the therapist to change this interaction.

As will be seen in later sections, we agree with Gurman and Kniskern that it is important to maintain a systemic framework rather than to look exclusively at either the patient or a particular dyad, as might be done within a behavioral framework. On the other hand, one of the areas of greatest convergence between our own views and those of the behaviorists concerns the importance of the presenting problem and its relation to the therapeutic contract. Jacobson (1978) has stated this position succinctly with regard to marital therapy:

> Couples enter into marital therapy with presenting complaints, which often amount to specific behaviors on the part of the partner which each spouse desires to be changed. If these complaints are not modified by concrete changes in these target behaviors as a function of therapy, it is problematic to argue that therapy was successful. To the extent that the alleviation of such complaints can be objectively measured, they are ideal outcome measures. (p. 400)

We would argue, as do the behaviorists, that therapy typically is presented as a method for reducing distress and eliminating problems. Other contracts, such as "enhancing individual freedom," are certainly possible but should not be misrepresented.

We also share the assumption of most behaviorists that "what works" in therapy can be identified and specified. The efforts of the behavioral marital therapists to isolate the "critical ingredients" in behavioral marital therapy seem particularly praiseworthy. There is tentative evidence that communication training is the most important ingredient in the treatment "packages" that also have included training in problem-solving and contingency contracting. It is perhaps ironic that, as Jacobson (1978) has noted, "It may be that the most effective element in the behavioral approach is the one which is the least unique to a behavioral approach" (p. 425).

From our perspective, the greatest deficiencies in behaviorally oriented research have derived from what appears to us to be an overvaluing of the laboratory method. This model of research has led to many of the problems for which the behaviorists have been criticized by Gurman, ourselves (Stanton & Todd, 1980), and others, for example, working with nonclinical or mildly disturbed populations, using volunteers rather than patients, conducting treatment with minimally trained therapists, devoting little effort to studying the effects of all the behavioral "technology" itself, giving insufficient attention to predicting who will drop out or refuse to cooperate with a structured behavioral format, and so forth.

Our difficulty with this emphasis also stems from a basic disagreement about innovation and the development of new techniques. As the following sections illustrate, we believe that life and research are inevitably messy and that it is particularly dangerous to attempt to reach premature closure and rigor. It seems unlikely to us that important new clinical techniques will originate in the laboratory or by revising a treatment manual. Instead, it seems more fruitful first to identify promising and potentially powerful new techniques in the clinical arena and then to attempt to specify therapeutic operations in detail and to isolate the "crucial ingredients."

2. Life—and Research—Cannot Be Simple

It has become a commonplace assumption that research on individual psychotherapy is inevitably complex (see S. L. Garfield, 1978; Kiesler, 1966; Parloff, Waskow, & Wolfe, 1978; Strupp, 1978). Some of these complexities, particularly the problem of multiple perspectives, have emerged only recently in the individual therapy research literature. Attempting to conduct research on marital and family therapy, by contrast, makes such difficulties immediately obvious. It may seem simple to measure change when there is only a single patient in therapy alone, but what happens when father and mother disagree about changes in the child, or even about the nature of the problem? The researcher in marital and family therapy is immediately faced with the problem of differentially weighting changes in individuals, family relationships, and larger systems. Further, within marital/family therapy certain outcomes (such as divorce) are value-laden, making it difficult to obtain an easy consensus as to whether the outcome is positive or negative.

The basic premises of systems theory imply that any attempt to measure the change process inevitably will be difficult. These difficulties are shared by individual psychotherapy research and even by more "scientific" areas such as drug research, but they have been less obvious in these research domains because the relevant observations have not been made. One obvious example is the potential change or deterioration in other family members either through "symptoms" or through shifts in relationships. A systems view also suggests that it is impossible to define in any mechanical way which individuals are likely to be affected since these effects depend on the natural linkages between components of the system and on which level of system happens to be critical in a given case (e.g., parent–child, extended family, family/school).

Other commonly accepted premises of systems theory seem to pose difficulties for the researcher that may be even more fundamental. One is the notion of first-order vs. second-order change (Watzlawick, Weakland, & Fisch, 1974). According to this view, apparent changes may produce new patterns that are "isomorphic" with the original pattern and thus at a higher level do not represent any basic change. Symptom substitution or developing new "patients" in the family are familiar examples, but other examples may be more subtle, such as moving from one extreme to another. Systems theorists have also begun to realize that change may be discontinuous and sudden, rather than gradual (Hoffman 1980, 1981) and that such change may require new mathematical treatment, such as "catastrophe theory" (Thom, 1975).

Our own systemic perspective also has led us to be suspicious of any presentation of therapy research that implies that the research or the treatment "stood still" during the life of the research. Instead, as examples from our own experience will show, research and treatment typically interact—evolving or "co-evolving" together. In the sections to follow, examples will be proferred with the hope of sensitizing the reader to these effects, whether they are acknowledged by particular researchers or not.

2.1. The Interaction between Research and Therapy

Participation in a research project, especially an outcome study, has an inevitable impact on the conduct of the therapy. The therapist cannot fail to be aware of the "public" nature of the results of treatment, which generally increases the pressure on the therapist. (See Todd, Berger, & Lande, 1982, for a candid discussion of these effects, as well as the effects on the clinical supervisor.) In particular, participation in a research project makes it less likely that patient attrition or ambiguous outcomes will go unchallenged.

In addition to the direct effects on therapy and the therapist, the research project typically has important effects on the treatment context. In our drug project,[3] for example, the urinalysis procedures at the drug treatment center were gradually tightened up—as were the program rules—because of the research; these changes, in turn, undoubtedly affected the treatment. Changes such as these might have occurred during a routine collaboration between family therapists and drug program staff, but there is little question that the research collaboration increased the motivation of the latter to cooperate with the therapists.

We also suspect that there were definite "reactive effects" on the family from

[3]This has been a collaborative effort between the Philadelphia Child Guidance Clinic and the Philadelphia VA Hospital Drug Dependence Treatment Center, entitled the "Addicts and Families Program."

participation in the research project. Our control group involved convening the family to watch anthropology movies, along with (a) receiving feedback about the addict's drug taking, (b) providing research data, and (c) being paid for participation. Each of these control group activities probably constituted an important intervention, and the cumulative effect had some positive impact on drug taking (Stanton, Todd, Steier, Van Deusen, Marder, Rosoff, Seaman, & Skibinski, 1980; Stanton, Todd, & Associates, 1982).

2.2. The Co-Evolution of Therapy and Research

As stated earlier, we believe that the specification of treatment methods and the isolation of crucial ingredients of treatment are worthwhile goals. This degree of specificity is only appropriate at a very late stage in the evolution of effective treatment methods. In most research presentations, the continued evolution of both research and treatment is typically de-emphasized, so that it appears that therapists and researchers knew exactly what they were doing from the start.

We have no reason to believe that our own experience has been atypical. An important example was the progressive evolution of the teatment (and research) goals. From the beginning, it was clear that reduction in illegal drug taking was a major goal, but it was unclear whether detoxification from methadone was feasible and desirable or whether it might interfere with the primary goal. The drug treatment program itself was quite ambivalent about methadone, viewing detoxification from methadone as an ideal, but probably unattainable, goal. By the end of the project, freedom from illegal *and* legal drugs (methadone) was a major goal of the therapy and the research project and was accepted as a realistic possibility by the drug program.[4] Without the clinical experience gained during the project it probably would have been impossible to resolve this issue.

Structural family therapy is probably second only to behavioral marital and family therapy in being explicit about its training procedures and treatment methods. The therapists in our project were well versed in structural family therapy and confident that it could be applied to heroin abuse in young adults. Despite the commitment to a well developed model, it still would have been premature at the beginning of the project to attempt to write a treatment "manual" or to slavishly follow one. Even now, after many years of accumulated experience and considerable effort in articulating our principles of treatment (Stanton & Todd, 1979; Stanton, Todd, & Associates, 1982), such a manual still seems to be an unrealistic goal. In fact, the very idea of a manual conflicts with one of our central clinical principles, that of therapist flexibility.

Kniskern and Gurman (1982) have identified the "crucial ingredients" question as a central one for structural family therapists, because of the propensity of structural therapists to borrow techniques from other approaches, even those that appear radically different. We believe that we have succeeded, to a moderate degree, in identifying common elements in cases that often appear superficially dissimilar. Again, this was a progressive evolution: We began with general principles, applied them to a large number of cases, and then looked for patterns in the differences that evolved in response to clinical feedback.

We would posit that some dependence on clinical data is inevitable and that it is particularly risky to rely solely on group data from research. Take, for example, the relatively well established conclusion that the presence of the father generally improves

[4]This evolution of treatment goals made it important for the research to examine possible differences in outcome for early and late cases; such an evaluation revealed no significant differences.

the outcome of family therapy. This effect is sufficiently potent to have emerged repeatedly in a number of studies. It nevertheless may be true, as clinical experience seems to indicate, that at times it may be counterproductive and even harmful to include the father, particularly in some situations of separation and divorce. Our major point is that this important question, while amenable to research verification, would never have emerged from a consideration limited to group effects. A continuous interplay between clinical data gathering and hypothesis generating, followed by validating research, seems the most productive strategy.

3. Inevitable Binds and Compromises

3.1. The Perfect Study is Probably Impossible

One important goal of the many reviewers of marital and family therapy research has been to increase the general awareness of issues of research design. The extent to which this effort has succeeded, however, is unclear, as is illustrated by an examination of trends in research "quality" by A. M. Williams and Miller (1981) which showed little evidence of progressive improvement in such endeavors over a period of years.

Such improvement is nevertheless a laudable goal. We are particularly impressed with the "design quality" criteria developed by Gurman and Kniskern (1981), which have been reproduced in Table 1. It is possible to design research studies that satisfy most of these criteria, although this usually can be done only through a major project requiring ambition and funding of a magnitude that has become increasingly difficult to obtain. Even if one succeeds in designing such a study with high marks for quality, it seems inevitable that it will fall short of achieving everything that might be desired. In this section, we will focus on several dilemmas regarding control groups and comparative designs. In the remainder of the chapter, we will offer our own admittedly imperfect recommendations regarding a wide variety of questions of research strategy, where it is obvious that choices and compromises must be made.

3.1.1. Denying (or Postponing) Treatment Is Problematic; Yet Alternatives Have Their Own Problems

Fiske, Hunt, Luborsky, Orne, Parloff, Reiser, and Tuma (1970) and Gurman and Kniskern (1981) have argued persuasively that the idea of the untreated control group is largely a myth, and that the problem cannot be circumvented by utilizing a wait-list control. That argument is strong by itself, but it is inconsequential in comparison to the increasing ethical and practical difficulties in utilizing designs involving such control groups. An increase in emphasis on consumer protection and informed consent has made it progressively more difficult to justify such a design in any clinical situation for which there is a treatment of presumed effectiveness (Winter & Kolevson, 1982).

Gurman and Kniskern (1981) have espoused the "treatment on demand" (TOD) design as their preferred alternative. In this design, which has been utilized in the Boston-New Haven collaborative study of depression (Di Mascio & Klerman, 1977) and in a similar study at the University of Wisconsin (Klein, Greist, Gurman, & Van Cura, 1978), patients in the comparison group are also assigned a therapist. They are told that they can have access to the therapist *on demand* whenever they request a session. In practice, any case demanding more than an established cutoff number of sessions would be dropped from the TOD condition. This design therefore yields four groups: (1) families or couples receiving treatment X; (2) TOD remainers, who never have requested any sessions; (3) TOD partial remainers, who have received sessions but not exceeded the cutoff number of sessions; (4) TOD dropouts, who have been dropped because they requested more than the established cutoff number of sessions.

This design has obvious appeal from the standpoint of allowing access to treatment, yet we find it difficult to defend as an adequate control group. Gurman and Kniskern (1981) claim that "TOD probably offers the closest approximation to a 'true' no-treatment condition that has yet emerged in psychotherapy research" (p. 747), yet the design has obvious inherent difficulties due to self-selection. The only comparison based on random assignment that is possible is the comparison between the treatment group (1) compared to the combination of all the TOD groups, groups (2), (3), and (4). The only advantages offered by TOD over the untreated control group (which Gurman and Kniskern criticize) are that subjects believe they are receiving treatment and that it is possible to measure how much of the treatment they actually seek. Otherwise, comparisons involving the various TOD groups are virtually uninterpretable, due to self-selection.

The other solution is to compare parallel treatment groups, with random assignment. The problem of the untreated control group is eliminated since all groups receive treatment. This design can take several forms. One is the comparison between two or more (presumably) equally valued treatments, for example, marital problem-solving training versus marital communication training, or behavioral marital therapy versus psychodynamic marital therapy. A second alternative, which we term the "add-on" design, adds

Table 1. Criteria for Rating Research Design Quality Used by Gurman and Kniskern (1978a)

1. *Controlled assignment to treatment conditions:* random assignment, matching of total groups or matching in pairs (5).[a]
2. *Pre-postmeasurement of change:* it is not uncommon (Gurman, 1973b; Wells *et al.*, 1972) for family therapy research to use postevaluations only (5).
3. *No contamination of major independent variables:* this includes therapists' experience level, number of therapists per treatment condition, and *relevant* therapeutic competence (e.g., a psychoanalyst using behavior therapy for the first time offers a poor test of the power of a behavioral method) (5).
4. *Appropriate statistical analysis* (1).
5. *Follow-up:* none (0), 1 to 3 months (1/2), 3 months or more (1).
6. *Treatments equally valued:* tremendous biases are often engendered for both therapists and patients when this criterion is not met (1).
7. *Treatment carried out as described or expected:* clear evidence (1), presumptive evidence (1/2).
8. *Multiple change indices* used (1).
9. *Multiple vantage points* used in assessing outcome (1).
10. *Outcome not limited to change in the "identified patient":* this criterion is perhaps uniquely required in marital/family therapy (1).
11. *Data on other concurrent treatment:* evidence of none or, if present, of its equivalence across groups (1); mention of such treatment without documentation of amount or equivalence (1/2).
12. *Equal treatment length* in comparative studies (1).
13. *Outcome assessment allows for both positive and negative change* (1).
14. *Therapist-investigator nonequivalence:* earlier reviews (Gurman, 1973b) had found the two to be the same person in about 75 percent of the studies examined (1).

[a]Design quality "points" achievable are noted in parentheses. Criterion scores were: 0 to 10, poor; 10½ to 15, fair; 15½ to 20, good; and 20½ to 26, very good.

a new treatment to a previously well established treatment package. In our own project, this meant adding family therapy to a multimodal methadone maintenance program; similarly, an approach like cognitive behavior therapy could be added to a standard chemotherapy regimen.

The "add-on" design has one drawback, the possibility of interaction between the new method and the existing treatment. In the examples given, it would take further research to establish the effectiveness of family therapy in a nonmethadone program or to show that cognitive behavior therapy would work without being combined with chemotherapy. Thus the two treatments might be either synergistic (rather than summative) or, in combination, could work to cancel out each others' effects.

Both of the parallel group designs, since they lack an untreated control group, have another potential drawback, particularly in the interpretation of a finding of "no difference" between approaches. Does the finding of no difference mean that the treatments were equally effective or equally ineffective? Much depends on one's interpretation of the existing body of research evidence. If one accepts, as is the premise of this chapter, that it is no longer necessary to prove the general effectiveness of marital and family therapy, then it is no longer necessary to include an untreated control group. Inclusion of a control group could therefore be considered unnecessarily wasteful and unfair to patients assigned to the control group.

3.1.2. It Is Difficult to Make Parallel Groups Truly Parallel

Although we favor using some variation of the comparative treatments or the "add-on" design, there are some practical problems in implementation. This is a critical problem, since the strength of the design depends on the comparability of the parallel treatments.

It obviously is important to attempt to ensure that all treatments are perceived as equally valued by the patients in the study. This typically is a problem with a "treatment as usual" condition, since patients in the experimental conditions may receive more attention and fanfare about innovative treatment methods. Expectations particular to the treatment setting also may be critical. A nonmethadone treatment would have a different perceived value in the context of a methadone maintenance program compared to the context of a drug-free therapeutic community. Similarly, patients coming to an agency well known for family therapy and receiving behavior therapy are not likely to value their treatment as highly as would be the case if the situation were reversed.

Therapist variables introduce additional problems both in differential expectations and different skill levels. It seems virtually impossible to have one therapist conduct two different treatments with equal expectations about the effectiveness of the treatments and equal skill in conducting them. For this reason, it seems imperative to have each treatment conducted by therapists with unquestionable competence in the given approach, as has been done in the landmark projects by Sloane, Staples, Cristol, Yorkston, and Whipple (1975) and in the family therapy field by Winter and Kolevson (1982).

Unequal time frames also present a vexing dilemma. As has been noted above, many family therapies are of rather brief duration, yet most individual and group psychotherapy approaches, and some marital and family therapy approaches, are presumed by their proponents to require significantly more time to be effective. No solution is completely satisfactory: It is not meaningful to limit arbitrarily to 10 sessions a therapy normally expected to require two years, yet it is difficult to compare two treatments with gross differences in duration and number of sessions. To us, it seems preferable to design treatment conditions that would be regarded as a "fair test" by the proponents of that approach; differences in duration then lend themselves to cost-effectiveness comparisons.

3.1.3. It Is Impossible to "Control" for Everything

Again, it is important to emphasize that there is no such thing as the perfect design or the ideal study. This is particularly so in regard to control groups and to comparisons across treatment conditions. One cannot "control" for every variable or contrast treatments on every potentially important dimension. In evaluating research, one must examine the logic of the control or standard treatment condition—what variables actually are being systematically compared? Similarly, in designing research, it is important to identify major variables that should take priority and variables that are likely to have particularly potent effects. It then becomes a matter of strategic choice whether to (a) systematically vary or control that variable, (b) attempt to hold that variable constant across conditions, or (c) measure existing variation in that variable and tease out the effects statistically. Many potentially interesting questions always will be left unanswered by any single study, no matter how comprehensive.

Our project illustrates all of these points. We utilized a control group in which the family was convened for 10 sessions to watch anthropology movies about families in other cultures. This procedure was given a therapeutic rationale: "We find that families which at times have difficulties can be helped by seeing how people in other cultures and societies live and work together, because it gives them a perspective." Families were paid on the same basis as our (presumably) most potent treatment condition, "paid" family therapy. They were systematically informed about the results of the addict's urine tests and were paid an amount that was contingent upon family member attendance and clean urines. (For further details, see Stanton *et al.*, 1980; Stanton, Steier, & Todd, 1982.)

In this one control group, we combined several factors that seemed potentially powerful in themselves, including (a) involving the family in treatment, (b) feedback on drug taking, and (c) contingent payment for involvement and success in keeping the addict "clean." To identify the contribution of each of these possible effects separately would have required an extremely elaborate and expensive design. (Simply to have included an unpaid movie group would have increased the total number of subjects by one-third and increased all costs proportionately). Our rationale was that for family therapy to be a viable approach it had to be effective above and beyond the cumulative effect of all these factors. Further teasing out of "critical ingredients" seemed premature until the overall effectiveness could be demonstrated.

Several other potentially important factors were held relatively constant by subject selection. These included sex (male), age (25 to 35), miltiary service (veteran), and household composition (in regular contact with two parents or parent-surrogates). Race seemed particularly important, so we selected an equal number of black and white subjects. Therapist variables also were held constant or matched, rather than systematically varied. Thus, we used only male therapists and attempted to match race of family and therapist (within the constraints of equal case loads). Treatment was limited to 10 sessions. Obviously there are a great many interesting research questions that cannot be answered by this one study, such as the extension to other populations, the comparative effectiveness of female therapists or a male-female team, and the effects of longer treatment.

Finally, there were other potentially important variables that were measured and then controlled statistically. These included such factors as history of drug use, employment and educational history, age, race, marital status, Vietnam service, frequency of contact with parents, and parental drinking problems. Whenever variables were identified that were significantly correlated with treatment outcome, we removed these effects statistically, using analysis of covariance techniques. Seven out of 16 covariates showed significant correlations with outcome measures: race; enrolled in school; father's education; parents living together; frequency of family contact; living in parents' home; parental drinking problem. It is particularly noteworthy that 4 of the 5 potential covariates relating to family of origin appeared on this list of significant predictors. We definitely recommend the use of covariates as a general research strategy and particularly suggest that future investigations of this patient population explore these particular variables.

4. Recommendations for the Future

In an era of increasingly scarce resources, it seems imperative that new research efforts make a maximum contribution to a growing body of knowledge. This is far from being the current state of affairs, as marital and family therapy research generally has been fragmented, all too often characterized by inadequate research design, and shown few relationships between studies. Although there is some utility in looking at broad trends and generalizations through comprehensive reviews, this represents a very poor rate of return on the time and money invested in individual research projects.

In addition to advocating tighter research design, in the same spirit as every other review, we can make specific recommendations for productive marital and family therapy research. Adopting these recommendations would go far toward increasing the utility of the research and creating a more systematic body of knowledge.

4.1. Be Clear about Ultimate and Subordinate Goals

Gurman and Kniskern (1981) have emphasized strongly the importance of ultimate and subordinate goals. Unfortunately, from our perspective, it seems to us that they have their priorities reversed.

Our view is that *the ultimate goal of therapy always should be the resolution of the presenting problem.* There are persuasive ethical, political, and scientific reasons for this stance. Any treatment offered for a psychiatric problem, such as depression, school phobia, or anorexia, should be judged by this primary criterion of symptom improvement. Any marital or family therapist (or psychoanalyst, for that matter) who is unwilling to adopt such a primary criterion should state this explicitly to his or her clients rather than imply that the treatment is intended to alleviate the symptom. If marital or family treatment can be shown to provide improvement in other family members *in addition* to symptomatic relief, that may provide additional support for these modalities. In our view, "better family communication" means little if a school phobic child still does not attend school or an anorectic girl continues to starve herself.

In general, it seems safe to assume that any goal that is specific to a particular "school" or method should be viewed as an intermediate goal rather than an ultimate goal. For example, it may be useful to hypothesize that better marital communication will lead to reduced depression or that greater assertiveness will lead to improvement in an anorectic girl. These are hypotheses that should be tested, rather than goals that should be substituted for the ultimate goal or weighted equally with it.

In this respect, it is well to remember that many "sacred cows" of the marital and family therapy field are being called into question by one or more prominent approaches. For example, better communication is not seen as a necessary or desirable goal by strategic therapists, who generally take the view that the important information is already being communicated and that one cannot *not* communicate (Haley, 1963). In a similar vein Madanes (1981) recently has described an approach that often utilizes "pretending" rather than "honesty." Finally, many therapists, such as the Milan group (Palazzoli-Selvini, Boscolo, Cecchin, & Prata, 1974, 1977, 1978, 1980), emphasize that change often occurs "off stage" and that it is not necessary for the therapist to know the reasons or the mechanisms for the changes that occur.

4.2. Multiple Outcome Measures Must Be Used

Although we regard measures of symptomatic improvement as the *sine qua non* of psychotherapy research, it is important to go beyond the use of a single indicator.

It now has become anachronistic even in the field of individual psychotherapy research to conduct research without employing multiple outcome measures from several perspectives. Hopefully this is even more obvious to those interested in marital and family therapy, who typically pride themselves in adopting a systemic framework.

To begin with, measurement of improvement in the identified patient is not a simple matter. As classic articles in the literature on individual psychotherapy research have shown (Bergin & Lambert, 1978; Cartwright, Kirtner, & Fiske, 1963; G. Garfield, Prager, & Bergin, 1971; Mintz, Auerbach, Luborsky, & Johnson, 1973), it can make a substantial difference who is asked (therapist, patient, relative) and how the data are collected (structured interview, behavioral checklist, global judgments of improvement).

Some of these difficulties can be eliminated or minimized by using objective, "hard" data to measure outcome (urine tests of drug taking, weight gain for anorectics). Unfortunately, not all presenting problems lend themselves to such simple measures. On any measure that is more subjective, a family systems perspective would not lead one to expect high levels of agreement among family members on what the problem is, how severe it is, or how much it improved. Todd (1973), for example, found major differences between fathers and mothers concerning number of problems identified, severity of initial problem, and degree of improvement, with fathers consistently minimizing the number and severity of problems and being more "middle of the road" about posttherapy changes.

Gurman and Kniskern (1981, p. 766) have developed a comprehensive schema for assessing therapeutic change at various system levels. They contend (and we concur) that an adequate comprehensive assessment should include assessment of changes in (a) individuals, (b) the marital relationship, and (c) the family as a whole. Other combinations are logically possible, but measuring every dyad, triad, etc., rapidly becomes prohibitive. It may be relevant from a given theoretical perspective to include other units for assessment—such as the grandparental generation in Bowenian research—but inclusion of the three system levels mentioned above is crucial for studies to be comparable.

The inclusion of multiple perspectives and measures immediately introduces the question of how different patterns of outcome should be weighted and combined. If an asthmatic child improves and the parental marriage deteriorates, should this be considered a success? Gurman and Kniskern (1981, pp. 765–766) go to considerable lengths to make explicit their assumptions about which types and combinations of positive change are most meaningful (e.g., "more positive change can be said to have occurred when improvement is noted on a total system level than on a single relationship level," p. 766) and assumptions about which forms of deterioration should be seen as most serious.

We already have noted our strong bias toward the use of symptom improvement as the primary criterion of success in any form of therapy. In using multiple measures, it is also important not to "water down" the evaluation of improvement by including insensitive or inappropriate measures. Many measures of marital or family improvement are too global and often are thinly disguised measures of satisfaction with therapy. We strongly believe that satisfaction with therapy or liking one's therapist never should be confused with success of therapy in achieving its stated goal. To use a medical analogy, successful open-heart surgery is not measured by how much the patients (or worse yet, the surviving relatives) like the surgeon.

Like Gurman and Kniskern (1981, p. 764) we are "adamantly middle of the road" on the subject of a core battery of outcome measures for marital and family research. It seems obvious that the field cannot progress without the inclusion of certain standardized measures to insure comparability across studies. The core battery approach was never intended to supplant measures of particular interest to a given researcher but rather to guarantee that additional new measures can be related to widely adopted measures that are not tied to a given theory.

Naturally it will be difficult to achieve the degree of consensus required for adoption of a core battery of measures, yet we believe this is an urgent priority and is closely related to the urgent need to operationalize key concepts pointed out in the next section. In fact our hopes and recommendations are even more ambitious, for we believe that maximum progress is possible only if a marital/family therapy core battery at least overlaps with that developed for individual psychotherapy (Waskow & Parloff, 1975). Only in this way will it be possible to accumulate accepted evidence for the effectiveness of marital and family therapy for problems that are not necessarily defined as relationship problems and to begin to evaluate the impact of individual psychotherapy on the larger system.

4.2.1. Recommendations for a "Core" Battery

We have attempted to evaluate the recommendations in the Waskow and Parloff (1975) volume from the standpoint of marital and family therapy research. We have divided these recommendations in the same way that Waskow and Parloff did, according to the "vantage point" from which the observations or ratings are made:

1. Independent Evaluator. In view of the predictable differences in outcome evaluation associated with the vantage point of the evaluator, it seems desirable to include a standard measure of psychiatric status, evaluated by an independent clinical interviewer. The best existing measure, which was recommended in the original "core battery" is the Psychiatric Status Schedule (Spitzer, Endicott, Fleiss, & Cohen, 1970). This measure would be applied only to the "identified patient" because of the time and expense involved in administration. Unfortunately, even this measure, which has been validated more extensively than most,

is not uniformly satisfactory, as it is only applicable for adult patients, and for adults is more relevant for patients with major psychiatric disorders rather than milder symptoms or relationship problems. Although it is too early to evaluate as a research instrument, the recently adopted *Diagnostic and Statistical Manual of Mental Disorders* (3rd ed.), popularly known as DSM-III (American Psychiatric Association, 1980), seems to offer promise. In particular, it covers all age ranges and all degrees of severity. It also allows estimates of the severity of psychosocial stresses and an index of the highest level of previous adaptive functioning, both of which may have importance in predicting the outcome of treatment.

2. Patient Measures. We are in agreement with the two major recommendations made by Waskow and Parloff (1975) for patient measures: (1) The Hopkins Symptoms Checklist (HSCL) is included as a measure of patient distress with particular symptoms (see H. V. Williams, Lipman, Rickels, Covi, Uhlenhuth, & Mattson, 1968). (2) "Target complaints" (Battle, Imber, Hohen-Saric, Stone, Nash, & Frank, 1966) are included because they allow specific target symptoms or problems to be identified, rather than relying on the standard list incorporated in the HCSL.

   As was the case with the interviewer measures, the greatest shortcoming of the recommended measures is their limited applicability when a child is the I.P. For such cases, we recommend the Child Behavior Checklist (Achenbach, 1979) instead of the HSCL. The "target complaints" instrument offers sufficient flexibility to allow the inclusion of complaints involving relationship problems and is not limited to individual symptoms.

3. Therapist Measures. In this area, we recommend the use of "target complaints," as rated by the therapist. We recommend the modified procedure utilized by Luborsky, Mintz, Auerbach, Christoph, Bachrach, Todd, Johnson, Cohen, and O'Brien (1980) in a major outcome research project. In this project, therapists were asked for two kinds of information: (a) specifying and rating the important problems as perceived by the therapist; (b) rating the severity of those target complaints identified by the patient. This two-stage process allows the therapist to specify what he considers the "real" problem, as well as proving an independent estimate of severity of the problems identified by the patient.

   We also agree with the recommendation of the Core Battery Selection Conference that there is a "need to develop a more adequate instrument to tap the specific and general, mediating and ultimate goals that a therapist sets for an individual patient or for groups of patients" (Waskow & Parloff, 1975, p. 297). This certainly is in line with our emphasis on distinguishing between ultimate and subordinate goals. Although there is no fully adequate instrument to measure the achievement of therapist goals, probably the most promising instrument is goal attainment scaling (Kiresuk & Sherman, 1968). We strongly recommend modifying this measure, or something similar, to make it more applicable to marital and family therapy.

4. "Significant Others." Fiske (1975) has described various strategies for the inclusion of "significant others" in the evaluation process. It is probably not surprising that the measures recommended for inclusion of significant others in individual psychotherapy research are the most disappointing to a marital and family therapist. This is clearly the area in which marital and family therapy researchers

can have the most impact in developing new measures and their efforts also should be useful in research on individual psychotherapy.

4.3. Operationalizing Key Concepts Should Be an Urgent Priority

The division of the fields of marital and family therapy into isolated "schools" or "camps" is a serious barrier to the overall advancement of a systematic body of knowledge. There are hopeful signs that later generations of students and researchers are noting more commonality than typically has been implied by the pioneers in these areas. For example, there is speculation that Minuchin's concepts of "enmeshment" and "disengagement" may relate to Bowen's key concepts of "fusion" and "differentiation of self." If such comparability could be established, or if the differences in these dimensions from different theories could be described operationally, this would have major implications for developing a more coherent body of knowledge.

A promising start in this direction has been made by Olson and his co-workers (Olson, Russell, & Sprenkle, 1979; Olson, Sprenkle, & Russell, 1979). As part of their "Circumplex Model," they have attempted to develop a single indicator of family cohesion that would pull together a number of related concepts in the literature: emotional bonding, independence, family boundaries, coalitions, time, space, friends, decision making, and interests and recreation. This is an extremely useful effort, although Bilbro and Dreyer (1981) have shown that the family cohesion measure currently has some severe methodological problems. In addition to empirical analyses, such as those done by Bilbro and Dreyer, there is also a critical need for theoretical analyses that would evaluate how adequately concepts from other theories are represented by a measure such as family cohesion.

4.4. Important Methodological Issues Need Investigation

In addition to operationalizing key concepts, there are important issues of therapeutic methodology within each major theoretical approach that are in urgent need of investigation. Closely related to these are issues revolving around training methods (Kniskern & Gurman, 1982). In the areas of both practice and training, there are often extreme differences in approach across "schools," with far-reaching practical significance.

Not all questions are of equal interest or significance within a given theoretical approach. It has been the consistent emphasis of this chapter that priorities must be set if research is to have the maximum payoff within realistic constraints. Kniskern and Gurman (1982) recently have identified major researchable questions within several major theoretical approaches to marital and family therapy. Some of these questions are included here to illustrate the major point that research priority should be given to the major questions of particular relevance to a given theoretical orientation. (To take an extreme example, it is pointless to wait for a behaviorally oriented researcher to investigate the effects of personal psychotherapy on the therapist's effectiveness; if such a study is ever performed, it most likely will be done from a psychodynamic viewpoint.)

Kniskern and Gurman have chosen representative examples from each of four major clusters of approaches: systems approaches, intergenerational approaches, behavioral approaches, and psychodynamic approaches. The school or schools chosen have been selected purely to illustrate the research hypotheses that can be drawn.

Within structural-strategic therapy, for example, there is a heavy emphasis on tasks and directives, yet little research to show whether extra-session tasks speed up therapy or increase generalization. The use of indirect methods and the lack of emphasis on insight may raise questions (at least for Kniskern and Gurman) of the generalizability of results. Since structural-strategic therapy is highly pragmatic and results in borrowing techniques from other approaches, the question of critical ingredients becomes particularly salient. With regard to training, there has been much more emphasis on technique factors than on therapist factors; empirical validation of this emphasis would have great practical significance.

Many of the intergenerational approaches place a heavy emphasis on cotherapy. As mentioned above, this is an expensive practice that thus far has not been validated empirically. Bowen theory, as a particular example of the intergenerational approach, raises other interesting research issues. Gurman (1978) has noted that the key concept of "differentiation of self," which seems so central to all of Bowen theory and practice, sorely needs validation. From the standpoint of practice, it also would be important to investigate the technique of working predominantly with one family member. In regard to training, the importance of having therapists work on their own families of origin clearly needs validation. To date, little research of any sort has been conducted on any of the intergenerational approaches.

Behavioral marital and family therapy have placed a relatively heavy emphasis on empirical validation. This has led to a greater possibility within this approach of beginning to ask questions concerning "crucial ingredients." There are questions concerning whether skill training is sufficient, by itself, for all couples and all parents; there are preliminary indications that such training alone will not be sufficient for more severely disturbed couples. The very specificity of behavioral methods also raises the issue of generalization of treatment effects (Forehand & Atkinson, 1977). This includes generalization to other settings, to other nontargeted problems, and to other family relationships. Therapist training also is an important issue; no other approach has so consistently implied that therapy could be conducted "by the book," yet there seems to be some increased awareness of the need for other approaches and the importance of nonspecific factors.

Group-analytic family therapy (Skynner, 1981), like most psychodynamic approaches, places a heavy emphasis on the therapist as the therapeutic instrument. This creates a critical need for investigation of the effects of the personality and psychopathology of the therapist as well as his or her training. How trainees should be selected and what forms of training they should receive are important questions.

4.5. Work with Well-Defined Populations

It is to be hoped that the field is progressing beyond questions such as "Does family therapy work?" or "What form of family therapy works the best?" to more refined questions of "What treatment approach (or combination of approaches) is most effective within this particular clinical situation?" For the last of these questions to be meaningful, however, it is important to have systematic ways for categorizing types of clinical situations.

It does not appear accidental that the most successful outcome research in marital and family therapy has been conducted with well defined populations or that these categorizations have been based on the symptomatology of the identified patient. (See Number 4 in the first section on conclusions from existing research, pp. 94–95.)

In this respect, it is worth examining further the notion of "homogeneity." We are familiar with the two major populations studied at the Philadelphia Child Guidance Clinic—families with psychosomatic children and families with a young adult male heroin addict—and we certainly have been struck by how homogenous each of these populations seems. It may be, as Haley (1980) suggests, that an additional reason for homogeneity is that each group comes from a similar stage in the family life cycle. Inclusion of adult-onset anorectics or drug-taking adolescents might have destroyed the homogeneity of each of these groups. It is tempting to speculate that some unprofitable research investigations of other clinical groups, such as schizophrenics or problem children, may have failed because they do not represent homogeneous entities.

We agree fully with Gurman and Kniskern (1981) that complete reliance on traditional psychiatric nosology is not very satisfactory, yet "it is clear that diagnostic procedures at a family system level are so poorly developed as to currently preclude routine sample definition with such strategies" (p. 754). Until such measures are better developed and more generally accepted, there seems little alternative but to begin with some uniform presenting problem and further refine the sample on the basis of family factors (e.g., life cycle stage, single parent, degree of marital conflict).

It is, of course, important to have a theory that helps to describe the patterns that exist and that distinguishes between differences that matter and those that are only variations of the same pattern. For example, in the psychosomatic research at Philadelphia Child Guidance Clinic, there appear to be strong similarities across psychosomatic problems (anorexia, asthma, diabetes), yet major differences between "brittle" diabetics and "behavioral" diabetics. These findings are based upon systematic observation of family interaction. Similarly, we saw strong similarities (and some differences) in the pattern of interactions of addicts' families from different ethnic groups. We saw little practical difference between families with an overinvolved mother-addict dyad compared to father-addict overinvolvement.

Another challenging task is to find valid indicators of the degree of difficulty of a given case. As mentioned earlier, this information may have important implications for the selection of particular techniques or approaches. Unfortunately, the degree of difficulty of a case may be a complex function of factors at several levels, including the presenting symptom, individual characteristics of the patient, the family system, and systems beyond the family. For example, prognosis in a case of school phobia probably is a function of at least the following: severity and persistence of the symptom; social and academic skills of the child; extrafamilial interests of the overinvolved parent; quality of the marital relationship and supports available to the overinvolved parent; quality of the school environment, such as the degree of actual danger extant. Factors such as these probably do not make extreme, qualitative differences between cases, but they have major impact on the length of treatment and the degree of success.

4.6. What Happens in Therapy?

4.6.1. How Can We Move Beyond a "Black Box" View?

We already have noted that the strongest research evidence has come from investigations of treatment methods that are relatively well defined, such as behavioral sex therapy, structural family therapy, and functional family therapy. Further movement in the direction of specificity seems important to the advancement of the field. We will touch briefly on several areas of research that would help us to move away from a view of therapy as a mysterious "black box."

Are the Practitioners Skilled? Specific evidence of the skills of the therapists studied is important in both single-method and comparative studies. In evaluating the effectiveness of a single method, it is important to have data on the kind and amount of training. For comparative studies, it is even more important that the practitioners are equally skilled. Measurement is not simple; measures such as years of experience are not particularly informative and typically have been poor predictors of success. The approach of using "certified experts" in a given technique is slightly better, but it still tells little about what these experts know and do and how they differ from other therapists. Further specification would include the actual content of the training and the evaluative mechanisms used to measure the acquisition of skills.

What Do Therapists Actually Do? An exciting, empirically based approach to the question of what therapists actually do is the investigation of process (Pinsof, 1981). It is based on the assumption that the best way of explicating similarities and differences across approaches is through the systematic study of videotaped samples of therapy. Although this approach is difficult and time-consuming, it may help to break down artificial distinctions between approaches.

The opposite approach is the construction of "manuals," such as have been heavily used by behaviorally oriented therapists. Even if an actual "recipe" cannot be written, it is useful to identify the basic elements of the therapeutic framework and to show that these elements can be communicated and taught to practitioners. Of course, even when this approach is adopted, it still is important to verify through the analysis of tapes that the approach is being followed and that other factors are not operating.

What Other Therapy/Therapist Factors Matter? Not surprisingly, given our structural-strategic orientation, we do not share the belief of Gurman and Kniskern (1978d) that therapist factors are the most important, compared to technique factors. We do, on the other hand, believe that a wide variety of nonspecific factors, such as therapist expectations, therapist self-confidence, and the utilization of a clear, explanatory framework (Frank, 1973; A. K. Shapiro & Morris, 1978), have important effects on therapy outcome. We would contend that these factors can be taught and systematically utilized to improve outcome.

Realistically, it seems safe to assume that therapist factors, method factors, and nonspecific factors all interact with each other (as well as with family characteristics). It seems foolish to think of factors such as empathy and warmth, or technical skill, operating in a vacuum. Instead each, in the presence of the other, may contribute to overall success.

5. Summary of Recommendations

In conclusion, we offer our "recipe" for successful research in marital and family therapy. Although no recommendations can guarantee success, adopting these guidelines should help to prevent uninterpretable results and to make good use of available resources for research. In short, the researcher should:

1. Begin with a well defined clinical population.
2. Compare a new method to a standard approach that is well established (and

hopefully empirically validated). This standard approach should be practiced by therapists who are skilled in applying it and who believe in its effectiveness.

3. Specify the new treatment method: How are therapists trained and what will they do? Document what they actually do, using videotapes and other evidence, such as session goals and patient feedback.
4. Use random assignment and the other crucial design features identified in the literature.
5. Carefully distinguish between ultimate goals and intervening goals. Test hypothesized connections between intervening and ultimate goals.
6. Employ multiple outcome measures, without obscuring the primary importance of the presenting problem.
7. Conduct periodic follow-up.

6. References

Achenbach, T. M. The child behavioral profile: An empirically based system for assessing children's behavioral problems and competencies. *International Journal of Mental Health*, 1979, *7*, 24–42.

American Psychiatric Association. *Diagnostic and statistical manual of mental disorders* (3rd ed.). Washington, D.C.: Author, 1980.

Barton, C., & Alexander, J. Functional family therapy. In A. Gurman & D. Kniskern (Eds.), *Handbook of family therapy*. New York: Brunner/Mazel, 1981.

Battle, C. C., Imber, S. D., Hoehn-Saric, R., Stone, A. R., Nash, E. R., & Frank, J. D. Target complaints as criteria of improvement. *American Journal of Psychotherapy*, 1966, *20*, 184–192.

Bergin, A. E., & Lambert, M. J. The evaluation of therapeutic outcome. In S. L. Garfield & A. E. Bergin (Eds.), *Handbook of psychotherapy and behavior change* (2nd ed.). New York: Wiley, 1978.

Bilbro, T., & Dreyer, A. A methodological study of a measure of family cohesion. *Family Process*, 1981, *20*, 419–427.

Cartwright, D. S., Kirtner, W. L., & Fiske, D. W. Method factors in changes associated with psychotherapy. *Journal of Abnormal and Social Psychology*, 1963, *66*, 164–175.

Colapinto, J. The relative value of empirical evidence. *Family Process*, 1979, *18*, 427–441.

DeWitt, K. N. The effectiveness of family therapy: A review of outcome research. *Archives of General Psychiatry*, 1978, *35*, 549–561.

DiMascio, A., & Klerman, G. *An appropriate control group for psychotherapy research in depression*. Paper presented at a meeting of the Society for Psychotherapy Research, Madison, Wisc., June 1977.

Fiske, D. W. The use of significant others in assessing the outcome of psychotherapy. In I. E. Waskow & M. B. Parloff (Eds.), *Psychotherapy change measures*. Rockville, Md.: National Institute of Mental Health, 1975.

Fiske, D. W., Hunt, H. F., Luborsky, L., Orne, M. T., Parloff, M. B., Reiser, M. F., & Tuma, A. H. Planning of research on effectiveness of psychotherapy. *Archives of General Psychiatry*, 1970, *22*, 22–32.

Forehand, R., & Atkinson, B. M. Generality of treatment effects with parents as therapists: A review of assessment and implementation procedures. *Behavior Therapy*, 1977, *8*, 575–593.

Frank, J. D. *Persuasion and healing* (2nd ed.). Baltimore: Johns Hopkins University Press, 1973.

Garfield, S., Prager, R., & Bergin, A. Evaluation of outcome in psychotherapy. *Journal of Consulting and Clinical Psychology*, 1971, *37*, 307–313.

Garfield, S. L. Research on client variables in psychotherapy. In S. L. Garfield & A. E. Bergin (Eds.), *Handbook of psychotherapy and behavior change* (2nd ed.). New York: Wiley, 1978.

Gurman, A. S. Contemporary marital therapies. In T. J. Paolino & B. S. McGrady (Eds.), *Marriage and marital therapy: Psychoanalytic, behavioral and systems theory perspectives*. New York: Brunner/Mazel, 1978.

Gurman, A. S., & Klein, M. H. The treatment of women in marital and family conflict: Recommendations for outcome evaluation. In A. Brodsky & R. Hare-Mustin (Eds.), *Research on psychotherapy with women*. New York: Guilford Press, 1980.

Gurman, A. S., & Kniskern, D. P. Behavioral marriage therapy: II. Empirical perspective. *Family Process,* 1978, *17,* 139–148. (a)

Gurman, A. S., & Kniskern, D. P. Deterioration in marital and family therapy: Empirical, clinical and conceptual issues. *Family Process,* 1978, *17,* 3–20. (b)

Gurman, A. S., & Kniskern, D. P. Research on marital and family therapy: Progress, perspective and prospect. In S. Garfield & A. Bergin (Eds.), *Handbook of psychotherapy and behavior change* (2nd ed.). New York: Wiley, 1978. (c)

Gurman, A. S., & Kniskern, D. P. Technolatry, methodolatry and results of family therapy. *Family Process,* 1978, *17,* 275–281. (d)

Gurman, A. S., & Kniskern, D. P. Family therapy outcome research: Knowns and unknowns. In A. Gurman & D. Kniskern (Eds.), *Handbook of family therapy.* New York: Brunner/Mazel, 1981.

Gurman, A. S., & Knudson, R. M. Behavioral marriage therapy: I. A psychodynamic-systems analysis and critique. *Family Process,* 1978, *17,* 121–138.

Gurman, A. S., Knudson, R. M., & Kniskern, D. P. Behavioral marriage therapy: IV. Take two aspirin and call us in the morning. *Family Process,* 1978, *17,* 165–180.

Haley, J. *Strategies of psychotherapy.* New York: Grune & Stratton, 1963.

Haley, J. *Leaving home.* New York: McGraw-Hill, 1980.

Hoffman, L. The family life cycle and discontinuous change. In E. Carter & M. Orfanidis (Eds.), *The family life cycle.* New York: Gardner Press, 1980.

Hoffman, L. *Foundations of family therapy: A conceptual framework for systems change.* New York: Basic Books, 1981.

Jacobson, N. S. A review of the research on the effectiveness of marital therapy. In T. J. Paolino & B. S. McCrady (Eds.), *Marriage and marital therapy: Psychoanalytic, behavioral and systems theory perspectives.* New York: Brunner/Mazel, 1978.

Jacobson, N. S., & Martin, B. Behavioral marriage therapy: Current status. *Psychological Bulletin,* 1976, *83,* 540–556.

Jacobson, N. S., & Weiss, R. L. Behavioral marriage therapy: III. Critique: The contents of Gurman *et al.* may be hazardous to our health. *Family Process,* 1978, *17,* 149–163.

Kiersuk, T. J., & Sherman, R. E. Goal attainment scaling: A general method for evaluating comprehensive community mental health programs. *Community Mental Health Journal,* 1968, *4,* 443–453.

Kiesler, D. J. Some myths of psychotherapy research and the search for a paradigm. *Psychological Bulletin,* 1966, *65,* 110–136.

Klein, M. H., Greist, J. H., Gurman, A. S., & Van Cura, L. *The psychotherapy of depression.* Research project, University of Wisconsin Medical School, 1978.

Kniskern, D. P., & Gurman, A. S. Research on training in marriage and family therapy: Status, issues and directions. In M. Andolfi & I. Zwerling (Eds.), *Dimensions of family therapy.* New York: Guilford Press, 1980.

Kniskern, D. P., & Gurman, A. Advances and prospects for family therapy research. In J. P. Vincent (Ed.), *Advances in family intervention, assessment and theory: An annual compilation of research.* Greenwich, Conn.: Jai Press, 1981.

Lebow, J. Issues in the assessment of outcome in family therapy. *Family Process,* 1981, *20,* 167–188.

Love, L. R., Kaswan, J., & Bugental, D. E. Differential effectiveness of three clinical interventions for different socioeconomic groupings. *Journal of Consulting and Clinical Psychology,* 1972, *39,* 347–360.

Luborsky, L., Mintz, J., Auerbach, A. H., Christoph, P., Bachrach, H., Todd, T., Johnson, M., Cohen, M., & O'Brien, C. P. Predicting the outcome of psychotherapy: Findings of the Penn Psychotherapy Project. *Archives of General Psychiatry,* 1980, *37,* 471–481.

Madanes, C. *Strategic family therapy.* San Francisco: Jossey-Bass, 1981.

Mintz, J., Auerbach, A., Luborsky, J., & Johnson, M. Patients', therapists', and observers' views of psychotherapy: A "Rashomon" experience or a reasonable consensus? *British Journal of Medical Psychology,* 1973, *46,* 83–89.

Minuchin, S., Baker, L., Rosman, B., Liebman, R., Milman, L., & Todd, T. A conceptual model of psychosomatic illness in children. *Archives of General Psychiatry,* 1975, *32,* 1031–1038.

Minuchin, S., Rosman, B. O., & Baker, L. *Psychosomatic families.* Cambridge: Harvard University Press, 1978.

Olson, D. H., Russell, C., & Sprenkle, D. Circumplex model of marital and family systems: II. Empirical studies and clinical intervention. In J. P. Vincent (Ed.), *Advances in family intervention, assessment and theory*. Greenwich, Conn.: Jai Press, 1979.

Olson, D. H., Sprenkle, D., & Russell, C. Circumplex model of marital and family systems: I. Cohesion and adaptability dimensions, family types and clinical applications. *Family Process*, 1979, *18*, 3–28.

Olson, D. H., Russell, C. S., & Sprenkle, D. H. Marital and family therapy: A decade review. *Journal of Marriage and the Family*, 1980, *42*, 973–993.

Palazzoli-Selvini, M., Boscolo, L., Cecchin, G. F., & Prata, G. The treatment of children through brief therapy of their parents. *Family Process*, 1974, *13*, 429–442.

Palazzoli-Selvini, M., Boscolo, L., Cecchin, G. F., & Prata, G. Family rituals: A powerful tool in family therapy. *Family Process*, 1977, *16*, 445–453.

Palazzoli-Selvini, M., Boscolo, L., Cecchin, G., & Prata, G. *Paradox and counter-paradox: A new model in the therapy of the family in schizophrenic transaction*. New York: Jason Aaronson, 1978.

Palazzoli-Selvini, M., Boscolo, L., Cecchin, G. F., & Prata, G. Hypothesizing—circularity—neutrality: Three guidelines for the conductor of the session. *Family Process*, 1980, *19*, 3–12.

Parloff, M. B., Waskow, I. E., & Wolfe, B. E. Research on therapist variables in relation to process and outcome. In S. L. Garfield & A. E. Bergin (Eds.), *Handbook of psychotherapy and behavior change* (2nd ed.). New York: Wiley, 1978.

Pinsof, W. Family therapy process research. In A. Gurman & D. Kniskern (Eds.), *Handbook of family therapy*. New York: Brunner/Mazel, 1981.

Shapiro, A. K., & Morris, L. A. The placebo effect in medical and psychological therapies. In S. L. Garfield & A. E. Bergin (Eds.), *Handbook of psychotherapy and behavior change* (2nd ed.). New York: Wiley, 1978.

Shapiro, R., & Budman, S. Defection, termination and continuation in family and individual therapy. *Family Process*, 1973, *12*, 55–67.

Skynner, A. C. An open-systems, group analytic approach to family therapy. In A. Gurman & D. Kniskern (Eds.), *Handbook of family therapy*. New York: Brunner/Mazel, 1981.

Sloane, R. B., Staples, F. R., Cristol, A. H., Yorkston, N. J., & Whipple, K. *Psychotherapy versus behavior therapy*. Cambridge: Harvard University Press, 1975.

Spitzer, R. L., Endicott, J., Fleiss, J. L., & Cohen, J. The psychiatric status schedule: A technique for evaluating psychopathology and impairment in role functioning. *Archives of General Psychiatry*, 1970, *23*, 41–55.

Stanton, M. D. Strategic approaches to family therapy. In A. S. Gurman & D. P. Kniskern (Eds.), *Handbook of family therapy*. New York: Brunner/Mazel, 1981.

Stanton, M. D., & Todd, T. C. Structural family therapy with drug addicts. In E. Kaufman & P. Kaufmann (Eds.), *The family therapy of drug and alcohol abuse*. New York: Gardner, 1979.

Stanton, M. D., & Todd, T. C. A critique of the Wells and Dezen review of the results of nonbehavioral family therapy. *Family Process*, 1980, *19*, 169–176.

Stanton, M. D., Todd, T. C., Heard, D. B., Kirschner, S., Kleiman, J. I., Mowatt, D. T., Riley, P., Scott, S. M., & Van Deusen, J. M. Heroin addiction as a family phenomenon: A new conceptual model. *American Journal of Drug and Alcohol Abuse*, 1978, *5*, 125–150.

Stanton, M. D., Todd, T. C., Steier, F., Van Deusen, J. M., Marder, L., Rosoff, R. J., Seaman, S. F., & Skibinski, E. *Family characteristics and family therapy of heroin addicts: Final report 1974–1978* (Grant No. R01 DA 01119). Report prepared for the National Institute on Drug Abuse (2nd printing), December 1980.

Stanton, M. D., Steier, F., & Todd, T. C. Paying families for attending sessions: Counteracting the dropout problem. *Journal of Marital and Family Therapy*, 1982, *8*, 371–373.

Stanton, M. D., Todd, T. C., & Associates. *The family therapy of drug abuse and addiction*. New York: Guilford, 1982.

Strupp, H. H. Psychotherapy research and practice: An overview. In S. L. Garfield & A. E. Bergin (Eds.), *Handbook of psychotherapy and behavior change* (2nd ed.). New York: Wiley, 1978.

Thom, R. *Structural stability and morphogenesis*, Reading, Mass.: Benjamin/Cummings, 1975.

Todd, T. C. *Family therapy evaluated*. Paper presented at a meeting of the Society for Psychotherapy Research, Philadelphia, Pa., June 1973.

Todd, T. C., Berger, H., & Lande, G. Supervisors' views on the special requirements of family therapy with drug abusers. In M. D. Stanton, T. C. Todd, & Associates, *The family therapy of drug abuse and addiction*. New York: Guilford, 1982.

Waskow, I. E., & Parloff, M. B. *Psychotherapy change measures*. Rockville, Md.: National Institute of Mental Health, 1975.

Watzlawick, P., Weakland, J., & Fisch, R. *Change: Principles of problem formation and problem resolution.* New York: Norton, 1974.

Wells, R. A., & Dezen, A. E. The results of family therapy revisited: The nonbehavioral methods. *Family Process,* 1978, *17,* 251–274. (a)

Wells, R. A., & Dezen, A. E. Ideologies, idols (and graven images?): Rejoinder to Gurman and Kniskern. *Family Process,* 1978, *17,* 283–286. (b)

Williams, A. M., & Miller, W. R. Evaluation and research on marital therapy. In G. P. Sholevar (Ed.), *The handbook of marriage and marital therapy.* New York: Spectrum, 1981.

Williams, H. V., Lipman, R., Rickels, K., Covi, L., Uhlenhuth, E., & Mattson, N. Replication of symptom distress factors in anxious neurotic outpatients. *Multivariate Behavioral Research,* 1968, *3,* 199–212.

Wincze, J. P., & Caird, W. K. The effects of systematic desensitization and video desensitization in the treatment of essential sexual dysfunction in women. *Behavior Therapy,* 1976, *7,* 335–342.

Winter, J. E., & Kolevzon, M. S. A conceptual framework for family therapy treatment and training research: Systems, strategic, communications. In C. H. Simpkinson (Ed.), *1980 Synopsis of family therapy practice.* Olney, Md.: Family Therapy Practice Network, 1982.

7

Training in Marriage and Family Therapy

ROBERT HENLEY WOODY AND
GWEN KATHLEEN WEBER

Independent innovation has been the hallmark of the early learning models and methods for education and training in marriage and family therapy.[1] Often the creative trainer became the model for the student, just as the original charismatic practitioner grasped the professional's interest in early practice.

Education and training programs have been notably lacking in therapeutic, scientific, and systemic developments. Kniskern and Gurman (1980) have stated: "After reviewing the literature on family therapy training, we have to confess our field's collective empirical ignorance about this topic" (p. 221).

Academic and institutional training programs are now working to establish viable training programs and curricula and there are educational and professional standards and legal sanctions being promulgated. The potential impact of the therapist on the lives of his or her clients makes it clear that professional controls must set some minimal competency level of training for family therapists. The development of family therapy education programs with standardized criteria for professional competence has become the primary development task of the family therapy movement of the 1980s.

The tremendous variety of formal institutional training programs now existing make the evaluation and standardization of family therapy training a complex and confusing task. It is difficult to create a multidisciplinary educational program that is applicable to all of the existing disciplines, for example, psychiatry, psychology, social work, counseling, and psychiatric nursing (Bloch, 1981). At the same time professionals are working to establish a new systematic epistemology that shifts to an ecosystem, biopsychosocial definition of illness, and the development and adoption of interventions that serve as a generic conceptual foundation for professional use.

[1]Herein, brevity dictates generic terminology. Unless stated specifically, "education" will encompass both "education and training" and "family therapy" will encompass both "marriage and family therapy."

ROBERT HENLEY WOODY • Department of Psychology, University of Nebraska at Omaha, Omaha, Nebraska 68182. **GWEN KATHLEEN WEBER** • Department of Psychiatry, C. Louis Meyer Children's Rehabilitation Institute, Omaha, Nebraska 68131.

This chapter discusses the dimensions and current issues of the existing "state of the art" of family therapy education. It considers the progress and development of educational programs in family therapy and the current issues and dilemmas that have thwarted or facilitated the educational processes. A didactic eclectic conceptual framework is presented that is applicable to either an academic or a clinical setting. It considers the role of the educator, supervisor, and peer group and the clinical training experiences in promoting the personal development, family awareness, and the processes that enhance the development of clinical therapy skills. The integration of these individualized learning experiences within the context of the educational framework is reviewed in recognizing the diverse learning methods necessary to facilitate this process. Lastly, this chapter reviews ethics and law as relevant to practice and concludes with speculations about the future.

1. Early Marriage and Family Therapy Education

Initially two major factors delayed the progressive development of family therapy education. First, most early family therapy training occurred in clinical settings, where trainers were more concerned with treatment methods and the student's personal development than in establishing educational foundations or a new profession. The student worked with his or her mentor or teacher, with "modeling" being the primary mode for learning. Such pioneers as Bowen, Ackerman, Bateson, Haley, Whitaker, Framo, and others each were independently establishing training experiences; most of these experiences were admittedly unclear as to the efficacy of the methods for practice and training. Haley (1969) commented: "When the unit of treatment shifted to the family, the disciplines became undisciplined" (p. 149).

Once the various trainers began sharing their efforts they realized great diversity existed among them. Ackerman (1970) observed:

> The most striking feature of our field today is the emergence of a bewildering array of diverse forms of family treatment. Each therapist seems to be doing "his own thing." We are faced squarely with the challenge to evaluate this diversity. Which of the differences are real? Which more apparent than real? Does the dramatic quality of these differences, in effect, obscure some basic sameness? Given choices, family therapists tend to polarize and specialize. In the final analysis each does what he likes to do and what he does best. (p. 123)

These numerous activities led to many creative training experiences; however, no effective means to compare, actually study, or integrate these efforts existed.

There also were practitioners who did not believe that skills in family therapy could be taught through a conceptual process due to the personal artistic nature of the practice. Whitaker (1976) stated: "By its very nature, it defies technical and theoretical components" (p. 156). Whitaker viewed the learning process to be similar to Zen, that being: "It increases courage and know-how to face impossible problems" (p. 158).

These early educational efforts were fragmented, inconclusive, and related specifically to the practice skills and the individual's personal development as a therapist. The various "theoretical orientations" usually were idiosyncratic according to the mentor-supervisor's clinical preferences.

There was also a question of whether to integrate family therapy into established professional disciplines or to exempt it (i.e., carve out a new discipline) that thwarted family therapy education further. Academic training programs in the traditional disciplines (e.g., psychiatry, psychology, and social work) questioned the extent of their interest and involvement in marriage and family therapy. Many have continued to question whether it is a practice modality, a theoretical orientation, a new orientation that seeks to become a distinct entity, or a new profession unique in itself. For example, Cooper, Rampage, and Soucy (1981) found those psychology faculty aligned with family therapy often perceived themselves as a minority or third-rate professors when compared to those in other traditional fields of study in psychology.

Each discipline originally gave its unique reasons to ''stand-off'' from family therapy evaluation in its respective academic programs. One basic factor was the multidisciplinary status of family therapy. No one discipline had ''ownership'' of family therapy; thus, there was hesitation about borrowing or integrating the eclectic theoretical models into a given profession's curriculum. Psychiatry remained committed to medical/clinical models that focused on individual disease and illness. Psychology's curriculum focused primarily on adult and child treatment modalities, which most often separated members of the family unit for treatment. Social work viewed the early family casework concepts as congruent with family therapy concepts—and indeed they were. Rather than providing professional leadership or integrating new concepts into existing curricula however, social work educators too often continued in the established curricula and ignored the family therapy movement. Or, if workers pursued the uniqueness of the new theories, they often departed from traditional professional education and realigned their allegiance to the family therapy movement apart from a social work professional identity (Weber, 1979).

In summary, early family therapy education efforts were delayed by: (1) the lack of leadership by any one professional discipline or early development of a separate professional entity; (2) the hesitation of academic settings to develop a curriculum in the area of family therapy; (3) the fragmentation of the early training programs based in clinical settings and the emphasis therein being to consider the personal, artistic development of therapy skills in the student; and (4) the diverse theoretical orientations, lack of a clear eclectic conceptual theory, and lack of a clear definition of the relationship of theory to the practice of family therapy.

2. Current Family Therapy Education Programs

More professionals have been seeking family therapy education than ever before, and more and more facilities are now offering a variety of learning experiences. In 1978–79, Bloch and Weiss (1981) found an estimated 4,140 students to be receiving long-term training (1 to 3 years or graduate programs) in marriage and family therapy. A total of approximately 18,000 were reported to have received at least brief family therapy ''enrichment'' educational experiences in credited or noncredited family therapy courses, workshops, and conferences, or were involved in one year extern training programs at family institutes in 1978–79. Approximately 60% of the total training sites listed in their master list of family therapy training programs in the United States were founded between 1971 and 1980 (i.e., 77 new university programs).

There is now a strong impetus to assess systematically the professional education in the field of marriage and family therapy. Professionals are moving toward achieving a greater level of consensus about the content and standards needed for a professional education base for the family therapist. Several factors have given an increased thrust for this movement.

The government now gives its official recognition to the emerging field of marriage and family therapy. First, seven states have successfully acquired licensure requirements for marriage and family therapists. Second, the federal government has authorized the Commission of Accreditation for Marriage and Family Therapy as the official organization to monitor and develop professional standards of quality marriage and family therapy education.

Professional organizations and associations also have contributed to the multidisciplinary support of family therapy. New associations, such as the American Family Therapy Association and American Board of Family Psychology, Inc., and the continued quality activities of the American Orthopsychiatric Association and American Association for Marriage and Family Therapy, each have provided a professional identity for the family therapist. Competency for practice seems to be an integral part of membership requirements, such as for "Clinical Member" status in the American Association for Marriage and Family Therapy.

3. Academic Degree Programs

Academic training for marriage and family therapy has been developed primarily in psychiatry, clinical psychology, guidance and counseling, social work, and home economics programs. Some of these curricula provide a specialization or sequence of study separate from the established basic course of professional study. Academic credits are not always given for the intern or extern programs that exist in institutions; however, their educational programs are as valid as those academically based ones.

Until recently there has been little information available about these programs or the extent of them. The recent studies of Bloch and Weiss (1981), Sugarman (1981), Cooper, Rampage, and Soucy (1981), and Weber (1979) provide some current identification of the training occurring throughout the nation.

3.1. Psychiatry Residency Programs

The Group for the Advancement of Psychiatry report of 1970 suggested that the future of psychiatry might be altered radically by a shift from individual to relational psychology as its theoretical understructure. The current training programs reflect some of this projected trend.

Sugarman's (1981) survey included 20% of the accredited graduate residency programs in psychiatry in the United States. It showed an increase in marriage and family therapy education. For example, 98% of the reporting programs *required* some family therapy training. Eighty-eight % of these programs required 100 to 650 hours of training.

Over one-half of the programs had a full-time faculty member as the designated head of the family therapy program. The preferred emphasis or objectives of the programs were to expand and change the theoretical views of the residents; providing specific interventions was a secondary goal. These often were accomplished through direct experiences however. Sixty-six % of the programs viewed themselves as being more practice oriented than theory oriented (34%). The eclectic and structural theoretical models were preferred by 91% of the programs. In conclusion, the practice of family therapy in both inpatient and outpatient cases had increased significantly as the treatment of choice.

3.2. Clinical Psychology Programs

Stanton (1975) observed that: "Only recently has acceptance of the family system's approach to therapy begun to creep into academic psychology departments" (p. 43). At that time, only 10 clinical programs offered family therapy training. Liddle (1976) wrote of his initial frustrations in his efforts to develop a family therapy curriculum in a psychology department. Cooper *et al.* (1981) noted that often the family therapy training in various psychology departments occupied a "third-class" status to the traditional curriculum.

The study by Cooper *et al.* (1981) considered family therapy training in academic programs that offer a PhD or PsyD in clinical psychology and are accredited by the American Psychological Association. Sixty-five % of the total programs were included. Only 18% of all of the available psychotherapy courses were identified as family therapy courses. Only 8% of the schools actually *required* a family treatment course. Thirty-nine % of the internship programs required any family therapy training. Ten % of the faculty members identified themselves as family-oriented psychologists and 32% of all of the programs had no faculty identified in the area of family therapy.

The findings revealed that a broad psychotherapeutic foundation (which included adult, child, group, and family curriculum) continued to be more the educational norm, as opposed to a concentration in any one specialization. The Cooper *et al.* study did show an interesting absence of a consistent relationship between the school's estimation of the importance of training in family therapy and the relevant number of courses offered in that area, which perhaps suggests the interest present to further develop family therapy curriculum in the future.

3.3. Graduate Social Work Programs

Most schools of social work in the nation offer family therapy education. Siporin (1980) received responses from 95% of all graduate schools of social work or social welfare in the United States in his study conducted in 1975–76. Ninety % of the schools reported that instruction was given on the specific content of marriage and family counseling/therapy in the required methods courses on social work practice, casework, or social treatment. Sixty-eight % of the schools gave elective courses on family therapy, 33% on marriage therapy, and 46% on combined marriage and family therapy. Eighty % of the respondents considered family therapy to be a legitimate area of practice specialization, and 67% accepted this categorization separately for marriage therapy. The social work faculty expressed the need for assistance in the content and instructional materials for these courses.

Weber's (1979) study included 82% of all accredited social work graduate programs in the United States. Ninety-six % of these schools reported that at least one graduate course on family therapy was offered. Only three schools reported no family therapy courses. All of the courses were identified as elective.

Presently, there are no guidelines or national standards for developing social work courses in family therapy. A comparative analysis of the courses' curricula found extreme diversity in their content. Some of the courses identified as family therapy emphasized the social, cultural, political, and economic aspects of family life and related social policy. Other courses were found to emphasize treatment and the clinical practice of family therapy. Many courses were generic and covered a broad spectrum of family theory and practice. Fifty-two % of the schools differentiated the meanings of family therapy, casework with families, and family counseling; however, a common definition was not evident. The current family therapy theories emphasized in the courses' contents were systems, communication, structural, behavioral, and interactional.

Fifty-nine % of the schools reported having only 1 professor teaching family therapy; 25% reported having 2 faculty; and 17% reported having 3 or more faculty. In personal interviews with 15 of these faculty, Weber identified their concerns of needing some professional or national direction for the educational experiences in family therapy.

While 40% of the schools provided practicum experiences in marriage and family therapy, the interface of these experiences with the curriculum content was viewed as problematic. The need for additional practicum sites, quality supervision in marraige and family therapy, and the coordination of these experiences with the school were common concerns expressed in the study. Weber concluded that while social workers are found to practice family therapy more than any other discipline, the educational preparation is not professionally based with well established training standards.

4. Institutional Training

Family therapy training has much of its heritage in institutionally based programs. A recent study of Bloch and Weiss (1981) sought to identify and categorize those programs currently existing across the nation. The respondents were categorized into one of two groups, according to their administrative auspices. Type I included institutions or programs that were involved exclusively in family therapy training. Type II programs were those embedded in a larger program, for example, academic departments. The programs were grouped into: (*A*) training; (*B*) enrichment; or (*AB*) mixed with both. The survey included 175 facilities; 128 were institutionally based programs.

The progressive growth of family therapy education was obvious. Eighty-nine % of the programs had been founded since 1961, with 60% being initiated since 1971. Since academic programs have increased at a proportionate ratio, the ratio of training programs in family institutes has remained nearly the same ratio, namely, 1:2, during the past 20 years.

Most of the institutional programs offered more than enrichment experiences only; other options were ongoing training through intensive on-site practicum experiences or external study programs. Little information was available from these institutions on the students' background and experiences. Many of them were receiving training as a part of the curriculum in a master's degree program. Most of the students were identified as having been a participant in workshops, conferences, and/or had family therapy courses in an academic or a graduate program. Bloch and Weiss (1981) believed that these "data make clear the necessity for professional standards that set some minimal acceptable level of training for family therapists" (p. 139).

Since the previous small apprentice-type programs have become more structured and institutionalized than in the past the potential for this is more likely to occur. Bloch (1981) commented:

> The implications are clear: that training in family therapy at a sophisticated level is now to be a regular part of the future training of psychiatrists, psychologists, social workers, and psychiatric nurses and that, in addition, as a second distinctive career line, there is a new profession of family therapist, with its own entry point and academic pathway. (p. 131)

They believed that as a consensus develops in the field about its theoretical base, clinical skills, and training procedures, family systems thinking will become more influential to the professionals.

5. Review of Existing Training Experiences

This review of the existing family therapy education programs supports the belief that there has been developmental progress but that there are many pressing educational concerns in need of resolution. In summary, the following observations are made:

1. Professionals and paraprofessionals have increased their participation in a variety of family therapy education and training programs. There is little information on the background, experience, or learning interests of these trainee-students. Likewise, there is a lack of information on the application or use of the training received.
2. The number of family therapy education programs has increased significantly in the past 20 years. These have progressively moved toward more formalized or structured experiences; however, no standardized criteria or levels of competence have been established and there seems to be a concomitant of qualitative inconsistency throughout the various programs.
3. Academic facilities have included an increased amount of family therapy education in their curricula. These courses and experiences are nearly all still electives; they typically include both clinical practice and courses. Some academic facilities have hesitated to develop curricula, although they have expressed an interest in marriage and family therapy education. The quality and extent of student supervision is a concern for many clinical settings. The interface of the family therapy curriculum with the existing traditional professional course content remains unclear, as does the relationship of academic marriage and family therapy graduate programs to the other professions or institutionally based training programs.
4. Family therapy practitioners presently have diverse backgrounds, experiences, and preparations. The few state licensure laws and other nonrequired clinical memberships (e.g., in the American Association of Marriage and Family Therapy, American Family Therapy Association, and American Association of Family Psychologists) are the only standards-setting procedures existing for the family therapy practitioner.
5. The multidisciplinary nature of family therapy practice has hampered the development of a professional leadership in family therapy. Thus far, the disciplines have tended to be undisciplined. This has effected the organizational base for practice and the development of a comprehensive body of knowledge. The formalization, standardization, and sanction of existing educational programs have been thwarted by this lack of professional leadership. How the current existing professional academic accrediting bodies will interact remains unclear.
6. Who may practice family therapy? There continue to be, classically, only voluntary criteria that define competency to practice as a "family therapist." The uniqueness and specific definition of family therapy has not been clearly delineated. There are no national sanctions that are enforceable to delineate and distinguish the qualified marriage and family therapist. There is little consumer protection vis-à-vis the professional's practice of family therapy.

7. To date, there is no comprehensive conceptual framework for family therapy that will support the formulation of a new professional body of knowledge. The foundation for practice is not yet complete and the need is self-evident for a comprehensive, generic framework that reflects an ecosystematic, biopsychosocial definition of family relationships and "illness."
8. The future role and function of the family in society is changing, as are typical family structures. The therapeutic services to enhance the diverse family forms is poorly developed theoretically. The field needs to develop a more comprehensive view of the varieties of family life and find alternative treatment methods to serve them.

6. Family Therapy Education: The Content

As family therapy moves toward professionalism, a comprehensive theoretical base of knowledge will be even more essential as a prerequisite for practice. These concepts must relate to the practice-realities experienced by the family therapist. The processes for teaching family therapy practice, as well as the selected content, have been a concern for trainers. A meaningful educational model must, therefore, meld theory into practice via a formal or classroom procedure. This section will discuss both the content base and supervisory processes or teaching methods available to promote learning.

6.1. Eclectic Theoretical Models

There has been an abundance of literature, research, and practice experiences published during the last decade. Unfortunately, there has been little organization to this myriad of information. The literature has progressed linearly without a comprehensive gestalt emerging from it. Russell (1976), viewing this as a primary concern for the field, stated:

> There is not enough theory building going on. The integrative development of formal theoretical bases leading to the construction of more systematic approaches in the treatment of disturbed families is not impressive. The single universal comprehensive theory of behavior, which would serve as an ironclad rationale for intervention into the family system, therefore, still evades us, as does an acceptable theory linking family process and the growth of individual family members' personalities. (p. 243)

LeVande (1976), a social work professor, requested a curriculum model:

> for the study of substantive and conceptual theories which pertained to the family as a total unit, in addition to or integrated with the study of practice theories and approaches to family intervention. (p. 292)

The existing diversity and disarray of those theories available has necessitated each trainer/educators relying upon his or her own preferences, knowledge, and experiences when developing educational content.

At this point, relevant research suggests preference for eclectic theoretical models. Cooper *et al.* (1981) found 63% of the clinical psychology programs used an "eclectic" theoretical orientation in their curricula. Fifty-five % of the clinical staff providing supervision to internships were eclectic. This was twice as great as any other orientation. Ninety-one % of those providing training in psychiatry residency programs viewed themselves being on the eclectic/structural end of the theoretical continuum (Sugarman, 1981). Many social work professors have relied upon eclectic-based texts and integrated basic systems, structural, communication, problem solving, and psychodynamic models into other traditional family casework concepts (Weber, 1979). Several authors have developed texts and references that reflect these (e.g., Goldenberg & Goldenberg, 1980; Jansen & Harris, 1981; Sedgewick, 1981; Waldron-Skinner, 1976).

Tomm and Wright (1979) developed a training model for family therapy students based on conceptual, perceptual, and executive skills. The model further exemplified the earlier teaching models developed by Cleghorn and Levin (1973). Both efforts were directed toward standardizing educational processes and used criterion based, measurable variables developed around functional areas. Students were to demonstrate skills that were paired with perceptual/conceptual skills and then matched with corresponding executive skills.

In brief, the Tomm-Wright model identifies four family therapist functions: (1) engagement; (2) problem identification; (3) change facilitation; and (4) termination. Each function has conceptual/perceptual and executive skills to be achieved. The conceptual skills are largely cognitive and include an understanding of the definitions and concepts incorporated within the model, general systems theories, communications theory, cybernetics, and social learning theory. These are largely perceptual skills that focus on the student's ability to: (1) perceive data; (2) accurately identify family and treatment behaviors; and (3) integrate them with the conceptual model used. The executive skills concentrate on the student's ability to execute and carry out treatment. These include the therapist's ability to use his or her own emotional reactions constructively by channeling them into specific therapeutic activity.

6.2. Educational Components

Family therapy training should be based upon some foundation concepts that are inherent to the program irrespective of the setting, experience of the student, and theoretical preferences of the trainer. These will be briefly discussed in the following section as content germane for the curriculum.

Family therapy focuses upon the influence of interrelationships. Systems theory provides the framework from which the family interactions can be understood. Early concepts developed by Wiener (1947), Von Bertalanffy (1950), Sullivan (1953), and Beier (1966), emphasized the mutual reciprocity of larger and smaller systems. For example, Bowen's (1966) family systems theory and Minuchin's (1974) structural family theory each have developed an approach that is applicable to understand the family relations and structures. Their respective theories provide guidelines for the practicing therapist to assess and develop treatment interventions that are intended to create systemic changes among the family members. Students of family therapy must orient their manner of thinking to focus on the relationships occurring within the family to be a circular, mutually sustaining process in a moment of time (rather than a sequential process through time).

Systems theory will likely continue to be a foundation theory for family therapy education. Bloch and Weiss (1981) state:

> As greater consensus develops in the field about its base of theory, clinical techniques, outcomes, and training procedures, family systems thinking will become more powerful and influential. (p. 146)

Many who have developed eclectic theories that have attempted to integrate several theoretical orientations have done so with the systems theory as their basic theory (e.g., Jansen & Harris, 1980; Sedgwick, 1981; Waldron-Skinner, 1976).

Students should learn to assess the family from a developmental model that considers the progression of the family through the family's life stages. The extent of the family's level of function and dysfunction should be considered in relation to the tasks presented in the particular life stage of the family. Each stage of the life cycle requires that specific tasks be successfully accomplished before the family progresses onto the next stage. Failure to perform the tasks can result in becoming fixated and problems or symptoms occur. Students need to consider the family's current functioning and/or dysfunction in relation to these tasks and life stages and learn to develop interventions that will move the family forward in this sequence of family life stages.

Family theories also emphasize the individuation processes of the family members as a primary function and task for the family to accomplish. The individual's symptoms, behaviors, or problems should be considered within the context of the family unit. Students need to learn how such symptoms may be reflective of family stress, conflict, or the internalization of other family breakdowns. The less effective the family, the more likely the family is to be limited in its capacities or resources to facilitate the individuation processes. The student needs to learn how accurately to assess and develop goals and strategies for the family that will alter the family system and that promote the growth and development of each individual in it.

Family therapy is problem focused. The ability to aggressively engage in problem-solving skills with a family must be a primary learning objective for the student in family therapy training. Skills that accurately assess the meaning or function of the problem for the family and the family system's response to it are crucial for the beginning therapist to acquire (e.g., enmeshed or disengaged relations, rigidity, regression, or internalization).

The conceptual orientation of the curriculum will influence how the desired problem resolution will be accomplished. Therapists and theories vary as to the best means to accomplish this. Some theories (e.g., problem-solving, learning, behavioral, communication) emphasize the new conceptual learning of problem-solving skills and processes as a major therapeutic objective, while other theories, especially those of the strategic therapists, use indirect, manipulative, or meta-communications to induce change for problem resolution.

The curriculum should include the study of specific treatment interventions of the role of the family therapist and skills that are congruent with the students' characteristics and capacities. The roles as a "conductor" or a "reactor" (as described by Ferber, Mendelsohn, & Napier, 1973) describe the degree of initiative or responsiveness that the therapist uses in relating with families in treatment. As a theory of action, the student must develop the capability to control or manage the treatment session, perceive the processes of verbal and nonverbal communications, and conceptually develop responses and interventions that promote the therapeutic relationship, as well as the use of self in effecting change with planned interventions.

6.3. Supervised Practice Experiences

As Haley (1969) noted, family therapy is a "therapy of action." The role of the therapist is complex and requires perceptual acumen, diagnostic formulations, and accurately developed interventions—all within the relationship context established with each family member.

Family therapy training programs must provide actual practice experiences as an integral component of the educational program for these skills to be competently developed. Students report these "learning by doing" experiences to be one of the more valuable components of their training. It enables them to acquire a personal understanding of the therapist role and skills, apply the theoretical concepts to real situations, and learn from their own individual characteristics and capacities in a treatment relationship.

Supervision should be provided to students during these initial practice experiences. Family therapists have been innovative in developing a number of various supervisory methods. These range from individual to peer group to team supervision, and often include "live supervision" that occurs with the supervisor or team actively involved in the training during the family therapy session (e.g., as cotherapist, an observer, or by videotape). Liddle and Halpin (1978) found the various supervisory models selected by the trainer to be more a "metaphor of one's beliefs, and values," as well as reflective of the supervisor's beliefs of how therapy should be conducted (rather than on a professionally based standard procedure).

Effective supervision for practice must have a reasonable theoretical base (Munson, 1980). The theory–technique integration process becomes a major objective of the supervisory process. Liddle and Halpin (1978) consistently found that the goals of training and supervision and the skills of the supervisor were dependent upon the theoretical orientation of the program. Irrespective of the models selected, the supervisors believed that all training should encompass technical and conceptual competencies as well as interpersonal skills.

Many have tried to develop learning objectives and procedural guides to evaluate the supervisory process and measure the student's learning. Tucker, Hart, and Liddle (1976), for example, established primary supervisory objectives that were:

(a) to elicit reactions of the co-therapists to each other,
(b) to analyze observed family dynamics as a group,
(c) to make generalizations about the observed family and family therapy in general,
(d) to plan for future sessions with the family, and
(e) to express and discuss reactions to and feelings about the supervision. (p. 272)

The learning objectives and expectations should be spelled out specifically in empirical terms that meet the specific needs of the student.

The nature of the supervisory relationship has been debated among family therapists. As with the model selected, it appears to be reflective of the supervisor's and program's values and orientation. The relationships vary in degree of egalitarian, hierarchial, or authoritarian characteristics. Early trainers, including Ackerman, Fogarty, Guerin, Bowen, and Ferber, believed the egalitarian supervisory relationships supported the student's and supervisor's willingness to be open about oneself and encouraged the personalization of the work. The boundaries among life, education, supervision, and therapy were deemed to be diffuse and supportive of democratic relations. Both the supervisor and the student experience the intense effects of this process and self-disclosure. Most of these supervisory processes are reflective of a psychodynamically oriented training framework.

Proponents from structural, behavioral, and cognitive therapies (e.g., Haley and Minuchin) differ in their views and argue that the supervisory relationship should be more hierarchical in character and that that relationship is developed, organized, and defined around the task of aiding the therapist-trainee to help the family. On this end of the continuum, the task, skills, and goal-oriented philosophy predominates in comparison to the other more personal, process-oriented philosophy.

6.4. Personal Awareness and Development

Most current training programs in marriage and family therapy include the student's study of his or her own family experiences and philosophies. Even though the interface of this potentially therapeutic process is unclear to the overall educational content and objectives, it nonetheless is viewed strongly by most family therapists as a viable element of the educational process.

Bowen (1971) was one of the first professors to have students formally study their own family of origin as part of their training experience. His psychiatry residents reported that the understanding of their own experiences with their families they acquired made it possible to better understand and relate to clinical families.

Schulman (1976) noted that her social work students found it difficult to differentiate their subjective reactions from the reality of what occurred in clinical experiences. The class members also sought to fit the given theoretical concepts into their practical experiences.

The subjective nature of family therapy creates the risk of the therapist's responding in ways that are influenced by his or her own past family experiences. The reactions, perceptions, and assessments potentially are influenced by personal past experiences and may result in distorted ''frames of reference'' through which the current family exchanges or relations are viewed.

The therapist has the potential to project or reexperience the past personal experiences onto the family in treatment. Old family-based conflicts, roles, positions, and sexual identities may result in the therapist's becoming entrapped or enmeshed into the clinical family group, becoming powerless to create change or objectively experience the existing family's dynamics.

The therapist can become caught in the ''pseudoneutrality'' of the family that keeps conflict covert or that maintains the family system. Fulweiler (1967) commented: ''If you have ever been married, or have ever been a child in a family, or have had *any* family experience at all, these people will catch your problems and demonstrate them for you and to you and through you'' (p. 320).

Framo (1975) also believes that family therapists continue to struggle with their own families of origin with their clinical families. He believes the first obligation of a family therapist is ''to improve his or her own functioning and get his own house in order'' (p. 116). To him, the personal side of being a family therapist is more important than the theories and techniques:

> Although all family therapists, I believe, continue to struggle with their own families of origin with their clinical families, some have mastered or resolved or have come to terms with their own past so that they can use the experience adaptively. Others, I fear, do use families in order to work out their own problems. (p. 26)

Numerous training programs include personal awareness experiences as part of the learning objectives, for example, Cleghorn and Levin (1973), Ferber and Mendelsohn (1973), Guldner (1978), and Carter and Orfanidis (1976). Many have observed the direct relationship between self-knowledge and clinical skills. Carter and Orfanidis (1976) stated:

> In our experience there and at other training centers where our staff teaches or has taught, there appears to be a relationship between work done by the therapist in his own family of origin and his clinical proficiency as a family therapist. (p. 194)

More than any other method of treatment, family therapy confronts the therapist with his or her own past or current family experiences. These should not be disregarded but be viewed as an inherent reality for the supervisor to consider in the student's development as a family therapist.

The criteria for student self-exploration are not clearly developed and supervisors have had to rely upon individual and group experiences to facilitate their innovative approaches for this. Siporin (1981) discussed the interface of the educational and therapeutic objectives of the family therapy curricula in social work. He viewed both developing technical competence and developing as a person as crucial elements of the education process:

> Learning about techniques is important, but of central importance is the student's work in formulating a personal philosophy of life: the standards, values, and precepts to live by and with which to make choices, meanings and assumptive beliefs to guide one's perceptions, emotions, and behavior. All of these are also very important in helping clients. (p. 24)

Waldron-Skinner (1976) also believed that the techniques for intervention were difficult to teach since they relied more on the empathic nature and idealogy of the therapist. She found:

> Whatever skills or techniques the family therapist may acquire, his personal style and value system will be the most important factors influencing his therapeutic work, for a family therapist is a human being skillful, not a skillful human being. (p. 151)

In conclusion, the family therapy educator should be mindful of the powerful impact the therapist's bias and personal life, including operational assumptions and values, have upon determining the therapeutic process and goals of the therapy process. Consideration of these individual qualities and life experiences needs to be an integral part of the total training program. These self-actualizing experiences should be fashioned to promote self-disclosure, guided self-development, and personal maturation—while remaining in an educational context of professional development and therapeutic competence.

Creating an effective balance between educational and therapeutic content has been a controversial issue for family therapists. There are those who disagree that subjective or personal experiences are relevant in becoming a competent family therapist. For example, Haley, Minuchin, Watzlawick, and others from the structural and behavioral models question the efficacy of any form of personal therapy or study of one's own family. They note that no empirical data validate the assumptions of their worth and believe that a task- or problem-oriented approach to student supervision is preferred. They strive for behavior techniques, strategies, and the use of directives or tasks as more favorable supervision tasks.

It is the authors' view that a holistic educational model is preferred, one that includes self-awareness and the potential for personal maturation as part of the learning experience. Given the use of individual relationships as a primary medium for therapeutic exchange, the therapist *must* differentiate between previous personal experiences and the "use of self" in a new family relationship in order to be effective as a therapist in charge of therapeutic processes at any given moment. The awarness of personal values, attitudes, and personal philosophies must be considered, especially as they influence one's therapeutic objectives and ethical base for practice.

In conclusion, the family therapy educational program must be specific in its goals and objectives. These should include both a professional theoretical orientation to the practice of family therapy and an individualized learning experience. Students need the opportunity to integrate their theoretical orientation into actual practice experiences and to develop further personal skills that reflect an objective use of "self as a therapist" in relationship to the family group. The ethical values and individual philosophies need to be identified and developed as a foundation for his or her own approach and devotion to the field.

7. Ethics and Law

Despite its critical role in the practice of marriage and family therapy, ethics and law is a commonly neglected area of training. A minority of training programs offer a specialized course, particularly in the legal aspects of a discipline with secondary reference to marriage and family therapy. A few training programs have arrangements with other disciplines (such as a college of law on the same campus) for students to elect specialized courses. Formal efforts between colleges of law and schools of social work have been acknowledge as being overall, unfruitful.

To date, the usual approach to ethical aspects is to include reference to ethics within a generic role-defining seminar and to study a single discipline's code of ethics. There is seldom concentration on: (1) ethics that pertain specifically to marriage and family therapy; or (2) ethical aspects of case handling.

The usual approach to the legal aspects of marriage and family therapy is even more vulnerable. Although well intentioned, professors with little or no formal training in legal aspects often are expected to deal with the subject within a practice-oriented course.

Part of the difficulty no doubt comes from the fact that thare are only limited materials available on the ethical aspects of marriage and family therapy. Within law, there is a similar lack of materials tailoring the law to marriage and family practitioners, but there is a plethora of legal materials on the components of family law (e.g., divorce, custody, and adoption) that would benefit the marriage and family therapist. In this instance, however, the training programs usually fail to direct the trainees toward this type of material with the consequence that the trainees often are left feeling incapable of reading, understanding, and applying legal information.

The context of this chapter does not allow for a review of academic ethical and legal information *per se*. Rather, the focus here will be on the critical areas that should be provided to trainees in marriage and family therapy.

In the realm of ethics, the framework should be predicated upon the code of ethics for the trainee's basic discipline (e.g., psychiatry, psychology, social work, counseling, or psychiatric nursing). At this point, there should then be a distinct move on to specialization. To be sure, a general training program cannot provide an in-depth exposure to all specializations, but it can adopt some sort of teaching strategy, such as an individual study method, that will accommodate each student's acquiring the kind of specialized case materials upon which the discipline's code of ethics can be superimposed. This would allow the trainee interested in marriage and family therapy to embrace the discipline's ethical code, but also make adaptations to his or her desired specialization.

In the realm of the law, matters become a bit more complex. It should go without saying that the trainee in marriage and family therapy cannot expect to comprehend the law in full. The objectives should be: (1) to appreciate the interface between law and professional practice; (2) to have knowledge of certain critical legal principles and practices that have relevance to marriage and family therapy clients; and (3) to be equipped to investigate the law for information pertinent to any given client. It is the latter objective that can be the primary thrust of a training program in marriage and family therapy.

To be able to investigate the law for information pertinent to any given client requires that the trainee be familiar with legal materials. In gaining the familiarity, there will be a concomitant development of knowledge of the interface between the law and the profession and of the legal principles and practices (e.g., how the legal system operates, crucial statutory law, and the common law principles that are applicable to marriage and family therapy). In other words, the first and second objectives are initiated in the course of learning how to investigate the law. An investigation requires an awareness of how to locate legal materials. (Most university libraries have a reference librarian who is assigned to the legal materials and to be available for lectures on legal research.) Finally, an investigation of the law can be attained through being able to interact effectively with members of the legal profession (experience supports the belief that attorneys usually are ready and willing to assist "outsiders" who have an ancillary connection to the courts, as would be the case with a marriage and family therapist working, for example, with an emotionally torn family).

Certain substantive areas of the law should be provided, at least in an overview fashion, to marriage and family therapy trainees. Among others these subjects include: (1) the nature of the legal system; (2) how to do rudimentary legal research; (3) trial practices (particularly how rules of evidence apply to expert testimony provided by marriage and family therapists); (4) criminal law (such as predicting dangerousness and the rights of criminals); (5) the uniqueness of the juvenile justice system; (6) rights of workers; and, foremost, (7) divorce and custody.

Intentionally not mentioned thus far are the areas that relate to professional practice. These include: (1) privileged communication; (2) standard of care; (3) malpractice; (4) duty to warn; and (5) predicting dangerousness. Each of these has been plagued by faulty information and misperceptions in most marriage and family therapy training programs.

Most marriage and family therapists probably believe that, since their clients want the therapy session to be treated confidentially, there is *privileged communication*. In other words, therapists typically believe that no one can make them break the confidential nature of the therapy sessions. Since privileged communication must be specified by state statutory law and therein must delineate the qualifications of the professional to whom it applies, such as licensed physicians and psychologists, there may be no legal privileged communication operating in marriage and family therapy. Further, there is the matter of the subpoena power of the court which requires even the professional relationship protected by privileged communication to be subverted to the social benefits derived from the professional giving testimony in a judicial proceeding. Awareness of this vulnerability is essential to all marriage and family therapists, yet it is seldom provided for in their training.

Each professional must maintain a *standard of care* for practice that is consonant with the average skill and knowledge possessed by professionals in like circumstances. It is easy to claim such a standard, but harder to prove that it has been maintained. For example, the traditional approach of using practitioners in the same geographical community as points of comparison rapidly is giving way to a national professional comparison. If there is any type of specialization (e.g., being certified by the Academy of Certified

Social Workers or being diplomated by the American Board of Professional Psychology), the standard is elevated. All too often the practitioner, be it marriage and family therapist or otherwise, neglects the establishment of a clear-cut standard of care. In so doing, he or she is highly vulnerable to criticism and/or legal action.

Malpractice is connected to standard of care. A failure to maintain an acceptable standard of care is the basis for a malpractice suit. While the courts typically seem to strain to honor professionalism, the practitioner must be careful not to be stripped of his or her professional vestments. For example, marriage and family therapists who practice an avant-garde set of techniques—for example, some form of nontraditional "encounter" approach—nonetheless probably will be compared to traditional psychodynamic practitioners in the event there is a legal action to defend against.

The *duty to warn* is a relatively new professional responsibility. It stems from court determinations that protecting society from danger is more important than allowing the privileged communication aligned with psychotherapy. It knows no disciplinary bounds and there is no legal exemption. It mandates that any professional who knows (or *should* know) that one of his or her clients poses a threat to the safety of another person has a *duty* to warn the endangered person. This warning could be given to the person or to a law enforcement source. Obviously there is a need to let clients know that everything said in therapy is not sacrosanct: there may be statements, such as threats of violence, that must be reported.

Through the courts, society is also moving toward supporting that the professionals must, in some circumstances, *predict dangerousness*. That is, the professional may be subject to legal actions if he or she fails to predict that a client will harm another person (i.e., the threat need not be explicit). This clearly is placing a responsibility on the shoulders of the professional that will be difficult, if not impossible, to perform flawlessly. Few training programs prepare trainees for the onerous task of predicting dangerousness. A failure to be prepared, however, could result in, for example, a wrongful-death legal action if a therapist's client kills another person and the therapist was in the position of predicting the potential violence.

All of the previously cited substantive areas and the areas of privileged communication, standard of care, malpractice, duty to warn, and predicting dangerousness should be inherent to all training programs for marriage and family therapists. Regrettably, to date there are few, if any, that adequately meet this challenge. The evidence seems clear that the future will bring an even greater demand on professionals to fulfill these areas. Time, therefore, is of the essence for training programs to make accommodations accordingly.

8. Conclusion

This chapter has provided a review of dimensions of training in marriage and family therapy. Although there is a trend toward developing teaching strategies that are tailored to marriage and family therapy *per se*, the "state of the art" remains rooted in traditional, often poorly defined, generic training models. Special emphasis has been placed on the importance of the trainee's using his or her self-understanding as a means for enhancing professional competency for marriage and family therapy. Ethical and legal factors have been underscored.

The future is likely to present professionals with stronger societal expectations for quality. This is already witnessed by legal liabilities and the scrutiny imposed by insurance companies being asked to pay for therapy. The implications for training embrace: (1) more formal structuring of academic and clinical experiences; and (2) tighter controls through licensing. There is a definite press on professionals in general and marriage and family therapists in particular to be qualified to safeguard the best interests of their clients. Inevitably, this will mean that training programs will have to attain a higher degree of efficacy than can be established to date. This is clearly the time for renovations and improvements in the training of marriage and family therapists.

9. References

Ackerman, N. Family psychotherapy today. *Family Process*, 1970, *9*, 123–126.

Adler, A. *Understanding human nature*. New York: Greenberg, 1946.

Beier, E. *The Silent Language of Psychotherapy*. Chicago: Aldine, 1966.

Bertalanffy, L. *General systems theory*. New York: Braziller, 1968.

Bloch, D. Family therapy training: The institutional base. *Family Process*, 1981, *20*, 131. (Editor's note).

Bloch, D., & Weiss, H. Training facilities in marital and family therapy. *Family Process*, 1981, *20*, 133–146.

Bowen, M. The use of family theory in clinical practice. *Comprehensive Psychiatry*, 1966, *7*, 345–374.

Bowen, M. Towards the differentiation of self in one's family of origin. In F. Andres & J. Lord (Eds.), *Georgetown family symposia* (Vol. 1). Washington, D.C.: Department of Psychiatry, Georgetown University, 1971, 70–86.

Bowen, M. *Family therapy in clinical practice*. New York: Jason Aronson, 1978.

Carter, R., & Olfanidis, M. Family therapy with one person and the family therapist's own family. In P. Guerin (Ed.), *Family therapy, theory and practice*. New York: Gardner, 1976.

Cleghorn, J., & Levin, S. Training family therapists by setting learning objectives. *American Journal of Orthopsychiatry*, 1973, *43*, 439–446.

Cooper, A., Rampage, C., & Soucy, G. Family therapy training in clinical psychology programs. *Family Process*, 1981, *20*, 155–166.

Ferber, A., Mendelsohn, M., & Napier, A. *The book of family therapy*. Boston: Houghton Mifflin, 1973.

Framo, J. Personal reflections of a family therapist. *Journal of Marriage and Family Counseling*, 1975, *1*, 15–28.

Fulweiler, C. No man's land, an interview. In J. Haley & L. Hoffman (Eds.), *Techniques of family therapy*. New York: Basic Books, 1967.

Goldenberg, I., & Goldenberg, H. *Family therapy: An overview*. Monterey, Calif.: Brooks/Cole, 1980.

Guldner, C. Family therapy for the trainee in family therapy. *Journal of Marriage and Family Counseling*, 1978, *4*, 127–132.

Haley, J. An editor's farewell. *Family Process*, 1969, *8*, 149–158.

Janzen, C., & Harris, O. *Family treatment in social work practice*. Itasca, Ill.: F. E. Peacock, 1980.

Kniskern, D., & Gurman, A. Research in training in marriage and family therapy: Status, issues and direction. In M. Andolfi & I. Zwerling (Eds.), *Dimensions of family therapy*. New York: Guilford Press, 1980.

LeVande, D. Family theory as a necessary component of family therapy. *Social Casework*, 1976, *57*, 291–295.

Liddle, H. The emotional and political hazards of teaching and learning family therapy. *Family Therapy*, 1978, *5*, 1–12.

Liddle, H., & Halpin, R. Family therapy training and supervision literature: A comparative review. *Journal of Marriage and Family Counseling*, 1978, *4*, 77–98.

Minuchin, S. *Families and family therapy*. Cambridge: Harvard University Press, 1974.

Munson, C. Supervising the family therapist. *Social Casework*, 1980, *61*, 169–170.

Russell, A. Contemporary concerns in family therapy. *Journal of Marriage and Family Counseling*, 1976, *2*, 243–249.

Schulman, G. Teaching family therapy to social work students. *Social Casework*, 1976, *57*, 448–457.

Sedgwick, R. *Family mental health: Theory and practice*. St. Louis: C. V. Mosby, 1981.

Siporin, M. Teaching family and marriage therapy. *Social Casework*, 1981, *62*, 20–29.

Stanton, M. Family therapy training: Academic and internship opportunities for psychologists. *Family Process*, 1975, *14*, 433–439.

Sugarman, S. Family therapy training in selected general psychiatry residency programs. *Family Process*, 1981, *20*, 147–154.

Sullivan, H. *The Interpersonal theory of psychiatry*. New York: Norton, 1953.

Tomm, K., & Wright, L. Training in family therapy: Perceptual, conceptual and executive skills. *Family Process,* 1979, *18,* 227–250.

Tucker, B., Hart, G., & Liddle, H. Supervision in family therapy: A developmental perspective. *Journal of Marriage and Family Counseling,* 1976, *2,* 270–276.

Von Bertalanffy, L. An outline of general systems theory. *British Journal of Philosophy,* 1950, *1,* 134–165.

Waldron-Skinner, S. *Family therapy: The treatment of natural systems.* London: Routledge & Kegan Paul, 1976.

Weber, G. *Family therapy education in schools of social work, a national survey.* Unpublished doctoral dissertation, University of Nebraska, 1979.

Whitaker, C. The hinderance of theory in clinical work. In P. Guerin (Ed.), *Family therapy, theory and practice.* New York: Gardner, 1976.

Wiener, N. Time, communication, and the nervous system. In R. W. Miner (Ed.), *Teleological mechanisms.* Annals of the New York Academy of Sciences, 1947, *50.*

Wiener, N. *Cybernetics* (2nd ed.). Cambridge: M.I.T. Press, 1961.

II

Therapeutic Systems

8

Family Systems Theory and Therapy

DANIEL V. PAPERO

"Family Systems Theory" refers to the work of Murray Bowen, M.D., of Georgetown University. Over the past three decades Dr. Bowen has been a pioneer in the study of the human family. The product of his work is the Bowen Family Systems Theory, more simply referred to as the Bowen Theory. Consisting of eight interlocking concepts, Bowen Theory addresses the emotional forces that shape the functioning of nuclear and extended families. A methodology for work with families has developed directly from Bowen Theory and within the general framework of the methodology are a number of general techniques. The methodology and techniques are family systems therapy. Bowen Family Systems Theory and Therapy are taught primarily at the Georgetown University Family Center, where Dr. Bowen has assembled a faculty and developed a series of training programs.

Kerr (1981) has reviewed extensively the development of the early family movement and of Bowen in particular. The awareness among mental health professionals of the family's importance to the recovery of a psychiatric patient grew in the late 1940s and early 1950s. Bowen's work with the family began in this period while he was on the staff of The Menninger Clinic from 1946 to 1954. He initially sought to improve the outcome of therapy by involving the family as well as the patient. A special study of the intense relationship between parents and young psychotic patients led to concurrent psychotherapy with the parents as well as the patient. Bowen's increasing experience with the family led him to formulate a hypothesis about the mother–patient relationship (Bowen, 1971). The interdependence of mother and patient was seen as a natural phenomenon arising out of the incomplete self of the mother incorporating the self of the developing fetus, resulting in an *emotional stuck-togetherness* or *fusion* (Kerr, 1981). This intense attachment between mother and child was believed to be of biological proportions, representing the basic process from which clinical schizophrenia later developed.

The hypothesis of the mother–child symbiosis became the basis of a formal research study. The work began in 1954 at the National Institute of Mental Health (NIMH) in Bethesda, Maryland. The symbiosis was seen as a reciprocal emotional responsiveness

DANIEL V. PAPERO • Veterans Administration Medical Center, Nashville, Tennessee 37203.

that neither desired but which blocked the efforts of either to function autonomously. Bowen believed that the intense relationship with the mother blunted the patient's natural movement toward growth and development. If the emotional interplay between mother and patient could be altered or reduced, the patient's development would continue (Bowen, 1971). Of particular importance in this hypothesis was the exclusion of stated or implied causality. The symbiosis was seen as a natural development for which neither party was to blame. Behavior could be attributed to the shifting emotional intensity of the relationship rather than to specific causes. Although this was not yet systems thinking, it defined a major systems premise, the avoidance of cause and effect thinking.

In the actual research project mothers and their schizophrenic offspring lived together on a research unit for extended periods of time. The first year of the project led to several important observations. Among the most important was the recognition that the mother–patient relationship was in fact part of a larger active and shifting unit. This observation led to the inclusion of fathers in the new families admitted to the project (Bowen, 1978a). A second shift involved the increasing use of family therapy rather than individual therapy or a combination of individual and family therapy because families progressed much faster in family therapy alone. It is difficult a quarter of a century after the event to understand the impact of these observations. Today the notion of family therapy is widely accepted, and there is a general awareness of a systems point of view. Bowen describes the effect of the research on his thinking.

> It was a shaky experience for one long schooled in psychoanalytic theory to become aware that all he had held to be factual and irrevocable was no more than another theoretical assumption and that psychoanalytic therapy was no longer *the* therapy but simply another method. (Bowen, 1971, p. 391)

The NIMH research project continued until 1959, when Bowen moved to the Department of Psychiatry at Georgetown University. In the late 1950s Bowen continued his research on schizophrenia but was already moving toward the development of a family theory that could account for the broad spectrum of human emotional illness. During this period the groundwork was laid for the ideas that became the initial concepts of Bowen Theory. Bowen (1971) reports that once the patterns of emotional process were seen in research families, it was possible to see similar patterns in all other families. Bowen's observations led him to believe that the difference between the psychoses and the neuroses was quantitative rather than qualitative. The important difference was the level of emotional force or intensity that propelled the process. This viewpoint led to an effort to place all human functioning on a continuum from the poorest to the highest. The outcome of the effort to evaluate the level of functioning of individuals was called the scale of differentiation (Kerr, 1981).

In the interval between 1957 and 1963 Bowen's thinking evolved rapidly toward the initial six interlocking concepts of the Bowen Theory, referred to at that point for the first time as *family systems theory*. Five of the concepts—triangles, nuclear family emotional process, family projection process, scale of differentiation, and multigenerational transmission process—were formulated directly by Bowen. The sixth concept, sibling position, fell into place with the publication of Toman's (1961) book, *Family Constellation: Its effects on personality and social behavior.*

The initial six concepts addressed essentially emotional process in the nuclear and extended families. Two additional concepts, emotional cutoff and societal regression, were added in 1975 (Bowen, 1976). These concepts further addressed the emotional process across the generations in a family and in society. These eight concepts that comprise the Bowen Theory will be discussed in greater detail later in the chapter.[1]

An important underpinning to Bowen Theory is the notion of systems thinking. The term *systems* refers to the patterns of automatic, predictable behavior among family members. The systems thinker concentrates on the facts of functioning in human relationships, that is, wnat happened and how, when, and where did it happen (Bowen, 1977). The effort of systems thinking is to see a broader picture of human functioning than that defined by the various perspectives on individual functioning. To help broaden the focus of research observers to see beyond conventional psychiatry, Bowen (1977) formulated a series of underlying assumptions: (a) that emotional illness is directly related to human biology, (b) that emotional illness is a multigenerational process, and (c) that there is great variance between what humans do and what they say they do. In addition, Bowen worked to define difficult concepts into functional facts. An example of this effort can be found in the definition of love as a relationship fact. He wrote, "I am not able to accurately define love, but it is a fact that statements to another important person about the presence or absence of love in self, or in the other, predictably results in an emotional reaction in the relationship" (Bowen, 1977, p. 187).

Systems thinking has been characterized by an effort to avoid cause and effect thinking. The effort to assign a single cause to an effect is inherent in human thinking. In very narrow limits there is some accuracy to this perspective. In terms of human emotional functioning it surfaces in the efforts to fix blame for misfortune or to see the "cause" of a problem in a single person's behavior. The systems viewpoint attempts to understand human behavior as the product of a balance of forces in the family. All systems theories operate with a notion of forces that oppose one another to create a dynamic balance or homeostasis. From this perspective change occurs as a result of a disruption of homeostasis when the system is stressed. All biological systems appear to have mechanisms that are activated to restore balance to the stressed system. Symptoms may emerge when these adaptive mechanisms are overloaded, and the symptom that appears frequently can be an exaggeration of the restorative mechanism itself (Kerr, 1981). The important idea, therefore, is that symptoms emerge during periods of system imbalance and often represent the overloading of a normal restorative mechanism.

Bowen (1972) describes two major forces continually in operation within the family. The first is the togetherness force, seen as rooted in the instinctual, patterned behavior of the species and a product of the emotional system within each individual. The togetherness force defines all family members as alike in terms of their basic perspectives, principles, and feelings. The togetherness force is manifested in the degree to which people adapt self to preserve harmony with another, the degree to which one person will assume responsibility for another and will define his or her role in life on the basis of relationship, rather than on principle, and the degree to which one automatically thinks of and defers to another before self. There are infinite variations and feeling tones that color the operation of the togetherness force in humans. The second major force, acting in opposition to the togetherness force, is a force toward individuation. The individuation force moves the individual toward the establishment of goals based on careful thought and

[1]In November 1980, Dr. Bowen announced his work toward the development of a ninth concept dealing with the functional aspect of human spirituality. The only formal presentation of this concept at this time is a videotape discussion produced by The Georgetown Family Center.

the development of principles and belief that guide the self through the major decisions of a lifetime. The individuation force is manifested in the degree to which a person assumes responsibility for his or her own happiness and direction in life and avoids the blaming of others for personal malaise or failure. The force toward individuation allows a person to experience genuine caring for another without the need to possess or function for the other person. The individuation force operates in the thinking center of the person.

The center of human emotional functioning is thought to be the limbic system, comprised of the limbic cortex and its connections to the brain stem. Ancestral, patterned, repetitive behaviors as well as the deep-seated, instinctual emotions that become visible in the aggressive, defensive, and mating behaviors of humans are believed to be largely controlled by the limbic system (MacLean, 1973). The thinking center is thought to consist largely of the neocortex and to deal primarily with perception and mental processing. When the two centers are not clearly and recognizably distinct to a person, they are referred to as *fused*. In a fused state the emotional system tends to override the thinking system. The result is the initiation of a semiautomatic pattern of behavior, the roots of which lie in the personal past of the individual and the evolutionary past of the species. Where there is less fusion of the thinking and emotional systems, the person is referred to as more differentiated. The more highly differentiated person is able to maintain the objectivity and careful thought of the thinking system for longer periods of time in spite of the emotional center's arousal and tendency toward automatic patterned response.

Early (1957) in his NIMH research, Bowen (1978a) noted that anxiety was easily transferred among members in a family. An increase in anxiety in a mother would produce a predictable psychotic reaction in a daughter. The emotional system is believed to be acutely sensitive to anxiety in self or another. The greater the degree of fusion between the emotional and thinking systems, the more the person responds in an emotionally programed manner to the presence of anxiety in another, particularly in a close network such as the family. The term *fusion* is extended in this sense to reciprocal emotional reactivity of one person to another in the presence of anxiety.

The idea of "emotional reactiveness" is basic and important. In 1974, Bowen (1978b) compared the family system to an electronic circuit in which each member is connected to every other member. Each person becomes a nodal point or an electronic center, receiving and transmitting impulses from and to the other points in the system or circuit. If the major impulses sent through the system are considered to be emotional, representing the operation of the togetherness force, then the reaction of any member upon receipt of an emotional impulse and the further impulse(s) he or she transmits in response can be accurately described as emotional reactions. The more the impulses are anxiety based, the greater anxious reaction they provoke. Bowen (1978b) also used the term "emotional reflex" to refer to the same phenomenon. This term conveys the automatic quality of the reaction occurring out of awareness of the person. As is the case with physical reflexes, the emotional reflex can be brought within limited observation and limited conscious control.

It is on this deep level that the togetherness force in humans appears to operate. To a greater or lesser degree fusion is characteristic of all people and of all families. Where it is active, persons remain focused on others in a reactive manner, losing sight of personal beliefs and goals. Decisions become based more on what another says or does rather than on the thought and beliefs of self. In intense variations, the fused family lives in a world of intense emotional reactivity manifested in the feeling based goal of happiness fueled by a chronic level of family anxiety. In such families relief from such intense feeling states becomes a primary pursuit.

The force toward individuation defines the person as autonomous and able to determine a responsible life course for self. Kerr describes the individuality force as "rooted in an instinctual drive to be a self-contained, independent organism, an individual in one's own right" (1981, p. 236). The force toward individuation automatically emerges when anxiety decreases in a person and a family. It is possible for the thinking system to work toward individuation during periods of anxiety provided the separation of the thinking and emotional systems can be maintained in spite of the pressure of anxiety.

The product of the togetherness force in a family is fusion. The product of the force toward individuation is differentiation. All families lie somewhere along the fusion–differentiation continuum. Bowen Theory suggests that families with a high degree of fusion are vulnerable to the development of major life problems (Bowen, 1966). Families with greater levels of differentiation are consequently less vulnerable. The pressure for closeness in a highly fused family automatically produces in some members a reactive pressure to distance from the intensity of the closeness. That reactivity to the intensity of the family togetherness force is not the same as differentiation but is itself governed by the family pressure toward closeness. If the anxiety that fuels the push for togetherness can be calmed, the reactive need to distance also decreases. Distancing, therefore, can be another manifestation of fusion.

The togetherness force and the individuation force are oppositional and proportional. When the family system is in equilibrium, it operates with a ratio of the two. The state of equilibrium can favor either togetherness or individuation but not both, and the ratio becomes the norm for the family in that particular homeostatic configuration. When the equilibrium is threatened by a surge of either force the other force moves to offset the surge in the opposite direction. The release of togetherness forces in response to anxiety triggers forces for individuation and vice versa. In 1974, Bowen (1978b) indicated that optimum functioning would occur when the forces are evenly balanced with neither overriding the other and the system having sufficient flexibility to adapt to change. Once, for example, anxiety has released the togetherness forces in the name of emotional closeness, "love," or kinship, the individuation forces counter in the name of principle, self-determination, or autonomy. If the togetherness forces prevail, the family moves a little closer to the fusion end of the continuum. The family operates with a new equilibrium with increased togetherness and decreased individuation. If anxiety is sustained, the process will repeat, with the outcome of the clash of forces determining whether a new family norm for the ratio of individuation–togetherness is established or not.

An important and difficult point to keep in mind is that the forces for togetherness and individuation operate continuously. How the individual manages self amidst these forces, particularly the degree to which he or she can maintain the separation of the thinking and emotional systems in the presence of anxiety, plays a major role in determining the movement of the family along the fusion–differentiation continuum. The thinking system values each force as basic and important. It also allows choice between the forces based on beliefs and the personal definition of responsibility. The emotional system automatically responds to each force, spawning endless cycles of closeness and distance. An emotional reaction that denies the existence of the togetherness forces (e.g., distance), leaves the person desirous of and allergic to closeness whenever it appears. Since Bowen Theory sees human dysfunction largely as a product of fusion, much of the work of therapy itself is directed toward the separation of the thinking and emotional systems in the person in the belief that the individual can use the thinking system to move toward an autonomous yet connected position in the family.

From the preceding discussion it should be evident that Bowen Theory assigns major importance to the role of anxiety in family dysfunction. The greater the level or intensity of anxiety, the greater the tendency toward fusion of the emotional and thinking systems and of the individual to the group. Families react intensely to anxiety and often will do almost anything to prevent or reduce its presence in the family. Sometimes this includes the abandonment of personal belief or conviction in order to preserve relationship harmony, a short-term decision to relieve anxiety that can lead to greater dysfunction in the long run.

Another important idea is that of *functioning position*. Kerr (1981) uses the analogy of an engine to illustrate the concept. A person unfamiliar with engines could, when presented with a carburetor, describe its interior and exterior with accuracy but could only speculate about its function. When presented with an engine minus its carburetor and asked to design a unit to make the engine work, a person could, by studying the engine, design a part to perform the carburetor's functions. In designing an operational carburetor, it would be necessary to understand its role or functioning position in the overall operation of the engine. Individual theories are akin to the description of the carburetor. They can be descriptively accurate but have no way to account for the function of the person in the relationship system.

Systems thinking permits a broad view of the relationship matrix and the functioning position of each person. There are people in families who provide the energy or drive to assure that things get done. Family members automatically turn to these doers in times of trouble and these resourceful people generally pull the family through the emotional quagmire. Others appear continually to be the focal point of family concern. The person in this position frequently develops a chronic dysfunction that worsens during periods of family stress. Yet others in the family appear to function independently of it and to be relatively unaffected by shifting emotional forces in others. In systems terms each of these people has a functioning position in the family that is instrumental in maintaining a particular family configuration across time and in sustaining the patterns of emotional reactivity of the family in response to stress.

In turning to Bowen Family Systems Theory, the importance of the term *theory* requires further consideration. There are eight major concepts in the Bowen Family Systems Theory. Each of these concepts points to a major level or component of family behavior. Within each concept are a range of variables. These eight concepts provide a coherent body of general propositions to account for the range of human emotional functioning. Implied in the use of the term *theory* is the assumption that the current group of propositions is not necessarily complete but represents the best current thinking, an established framework within which known facts can be explained. The Bowen Theory is subject to continued refinement and expansion. In addition, the use of *theory* indicates the core of family systems therapy, the theoretical orientation and development of the therapist which defines both methodology and technique.

1. Bowen Family Systems Theory

The initial six concepts (triangles, nuclear family emotional process, family projection process, differentiation of self, multigenerational transmission process, and sibling position) were sufficiently clear and defined by 1963 that Bowen could call them *family systems theory* (Kerr, 1981). The concepts were published three years later (Bowen, 1966). The sixth concept, sibling position, took shape when Toman's (1961) book, *Family Constellation*, gave depth and structure to the concept. The seventh and eighth concepts (emotional cutoff, societal regression) were added to Bowen Theory in 1976. Each of the concepts will be discussed in some detail in the following text.

1.1. Triangles

The concept of the triangle addresses the behavior of the two-person relationship when stressed. When anxiety is low, a two-person, togetherness-oriented relationship can appear stable with a warm, positive feeling tone. With an increase in anxiety, tension in the relationship increases and may appear as conflict, distance, or some other form of relationship discomfort. Characteristically, one of the pair is more uncomfortable than the other. This discomfort intensifies if the mechanisms within the twosome (distance, conflict, the effort to talk it out, etc.) do not succeed in containing and reducing anxiety. If the level of anxiety becomes great enough, one partner, generally the least comfortable, automatically will move to form a new relationship with a significant outsider. Important variables that affect the level of anxiety required to trigger this response include the degree of togetherness forces and fusion in the pair and the level of chronic anxiety in the relationship system.

The original partner is now placed in the outside position to this new twosome. The move can either bring relief or further increase anxiety within the relationship system. The original partner, now the outsider, may be relieved no longer to be the object of the other's anxious efforts to restore harmony and the uncomfortable partner may find solace in the intensity of the new relationship. On the other hand the outsider may see the partner's new involvement as a rejection and move to restore the original twosome. For example, the original partner may make a peace overture of some sort, acknowledging his or her error and promising to make amends. In extreme situations the original partner may threaten to harm self or another if the original twosome is not restored. If either of the new twosome resists this move, further tension can result. Once again important variables in determining whether the triangle brings relief or further tension are the degree of fusion, the level of chronic anxiety, and the intensity of acute anxiety in the relationship.

In a triangle there is always a twosome and an outsider. When anxiety is low, the twosome is generally comfortable. The outsider experiences varying degrees of discomfort and may seek to involve one of the twosome in a relationship. When anxiety is high, the outsider occupies the preferred position, relatively free from the pressure of the twosome. With moderate anxiety, the triangle tends to have two comfortable sides and one conflictual side. The comfortable and conflictual side may change or the triangle may become fixed in a characteristic configuration. In a mother–father–child triangle, for example, tension may develop in the marital pair with the greater discomfort located in the mother. She in turn manages her anxiety by focusing on the child. She may become exceedingly protective of the child, her worry about the child's health may intensify, or she may become openly critical and fall into conflict with the child. The tension in the marital relationship dissipates as the intensity of the mother–child relationship increases. If, for example, the mother–child relationship takes on a conflictual tone, the father then may intervene with the child to correct "disrespect" toward the mother. The tension then shifts to the father–child axis and cools some with the mother. The mother, however, then may intervene with the father "to correct his excesses" with the child. At that point the tension once again has gone full circle back to the marital pair where it began. In contrast the tension in some triangles remains fixed in a particular relationship, predominantly, in the marital pair or between either parent and child. The other two sides of the triangle remain relatively peaceful.

The movements of people within the triangle are automatic and generally without intellectual awareness. There are two important variables in triangles (Bowen, 1975). The first deals with the degree of fusion in the family. The second involves the level of anxiety or emotional tension in the system. The higher the degree of fusion, the more intense triangling becomes. If anxiety is high enough, it cannot be contained within a single triangle. It spills over, so to speak, into the series of interlocking triangles that comprise the family system as more and more people become involved in it. At times it can spill over to involve friends, clergy, or even social institutions such as the court system or the network of professional helpers. In this manner an entire family can react to and focus upon a dysfunctional member in times of stress. For example, an intensification of anxiety in a marital relationship may appear as a drinking problem in the husband. The other partner may involve their oldest daughter to help solve what becomes defined as an alcohol problem. The involvement of the daughter in the triangle with her parents may create anxiety in her own marriage. The anxiety in the marriage may spread to an uninvolved child, who may suddenly develop a problem at school that comes to the attention of a school social worker. In this manner a surge of anxiety anywhere in the family can spread and intensify through the matrix of interlocking triangles across family generations and boundaries to involve a professional helper. Characteristically, however, the family will define the problem in terms of a person rather than in terms of family tension involving them all.

In summary, the concept of the triangle addresses the automatic movement of individuals to maintain the degree of closeness/distance that allows them the greatest degree of freedom from anxiety. The operation of interlocking triangles results in patterns of emotional reactivity in the family that can be identified.

1.2. Nuclear Family Emotional Process

There are four mechanisms or patterns of behavior that come into effect to contain anxiety in the nuclear family. A particular family may use one mechanism predominantly or a mixture of all four. Each mechanism can absorb or bind an amount of anxiety in a relationship. When the anxiety level surpasses the amount that can be absorbed by the mechanism, the mechanism itself may become symptomatic, that is, it will be seen by others as the cause of the problem rather than the anxiety that drives it. At that point the pattern may generate more anxiety than it binds. Chronic anxiety in a family often is manifested in the continual usage of one or more of these patterns of behavior to maintain equilibrium. Where mechanisms are in continual use, small increases in the level of chronic anxiety or numerous waves of acute anxiety can produce dysfunction. On the other hand in a calm family the mechanisms may be noticeable only during periods of stress. Each of the four patterns of behavior, emotional distance, marital conflict, dysfunction in a spouse, and the impairment of a child or children, will be discussed in the following paragraphs.

1.2.1. Emotional Distance

The term *emotional distance* refers to the reactive efforts of people to find relief from the emotional discomfort of too much closeness. The intensity of the closeness can be either negatively or positively toned, generally the former, but in either event the distancing represents a reaction to the discomfort of an intense emotional contact with the other. Emotional distance can be achieved either through actual physical distance (literally avoiding the other) or through internal mechanisms in each person that work against emotional contact. In either case viable emotional contact with the other is reduced or closed off. It should be noted that this distancing is automatic and based in emotional reactivity. It usually results in more distance than people want. When the discomfort of emotional distance is great enough, people seek closeness elsewhere in the pattern of the triangle described above. This can take the form of an affair or a major emotional investment in a career or a cause, or the distance may shift into a child focus or some other mechanism. What people actually are avoiding is their own discomfort or reactivity to each other. At the same time they tend to view the other, rather than their own reactivity, as the "cause" of their discomfort (Kerr, 1981).

1.2.2. Marital Conflict

Marital conflict represents a high degree of emotional reactivity in each partner to the other. Partners in marital conflict tend to spend much of their thinking time focused on the "unreasonable" and "uncaring" qualities of the other. Each tends to be firmly convinced that fault lies primarily with the other and works hard to convince the partner to change. During the conflict phases the partners can debate in great detail minute and, to the outsider, unimportant aspects of the current issue between them. The conflict often is followed by distance which each justifies on the basis of the other's behavior. These distanced periods often are spent reviewing arguments, preparing new lines of attack, and carefully monitoring the partner for new evidence of obstinacy and fault. There also are occasional brief periods of closeness and warmth. These periods equal in positive intensity the negative intensity of the conflict phases. This closeness is labile, however. Any of a range of trigger behaviors can set either partner into the conflict mode to which the other reacts at once.

When the anxiety no longer can be contained by the cycle of conflict and distance, the predictable effort to involve an outsider follows. Therapy often will be sought, although a range of outside involvements is possible. In therapy the couple will attempt to continue their debates at great length, as if the therapist were some sort of judge who ultimately could determine the innocence of one and the guilt of the other. Logical resolution of an issue hardly settles matters since the conflictual couple promptly will produce a new issue. The focusing of such emotional intensity on the partner can relieve a child who might otherwise become its target. It is possible for children to grow up in conflictual families with relative lack of impairment. If marital conflict is unable to regulate sufficiently anxiety in the marital pair, other mechanisms automatically come into play which can involve a child in the process.

1.2.3. Dysfunction in a Spouse

It is common for spouses to become adaptive to each other. There are continual compromises in which a partner yields to the wishes of the other to preserve relationship harmony. Over time these can create a pattern of one spouse gradually functioning with increasing responsibility for the other, who gradually yields responsibility for self. The result is an overfunctional–underfunctional reciprocity. The pressures toward this outcome can come from both partners. The overfunctioning spouse may have been accustomed to deciding for others in his or her family of origin, while the underfunctioning one may have a tendency to avoid the responsibility of decision making. These roles naturally blend together in the marriage to form a pattern of reciprocity. If stress is moderate, this mechanism can work quite well to contain anxiety. When anxiety is intense, however, the pattern can lead to the appearance of a symptom in the spouse who had yielded adaptively the greater sense of self to preserve harmony in the relationship. It can happen that the more adaptive spouse appears in the overfunctional position attempting to manage the life of the other. When stressed beyond tolerance, however, the apparent overfunctioner will collapse, often suddenly, into dysfunction. This collapse often is accompanied by a dramatic improvement in the partner's functioning. More typically, the more adaptive one develops symptoms that gradually can grow in severity when the family is anxious.

As in all patterns or mechanisms in the family, the greater the level of fusion in the family, the less reserves the family has to meet new stresses and the greater the likelihood of serious dysfunction. It is important to emphasize that the overfunctional– underfunctional pattern can be adaptive in a family and does not represent pathology in either partner. It is the presence of acute or chronic anxiety of sufficient intensity that leads to the emergence of symptoms. The appearance of the symptom marks the operation of the reciprocal mechanism in a field of high anxiety. The maintenance of the symptom across time, however, can result in new roles for family members that actually can decrease relationship tension in the family (Kerr, 1981). For example, the caretaking and nursing postures that develop in response to the dysfunctional person actually can ease relationship tension. The outcome presents an interesting paradox. Although the symptom marks an increased anxiety in the family and itself can contribute to a higher level of chronic anxiety, it also provides further devices that help to contain the anxiety and allow others in the family to continue their general level of functioning.

1.2.4. Impairment of Children (The Child Focus)

The fourth nuclear family process involves the shifting of parental anxiety toward one or more children. The other three processes can occur with little involvement of a child. In the child focus, however, parental emotional intensity is directed toward or focused upon a particular child. The process appears to work through the mother, who anxiously worries about the child. This maternal concern often becomes evident in a highly protective posture toward the child and a tendency to act and decide for the child. It may take the form of great concern about the child's health, with much attention to symptoms and heavy involvement of the medical community in the effort to track down and relieve the child's problem. This process can occur without any evidence of a problem in the child, although in a high anxiety field the child may reciprocate with behavior that justifies the mother's fears. The process also can involve a child with a clear handicap, for example a birth defect or a learning disability. The father characteristically supports the mother in her focus or withdraws from it. Either move frees him from the intensity of his spouse's anxiety.

It is important to note that at least initially this process is driven by anxiety in the parent rather than a problem in the child. The child in this position develops a heightened sensitivity to emotional forces in the family and particularly to emotionality in the mother. In the early developmental stages of the process, the anxiety is located in the parent. Later, the forces can be activated by anxiety in either the mother or the child. The outcome for the child is a higher degree of emotional and intellectual systems fusion than that of less involved siblings. In its more intense forms it may be difficult for the child to function away from the parent. The child can come to seek out closeness and at the same time react intensely to it, making other life relationships more intense and difficult.

The focus of parental anxiety on a child exists in all families to a degree. It is such a common phenomenon that it remains unnoticed except when the anxiety that fuels it is intense enough that a symptom results. Even where the child focus is not a primary means of anxiety absorption in the nuclear family, it is important to the development of the family across the generations. The third concept of the Bowen Theory, the family projection process, discusses this idea more fully.

1.3. Family Projection Process

Parental reactions and behaviors are not the same toward each child no matter how much the parents insist they treat each child equally. Those differences in parental behavior have important implications for the functioning of the children involved. The child focus mechanism describes the funneling of parental anxiety to a child. In any generation of siblings there also are children who remain less focused upon or even outside the child focus mechanism. Children who are the object of parental focus tend to develop greater fusion of thinking and emotion than their siblings and consequently remain more vulnerable than those siblings to anxiety and the operation of emotional forces.

The projection process is rooted in the parent's anxiety about the child, often present even before the child's birth. The mother's anxiety appears to be more influential than that of the father. The roots of maternal anxiety may lie in the past generations, in the marital relationship, or elsewhere. Anxious parents behave in a manner to justify parental worry. Once established, the pattern is reciprocal, and either parent or child can provoke the automatic pattern of response in the other. As previously noted in the description of the child focus, the process develops with or without an overt symptom in the child, although the presence of a defect or symptom adds impetus.

On a more general level the concept addresses the way in which parental fusion or undifferentiation is transmitted across the generations. How the parents behave, what they actually stand for in terms of their behavior is more important than what they say they believe. The parents, for example, may see a child as more sensitive or more delicate than their other children. The parents, generally through the mother, operate on their perception of the child as fragile. The father may work to "toughen up" the child, while the mother "protects" the child from the father and the world. The child begins to act in a manner that confirms the parental fears and the process can intensify. In short, the parents' emotionally shaped perception of what the child is like eventually becomes reality to the child, even though it may have had little or no basis originally (Kerr, 1981).

The same parents may behave quite differently with other children in the family. Free of the anxiety that shapes their actions toward the focused child, the parents are better able to allow the other siblings to develop their own direction in life. The parents automatically allow the other children room to grow without the anxious constraints that mark their efforts with the focused child. In return these siblings are better able to recognize and learn from their parents' strengths, while the focused child learns more about the parents' weaknesses.

When chronic anxiety and fusion are high in a family, all children are touched by the projection process to a certain degree. Even where chronic anxiety and fusion are intense, however, some children are more heavily involved in the projection process than are their siblings. Children less involved in the projection process emerge with greater ability to maintain the separation of thinking and emotion in self. Those children least involved in the projection process may be less vulnerable to fusion even than their parents. In summary, as a result of the projection process siblings emerge with varying degrees of vulnerability to fusion and with varying capacities for functioning in a given emotional system.

1.4. Differentiation of Self

No other concept in Bowen Theory is so important nor so often discussed and associated with Bowen's work as differentiation of self. It is the cornerstone of family systems theory and therapy.

The notion of the family as an emotional unit is fundamental to the concept of differentiation. In this framework *emotion* refers to forces deeply rooted in the individual and the family group. Feelings, for example, anger, sorrow, and joy, are seen as the very surface of deeper and more basic emotions. The center of human emotional functioning lies in the brain stem and limbic cortex. MacLean's research indicates that much patterned, repetitive behavior is influenced by the brain stem, the inheritance from our evolutionary predecessors (MacLean, 1973). MacLean hypothesizes that the brain stem, the counterpart of the reptilian brain in mammals, is the center for genetically constituted forms of behavior, for example, home site selection, establishment of territory, engaging in various types of display, hunting, homing, breeding, mating, imprinting, forming social hierarchies, and choosing leaders. The limbic cortex represents a newer evolutionary development. It has similar features in all mammals and has strong connections with the hypothalamus which plays a basic role in emotional expression (MacLean, 1973). MacLean's research indicates that the limbic system plays an important role in elaborating emotional feelings that guide behavior with respect to the two basic life principles of self-preservation and preservation of the species. In particular the limbic system appears to control the emotional states that lead to display of fearful behavior, aggression, and the behaviors of sexual arousal. At this level the term *emotional* is akin to *instinctual* and refers to the processes in the human brain that trigger the onset of patterned, genetically influenced if not determined behavior related to self-preservation and procreation. In social groups, however, the unfolding of patterned behavior in one individual appears to trigger other patterns in different individuals. In the human family people are acutely sensitive to the movements and behavior of others. In persons with low levels of differentiation much of life is spent monitoring and sensing the feelings and behavior of others. Along with such monitoring is a fairly high degree of reactive behavior, a semi-automatic unfolding of emotionally based response patterns. A more differentiated person is less caught up in the monitoring of others, has more energy that can be used for self in life, and is less reactive to the behavior of others.

Another element of emotionality has to do with anxiety in the person and in the family. Anxiety acts to trigger emotionally driven behavior. Some families operate with relatively high levels of chronic anxiety. In such families people fear anxiety and act to avoid it at all costs. In the process individuals compromise basic life principles and attempt to "walk on eggshells" in an effort to avoid triggering anxiety in self or in an important other. The very effort to avoid anxiety creates an anxious climate in the family. Acute anxiety, on the other hand, generally is related to an actual event in the family or the world, for example a death, a birth, or the loss of a job. In a family with a high level of chronic anxiety, an episode of acute anxiety can result in the development of some sort of fairly serious dysfunction in the family. It is as if there is insufficient reserve capacity in the family to meet the new wave of anxiety and collapse results. Less chronically anxious families meet the acute anxiety with less intense disruption and dysfunctions in life.

The broad substratum of ancestral, reactive behavior and response and the level of chronic anxiety that the family creates and inherits from its more immediate past create the family emotional unit. The family exerts a strong influence on individuals to behave in ways that maintain the emotional stability of the unit. In each individual there are genetic and feeling factors that move to acknowledge and act upon the family emotional pull. Bowen has called the sum total of these internal forces the *togetherness force* representing one of the two major forces in the individual.

It is against the backdrop of this potentially strong interplay between family and individual that the idea of differentiation becomes clearer. Borrowed from biology, the term represents a process analogous to that found in cellular development. From essentially the same material cells develop, or differentiate, to perform autonomous yet related functions in the organism. The analogy serves the family framework well, where the goal is for the individual to remain in viable emotional contact with the family yet develop the ability to function with responsible autonomy.

The basic level of differentiation of self is manifested in the degree to which a person manages across life to keep thinking and emotional systems separate, to retain choice about whether one acts in the influence of the thinking or emotional systems in a particular situation, and to set a life course based on careful thought and values that stem from such thought. This basic level of differentiation is also called the *solid self.* Bowen Theory suggests that the solid self develops and tends to become fixed early in life. It can be increased in later life through discplined effort, which lies at the heart of family systems therapy. To the degree that a family member can maintain the separation of thinking and emotional systems and can guide personal behavior with carefully thought out beliefs and principles in a highly anxious field, he or she displays a personal level or degree of differentiation.

The functional level of differentiation refers to shifts in the degree of fusion between the emotional and intellectual systems that are based in fluctuations in the level of anxiety the person experiences (Kerr, 1981). Another term for the functional level of differentiation is the *pseudoself.* Unlike the solid self, the pseudoself is relationship-based and its values are susceptible to relationship pressure. The pseudoself is group oriented, reactive, and easily altered under pressure. When relatively calm, a person may function with quite a bit of choice between thinking and emotional systems. Pseudoself and solid self levels emerge in the intensity of personal and relationship based anxiety. The *pseudoself* covets approval and the person appears to function well when receiving relationship-based approval. In the face of disapproval, however, pseudoself-based functioning can decline rapidly or radically change to conform to the demands of the relationship. In the same climate the solid self continues to define belief. The individual acts according to belief, risking disapproval from important others.

The functional level of differentiation can improve or deteriorate in response to relationship variables. It is relatively frequent, for example, to see a person who had been floundering appear to blossom with dramatic improvement in functioning after a divorce. In the same fashion, one occasionally sees the level of functioning drop when a person enters an intense relationship or marriage. In such shifts there is no change in the basic level of differentiation. The functional level of differentiation, based primarily on the level of personal anxiety, is the area of change.

People marry others with about the same level of differentiation as themselves. Through the family projection process they produce children with a somewhat lower level of differentiation than themselves. They also produce offspring less involved in the child focus mechanism whose level of differentiation is similar to or even somewhat higher than that of the parents. Each generation, therefore, has representatives of a process toward lower and toward higher levels of differentiation. Across time different branches of a family may develop toward greater or less vulnerability to dysfunction. This process is the subject of the multigenerational transmission process.

1.5. The Multigenerational Transmission Process

The concept of the multigenerational transmission process expands the perspective of the family as an emotional unit from the nuclear to the multigenerational family (Kerr, 1981). The family projection process, described earlier, and the idea that a person marries someone with the same level of basic differentiation as self are viewed from a multigenerational perspective. From this viewpoint, severe dysfunction is seen as the outcome of the operation of the family emotional system across time. A key element is movement of certain lines of the family toward increasingly lower levels of differentiation. The primary components of this trend are the family projection process and the selection of a spouse with a level of differentiation similar to one's own. The family projection process leads to a lower level of differentiation in each generation. The marriage of spouses with a similar level of differentiation passes the lowered level into the next generation.

As each generation of a line moving toward lower differentiation is produced, it becomes increasingly vulnerable to anxiety and fusion. Balancing mechanisms are used more intensely as each generation attempts to cope with the tightening circle of anxiety. In effect the compromise each generation arrives at is the use of those mechanisms that handicap the fewest people while allowing the rest to function relatively well. The appearance of a serious dysfunction in a family represents the end result of a series of compromises made by different generations in an effort to retain the functioning and comfort levels of as many people as possible. Although the lines of decreasing levels of differentiation across time are vulnerable to increasing dysfunction, one should not forget that each generation produces lines moving toward improved functioning as well in a balanced natural process.

The force of the transmission process in the family is variable. In families where most of the tension is absorbed in the focus on a child, the pace may be rather rapid. The use of the other mechanisms, for example, conflict, distance, or dysfunction, can slow the process. There also may be generations that live relatively free from external anxiety. In such fortunate generations the basic process remains dormant until a new surge of anxiety disrupts the status quo. Another factor influencing the development and pace of the transmission process is the degree of contact the person maintains to preceding family generations. The term *emotional cutoff* is used to refer to the process of avoiding emotionally charged areas between the generations (Kerr, 1981). The greater the degree of emotional cutoff, the greater the likelihood of more rapid development of the transmission process. The notion of emotional cutoff is so important that an entire concept has been given over to it.

1.6. Emotional Cutoff

Reactivity to relationship fusion lies at the root of emotional cutoff. The mechanisms of cutoff can be external or internal. The individual may live far from the family and carefully structure "duty visits" once or twice a year. Or the person may live in close proximity to the family and use a series of internal mechanisms to shut off emotional contact. The overall outcome of either set of mechanisms is the avoidance of any highly emotional area of family past or present. People distance themselves from the family to avoid emotional intensity, yet their reactive need for closeness and intense emotionality leads them into relationships to which they are equally reactive. When the intensity of the current relationship produces sufficient discomfort, the cutoff mechanism is again activated. People can cut off from the intensity of a marriage into an affair or into an intense psychotherapeutic relationship or into religion, and so forth. The emotional forces in the cutoff become active in all of life's relationships, emerging when emotional discomfort reaches a certain level in a given relationship. The cutoff is the product of both the intense emotional togetherness needs programmed in the relationship to the parents and the reactivity of people to that closeness. The emotional cutoff reflects a problem, solves a problem and creates a problem (Kerr, 1981). It reflects the problem of fusion with the parents and solves it by avoiding emotional contact with the past. It creates a new problem in that it isolates and alienates people, leaving them vulnerable to equally intense fusions and reactivity in other relationship systems.

1.7. Sibling Position

In 1961, Toman published his classic study on sibling position and birth order characteristics in families entitled *Family Constellation: Its effects on personality and social behavior*. Based on data collected in both the United States and Europe, the study presented behavior profiles of the characteristics of individuals occupying specific sibling positions in families. With Toman's profiles, it became possible to open a new area of predictability about the person's functioning in a family and in life. Many forces shaping, for instance, the behavior of a first born son or daughter are similar across families. By comparing a person's actual behavior with that predicted by Toman's profiles it becomes possible to note these and other forces at work that deflect development from the expected course. This, in turn, offers new insights into areas of family functioning.

Toman's work consolidated and clarified an entire area of Bowen's thinking. The information provided by the sibling position profiles, when combined with concept of the triangle, made it possible to see the mechanisms of the nuclear family more clearly than previously. The profiles made it possible to account for some of the interactional characteristics of marital partners, linking those characteristics with behavior originating in the family of origin. It was also possible to use sibling position profiles to reconstruct the functioning characteristics of long dead generations by combining profile information and known facts about the family to arrive at a broad view of family functioning across the generations, a major step in the development of the concept of the multigenerational transmission process.

1.8. Emotional Forces in Society

The eighth concept in the Bowen Family Systems Theory is an extension of thinking to the emotional forces operating in society. Essentially these forces are quite like those of the family, that is, the togetherness force and the individuation force. As in the family, the critical factor is the intensity of anxiety in society at a given point in time. The greater the level of anxiety, the more intense the togetherness operates with a corresponding erosion of the force toward individuation. In 1974, Bowen (1978b, p. 272) postulated that "man's increasing anxiety is a product of population explosion, the disappearance of new habitable land to colonize, the approaching depletion of raw materials necessary to sustain life, and growing awareness that 'spaceship earth' cannot indefinitely support human life in the style to which man and his technology have become accustomed."

Bowen became interested in the way anxious parents deal with teenage behavior problems and the way society through its representatives deals with the same problem. Anxious parents as well as anxious public officials lose sight of beliefs and principles with regard to their problem children. Decisions tend to reflect efforts to relieve anxious discomfort rather than adherence to carefully established principles. In the face of the teenager's anxious demand for rights, some parents lose their ability to think the situation through in terms of their own beliefs. Unclear about where they stand, the parents either become overly permissive in an effort to appease the child or react with a harshness not merited by the situation. The child becomes adept at exploiting the parents' anxious insecurity and they respond with greater demands for the child to be different. The cycle of acting-out and appeasement or repression can escalate into chaos. The efforts of public officials—judges, teachers, police, and probation officers—mirror those of the parents in dealing with the out-of-control teenager.

Bowen's observations have led him to believe that the functional level of differentiation in society has decreased in the past 25 years (Bowen, 1977). The anxiety that has driven societal regression, as Bowen originally described the process, stems from increasing population growth with increasingly limited resources. This has made it difficult for people to use new frontiers to distance from the closeness of population growth. The rising level of anxiety in society has led to a surge of a togetherness orientation, which in turn creates greater discomfort and further anxiety.

The anxious social climate has intensified the operation of the societal projection process (Bowen, 1977). In this process two people or groups of people join together and enhance their own functioning at the expense of a third party. The more this process is active, the more the emotional system in society comes to absorb or bind anxiety in the process. This is similar to what happens in the family projection process. In the process the twosome can force the third into submission; it can be cooperative with each side fitting the expectation of the other or the scapegoated party can force the other two to treat him or her as impaired. Each position is functional in the anxious system, that is, it plays a specific role in the management of anxiety. It is not possible to reduce the intensity of the projection process without first reducing the anxiety that propels it.

Alternating periods of societal anxiety and calm appear common in the course of human development. The emotional climate and processes of society represent yet another element in the emotional climate of the family.[2] The anxious society, like the anxious family, has difficulty resolving its problems without polarization around an issue, cutoff, reciprocal over-and-underfunctioning, and so forth. The result is a series of crises, generally resolved on the basis of restoring comfort rather than a thoughtful approach based upon principles and a degree of respect for differing viewpoints.

2. Bowen Family Systems Therapy

Therapy begins with the family evaluation. The family evaluation is conducted in four main areas: (1) the development and treatment history of the presenting problems; (2) the history of the nuclear family; (3) the history of the husband's extended family; and (4) the history of the wife's extended family. The information is recorded as collected on a multigenerational family diagram, a tool that in effect becomes the therapist's roadmap of family emotional process.

The initial step focuses on the history of the presenting problem. This involves identifying who has the symptom, when and in what environment it originated, how it has developed and been treated, and what has been the response to treatment. The type and location of the symptom provides initial information on the mechanisms and forces at work in the family. Exact dates are important, since they can be correlated with other information to determine their relationship to the family nodal events, namely, events that mark a significant alteration of family functioning. There is a strong family tendency to forget or overlook important dates and correlations. The therapist may have to be persistent and organized to gather all the pertinent information.

The history of the nuclear family begins when the couple first met. Their ages, level of functioning at the time, the length and nature of the courtship, the thinking of each that resulted in the decision to marry, and the reaction of their respective families to the marriage are all important areas. The birth dates, health, and growth histories of their children are collected, together with some information about family tensions before, during, and after the birth. Location changes by the family are important. Whether such moves have altered the relative distance to the families of origin or have preceded or followed a nodal event in the family should be determined. The therapist inquires about what has helped stabilize the nuclear family during periods of stress and what appears to have contributed to periods of family disruption. No single event is generally of critical importance, yet the overall picture aids the recognition and assessment of forces at work in the family and the nuclear family processes employed to maintain family equilibrium.

The history of each spouse's extended family takes the data collection backward in time to preceding generations. As in the nuclear family history, the effort is to collect information on people in the extended family. Birth dates, death dates, basic level of health, and life accomplishments create a picture of each individual's functioning. Questions can be addressed to relationship patterns within and between generations. The role and intensity of cutoff as a factor in the family is looked at. Sibling position information also is important. As in the nuclear family history, geographical location and family moves are significant. Attention is directed to determining which people have been most

[2]Readers interested in levels of system, for example, the family or societal level, may find the following recent book of interest: Scheflen, A. E. *Levels of Schizophrenia*. New York: Brunner/Mazel, 1981.

caught up in the family emotional processes and which have been less involved. The goal is a broad view of family functioning across time with an effort to understand the emotional forces and mechanisms that have led to the current situation.

In the concluding phase of the family evaluation the interviewer works with the family to define the direction of their efforts. The focus is quietly directed away from the symptom toward the emotional processes in the family. Often simply the suggestion that family members work to gain a little more objectivity about the situation will start people in the right direction. On some level family members know that their own personal reactivity contributes to the ongoing tension in the family, but this knowledge gets lost in the automatic responses they make to emotionality in others. The therapist can highlight the role of reactivity in maintaining family tension and can reflect upon the degree to which blaming others for the problem hinders progress toward its resolution.

The actual therapy flows from the Bowen Family Systems Theory. There are three major variables to consider, each defined by Bowen Theory. First is the basic level of differentiation of the person or persons involved. The degree to which a person has the ability to maintain separation between the emotional and intellectual systems and the degree to which a person is fused into the family emotional system determine to a large degree the ability to hear and understand the therapist's questions and the degree of difficulty in thinking nonreactively about the situation. A second major variable is the intensity of the anxiety in the family system. The greater the degree of anxiety, the more intense the symptom presentation. With intense acute anxiety, symptom control and even disappearance can be achieved, sometimes quickly, by reduction in the level of anxiety in the family. Symptoms rooted in the chronic anxiety of a family present a more difficult situation, as symptom mechanisms shift in and out of dormancy in response to subtle and slight shifts in anxiety. The third major variable has to do with the mechanisms used to manage or "bind" anxiety. Some families rely predominantly on a single mechanism, for example, marital conflict or dysfunction in a spouse, to keep anxiety within manageable limits. Other families use all mechanisms.

An important initial goal of therapy is derived from the theoretical position that the symptom mechanism in the family is emotionally driven and sustained by the family's level of anxiety. A reduction in family anxiety automatically will lead to an improvement in the functional differentiation of the people involved and the reduction or disappearance of symptomatic behavior. The initial efforts of the therapist are to manage self and approach the family in such a way that the acute anxiety driving the immediate presenting problem begins to dissipate. Anything that helps people think clearly and calmly about the situation can greatly help to reduce anxiety.

A basic guiding concept stems from Bowen's early thinking about triangles. A tense system between two people will resolve itself in the presence of a third person who can avoid emotional participation with either while still relating actively to both (Bowen, 1971). This theoretical position led to the method of seeing the marital unit together with the therapist occupying the third position in the triangle. This has remained a basic method of Bowen Family Systems Therapy. Further work and experience at "staying out of the triangle," as the effort to avoid emotional participation with either side while relating actively to both is called, has led to a refinement of the method to allow the therapist to see only one member of a family and remain detriangled.

The actual techniques used to stay out of the triangle vary widely from person to person. All include in some form or another a continual effort by the therapist to define his or her own position in the family emotional system and to communicate that position to all concerned. Questions and comments directed to the emotional climate rather than the issues of the family, the use of a gentle humor that aims at the often unacknowledged, sometimes paradoxical counterbalancing side of a person's emotional statement, and above all the effort of the therapist to maintain his or her own level of differentiation in the emotional climate of the family are common elements of detriangling techniques.

The distinction between content and process is important and somewhat difficult to grasp. The distinction is between what the family talks about or presents to others as the problem (content) and the postures or movements each family member makes in the anxiety driven reactive patterns of the family (process). On the one hand the distinction is somewhat artificial. Most family movement occurs around some content or issue. On the other, the more the therapist can direct his or her thinking and questions toward the process of the family, the clearer the roles of family members in the problem become. This is, in fact, movement toward a systems perspective with the family.

The effort to stay out of the triangle is continual and is the major principle guiding anxiety reduction. With a decrease in anxiety, the symptomatic behavior may decline or disappear altogether. The disappearance of a symptom should not be taken to indicate that the family has changed. With fluctuations in levels of acute anxiety, symptom patterns spring to life and return to dormancy in a continual flow. The degree of togetherness or fusion of family members remains unchanged in this process. The sustained reduction in anxiety makes it possible for motivated individuals to begin the slow process of differentiation. The idea is basically to substitute a controlled effort at differentiation for the intense anxiety of the fused system.

In 1968, following Bowen's presentation of his work on his own family to a group of well known family therapists, he reported a remarkable occurence among the psychiatric residents he was teaching. Essentially he observed that these residents were making efforts in their own families of origin and were making progress in their nuclear families and in their clinical work that equalled or surpassed that of residents seen in weekly family therapy with their spouses. From this observation there developed the method of training and therapy for which the Georgetown Family Center is best known, the effort to become more differentiated in one's family of origin.

The basic theoretical premise of this effort is that much of human dysfunction arises from the degree of undifferentiation or unresolved emotional attachment to the family of origin (Bowen, 1974). Therefore a major goal of therapy is to assist a person's movement toward greater differentiation of self. The fortuitous realization that quicker progress could be made working directly in the family of origin rather than in the nuclear family shaped the process known as "coaching." The initial sessions are spent with a person teaching the basic concepts of family systems theory, and the individual is encouraged to begin to study and learn about his or her own role in the family of origin. Among the initial goals is the effort to regain contact with the family of origin where such contact has been lost or eroded across time. The point is to reestablish reasonable emotional contact with the family, to open up, in effect, the relationship system. An open relationship system in a family is very effective in reducing the level of family anxiety although it does not increase the level of differentiation in the family.

The effort to establish emotional contact with the family of origin is important in another sense. The effort to differentiate a self requires that a person become a better observer of him or herself in the family and learn to control his or her own emotional reactiveness. It is important to visit the family frequently, particularly at times of emotional activity (e.g., around a birth, death, illness, marriage, etc.). The better a person becomes at observation, the greater objectivity is gained. It becomes possible to see parents as people rather than as "emotionally endowed images" (Bowen, 1978b, p. 531). It is possible to reduce one's own judgmental tendencies and to become less critical of others in the family. To that end Bowen has suggested the task of developing a person-to-person relationship with each living member of the extended family. Although this is an unattainable goal, in the process people can learn much about the forces that operate in the family to pull people together or to push them apart during periods of anxiety. One learns about the operation of emotional systems, particularly those to which one belongs, and along the way can learn much about his or her own behavior in an emotional field. A variation of this task is to develop a person-to-person relationship with each parent. In this effort all the emotional problems of the parents and of the family become evident. There are, however, numerous roadblocks as one approaches the task. At these points the "coach," who has worked with his or her own family already, is invaluable in providing suggestions to move the work along and to avoid the more obvious pitfalls.

The efforts to connect with the family, to become more observant and less reactive, and to work toward person-to-person relationships serve to reactivate the emotional system and to bring the person back into the family emotional field. At this point it is possible to see the triangles in the family that have shaped one's own development and to work to change self in them. The effort to detriangle self in the family is essentially the same as has been described earlier in working with a two-person relationship. The goal is to relate actively to both sides of the triangle without siding with either. Detriangling is attained when one can stay in contact with an emotional issue involving two other people and self and always have a neutral response that avoids taking sides, attacking others, or defending self. A single success at detriangling is not equivalent to differentiation. Generally the person with the goal of greater differentiation learns to recognize and guide him or herself through many family triangles. Each effort contributes another piece toward understanding family processes and one's own role in them.

Ultimately the effort leads to the attempt to alter one's own behavior in the reactive patterns of the family. In this task there is no substitute for the difficult work of discovering what one's beliefs and principles are and using those beliefs to guide oneself through the family emotional system. In recent years trainees at Georgetown have been assigned the task of writing down what their beliefs are and from whom they got them. This apparently simple exercise quickly highlights how few firm beliefs or principles many people have. It also illuminates the degree to which a personal belief system is assumed from important others with little thought oneself. However one chooses to work on the project of defining personal beliefs, it is an important ingredient of the work toward greater differentiation of self. Once one knows where one stands in terms of belief in a given family situation, it becomes necessary to make one's position clear to others in the family and to maintain it through the intensity of the family's reaction. The knowledge of triangles is invaluable at this stage. There is neither a "recipe" nor a clear timetable for the work on differentiation. Some people appear to progress rapidly; others work diligently for long periods with slight gain. On the other hand, even a small decrease in emotional reactivity can make a great difference in a person's functioning and in the emotional climate of a family.

In the process of therapy it is not always easy nor even initially advisable to direct people toward their extended families. Motivation is important and many people simply are neither interested nor see the point in reinvolving themselves with their families. In other instances anxiety may be so intense in the nuclear family that people cannot direct their attention elsewhere. An anxiety driven approach to the extended family can backfire and create further difficulties. It is important that the therapist be aware of and greatly respect the strength of family emotional processes across the generations. A person's moving back into a family emotional system after years of cutoff, particularly if based on the intention "to set this family straight," can activate intense reactions that may block further progress for years to come.

A more suitable goal when approaching extended family is to attempt to learn about family processes, especially one's own role in them. One works to become more observant of oneself and others in the family. It is especially important to observe one's own emotional reactivity to other people. The task resembles a research project to determine one's own behavior which contributes to the reactive patterns of the family. The more a person can assume an observant, nonjudgmental research posture, the greater the learning is likely to become. Bowen Family Systems Therapy is rooted in the theoretical perspective and development of the therapist. The development of a solid theoretical perspective depends upon both the training of the therapist and the experience he or she has gained in his or her own family of origin. The clinical family cannot progress beyond the therapist's own level of differentiation. If the therapist becomes fused with the family, he or she will tend not to recognize a family member's effort toward differentiation. The therapist's own anxious reactivity at that point will work against the effort to foster differentiation. The therapy may bog down in an anxious pattern or a family with strong motivation may drop out to find someone better able to work with them.

The discussion of Bowen Family Systems Therapy should not conclude without the focus returning again to theory. The force toward differentiation is seen as natural and inherent in humans. No matter how an anxious family clings together or reacts to the strength of the togetherness forces within it, the force toward individuation is present as well. The therapist's job is to work with the family in a way that will allow the natural corrective and counterbalancing force toward differentiation to emerge. In this sense the family always has had the power to heal itself.

3. Summary

The goal of this chapter has been to discuss the development, the theoretical concepts, and the application of Bowen Family Systems Theory and Therapy. Systems thinking and the eight concepts of the Bowen Theory have been discussed in detail, since therapeutic method and technique are based upon them. The final section has presented the general guidelines of Bowen Family Systems Therapy, including therapeutic methods and techniques.

4. References

Bowen, M. The use of family theory in clinical practice. *Comprehensive Psychiatry*, 1966, *7*, 345–374.

Bowen, M. Family therapy and family group therapy. In H. Kaplan & B. Sadock (Eds.), *Comprehensive group psychotherapy*. Baltimore: Williams & Wilkins, 1971.

Bowen, M. Toward the differentiation of a self in one's own family. In J. Framo (Ed.), *Family interaction*. New York: Springer, 1972.

Bowen, M. Family therapy after twenty years. In S. Arieti (Ed.), *American handbook of psychiatry* (Vol. 5). New York: Basic Books, 1975.

Bowen, M. Theory in the practice of psychotherapy. In P. Guerin (Ed.), *Family therapy*. New York: Gardner, 1976.

Bowen, M. Family systems theory and society. In J. P. Lorio & L. McClenathan (Eds.), *Georgetown family symposia: Volume II (1973–1974)*. Washington, D.C.: Georgetown Family Center, 1977.

Bowen, M. Treatment of family groups with a schizophrenic member. In M. Bowen, *Family therapy in clinical practice*. New York: Aronson, 1978. (a)

Bowen, M. Societal regression as viewed through family systems theory. In M. Bowen, *Family therapy in clinical practice*. New York: Aronson, 1978. (b)

Kerr, M. E. Family systems theory and therapy. In A. Gurman & D. P. Kniskern (Eds.), *Handbook of family therapy*. New York: Brunner/Mazel, 1981.

MacLean, P. D. Man's reptilian and limbic inheritance. In T. J. Boag & D. Campbell (Eds.), *A triune concept of the brain and behavior*. Toronto: University of Toronto Press, 1973.

Toman, W. *Family constellation: Its effects on personality and social behavior*. New York: Springer, 1961.

9

Structural Family Therapy

JOHN B. ROSENBERG

In the relatively brief 25 to 30 year history of family therapy, eight theoretical approaches have emerged (Kaslow, 1981).[1] Although each struggles to claim its uniqueness, a thorough examination of the various schools suggests much in common among them. All, for example, clearly subscribe to a systems approach and most would seem to begin family therapy with a focus on the presenting symptom (Wynne, in Gurman & Kniskern, 1981). On the other hand, each approach has contributed significantly to the body of information concerning theory and technique in understanding and working with troubled families. Although a combination of approaches utilizing an integrative approach has been advocated by some (Duhl & Duhl, 1981; Kaslow, 1981; Lazarus, 1981; Stanton, 1981a) in order to cull the best of the various schools, it is first imperative that one familiarize oneself with each theoretical orientation. The purpose of this chapter is to help the reader to understand fully and feel at home with the theory and technique developed within the school known as Structural Family Therapy. Case histories will be presented along with actual transcripts from early diagnostic sessions to illustrate just how one approaches a family from the structural perspective.

1. Historical Background

Minuchin and his colleagues developed the structural approach while working with a delinquent male population in the mid-sixties. This early work, which involved families of boys in residence at the Wiltwyck School for Boys in New York, appears to be the earliest attempt at using a family approach to handling difficult to manage youngsters. Because of the severity of the problems and because many of the families were extremely disorganized, the focus was on developing a way of bringing about behavioral change in a relatively brief period of time. Following the success of these early efforts, Salvador Minuchin and Braulio Montalvo came to Philadelphia to continue their work and expand their approach to the area of psychosomatic illness. Coming to the Child Guidance Clinic

[1]Psychoanalytic, Bowenian, Contextual, Experiential, Strategic, Structural, Communication, and Behavioral.

JOHN B. ROSENBERG • Philadelphia Child Guidance Clinic, Philadelphia, Pennsylvania 19104.

and teaming with Dr. Lester Baker, a pediatric endocrinologist at the Children's Hospital of Philadelphia, they began to investigate actively the role of family stress in the incidence of diabetes in children. It had become apparent that some of the diabetic patients at Children's Hospital were being hospitalized almost monthly for management of their diabetic acidosis, a life threatening condition. When there were no organic factors found during the hospitalization to explain the acidosis, the team of pediatricians and psychiatrists involved began to explore emotional factors that might have contributed to the repeated attacks.

Several of these early patients were at the time in individual therapy and some even had been hospitalized in intermediate acute care facilities. What became apparent was that they seemed to respond positively while in the hospital and seemed to benefit from individual psychotherapy, yet when they returned to their homes, they responded less positively to the medications given and soon wound up in the hospital emergency room. In short, the diabetes was under control when the youngster was in an institution and was running out of control when the child returned to his home. With this in mind, the research team set out to find the "mediating mechanism by which emotional arousal could be translated into diabetic acidosis" (Minuchin, Rosman, & Baker, 1978). The results of these early studies are most interesting in that they represent the first evidence of a direct link between stress within a system and the resultant physiological effects upon a child with primary psychosomatic illness. The reader is encouraged to review these early studies (Baker, Minuchin, & Rosman, 1974; Minuchin, Baker, Rosman, Liebman, Milman, & Todd, 1975; Minuchin *et al.*, 1978).

The findings from the early psychosomatic research pinpointed certain family characteristics (enmeshment, overprotectiveness, rigidity, and lack of conflict resolution) as existing to a much greater degree in families with psychosomatic children. In addition, it was found that children in these families seemed to jump right into any parental conflict. There clearly exists a two-way street in such families with parents creating stressful situations for the child and the child obliging by leaping into troubled waters. Thus the system is formed and maintained by all family members.

From these early roots in working with disorganized and psychosomatic families, the structural approach has been expanded and adapted to a variety of symptoms and family problems. Although the early and ongoing work with families of anorectic youngsters and addicted young adults has and is being reported in the literature, the current thrust is to study family interactional patterns and their effects upon social problems such as divorce, and physical illness such as hemophilia and sickle cell anemia.

2. Theoretical Orientation

As Minuchin states, "The structural approach to families is based on the concept that a family is more than the individual biopsychodynamics of its members. Family members relate according to certain arrangements, which govern their transactions. These arrangements, though usually not explicitly stated or even recognized, form a whole: the structure of the family. The reality of the structure is of a different order from the reality of the individual members" (Minuchin, 1974).

The structural approach in working with families suggests that each family unit either functions along normal developmental lines as outlined by Barcai (1981) or encounters difficulty in negotiating the expected life cycle crises. When a family runs into difficulty, one can assume that it is operating within a dysfunctional structure and one must then begin to assess or diagnose this system. Generally, family members tend to be overinvolved with one another, intrusive into the life space of a member, and too much into one another's skin. This has been referred to in Minuchin's writings as enmeshment and is a major component in some dysfunctional families. An example of this might be the mother who constantly protects and shelters her daughter from accepting more responsibility because the mother is afraid that if she allows her daughter to operate more independently she might fail. Such a failure would be hard for the mother to tolerate since she sees so much of herself in her daughter. One frequently catches glimpses of this in an interview when the mother either answers questions posed to her daughter or moves her lips in concert with the daughter's.

The other category of family dysfunction described by Minuchin is one in which there is little cohesiveness among and between family members. This end of the continuum is referred to as disengagement and reflects rather rigid and separate boundaries between family members. In an arrangement where members seem to have little to do with one another, one frequently finds a father who may be quite peripheral to the children and a mother who is more involved with her own life and less concerned with the well-being of the children. In such a family, each goes his own way until a major crisis develops and forces the family into therapy. It might be added that relatively few families actually appear as disengaged and that the vast majority fall somewhere in between the two extremes with characteristics of each. A notable exception to this are the psychosomatic families who tend to be conflict avoiders and quite enmeshed (Minuchin *et al.*, 1978).

The above discussion deals with an important area of structural family theory, namely the use of boundaries. There have to be generational divisions or boundaries to enable parents to operate successfully as the family executors. In order for a family to function satisfactorily, each subsystem, be it marital, parental, or sibling, and each person within his respective subsystem must have space. When one enters overwhelmingly into the life-space of another or when one is totally uninvolved with the affairs of another family member, dysfunction occurs. It is this boundary issue that allows for problems in enmeshment and disengagement and it is this that must be restructured in this approach to family therapy.

Although the above discussion deals with categories of dysfunctional families, more needs to be said about the rationale for viewing systems in this manner. Theoretically speaking, a family unit must have, as any well functioning system, executives and workers, chiefs and Indians, and decision makers and followers of those decisions. When the decision making occurs at both levels, that is, by parent and by child, the stage is set for triangulation. This term applies to a situation in which three people are vying for power within a framework. Illustratively, one can imagine three people with equal amounts of decision-making ability and clout trying to come to an agreement on anything. It is just not likely to happen. A family system functions best when parents operate as the executives and children function at a different and less powerful generational level. In order for this to occur, it is of paramount importance that the parents operate as a cohesive unit, at least on important and ongoing issues. From a developmental life cycle perspective it is most critical that the parents first form a unit as husband and wife. As this develops early in marriage and as trust and cooperation build, the marital unit can then, upon the introduction of the first child, start to work in concert as a parental unit as well. When the parents support one another at this level, there is a greater likelihood of positive family functioning. When there is trouble within the marital subsystem, this same couple is likely to encounter difficulty in operating within the parental subsystem. Therefore, from a structural perspective, one would say that well functioning families require as a minimum a well oiled and smooth operating set of parents.

3. Techniques of Change

To feel the force of a family system one has only to probe. The simplest questions posed by the therapist during the initial session frequently arouse powerful reactions on the part of some of the members. By closely observing the interactions and by consciously focusing on the process of the interactions rather than on the content of the verbalizations, the therapist can gain valuable diagnostic information. It is this information that allows the therapist to assess the structure of the family and begin to plan a strategy culminating in a constructive reorganization of structures.

The steps toward change involve unbalancing or a dissolution of the homeostatic balance of the unit, followed by a period of reorganization around a healthier means of communicating. This change, which centers on the structure and manner in which people respond to one another and not on the issues discussed, will allow for growth in interpersonal responsiveness to fellow family members. The concepts that have to be dealt with successfully in such a restructuring include joining, unbalancing, boundary making, relabeling, and reinforcing of the structural changes that have occurred. Some of these will be described in the early part of this paper and others will be illustrated in the case material presented.

3.1. Joining

Although joining is a central concept of structural family therapy it is frequently misinterpreted to be a beginning maneuver where the therapist seeks to establish rapport with the family. Joining goes well beyond this and occurs as a part of each family session. It calls for the therapist to connect with family members on an ongoing basis by emphasizing "the aspects of his personality and experience that are syntonic with the family's" (Minuchin, 1974). There are different times during sessions when the therapist may choose to join a member who is feeling excluded or threatened at the time. To think that one can devote the opening 10 minutes of an initial session to small talk and then proceed as if the family is hooked is a grave error. The hooking process is a continual one and requires attention each time the therapist meets with the family.

I recently had the opportunity to observe a trainee working with a family consisting of a rather large father who worked as a chef, the mother, a housewife, and daughters 17 and 14, the latter the index patient with a presenting problem of poor school performance and general immaturity. As I observed behind a one-way mirror, it was evident that father was overpowering and resistant to any of the therapist's interventions. Father made several references to therapists not being too smart and not really able to solve even some of their own problems. He clearly wanted to pull the therapist into a power struggle which he, of course, would win. The therapist had not effectively joined the father who was the power in the system. Before entering the room to rescue the situation I knew that I would have to join father successfully before any "therapy" could transpire. As I entered the room father greeted me with "Hi, Doc, want to tell me your problems?" I immediately told him I was having a terrible problem with trying to bake breads. The next few minutes were spent by my complaining how it was absolutely impossible ever to get yeast to rise. I added that my three attempts at baking bread were all disasters since the breads came out of the oven like bricks. As I appeared down and dissatisfied with my culinary performances, father came to my rescue by being supportive and offering some excellent suggestions. After a few minutes, I told him that we could discuss my baking at a later time since he was not coming to the clinic to help me with my problems. Immediately the tone of the session changed dramatically as father now felt competent, less threatened, and ready to discuss family concerns. Joining had taken place. As father was now more comfortable, the rest of the family followed his lead and became involved in the ensuing discussion. It might be said that when a family or family member is resistant or battling the therapist for power and control, joining has not occurred.

There are several ways to join systems. In some instances it occurs quickly. I have seen some families that have spoken words in Yiddish very early in the therapy. This seemed to me a test of my ability to understand them, that is, if I could speak the language I could understand their pain. My response in Yiddish and a few brief words about my grandmother and her teaching of the language during my childhood seemed to cement a working relationship almost immediately. For me, other ways of joining include finding areas of interest of the various members and spending some time talking about these. An acceptance and even identification with some of the family values also helps to cement a working relationship. A parent might refer nostalgically to the good old days when parents knew how to teach their kids respect and might talk of how things were much better then. To reinforce such recollections helps the joining process.

Just how one joins is less important than the fact that the therapist does connect. Although the specific techniques tend to be idiosyncratic, certain strategies for joining can be taught and will be presented in the case material that follows. The goal of joining is to allow the family to feel comfortable, less threatened, and confident that you really understand and therefore can help. Joining is a necessary condition for trust and without trust no significant change in the family system can occur.

Throughout this chapter I will refer to a most interesting family I treated over a period of two years. The presenting problem was serious concern over the worsening behavior of a 14-year-old boy who was being asked to leave a school for emotionally disturbed children. When father called, he informed me that he had taken his son for several evaluations and that the consensus was for placement in a state residential facility for severely disturbed children. Father seemed most concerned that his boy had stopped speaking nine months earlier and was withdrawing to a considerable extent. I sensed from our phone conversation that he had lost confidence in professionals and was coming only because the head of the adolescent unit that his son was scheduled to enter shortly had referred them to me for a consultation. Earlier I had presented a lecture to his staff on elective mutism, an interest of mine, and it was thought that a consultation around this issue prior to commitment would be helpful. The following few minutes of the initial interview in what was agreed upon as the first of a three-session consultation illustrate an early attempt to join the family prior to exploring the family system.

ROSENBERG: (*Turning to the youngest child after having greeted the parents in the waiting room before the family came into the therapy room*) Do you prefer to be called Elizabeth Ann?
BETTY ANN: I don't care.
FATHER: I guess that's a problem, too. She's had too many different names.
ROSENBERG: Too many different names?

BETTY ANN: Tiring.

ROSENBERG: Do you prefer to be called Betty Ann? (*Affirmative nod*) OK, we'll call you Betty Ann. How old are you, Betty Ann?

BETTY ANN: Twelve.

ROSENBERG: You're 12. And what grade are you in?

BETTY ANN: Seventh.

ROSENBERG: And you are 16, Judy?

JUDY: Uh-huh.

ROSENBERG: And, Robert, how old are you?

ROBERT: (*In a whisper*) Fourteen.

ROSENBERG: (*In a whisper to Robert*) Fourteen, OK.

ROSENBERG: What grade are you in, Judy?

JUDY: Eleventh.

ROSENBERG: (*To the parents*) OK, you're here. You've been through the mill. You've been to thousands of places, you've gone through thousands of things, and now you're coming to one more place. When I talked to you over the phone (*turning to father*), I got the feeling you had just about had it.

MOTHER: Yes, that's true.

ROSENBERG: Before, when I talked briefly to your husband in the waiting room, he said "Remember, just three visits," so I feel like you've really, really been through it. And I can't blame you. It must have been rough, a very rough time.

The above introduction illustrates the therapist's wanting to join the family before continuing. After an attempt was made to connect briefly with each of the children, the therapist turned to the parents and shared their concerns. His statements let them know that he felt for them in their sorrow and concern for their son. He also indicated to them through exaggeration that he knew they were fed up with professionals and was asking indirectly that they give it one more chance. The beginning of the joining process with Robert also was begun when the therapist responded to his whisper with a whisper of his own. The message was that he was ready to meet Robert at his point of entry.

3.2. Resistance

Although it is common practice for therapists to view early drop-out from treatment as the client's unwillingness to deal with unpleasant and difficult issues, the structural therapist sees himself responsible for selling a family on the need to continue in therapy. The initial phone call and first appointment are evidences that the family desires help. It is therefore up to the therapist to acknowledge the family's wanting help and to convince them that they can benefit from therapy.

Very often, families drop out of treatment because they do not develop an early confidence in the therapist. This may happen for a variety of reasons. It may be that the therapist does not adequately join the family or that the therapist moves too fast. I recently supervised a trainee who was attempting to push for structural change by having parents shift seats and deal with each other over rather conflictual material. My advice to the trainee via the phone into the family room was that he was doing very nice work for the ninth session, but that he was to remember that this was the initial interview. It has to be assumed that a family entering therapy is anxious, apprehensive, and guarded against any intrusions or unbalancing acts. To move in this direction before the stage is set is encouraging resistance and therapy drop-out.

Other times families will leave therapy when they feel the therapist is leaving the presenting problem and moving to other "nonrelated" issues prematurely (Rosenberg, 1978). The idea of remaining with the presenting problem until resolution offers the therapist added leverage and is helpful in keeping the family engaged. This approach is subscribed to by the Behavioral and Strategic schools as well.

There are many techniques that can reduce the drop-out rate in family therapy. In being cognizant of family structures and power, the structural therapist needs to recognize quickly the importance of hooking the parents. The goal of the initial session has to be to join the family successfully, especially the parents, and to convey to them that (1) you understand them and can relate to their concerns and (2) you can help them. Should either of these conditions not be met, it is probable that therapy will be discontinued. When both conditions are met, the continuation rate is high, regardless of socioeconomic class.

There are various means of hooking a family through a reading of their structure. As Whitaker so clearly states (1981), since mothers usually make the initial inquiry, it is incumbent upon the therapist to begin most sessions, at least the first one, by going directly to father. Since it can be assumed that he usually is less enamored with the notion of therapy, resistance can be lessened by addressing his concerns first and playing to his power.

3.3. Relabeling

To be truly effective as a therapist, one must be a good salesperson. Most often a family presents with a problem that is but a symptom of a dysfunctional system. To move the family from their point of entry to a readiness for structural change, the therapist must first sell them on the need to look elsewhere for the solution to the index patient's problem. As the therapist is able to help the family see alternate ways of perceiving the problem and therefore additional solutions, his power and influence will be enhanced.

At the onset of therapy the therapist frequently needs to change the family's perception of the problem, that is, the problem is really *Y* rather than *X* as you had thought. The therapist then uses the initial session to reframe the problem to a point that is more workable. The following example illustrates this.

The parents of 14-year-old Robert, mentioned earlier, were most concerned that their son had stopped speaking approximately nine months earlier. A consultation prior to admitting the youngster to a residential facility was begun with the major focus on the problem of elective mutism. As the initial session progressed, consisting of father, mother, 16-year-old Judy, 14-year-old Robert, and 12 year old Elizabeth, it became apparent that Robert's not talking was very much a part of the family's pattern of nonverbal communication. The following excerpts illustrate the therapist's efforts to relabel the problem from not talking in the index patient, to signaling rather than verbally communicating within this system.

In the following sequences, the therapist spreads the problem from Robert's elective mutism to the family's use of gesture in lieu of spoken language. These segments occur at different points in the first interview.

ROSENBERG: How about you, Betty? How do you do in school?
BETTY ANN: (*Made a noise*)
ROSENBERG: (*Imitated the noise*) What does that mean?
BETTY ANN: It's OK.
ROSENBERG: It's OK?
BETTY ANN: Yeah.

ROSENBERG: You do OK in school?

BETTY ANN: Oh, not really.

ROSENBERG: Not really? Mom's shaking her head, what does that mean?

MOTHER: She does all right.

A few minutes further into the session the therapist again identifies and accentuates the nonverbal interactions.

MOTHER: Well, I think she used to stay in the house a lot before we moved too.

FATHER: Yeah, but at least she would ride her bike once in a while. Of course that was a problem too because with the bike . . . I had to make an arrangement there to get the bike out from the basement.

ROSENBERG: (*To Betty Ann*) I wonder what that means? You were moving your head when your dad was talking. Can you tell him what that means? Can you, Betty? Because I'm not sure. I don't know if your dad is sure.

BETTY ANN: (*Silence*)

FATHER: What are you agreeing with? That you would go out if you could get your bike back, right?

BETTY ANN: Uh-huh. By myself.

As the family is directed toward exploring some of Judy's concerns, the following develops:

JUDY: Sometimes I wish she would talk more and other times it don't bother me.

MOTHER: Well, if you start a conversation—if you really want to tell me something—then we talk.

JUDY: Uh-huh.

ROSENBERG: Do you know what I think, Judy?

JUDY: What?

ROSENBERG: I think that it would be very good for you to tell your mom what it's like for you, because I have the feeling that this has been bothering you a little bit, OK? Is it your dad too? Your mom and your dad, or just your mom? . . . Everybody, did you ever notice, everybody shakes heads! Everything is in signals! You were talking before (*to father*), and Betty Ann was going like this (*therapist demonstrates*). (*Everyone laughs*). . . . And you were talking before (to mother) and Robert was either whispering or hiding under his coat. And while you're talking (*to father*), Judy is shaking this way. Everybody signals, either with their heads, or before Robert was going like this, with his hands. Everybody communicates, but not through talking! You have the most communicative family that I have ever in my life seen. Everybody gets through to everybody else, but nobody talks!

JUDY: That's true.

MOTHER: Especially with us two. We don't really even have to talk. It's just, like if before he even finishes his sentence, you know, he says one word, and I answer. Because I know exactly what he's going to ask.

ROSENBERG: That's frightening! (*Everyone laughs*) I thought you were going to say something else; I thought you were going to say that he says one word, and then stops and you know exactly what he's saying, then you answer him with one word, and then it goes on.

MOTHER: We really do sometimes.

ROSENBERG: Really?

MOTHER: Almost.

ROSENBERG: I'll bet you have the quietest household, maybe in the whole world!

MOTHER: We do, like even when we are riding in the car. I don't think anyone says a word until we are there.

ROSENBERG: (*Very emphatically*) Nobody talks?

MOTHER and JUDY: No, No.

ROSENBERG: So this is a real event for you?

FATHER: Except when we do talk we practically have accidents because I miss my signals. (*All laugh*)

ROSENBERG: So when you talk you get in big trouble, huh? Maybe it's better not to talk. (*Turning to Robert*) Stay quiet. (*He nods and smiles*)

Another example of a need to relabel is the following:

> In a family consisting at this time of mother and her 15-year-old son, where two other siblings have left the house and father had died suddenly three years prior to the beginning of therapy, mother complained that her son was delinquent, hyperactive, and out of control. This followed an incident where the boy, acting alone, entered an unfinished construction site and threw paint on the walls of one of the housing units. For mother to continue to view her son as out of control and in need of diagnosis would go nowhere, although this is what she had requested. (It had unfortunately been supported by a therapist mother had seen on an individual basis.) Mother's viewing her son as vulnerable and at risk would limit her in making efforts to have him improve his behavior. We find that to focus on strengths rather than weakness creates a much healthier atmosphere for positive change. Therefore, there had to be an attempt in the initial session to relabel the problem. As the session progressed, the therapist seized upon the theme of loss as the youngster spoke of his father's death, his older brother's move from the area, and his sister's recent departure for college. The therapist then developed the position that the boy was not delinquent, out of control, or hyperactive, but rather was sad, lonely, and abandoned. At this point, the boy acknowledged this by starting to cry and mother was encouraged to try to understand better her son's behavior in light of his rather sad affect. As the session ended, mother began to view her son in a different light and became more understanding and emotionally involved. Relabeling had taken place since mother was now able to see her son as depressed and needing her. As she accepted this in the session,she stopped referring to him as she had earlier and no longer requested a diagnosis. Therapy could now progress as the problem had been relabeled and was perceived differently by mother, therefore leading to constructive solutions to it.

3.4. Enactment

To reconstruct disputes and family problems that have occurred outside the therapy session has always been problematic. Too often the therapist is in the position of having to decide what factors led up to the conflict situation and then looking for solutions to the interactions that were so nonproductive. An important contribution of the structural family therapy model is the enactment, which is a technique designed to bring the conflict and presenting problem into the family session so that the therapy hour can become a laboratory to study dysfunctions within the system. The therapist then can get an inside view of the structures that have not been effective and can begin to push for structural change within the framework of the enactment.

A common example of the enactment is the situation where a parent states that a youngster is running out of control. To talk about the child's problem is not always immediately helpful since the child may be quiet during this discussion (or a younger child even may be running around the therapy room as the parent discusses this behavior). It is then up to the therapist to imagine what may transpire at home vis-à-vis this behavior. The goal in such a situation is to bring the behavior into the session so that it can be observed by the therapist and structural interventions can be made.

I remember a situation with a mother and 2½-year-old daughter, where mother complained that her daughter was constantly having tantrums and embarrassing her in stores, in front of grandparents, on buses, and so forth. During our first few sessions the child was as sweet and as well mannered as can be imagined. Mother would talk about her child's awful behavior and then seem somewhat uncomfortable because the girl would be reasonable and behaved during the session. At home and elsewhere the tantrums continued. I realized that I would have to encourage a tantrum in the session in order to help assess what was happening and to help the mother manage the child more effectively. During the third or fourth session I had my golden opportunity. The child seemed a bit feisty at the start of the session and shortly into the hour asked that mother give her some chewing gum. As mother reached into her purse for the gum, I asked that she not give any gum to her daughter since lunchtime was approaching and gum might ruin her appetite. Mother, following my cue, withheld the gum and the kid began to protest. As mother started to give her the gum to quiet her down, I again asked her not to. Within a few seconds the child was beginning to whimper, then crying and begging for the gum. Clearly the power struggle was taking shape and it was imperative that mother engage her child in battle and come out victorious. It sounds silly, doesn't it? Yet there clearly was a power struggle taking shape and the battle needed to continue. Within another minute or two, the child was crying loudly, falling to the floor, and undressing herself. As mother seemed rattled I talked to her in a calm voice telling her that she could give the gum to her daughter to hold until after lunch—after the crying and tantrum behavior stopped. Twenty minutes into the tantrum I left the room briefly to get a cup of coffee for mother and for me since the noise was deafening and we had to keep our respective cool. We timed the little girl and after 33 minutes, she came to a whimpering stop. Initially, mother had viewed her as weak, but during our session I pointed out that weak and fragile kids do not hold out for more than two minutes. As mother came to view her daughter as manipulative rather than weak, she found it easier to relax and to talk to me during the session. As the girl stopped crying and got dressed, mother calmly said that she was proud of her daughter stopping the tantrum and that the gum was now hers to hold until later. Both mother and I were exhausted at the end of the session but the little girl seemed just fine. An enactment had occurred and mother asserted her control, something that had not often happened at home. In short, the generational boundaries were drawn, mother was in charge and her daughter was comfortable in knowing that someone could handle her. Enactments in dealing with tantrum behavior in young children are always successful. In fact, this is the only condition in which I will offer the parents a money-back guarantee if the behavior cannot be readily controlled. Mother came in the following week to tell me that there was only one brief tantrum during the week and that her apparent indifference led her child to abandon the tantrum in about five minutes. (Behaviorists call this a lack of reinforcement which leads to extinction of the behavior.) Two additional sessions spaced over four weeks showed no additional tantrums and the case thus was closed.

The goal of a successful enactment is to exacerbate conflict within the therapy session so that structures can be studied and modified in a way that the presenting problem will be reduced in potency. Enactments also serve to create boundaries around family subsystems and to change proximity of members within the family unit.

4. Role of the Therapist

Although various theoretical approaches encourage the therapist to be reflective, passive, and, generally, nondirective, the structural approach to family therapy focuses on directing and reorganizing in a more assertive manner. The therapist frequently must interrupt a conversation, push for conflict through an enactment, and often build up or even put down a given member in order to unbalance a system. The role is a tough one since the therapist controls the rhythm of the session and sometimes even may act in an inconsistent manner within the course of it. For example, he initially may support an obnoxious 16-year-old in order to join the youngster and gain some leverage, only to support the parents in setting limits and encouraging them to get tough with their son later in the session.

The structural family therapist must operate freely. He has to join the system but also must retreat quickly, lest he be inducted by the power of the system. The therapist has to have a game plan prior to the start of the session and this plan is based on the knowledge of structures as well as early hypotheses concerning this family and the relationship of the presenting problem to the dynamics of this system.

The analogy of a Saturday afternoon football game makes this easier to understand. The coach must prepare his quarterback (his director, therapist) to outthink and outmaneuver the opposition. There must be a game plan developed that will allow the quarterback to enter the game ready to deal with what he expects from the opponents. We can think of this as a working hypothesis that is designed beforehand but often must be revised as the session progresses. From a structural therapy perspective, the therapist might assume that an adolescent son's disrespect for mother stems from father's anger toward mother and license he has given his son to go after her. This is a hypothesis that the therapist is working with as he begins to probe the system, that is, the game plan. As he gets to know the family during the first two sessions it becomes apparent that mother seems to gain some enjoyment from the constant battling with her son and that, in fact, dad tries to make peace between the warring parties. As go-between, he becomes frustrated and angered and then goes after both mother and son. The defense is now looking a bit different and so the quarterback must call an audible (as the team approaches the line of scrimmage, the therapist gives a verbal signal that informs his side that the play must now be different as a result of some changes in what was expected from the opposition).

If adequate joining has occurred between therapist and family, and if the family develops confidence in the person and the treatment, then the techniques of the therapist described throughout this chapter will be accepted by the family. Perhaps the most difficult aspect of this approach to teach is training the inexperienced (or sometimes experienced nonstructural therapist) to sit back and *direct* the interactions in a direction the therapist feels the family should proceed. The tendency has been to go with the family indefinitely, not to interrupt, to pick up on their content and thus to follow many false leads. That one should have one's own active agenda when working with a family is not easy to teach. It is one of those things that needs almost to be accepted and then practiced. As the experiences mount, the therapist develops greater confidence in the approach being described. As therapy progresses, the therapist should have an ongoing agenda dealing with family interactions. He should direct these interactions but does not necessarily have to be verbally active at all times. The goal should be to become increasingly less central as therapy progresses. Many families will use the therapist as a central switchboard during the earliest phases of treatment and this is acceptable in order to aid the joining process. The therapist, however, should be working toward encouraging family members to deal with one another with increasing frequency. Ideally, as the family approaches termination, the therapist should be relatively inactive, except at those times when he chooses to highlight and/or reinforce certain changed patterns of interaction.

4.1. Emphasis on Process

One of the more significant aspects of structural family therapy is its focus on interactional process rather than solely on content. In order for a restructuring of the family to occur, the therapist must constantly be tuned in to patterns of response rather than what the response might be. For example, when a mother enters the first session telling the therapist the bad deeds her son has done, what is important is not what she is saying, but that she is lecturing about the youngster in a manner that undoubtedly has been repeated at home and elsewhere several hundred times. This unproductive and limiting communication must be changed so that more effective communication can begin. If the son looks down, feeling he is on the hot seat, and the father appears peripheral, the therapist needs to swing into action by unbalancing the system. One early way might be to encourage father to talk to his son about what has happened at home. In pushing father and son to respond to each other, the son now is involved and must be accountable for his actions, and the father is no longer peripheral. Mother is also forced to respond differently since she now sees her husband getting involved with his son, something that she perhaps has wanted to happen for years. In this rather brief example, the reader can see how focusing on process rather than content begins to lead the family to new ways of interacting and thus to restructuring, which is so necessary for change to occur. As change begins to take place the therapist reinforces the new patterns of responding that over time will lead to more constructive family structures. In the above situation, the family may report after several sessions that father is taking more of an active interest in his son and that mother and son seem less antagonistic toward one another. A frequent by-product of this is an improved relationship in the marital dyad since there is less tension between the parents over the son's behavior and since father is now less peripheral. The likelihood is that mother is now somewhat more relaxed and feeling more positively toward her spouse. Positive structural changes such as this tend to be self reinforcing, that is, families will tend to repeat those behaviors acquired in therapy if the newly learned interactions work. If father's more active role keeps the son acting more appropriately and lessens arguments between father and mother, father is likely to continue to act this way.

It is difficult for the student to learn to concentrate on process. It runs counter to all we ever have learned about doing therapy: never interrupting a patient's train of thought and helping a person to explore further his thoughts and feelings. Unfortunately, if we follow content we will find ourselves taken down the garden path with regularity. Rather, we need to look for interactions that are counterproductive and point these out to family members so they can develop, with the therapist's assistance, alternate ways of dealing with these heretofore dysfunctional communication patterns. In doing so, the therapist must be cognizant of existing structures as well as how structures might be modified.

4.2. Length of Therapy

Structural family therapy tends to be shorter in duration than most approaches to family therapy, the exception being strategic therapy, where "therapists prefer to keep therapy brief and to terminate as soon as possible following positive change in the presenting problem" (Stanton, 1981b). The structural viewpoint would suggest that although the symptom sometimes drops out after the first few sessions, structural change must occur in order to prevent its recurrence. Evidence for this stance can be found in some of the early work using a behavioral paradigm in the treatment of anorexia nervosa.

This work by Brady and Rieger (1975) found that a behavioral approach was successful in helping anorectics gain weight and leave the hospital. However, the improvement was not sustained after the patients returned to their environment. This is presumed to have occurred because no significant change in the family structure had taken place (Minuchin *et al.*, 1978).

The structural therapist, therefore, works toward symptom removal as quickly as possible, but is at the same time looking to restructure the family so that the changes are more likely to hold. In reviewing my records for the past several years, I found that the average number of sessions per family was 17, with the typical time in therapy ranging from three to seven months. In this time frame, family structures can be successfully modified. One even can speculate that changes that do not occur within this amount of time are not likely to occur at all. (It must be pointed out that there are some situations that are extremely difficult and long standing, and in such cases therapy may run considerably longer.) Rather than continue indefinitely in therapy with families, the structural family therapist is more likely to terminate at a point where the presenting problem has been alleviated and the family structure has been altered sufficiently to allow for more effective problem-solving behavior. At termination, families are encouraged to be more reliant on their own resources and to reenter therapy only when absolutely necessary. When families return after an absence from therapy, they most often require only a few sessions to regain their confidence and ability to function satisfactorily. It is as though they sometimes require a booster shot to stave off problems that have occurred previously.

The following case history is presented to give the reader a clearer picture of some specific interventions a structural therapist makes. Continuing explanations of the interventions allow the reader an opportunity to travel through the session as though sitting behind the one-way screen with the therapist offering a running commentary on his work. The case chosen is that of an 18-year-old boy entering the Philadelphia Child Guidance Clinic Outpatient Department on an emergency basis. This case was chosen to illustrate the structural model in treating an adolescent with an acute psychotic break. Little has been said about this type of an approach in the presenting problem of psychosis, therefore, this is being offered to expand the readers understanding of the applicability of the structural family therapy approach.

Case History. Larry, who presented as a tall, well-built 18-year-old was brought to the clinic by his parents who were most concerned with what they described as strange behavior. According to the parents, their son, following graduation from high school 10 days earlier, began to engage in very atypical behavior that included seeming disoriented, getting in a fight (this had never happened to him), wanting to return to a friend's house late in the evening after a party to take repeated showers, and roaming around his house nude. Following a visit to the family physician, Larry was hospitalized for a three-day observation period at which time he became paranoid and difficult to control in the general hospital setting. Mother was asked to sleep in his room and she later reported that he thought the nurses were trying to poison him. He refused to allow an EMI scan and resisted blood tests, stating that the nurses were preparing to put air bubbles in his veins in an attempt to kill him. All hospital tests proved negative, including a brain scan later performed on an outpatient basis.

The following is a transcript of the second meeting held with this family one day after the emergency consultation. Because a bed in our inpatient unit was not available for several days, it was decided that the family should be seen the next day. Present for the session were father and mother, their 21-year-old daughter, and Larry. The therapists present were Dr. Thomas Shettle, a first-year resident, and the author. The interview selected includes the techniques discussed above and proceeds slowly and methodically toward a change in family structure. The therapist realized early in the interview (and from the previous day's session) that father and son were similar in many ways and somehow must be connected more closely within the session if a positive change in Larry's behavior were to occur. As will be seen in the interview, mother, who had been most involved in Larry's problem—at times overly involved—needed to be encouraged to pull back somewhat so that father could become more engaged with his son.

At the start of each session the therapist must have a goal and must proceed accordingly. The goal of this second session in the two-day period was to continue to get a clearer diagnostic picture, to develop further the joining process, and to begin to push gently for a structural change that would allow Larry to commuicate his concerns and reestablish contact with his peripheral, but very much involved, father. As the session develops, the reader can see another goal, namely, the reinforcement of appropriate statements and behaviors in Larry and his father, and an attempt to extinguish behaviors from Larry that seem nonproductive. The session begins with Dr. Shettle making some joining statements to sister Diane, who was not present the day before, and to Larry. The author is observing behind a one-way screen at the start of the session.

SHETTLE: I thought you were the one to ask her something. Why don't you ask your sister something? (*Silence*)

SHETTLE: I think it would be good for you to talk to your sister for a moment or two.

DIANE: (*To Larry*) What would you like to say?

SHETTLE: What would you like to say? (*Silence*)

SHETTLE: Go ahead, what would you like to say to your sister? (*Very long pause*) Maybe Diane should ask you something and you could respond to her?

DIANE: Do you want me to ask you something? OK . . . uhm . . . would you like to go swimming on Sunday?

LARRY: Yeah.

DIANE: With all the kids down the shore?

LARRY: Yeah.

SHETTLE: You were talking to Diane, why don't you talk to her; I'm not in this conversation.

DIANE: OK, we can take a lunch down there. Would you like that? (*Long pause*)

SHETTLE: (*Larry looking at Dr. Shettle*) There's Diane, talk to Diane.

DIANE: (*Long pause*) We can ride the waves and then on the way home we can stop for custard.

SHETTLE: You really have to tell her yes or no. I can't help you out here.

LARRY: Yeah.

DIANE: Yes? Or would you like to do something else? (*Long pause*)

LARRY: Doctor, when I came here, right? And you had signed a piece of paper, right?

SHETTLE: Uh-huh.

LARRY: And when she checked it she says "Oh, uh, this doctor's name isn't on the list." I didn't know what the cashier was talking about.

SHETTLE: Uh-huh. You mean you came in today at the Admissions desk?

DIANE: The cashier, she looked for your name on the list and she said he's a newer doctor and his name isn't placed up here yet.

SHETTLE: Right. I officially started here on the 18th and the new published listing doesn't come out until July 1st. So the woman at the cashier's desk may not have had my name on her list yet. Most likely she has you listed under Dr. Rosenberg's name because you're part of his case load. He just called me in to work with him so that's the explanation for that. That was upsetting to you a little bit, that I wasn't on her list?

LARRY: Yeah.

SHETTLE: Well, that's understandable. That's understandable.

LARRY: Doctor, I came here to see you again like you said and, uh, I want to know what you think I should do.

SHETTLE: OK, well, I think Dr. Rosenberg and I had spoken to you and your family yesterday and we thought it might be helpful for you to come into the hospital for a while, for a short time. When we have the first available bed that's when you could come in. I wanted to tell you that at morning report the staff said that the first available bed might be Monday, and it might not be until Tuesday or Wednesday. The exact date wasn't really clear. Is that OK with you? (*Silence*)

SHETTLE: Is that OK with you, Larry? The suggestion that you come into the hospital? (*Enter Dr. Rosenberg*)

SHETTLE: Larry's much improved today over yesterday. He was just asking . . . he was a little worried when they came in to the cashier . . .

ROSENBERG: I heard.

SHETTLE: Oh, you heard, you were there. OK. (*Indicates observation room*)

ROSENBERG: They didn't know which of us to put on the piece of paper. When that happens, we're all in big trouble. (*Laughter*)

It seems that Larry is unduly concerned about having two therapists' names on the cashier's sheet. To get into a discussion about this is not very helpful since it only dwells on his weakness and confusion. Rather, the attempt was to use humor to put this issue aside and continue with the session.

ROSENBERG: Diane, Hi. You weren't here yesterday, and so we didn't meet. So, hello. (*To Dr. Shettle*) You were asking Larry about his coming here?

SHETTLE: Oh, I just mentioned that Larry had asked when he would be coming in and the staff said there may or may not be a bed on Monday. It may not be until Tuesday, or even at the latest Wednesday. So that the actual admission will have to be played by ear.

ROSENBERG: (*To Larry*) How does that sound to you?

LARRY: (*Long pause*)

ROSENBERG: How does that sound to you? If there isn't a bed Monday you may have to wait till Tuesday, or maybe even Wednesday. That's about four days. Is that OK with you? What do you think, Larry?

LARRY: (*Pause*) That's not why I came here. I know I came here and my parents signed me out and they asked for my doctor and they said his name wasn't on the list, so I just showed them a piece of paper.

SHETTLE: What we explained. I apologize, I'm sorry that I wasn't on the list.

ROSENBERG: (*To Larry*) See, most people have only one doctor's name on the list, you're lucky you have two—OK, so you've got two of us and most other people only have one. So you're in very good shape, you're lucky; you lucked-out.

MOTHER: (*To Larry*) You're special.

ROSENBERG: (*To Larry*) Don't you think that's pretty good? If I went someplace and instead of getting one doctor I had two I'd feel great!

LARRY: Yeah.

ROSENBERG: You don't realize how lucky you are! You look worried about it and you should be thrilled! You don't realize how lucky you are. You got two guys working with you and the others only have one! . . . What do you think about coming into the hospital? Coming in here next week? We talked about it a little bit yesterday, we're talking about it a little more today. . . . What do you think?

At this point it is becoming evident that Larry uses his "psychopathology" to escape issues. When asked about coming into the hospital, he returned to the earlier mentioned concern of his that two doctor's names appeared on the cashier's sheet. This pattern will occur again during this session. Again, the therapist's attempt is to treat this with humor and move on to issues that need to be resolved.

LARRY: I was just, y'know, when I came here I uh . . . (*Long pause*)

ROSENBERG: Would you like to come in here next week so we can get a better chance to help you out?

LARRY: Yeah.

ROSENBERG: 'Cause you were saying yesterday that you felt confused. And you were worried about what was happening with you. You were also saying you like the old Larry better and that was the way you wanted to be, remember?

LARRY: Yeah.

ROSENBERG: So, that if you came in here, we have a hospital in this building, and maybe if you could stay here for a little while, we're not talking about six months or a year, maybe two weeks, maybe three weeks, until things get better, maybe even four weeks. Then your mom and dad, and your sisters and brothers would be visiting you. They'd be coming in and seeing you and maybe things could get straightened out so that you wouldn't be so confused. How does that sound to you? (Pause) You're looking at your dad, huh? What do you think about that?

Here we have an early reading of the family structure. When in trouble, Larry makes eye contact with his father. One can begin to feel the tie-in between the two. Also, both have seemed quite nonverbal up to this point in the session. My speculation is that I have to reach Larry through his dad. Both are appearing as somewhat peripheral to the other members of the family and somewhat distanced during the session. The immediate objective is to reach out to father in order to support him and enable him to help his son.

MOTHER: I think it's great! Gonna help Larry get back to the old Larry, I think it's just great!

ROSENBERG: (*To father*) Do you feel the same way?

FATHER: Yeah, I think it would be good for him.

ROSENBERG: (*To Larry*) Then we'll get you back on the farm again.

DIANE: He was back there today.

ROSENBERG: Really? (*To Larry*) What were you doing?

LARRY: Making crates, working.

Here the therapist senses some enthusiasm in Larry and joins around crate-making. Process rather than the content is most important here.

ROSENBERG: So, you were working this morning?

LARRY: Yeah.

MOTHER: Putting crates together.

Notice the tendency for mother to respond for Larry. An immediate objective is to ease her out of this tendency in order that later on father can begin to deal with his son.

ROSENBERG: How do you make a crate? Is it hard to do?

MOTHER: They're wooden crates and they come all opened up and . . . (*Describes crate-making*)

ROSENBERG: (To Larry) What do you do to them?

LARRY: Just make them, put them on a flat-bed tractor.

ROSENBERG: Yeah? Did you put stuff in them?

LARRY: Cabbage, yeah.

MOTHER: He was just . . . (*Cut off by Dr. Rosenberg*)

ROSENBERG: Cabbage? Do you pick the cabbage by hand?

LARRY: With a knife.

ROSENBERG: And then you load them into the crates? And then what do you do when you have the crates all loaded up?
LARRY: Stack them.
ROSENBERG: Then what do you do when you have them all loaded up?
LARRY: Put them on a truck.
ROSENBERG: And then take them to your produce place?
MOTHER: Yeah.
LARRY: Yeah.
ROSENBERG: So you're working tonight, huh, how does it feel to be working?
LARRY: OK.
ROSENBERG: Because you were saying yesterday that's something you really want to do. That's great.

A major technique is to reinforce changes that have taken place, no matter how unimportant they may seem. The goal throughout is to ignore undesirable behaviors (talk of sign-in sheet, two doctors) and pick up on and reinforce desirable behaviors such as Larry's having worked this morning and having permitted an EMI scan to be done on an outpatient basis. He had resisted this when hospitalized the previous week fearing someone was trying to kill him.

MOTHER: He also took his CAT scan today. They said it was OK.
ROSENBERG: (*To Larry*) So you handled that nicely, great. You must be feeling a lot better today.
LARRY: Yeah.
ROSENBERG: You're sure as hell looking better. (*To parents*) Don't you think? Yesterday he looked awful, today he's back to the good-looking kid that he was in the picture you showed me.
FATHER: Yeah, he's looking better.

At this point in the session, the therapist turns from issues concerning Larry to some questioning of Diane, her college problems (they're quite minor), issues within the family, and so forth. The objective is to develop a rhythm within the session. One needs to give the family a breather so that the session consists of joining and then moving in on weighty issues followed by retreat into insignificant topics. As the tension lessens and family members relax, the therapist then can return to the important issues. The next several minutes, not included here, seek to lessen tensions while still giving the therapist data on the existing structures.

We continue with the session several minutes later as the questioning of Larry continues. The discussion centers around Larry's job on the family farm

ROSENBERG: How many hours a week do you work there?
LARRY: Oh, I can work 15 hours a day—sometimes 12 or 15 hours a day on a summer day.
ROSENBERG: Really?
MOTHER: Yes, he does.
ROSENBERG: Wow.
MOTHER: From 7 in the morning till 9, 10 at night.
ROSENBERG: Do you make a lot of money?
LARRY: Yeah.
ROSENBERG: Are you going to build up your bank account again?
LARRY: (*Pause*)
ROSENBERG: It sounds like it was up really high.

Here the therapist again begins to push. Earlier in the year Larry's bank account was several thousand dollars; however, a car wreck and some drinking and drug-related expenses rapidly depleted it. Parents had mentioned in the previous session that this was a charged topic.

LARRY: (*Pause*)
ROSENBERG: Yeah?
LARRY: Yeah.
ROSENBERG: Then you got sort of wiped out a little bit? Making a comeback?
LARRY: (*Silence*)
ROSENBERG: What do you think?
LARRY: (*Silence*)

It is becoming increasingly apparent that Larry is not about to let the therapist enter his space. His pauses are frequent and relatively long and his eye contact is minimal. At this point I have decided to pull back and try to get at some systems issues. This is where I begin my ''fishing'' expedition. I don't know what will turn up but strongly suspect something powerful is going on in the family and that it will come to the fore.

ROSENBERG: You look at your mom and dad all the time, how come? Are you waiting for them to answer? (*To the parents*) Have you had any major difficulties with any of the kids? Either Larry or any of the others that you wanted to talk about as long as you're here?
FATHER: No.
MOTHER: They're all very good children—no problem with any of them.
ROSENBERG: That's great. Do the kids see it the same way?
DIANE: Yeah, (ha, ha) well, I don't know, I'd say nothing really difficult.
ROSENBERG: Nothing major, any minor ones? Every family in the world has. . . .
DIANE: Every family in the world has somebody that flies off the handle every once in awhile.
ROSENBERG: How badly does mom fly off the handle? You can talk, she's not listening.

One can push much more with the use of humor. Here Diane becomes freer to talk since she is told that mother is not listening.

DIANE: Yeah, she'll go off once in a while, but not too often.
ROSENBERG: Can you handle her when she goes off the handle?
DIANE: Yeah, I've sort of gotten used to it now.
ROSENBERG: How do you deal with her?
DIANE: How do I deal with her? Oh, I sort of just take it in stride, it doesn't really bother me.
ROSENBERG: Not at all?
DIANE: No, once in a while if it's something that pertains directly to me, or if it is derogatory to me, that'll affect me, but it easily wears off after a day or so.
ROSENBERG: How about you, Larry, how do you handle your mom when she flies off the handle?

Here the therapist employs a behavioral paradigm, that of successive approximations. It is as though one were building a hierarchy in treating a phobia. The least anxiety producing situation is having Diane talk about mother. This leads to Larry commenting on mom, then Diane talking about dad and, finally, Larry talking about dad, probably the most anxiety laden connection (Rosenberg & Lindblad, 1978).

LARRY: She's OK, she's . . .
ROSENBERG: I didn't ask you if she's OK. How do you handle her when she flies off? (*Laughter*)
LARRY: I listen to her.
ROSENBERG: Do you?
LARRY: Uh-huh.
ROSENBERG: Is it hard to listen to her sometimes? Does she really get hyper?
LARRY: Yeah, once in awhile.

ROSENBERG: Well, how do you deal with her when she's like that?
LARRY: (*Long pause*)
ROSENBERG: Diane is saying that she can handle her and I'm wondering if you can handle her?
LARRY: Yeah, I can handle my mother.
ROSENBERG: You can?
LARRY: Uh-huh.
ROSENBERG: She's not that tough to handle?
MOTHER: (*Chuckle*)
ROSENBERG: How about your dad, Diane. How do you handle him?
DIANE: How do I handle him?
ROSENBERG: Yeah.
DIANE: He doesn't really say too much. Once in a while he'll yell but he listens.
ROSENBERG: Is he a tough guy to deal with?
DIANE: Once in a while, yeah, but usually I just turn the other way. . . . I just wait until he cools down.
ROSENBERG: He then cools down?
DIANE: Yeah.
ROSENBERG: So you know he's going to explode, and after he explodes he bounces off the ceiling and then he settles down?
DIANE: Yeah, something like that.
ROSENBERG: (*To Larry*) Can you handle your dad?
LARRY: Yeah, I can handle my dad.
ROSENBERG: How do you deal with him?
LARRY: By listening to him.
ROSENBERG: What do you do when he gets really mad?
LARRY: He's smiling. I ain't saying nothing. (*Laughter from everyone*)
ROSENBERG: What do you do when your dad really gets angry at you?
LARRY: I help him out.
ROSENBERG: How do you do that?
LARRY: (*Silence*)
ROSENBERG: How do you help him out Larry?
LARRY: (*Silence*)
ROSENBERG: He's waiting to hear how you handle him, how do you do it?
LARRY: (*Silence*)
ROSENBERG: (*To Dr. Shettle*) Do you think I'm asking an unfair question?

Here the therapists talk to one another in a manner that will allow them to get at important issues without having to confront the family. All are free to listen to what the therapists are saying and no one needs to become defensive.

SHETTLE: I don't know. There's a resistance to talk in here, to explain it. He doesn't want to let the secret out.
ROSENBERG: Do you think it's a good thing that he's just going to hold it in?
SHETTLE: That's the thing, you see if he lets us in on his secrets he won't be able to control his dad anymore. It's important to be able to keep control of that, huh? (*To Larry*)
LARRY: Yeah.
SHETTLE: And mom too, probably, huh?
ROSENBERG: I just wonder if mom's easier to handle in this family than dad is.
SHETTLE: I don't know. Who's easier to handle, Larry?
MOTHER: Mom's the discipliner. He gets away with things with his dad.
ROSENBERG: You mean dad's the soft touch?
LARRY: Yeah. No.
ROSENBERG: You can tell us. He's the easy guy in the family? Is he a marshmallow?

LARRY: No, he ain't a marshmallow.

ROSENBERG: If your family is like most other families, and I think you probably are, there are a lot of things that come up from time to time that really get to be problems. Maybe they're not major, but after a long period of time, they get to be. And there may now be some things going on in your family that maybe the kids have been thinking about or maybe, Larry, that you've been thinking about, that you've not shared with dad or mom; maybe stuff that sort of bugs you, you know, that sort of gets to you after a while. Maybe you can help them be better parents by letting them know what's really been getting to you, you know? Because all parents bug their kids. Don't you think? My kids tell me all the time that I bug them, so I just assume that that always happens. So, maybe the two of you have to find out from the other kids too, not just from Larry, what kinds of things are going on, so that maybe you could react a little bit differently to them. Because it sounds like it's been rough for you around the house, and things have been very stressful. And not just the last 10 days—they've been extra hard for you. But I think maybe the last 10 months. A lot of stress in the whole family. Maybe those are things that need to be explored a little bit more and looked into. You were away much of the year, Diane, weren't you? Did you live at college?

The fishing expedition continues. Also, in the above the therapist normalizes family problems to minimize the threat to this family unit.

DIANE: No, I was home.

MOTHER: She commutes every day.

ROSENBERG: What did you think, Diane, about what was going on in the family over the last year?

DIANE: Over the last year?

ROSENBERG: Uh-huh.

DIANE: (*Deep breath, sigh*) Well, uh, our family is . . . is very quiet and not too much is . . . well, you know, we have times when we joke around. I think if we could talk more, we'd all feel a lot better. It's been very stressful because my father was sick last summer. And then we had my sister's wedding a month later.

At last there seems to be a major issue—father's illness. Since Larry's problem with truanting school and fairly heavy drinking began approximately 10 months ago, it looks as though we may have discovered an important tie between Larry and his father. The objective now is to explore this issue fully along structural lines, that is, father's illness and its affect upon Larry's behavior.

ROSENBERG: What was your dad sick with?

LARRY: High blood pressure.

DIANE: He had high blood pressure.

MOTHER: His blood pressure was 300 over 160. He takes 14 pills a day to control it.

ROSENBERG: Was there anything last summer that happened to you, or was it just discovered?

FATHER: Oh, I just discovered that it was high, I started off on dyazide and I . . . I don't know if you're familiar with . . . I was taking aldomet medicine and I had a terrible reaction to it.

MOTHER: We almost lost him.

ROSENBERG: Really?

FATHER: Yeah.

MOTHER: Because the doctor gave him too big of a dose, he was giving him 1,000 mgs a day, and it like poisoned . . . he turned all blue, it affected his kidneys, his lungs, his liver. . . . He was in postintensive care for a week, and under oxygen; he couldn't breathe anymore.

ROSENBERG: Oh, wow.

FATHER: And I just went to the doctor this past Wednesday and it's the first time since last June that it's been fairly low. It was 130 over 80, which is, the doctor was well pleased with that, that's . . .

ROSENBERG: Solidly average.
FATHER: Yeah, but I'm still taking 14 pills a day, 5 different kinds of medicine.
MOTHER: The two or three days that Larry was in the hospital his blood pressure kept fluctuating. It would be normal, then it would go up like 160 over 110.
SHETTLE: Larry's you're talking about?
EVERYONE: Yes.

Here again we see the strong bond between Larry and his father. The steep rise in Larry's blood pressure during his recent hospitalization is a way of his identifying with father through his father's illness. The hypothesis that one needs to approach Larry through his father is again confirmed.

MOTHER: Like I said, we was preparing for Linda's wedding at the same time. He got sick; he was in the whole month of July, and August, and Linda got married the first week in September, and . . . a lot of tension.
ROSENBERG: Very close to your dad?
LARRY: Yeah, I'm *very* close to my dad.
ROSENBERG: I bet you were *panicked* last summer!
LARRY: Yeah, I was.
ROSENBERG: You must have been scared to death!
LARRY: (*Silence*)
SHETTLE: Did you ever tell your dad that? How frightened you were about his condition?
LARRY: Yeah.
SHETTLE: You told him?
LARRY: Yeah.
SHETTLE: Well, that's good, I think he needs that. I think he needs to know that you're concerned right now.
ROSENBERG: This is starting to make sense. You thought your dad was going to die?
LARRY: No.
ROSENBERG: From what your mom said, I'll bet she worried about that, didn't you?
MOTHER: Sure did.
ROSENBERG: You're very close to your dad. You must have been *absolutely panicked*. Were you panicked, Diane?
DIANE: Yes.
ROSENBERG: The whole family was?
DIANE: Yes. He was never really sick before, and this happened just like that.
ROSENBERG: He was always the rock in the family, sort of the pillar that everybody could lean against, and now all of a sudden everyone found out that dad was really very sick.
DIANE: Yeah.
ROSENBERG: That was last summer?
MOTHER: July.
FATHER: July, yeah, end of July.
ROSENBERG: Is that when you started to do yourself in? You started drinking and stuff?
LARRY: A little bit, yeah.
ROSENBERG: You figured if your dad was in trouble, screw it all, you might as well just tear loose?
LARRY: No, that's not how I feel.
ROSENBERG: Sometimes people feel that way. Sometimes guys your age do things like that, you know? They're very close to their father and their father gets very sick and they worry and panic and all of a sudden they say "screw the world, I'm just going to go do anything, who cares?" Is it that way with you?
LARRY: No.
ROSENBERG: What was it like for you?
LARRY: (*Long silence*)

ROSENBERG: Did you ever tell anybody you were upset?

LARRY: Yeah.

ROSENBERG: Who'd you talk to about it?

LARRY: A lot of people. My sisters.

ROSENBERG: (*To Diane*) Did you feel Larry was very open about his concern over his dad's health?

DIANE: No.

ROSENBERG: Kept it all inside?

DIANE: Uh-huh.

MOTHER: Uh-huh, he never said nothing.

ROSENBERG: That's a problem. He's like his dad in a lot of ways. His dad was saying yesterday he doesn't say a thing. He keeps everything to himself.

MOTHER: Yes, his father is very quiet. Mealtimes at our house are very quiet.

ROSENBERG: Because Larry's the first-born son he feels he has to be like his dad and be quiet too. . . . So, everybody was able to talk about how scared they were and what was going on with dad while he was in the hospital?

MOTHER: Not really, like Diane said, nobody talks out to each other, everybody keeps their problems to themselves.

ROSENBERG: Not too good, is it?

FATHER: No.

MOTHER: No, it really isn't.

ROSENBERG: Maybe the two of you could help your kids to be able to talk a little bit more about important things in the family. Can't think of anything more important than your health. Are you worried about it now?

FATHER: About my health?

ROSENBERG: Or are you feeling a whole lot better?

FATHER: Oh, I feel pretty good now, better than I have in a long time. Naturally, when you go to the doctor if your blood pressure is near normal . . . I think he's still concerned about it but not as much as before. Because for about three or four months when I first started taking medicine they still couldn't take it down. But, now it's pretty good, the doctor was well pleased with it.

ROSENBERG: So, this whole thing, then, lasted about four or five months, until things were really under control?

FATHER: Oh, yeah, really.

ROSENBERG: So, it was a very stressful year for a lot of reasons. Is this the toughest year you've all had?

MOTHER: Yeah, I would say.

FATHER: Yeah, probably, I would say so.

At this point the therapists leave the room so they can observe and discuss strategies. The family is asked to discuss family issues that have been problematic over the past few months.

As the therapists observe, it becomes increasingly apparent that mother takes over and initiates questioning with Larry while tending to infantilize him.

An objective upon entering the room was to encourage and reinforce verbal communication between father and son and to gracefully exclude mother. It was hypothesized that a strong father–son tie would help Larry to become more responsible and act in a less disturbed manner. The therapists returned after about five minutes and immediately began to work on the father–son dyad.

As we reenter the room, we rearrange the seating so father and son are close and removed spacially from the rest of the family. The earlier seating had been according to the arrangement in Figure 1.

As the therapists entered, the seating was changed to the arrangement as seen in Figure 2.

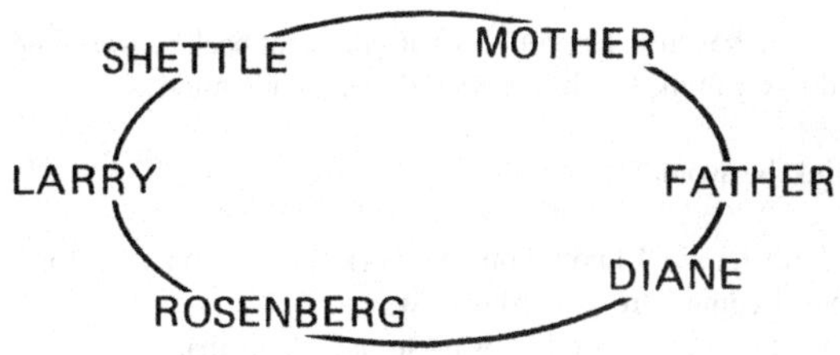

Figure 1

ROSENBERG: (*To Father*) Would you do me a favor? Would you change seats and sit next to Larry? You are starting to find out from him what some of his concerns are and I think it's important. Could you continue?

FATHER: (*Changes seat and looks at son*) Uh-huh. So, that's what's bothering you a little bit.

LARRY: Yeah.

FATHER: Well, can't you keep working there? If you want?

LARRY: Yeah. (*Pause*) When we were home last night, right? I . . . I just couldn't take the pressure like now. I'm just not a pressure person and our family's like that. We're all close, and it's hard for me to talk when nobody else is talking.

ROSENBERG: You're talking fine to your dad. Your dad was telling you some things. You're talking fine, keep up, don't stop.

The unbalancing has begun and father and son are now relating at a verbal level. At one point, mother begins to enter and the therapist gently touches her knee and nonverbally requests that she not enter into the discussion. Again, Larry's positive behaviors are being reinforced.

FATHER: So what do you want to do, do you want to work for Uncle Joe?

LARRY: Yeah. I want to work for Uncle Joe.

FATHER: Do you want to buy the stand, is that what you want to do?

LARRY: Yeah, that's what I want to do, yeah.

FATHER: That's all right with me, all right? But you'd have to work that out with Uncle Joe, right?

LARRY: Yeah.

FATHER: And Uncle Joe got a little bit disturbed because you were drinking too much, right? And that's why he told you he wasn't going to help you out with the stand anymore, right?

LARRY: Yeah that's right.

FATHER: So what's . . . what do you think is best? What do you think you need to do?

LARRY: I . . . I don't want to hurt you, and I want to help you.

FATHER: OK, that's good. What do you want to do, I mean? In other words, you think if you stopped drinking and . . .

LARRY: I haven't been drinking.

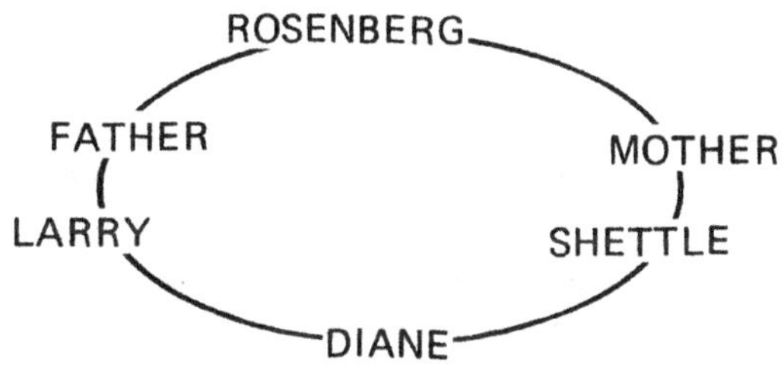

Figure 2

FATHER: No, I know you haven't. Do you think if you went back to work and if you went back to the old Larry, do you think Uncle Joe would change his mind, or . . . ? Huh?

LARRY: Yeah.

FATHER: Do you think he would?

LARRY: Yeah.

FATHER: Maybe. I don't know. I know you can work there if you want for the summer.

LARRY: Doctor, when I came here yesterday, I was . . .

ROSENBERG: Wait, wait, wait . . . I don't want to talk about that.

Here Larry begins to return to his earlier talk about two doctors at the sign-in desk and the therapist does not allow him to continue. The discussion is kept between Larry and his dad.

FATHER: Maybe if you want to you can try . . . what do you think?

LARRY: Yeah.

FATHER: You think you'd like to try?

LARRY: Yeah.

FATHER: OK.

ROSENBERG: I'll tell you what I don't understand. Everybody says you're quiet, and you talk beautifully to your son. And he responds very nicely to you.

FATHER: I usually don't talk that much, heh-heh-heh.

ROSENBERG: You did a hell of a job, you know. Do you know what I think has happened? In your family I think over the years Dad has been very quiet, and because he's been so quiet, Mom has really jumped in and worked overtime, and worked very, very hard to keep things going. And the more you've done that, the more quiet Dad has become. And I think because Larry is so much like his dad, Larry, too, has become very, very quiet, and I think that whole thing needs to change. And the way you could help him is everytime you're ready to jump in, sort of bite your tongue a little bit and let your husband take over with him, because a boy Larry's age really needs to respond in a lot of ways to his dad, see? And while you've been doing a good job, you've been doing it for a long time, now you can relax a little bit.

Changes in structure have started to occur physically and verbally. Here an explanation is given with the intent being to encourage further participation by father and less intrusiveness by mother. It is most helpful when interactional sequences are identified, so that in subsequent interactions, family members can be aware and thus can modify their dysfunctional statements and actions.

ROSENBERG: See, I think he handles him beautifully.

MOTHER: Yeah, I know he does, he can handle him better than I can. But, he leaves it up to me.

FATHER: I'm not usually home.

EVERYONE: (*Laughing at his excuse*)

ROSENBERG: Oh, that we don't accept at all. I think you need to turn it back, and don't bail your husband out so quickly, because I think that he and Larry really need to talk some of these things out.

LARRY: That . . . that is one problem in our family, I really think lately.

ROSENBERG: What, Larry?

LARRY: Communication.

ROSENBERG: You're absolutely right! But that's something that can change. Right?

LARRY: Yeah.

Here, for the first time in the session, Larry offers some unsolicited observations on the family. The change in structure is beginning to produce tangible results.

ROSENBERG: When it changes I think things are going to go better for you. And for your dad. And I think that when there are things that you want to find out about your son, talk to him very naturally, like you did now, because he responds beautifully to you.

FATHER: He wouldn't eat last night until everybody left the table and I sat down with him. . . .

MOTHER: Just, just him and his father, and then he ate two dishes.

Mother is now beginning to support the new structure. Earlier she spoke of father not being available. Now she speaks positively of father's involvement with his son.

ROSENBERG: Exactly what I'm talking about. He talks a whole lot better to you than he does to either of us. When we were in the other room we were saying "look how Larry opens up when he and his dad start talking. His dad really has the key to him." We ask him questions and he doesn't say anything.

FATHER: I was kind of following your leads . . . ha-ha.

ROSENBERG: You're doing a hell of a better job than we are, I'll tell you. Keep it up. I think he idolizes you.

The therapist continued to join and reinforce father's increased interest and verbal behavior. Notice how father is beginning to become more assertive.

FATHER: One thing, when he was younger we used to go fishing a lot in the summer. When he started working that kind of fell by the wayside, right?

LARRY: Yeah. I was staying over at grandmom's and wasn't seeing my father as much, and last night when we went home we just talked.

FATHER: We still go hunting quite a bit together, that hasn't changed.

ROSENBERG: When was the last time you guys went fishing?

LARRY: Couple of years ago, couple of summers.

FATHER: Couple of years ago.

LARRY: I really got into a lot of heavy work these last two summers building up the trade.

ROSENBERG: Well, that's good, but you can certainly take a day off to go fishing once in a while.

LARRY: Well, that's a lot of work itself. (*Joking, all laugh*)

ROSENBERG: What kind of fishing do you do?

FATHER: Fresh-water fishing, mostly.

ROSENBERG: Mostly trout?

FATHER: Bass, pickerel. But I haven't gone yet this year myself, with anybody.

MOTHER: That's the problem, you just got to take the time and go.

FATHER: I always enjoyed it, in fact I haven't taken my younger son this year either.

SHETTLE: Kevin?

FATHER: Yes, Kevin.

SHETTLE: Is there some chance that you could go fishing this weekend?

FATHER: This weekend, yeah, we could go somehow.

ROSENBERG: (*To Larry*) Unless you're working too hard.

FATHER: Ha-ha-ha.

FATHER: He was making crates this morning, ask Diane, she took them over.

DIANE: He was going like wildfire.

ROSENBERG: Too busy to take off and do some fishing?

MOTHER: No, I'm sure he could . . . well, Lar?

LARRY: Yeah.

ROSENBERG: That's what I'd do this weekend. If it were up to me. I'd rather be playing around with bass than with crates.

EVERYONE: (*Laughter*)

ROSENBERG: You can do whatever you want to do. Anyhow, we're going to have to stop. You look a whole lot better today than you were looking yesterday. I think you're on your way to turning this thing around. Do you feel that way?

LARRY: No, I don't feel that way.

ROSENBERG: You feel like you've still got a long way to go, huh?
LARRY: (*No answer*)
FATHER: You don't think you feel better today than yesterday?
LARRY: Yeah, I feel better.

When I ask Larry if he feels better, he says no. When father asks him, he responds more positively. This clearly illustrates the issue and the power of father in helping his son. The process of positive interaction and communication between father and Larry has begun. The task suggested, that they go fishing over the weekend, was designed to encourage further the structural change that was begun during this session.

FATHER: So, you think you're on the road to being the old Larry again? Huh? Or not? Do you? Had a rough time getting to sleep last night, right?
LARRY: Yeah.
FATHER: Do you think tonight will be better? I think so.

The session presented illustrates many of the techniques of structural family therapy discussed earlier. Joining took place on a continuing basis, an enactment between Larry and father was used in order to strengthen this dyad and weaken mother's overinvolvement, and this unbalancing led to a more healthy communication pattern involving both parents and son. Although Larry's presenting problem was one of an acute psychotic break, this behavior was relabeled to being an acting-out problem related to concern about father's illness and an inability to express these concerns.

Reinforcement of positive, healthy behaviors led to more appropriate statements and affect, while less attention to pathological statements reduced the incidence of these nonproductive exchanges.

The key to the session was the major structural change of having father begin to deal directly and more assertively with his son. The change in Larry's responses, when father became more involved, is most striking. The quality of their interactions was most rewarding to observe.

During the two session consultation, significant structural changes took place. As mother pulled back and supported her husband's more active role, the infantilization of Larry greatly diminished and more was now being expected of him. Also, the marital dyad seemed now to be functioning more efficiently, that is, parents were more united and therefore fewer marital tensions existed (Rosenberg, 1983).

On Monday morning, three days after the interview, the family came to the inpatient unit to have Larry admitted. The youngster's behavior had improved so significantly that the staff felt that Larry should not be admitted. The decision was made to continue to treat the family on an outpatient basis.

ACKNOWLEDGMENTS

The author wishes to thank Suzanne B. Perot, Ph.D., Kenneth Covelman, Ph.D., and M. Duncan Stanton, Ph.D. for their helpful suggestions in the preparation of this manuscript.

5. References

Baker, L., Minuchin, S., & Rosman, B. The use of beta-adrenergic blockade in the treatment of psychosomatic aspects of juvenile diabetes mellitus. In A. Smart (Ed.), *Advances in beta-adrenergic blocking therapy*. Princeton, N.J.: Excerpta Medica, 1974.

Barcai, A. Normative family development. *Journal of Marital and Family Therapy,* 1981, *7,* 353–359.

Brady, J. P., & Rieger, W. Behavioral treatment in anorexia nervosa. In T. Thompson & W. S. Dockens, III (Eds.), *Applications of behavior modification.* New York: Academic Press, 1975.

Duhl, B. S., & Duhl, F. J. *Integrative family therapy.* In A. Gurman & D. Kniskern (Eds.), *Handbook of family therapy.* New York: Brunner/Mazel, 1981.

Gurman, A., & Kniskern, D. (Eds.), *Handbook of family therapy.* New York: Brunner/Mazel, 1981.

Kaslow, F. A diaclectic approach to family therapy and practice: Selectivity and synthesis. *Journal of Marital and Family Therapy,* 1981, *7,* 345–351.

Lazarus, A. *The practice of multi-model therapy.* New York: McGraw-Hill, 1981.

Minuchin, S. *Families and family therapy.* Cambridge: Harvard University Press, 1974.

Minuchin, S., Baker, L., Rosman B. L., Liebman, R., Milman, L., & Todd, T. C. A conceptual model of psychosomatic illness in children. *Archives of General Psychiatry,* 1975, *32,* 1031–1038.

Minuchin, S., Rosman, B. L., & Baker, L. *Psychosomatic families: Anorexia nervosa in context.* Cambridge: Harvard University Press, 1978.

Rosenberg, J. B. Two is better than one: Use of behavioral techniques within a structural family therapy model. *Journal of Marriage and Family Counseling,* 1978, *4,* 31–39.

Rosenberg, J. B. A behavioral/structural approach to marital therapy. Submitted for publication, 1983.

Rosenberg, J. B., & Lindblad, M. Behavior therapy in a family context: Treating elective mutism. *Family Process,* 1978, *17,* 77–82.

Stanton, M. D. Marital therapy from a structural/strategic viewpoint. In G. P. Sholevar (Ed.), *The handbook of marriage and marital therapy.* Jamaica, N.Y.: S.P. Medical and Scientific Books, 1981. (a)

Stanton, M. D. Strategic approaches to family therapy. In A. Gurman & D. Kniskern (Eds.), *Handbook of family therapy.* New York. Brunner/Mazel, 1981. (b)

Whitaker, C. Symbolic-experiential family therapy. In A. Gurman & D. Kniskern (Eds.), *Handbook of family therapy.* New York: Brunner/Mazel, 1981.

Wynne, L. C. In A. Gurman & D. Kniskern (Eds.), *Handbook of family therapy.* New York: Brunner/Mazel, 1981.

10

Contextual Family and Marital Therapy

DAVID N. ULRICH

1. Conceptual Therapy

"Contextual therapy" is the name chosen by Ivan Boszormenyi-Nagy for the approach he and his associates have developed. The contextual approach to therapy may provide a model for general health care delivery as well as for family, marital, individual, or otherwise designated therapeutic frames. Such distinctions as *marital* or *family* therapy may seem as limited as the term *identified patient,* when the implications of a comprehensive approach are grasped. Potential for a comprehensive approach is provided by the basic premise of contextual therapy; that is, the extension of equal concern to all those who may be affected by treatment, taking into account their basic welfare interests as perceived by themselves and by others. This premise may be considered "ethical" in the sense of providing a basic commitment for the therapist and a direction for those engaged in therapy. This ethical orientation emerged on a step-by-step basis as parents, and then other family members, were brought into treatment along with hospitalized schizophrenics, and the experience thereby gained was extended to outpatient work.

As this orientation was developed, it began to appear that what affects relationships can be sorted into four dimensions:

The Dimension of Fact. The first of these dimensions is the realm of fact. Being born of a given ethnic background is a fact; being the second generation born in the United States is a fact, and such facts bear significantly on relationships. Having to assume care of a family at 17 because of a father's death or disappearance is a significant fact, one that may affect the lives of several generations.

The Psychological Dimension. The second dimension is the psychological realm, one whose boundaries of course are not entirely distinct. What happens internally often is conceptualized by family therapists as a "subsystem" of the "family system." It would belong in the realm of psychology, for instance, whether one perceived the fact of father's death as a crippling blow, or the fact of one's ethnicity as grounds for expecting less, or

DAVID N. ULRICH • 337 Thornridge Drive, Stamford, Connecticut 06903.

more, from life than one's fellow human beings. The defenses, of course, lie within the realm of psychology; fact can be repressed, denied, or avoided, or the unconscious perception of one's inner state can be projected onto someone else, so the facts are distorted.

Of special significance to contextual therapy, within the psychological realm, is the process described by such terms as *substitution, displacement,* or *transference*. The rage felt toward a father can be displaced on a son; the son is only a symbol for the hated father, but this does not diminish the rage. The son becomes a substitute victim without knowing why. Or the attitudes toward the father may be displaced on the therapist, and this substitutive process may be utilized as the major tool of psychoanalytic therapy. In contrast, contextual therapy is oriented toward directing attitudes and affects toward the original persons.

As psychoanalysis and psychodynamic therapy evolved, their theorists made various attempts at reductionism, such as seeking to account for relational phenomena, even at the level of international tensions, as manifestations of the intrapsychic. As family therapy evolved, some of its theorists made vigorous efforts to push the pendulum to the other extreme. It became modish either to treat all intrapsychic process as manifestations of systemic events or to reject the intrapsychic as irrelevant. The contextual approach holds that nothing is gained and much is lost by such reductionism.

The Transactional Dimension. The third dimension includes everything that can be loosely embraced by the term *transactional.* Triangles, coalitions, distance and pursuit, applications of power, interruption of feedback—the phenomena that have become the focus of much family work—may be considered as aspects of this dimension.

The Ethical Dimension. The contextual approach assigns separate status to the ethical dimension; it cannot be reduced to any of the others. It must be spelled out in quite specific terms because it provides direction for the therapeutic methods and leverages of contextual therapy. As stated, contextual therapy means a commitment by the therapist to extend equal therapeutic concern to all those who may be affected by treatment. This also means focusing on the balance of fairness in relationships among people.

This is a matter with which, in fact, most people are intensely concerned. If one listens to a wife's account of how her marriage has deteriorated over the years, her complaint may have to do with her husband's indifference to her, to his failure to listen. But being heard is not merely a pleasure in itself; one usually wants to be heard because one is trying to get a point across. When one asks the wife to specify how her husband's indifference to her was manifested, she does not stop at a description of how he would walk out or watch television when she tried to talk. The response is almost certain to be a chronicle of what she did for him and what he failed to do for her, what he did to her, what he took away from her. Her pain goes along with her sense that their relationship has been continually out of balance, that is, inequitable. It is this to which she wants him to listen.

The issue of fairness, or equitability, is present in all relationships, but it goes deeper in families because family relationships are inescapable; they last longer. The questions of fairness may persist even through successive generations. Death may highlight, rather than terminate such questions, as the squabbling over the property of the dead so often attests. Divorce, especially when children are involved, may prove to be only a partial escape from the ongoing issues of fairness. Walking out for good does not settle accounts; it only leaves them up in the air for good, with inevitable consequences on all sides.

To assess the question of fairness, we start with the recognition that each person has "basic welfare interests," including survival, growth, and relatedness. The child does not merely have a "need" to receive or give affection; the exchange of affection contributes to the child's growth and relatedness and is therefore relevant to the child's basic interests.

The interests of each family member will be recognized and fulfilled if there is fairness of exchange, which can also be called reciprocity or balance of give and take. Of course we are not speaking here in terms of a strict bookkeeping system of accounts. If the husband objects that his wife failed to make her last car payment on time and he had to do it for her, this is bookkeeping in a very limited sense. We are speaking rather of the ebb and flow of give and take in a relationship over time, whereby each partner may come to feel that however much he or she has invested in the relationship, the other has more or less kept pace. At any given time, the balance may go to one side or the other, for example, the wife who limits herself to a secretarial job so her husband can finish law school. Her expectation is that what she has invested in the common fund eventually will be replaced, to the enrichment of both.

No one person is in a position to assess whether the long-term balance of fairness has been maintained. Subjective perceptions vary widely. The husband who insists that he is fulfilling his obligations by bringing home paychecks is not yet facing the issue of fairness in the relationship; he is simply expressing an attitude. Some of the fiercest marital disputes may have to do with issues such as this. But such disputes can be productive. Often it is only through the active antithesis of individual points of view that the sense finally will emerge that everyone's interests have been considered.

For one spouse to assume that the marriage vows or the partner's repeated assurances of love and devotion automatically set up guarantees of fairness would be magical thinking. In reality the balance is seldom perfect, and the work of facing and redressing imbalances must be done if the marriage is to be kept alive. Yet, no matter how much the issues of fairness may be avoided or denied, they remain, and they somehow will become manifest. They are not simply subjective phenomena; they are existentially given.

1.1. Trustworthiness of Relationship

As the members of a family work at give and take, a growing trustworthiness of relationship gradually emerges, fueled by concern over the welfare of the others. We refer to moves toward trust as "rejunctive," and moves away from it as "disjunctive." Without ignoring the importance of affection, or overlooking the ever-present element of power, we hold that trustworthiness is the critical element in holding relationships together. Looking at the question of trust in terms of the individual, Erik Erikson (1968) has taken the position that "basic trust" is the cornerstone of a vital personality. Using the term *confident expectation* as more or less the equivalent of Erikson's "basic trust," Margaret Mahler (1979) has observed that the infant's confident expectation of need fulfilling and limit setting by the parents is what keeps the infant from being traumatically overwhelmed by its own needs and provides the base for integrated growth. Without being so specific about the trust aspect, Kohut (1977) makes it clear enough that if the parents' narcissistic needs interfere with balanced giving and withholding, the child's cohesive sense of self may be impaired.

In the relational context, we look not only at whether the child has developed "basic trust" in the parents, but also at whether the reciprocity among family members is such as to foster growing trustworthiness in the relationships. This issue is sometimes put to its first crucial test during the child's adolescence, when new strivings toward autonomy may place severe stress on the existing balances.

1.2. The Ledger

The concept of *ledger* is implicit in considerations of trustworthiness. As noted, we do not mean *ledger* in a strict bookkeeping sense, but in a deeper sense of whether the investment of one partner has over time balanced that of the others. The contextual therapist will give this question a critical place in assessing the health of the family. If one member remains stuck in a ''down'' position vis-à-vis the family ledger, this affects the adjustment of all family members. If, for instance, one daughter remains at home permanently in order to meet her parents' needs, she may give her siblings the gift of what resembles freedom, but it is not quite real. The daughter pays out too much in filial devotion and sacrifices herself. At the same time, the parents' lives get stuck in the sense that they are not doing what they should for themselves, and the sacrificial sibling has robbed the others of their fair share of filial responsibility. Their seeming autonomy therefore is built on a shaky base, and their guilt and immaturity eventually may intrude into their lives through marital breakdown or other symptomatic problems. Thus the costs of a permanent ledger imbalance eventually may manifest themselves in the lives of all the people who have colluded in keeping the accounts stuck.

1.3. Accountability

Both implicity and explicitly, concepts of fairness and ledger lead to the matter of accountability. Each partner to the relationship pattern is accountable for keeping his or her input actively keyed to the interests of the others. This includes, of course, the recognition that everyone's interests shift as they pass through the various stages of their own life cycle. A structural component is involved here; a parent, for example, is accountable for protecting a child's welfare in the face of crazy behavior from the other parent. A mother is accountable for stepping back at the appropriate time to allow her daughter more autonomy. A husband is accountable for balancing his investment in his work and his family.

The question of accountability is related to the issue of guilt. Freud and his successors observed that guilt may be neurotic, and neurotic guilt may be crippling. This has sometimes been misconstrued to mean that guilt should be banished in the name of mental health. If, however, people have failed to be accountable when the situation calls for them to face issues, they become existentially guilty whether they feel subjectively guilty or not, and the absence of subjective guilt itself may be pathological. The solution for existential guilt is to face the imbalances in the relational accounts.

1.4. Merit and Entitlement

Someone who is prompted by concern for the welfare of others in a reciprocal context will do many things by which he or she acquires merit. The concept of merit has specific importance because it is the key to the contextual definition of entitlement. As we use the term *entitlement,* it does not carry primary connotations of exercise of power to claim a bigger piece of the pie, although of course any entitlement may wither if one does not assert a claim to it. What we mean by entitlement is the accumulation of merit. The entitled person is one who has performed enough acts of merit, that is, invested enough in the relationship, to stand in a favorable position vis-à-vis the ledger. This is, of course, the genuine antidote to guilt. We hold that entitlement is necessary to individuation. To face one's accountability and do those things that ought to be done is vital to an adequate sense of self. We hold that entitlement both enriches and liberates, conferring freedom from stuck relating. One who has paid the tab is free to leave the tavern; one who has kept his relational accounts balanced is free to move on to new aspects of the relationship or, with the passage of time, to move into new relationships; for example, the son is free to become a husband. As we shall spell out later, entitlement also confers freedom from excessive burdens of legacy which, if they are not thrown off, can impose crippling restraints on life and growth.

According to the contextual view of relational dynamics, the process of gaining liberation through entitlement is not contingent upon one's contribution's being reciprocated or even acknowledged. The daughter who gives up her vacation in order to attend her terminally ill parent in the hospital is acquiring entitlement, even if the parent is too sick or otherwise immobilized to offer thanks. The son who seeks out a way to "get through" to a chronically angry and embittered parent is acquiring entitlement, whether the parent responds or not. It makes a lasting difference if one can say "I tried." The spouse who commits himself or herself to being straight with the partner is in a far better position to assess the relationship than one who has made a commitment only to prolonging a quarrel.

1.5. Multigenerational Aspects

The contextual therapist works habitually in a context of at least three generations and usually more. This may seem complicated at first. But what turns out is that knowing what happened before makes it easier to see how things fit together in the here and now, and how the future will be affected. The net result can be a substantial economy of time and effort.

1.6. Parenting

We take, as a pivotal point of reference, the responsibility of parents for the generations succeeding them. In a given family, the emotional involvement of one spouse with the other may appear to be far more intense than that of either spouse with the children. This becomes visible when the husband and wife ignore the impact on the children of their fighting with each other. It is, however, obviously far more usual for one parent to break off with the other than to break off with the children. The ties of common biological rootedness usually will endure long after the ties of marriage have been dissolved.

Along the power dimension, the parents of young children usually have the upper hand. In ethical terms, this very imbalance of power makes it all the more compelling for the parents to be actively aware of what they owe the child in providing for its survival, growth, and ability to relate to others. If parents exercise their power well enough, this actively sets up the basis for expanding trust among future generations. If parents exploit what has been entrusted to them, then the basis for trust among future generations in the family will be weakened or even destroyed.

Suppose, for example, that an immigrant father of seven children humiliates and impoverishes his family by turning into a drunk and a drifter. His oldest daughter, fiercely imbued with a legacy of lost decency, sets out on an iron-fisted campaign, not merely to salvage the family but to elevate it. She succeeds, but only by driving her siblings so hard that their chance for ordinary relating is cut off. In the push to excel, their efforts to reach out to one another, or to anyone outside the family, on ordinary human terms, are disrupted. They, in turn, feel betrayed. One eventually expresses this through suicide, another through severe learning impairment. The linkage between the earlier and later betrayals is clear and direct. Conversely, within this picture, one can find enough evidence of human concern and caring to provide the necessary leverage for new moves toward restoration of trust.

1.7. Being a Child

The child at birth acquires a legacy that stems from the common biological roots with both parents and their families. The child is born into a set of expectations derived from its ethnic and cultural background, from the unique patterning of the family, and from the position as boy or girl, first or later sibling. The child senses that it has a place in a family, and out of this sense of legacy emerges the child's loyalty to the family.

Loyalty. Initially, the child owes loyalty to the natural parent because of its legacy, that is, through the existential fact of being born of that parent. We know that adopted children tend to make a place in their thinking, and in their selves, for the natural parent, even if the place is filled only by a sense of mystery. We know that children who were abandoned by one parent soon after birth may engage in a lifelong search for the missing mother or father. Existentially, such children are placed in a position of split loyalty between the natural and substitute parent, whether the substitute parent acknowledges it or not.

In the ordinary course of events, the child's loyalty is reinforced by the parents' nurturance in a context of balanced giving and withholding. If the parent cannot maintain a fair balance, then the child's potential for loyalty and for trustworthy relating may be impaired.

The child's loyalty is a contribution to the family. It serves as a "reservoir of trust" that the child extends to its parents, siblings, grandparents, and others. In a well functioning family, the child's contribution of loyalty is a source of enrichment for everyone who comes in contact with it. In families where there is marital conflict, parental depression, or other evidence of trouble, children will tap their reservoir of trust in their effort to help. They may attempt to deflect the parental conflict onto themselves or by various means, including delinquency and suicide, to compel the parents to change their pattern. Regardless of what they may attempt, children usually find themselves powerless to effect any major change. This discovery is coming to be recognized as one of the crippling impediments to a child's adequate sense of self.

In working with a family, especially with parent–child relationships, it is unsound ever to assume that the deepest level in the family is adversary. No matter how hostile the parent may be to the child, or the child to the parent, their exchanges probably are occurring in a context that includes deeper substrata of connectedness. Clinically, this comes to light when a psychotic mother who has been demanding that her child be placed, lashes out at anyone who tries to act seriously on her request, or when a child who has been reviling a parent pauses to attack anyone else, including the therapist, who has spoken against the parent. The therapist thus is rudely reminded of being a stranger. Often the child's hostility will prove, on closer examination, to be a way of expressing loyalty to the parent, because its essential aim is to correct an imbalance in the family ledger of accounts.

1.8. Legacy

Reference has been made to the significance of the child's birth, the fact of being born into a particular family, with its own mix of ethnic and cultural expectations and its own unique set of family expectations. Elsewhere such a set of expectations has sometimes been referred to as a family "myth" or "legend." We use the term *legacy* in part because it conveys the sense of a binding force. The child is not simply accepting a myth; by the fact of being born into the family, he or she is held by multigenerational imperatives that state what is expected: what he or she will owe, what he or she is owed. A vivid example is the child born into the expectation that he or she will avoid public school and become a thief in order to pay his or her due to the family. For the child to throw off this legacy is to make a wrenching move away from his or her own roots.

1.9. Legacy and the Ledger

We have spoken of the ledger of relational accounts and how it is affected by acts of merit. But legacy may have an even deeper impact on the ledger. Legacy dictates certain debts and entitlements. For example, a son whose familial legacy is one of mistrust among family members, angrily confronts his wife every time she spends any money without his prior approval. He is convinced, and he tries to convince her, that her untrustworthy, spendthrift behavior is going to bankrupt them. In fact, she is carrying a full-time job in addition to working as wife and mother. Her buying a dress or a lunch may throw off the week's budget, but she is helping her husband stay solvent. Her response to his anger is to be fearful of him—a response that has its own legacy aspects. She conceals her purchases, and he discovers her concealments. His mistrust of her, and her response, become corrosive enough to destroy the marriage.

In analytic terms, one could evaluate the husband as having a penurious character disorder—or her as having a marked tendency toward the hysteric. In ledger terms, he is still making payments to his mother by acting on what was in this case her quite explicit injunction that he was not to trust his wife. This throws the relational ledger with his wife irretrievably out of balance. He is, of course, trapped by his legacy and by his loyalty to it. He is paying his parents far more than he owes them and robbing his wife in the process. Through a creative reassessment of all his relationships, he might have worked his way to a better balance, paying off legitimate filial debts without short shrifting his wife. But his entrapment appeared to be too profound. Conversely, when the legacy is one of sharing between partners, the son or daughter will be inclined to trust the contribution of the spouse, and the relational ledger will remain more or less in balance as long as the trust is reciprocal.

We referred above to a "creative reassessment." There were plenty of realistic ways in which the husband could discharge his filial debts; he could, and did, for instance, help his parents to keep their finances in order and their house and yard in repair. He also brought grandchildren into their lives. The fact that he himself was functioning well—succeeding at work, maintaining a marriage, engaging in community affairs—did, or at least could have, brought enrichment into his parents' lives; certainly he was no burden to them. All of these efforts contributed to his entitlement vis-à-vis his parents. At any time, he could have said, "I'm doing enough for you; I've earned the freedom to use my own judgment about my wife." This kind of separation did not take place, but the resources were at hand for him to free himself from the chains of legacy.

Had he been able to do so, his children would have benefited. They would not, in turn, have to struggle with the legacy of mistrust, which already was permeating their attitudes toward each of their parents. The older child, for instance, was torn by wondering why mother did not do things the way father needed them done and why father got so angry about it all. Through the son's failure to claim his own entitlement vis-à-vis his parents, the legacy that had bound him already was beginning to bind his children.

1.10. Ritual Disagreement

In many instances, couples enter treatment focusing on some complaint that proves to be a perfect stalemate. She cannot enjoy his touch until he talks to her; to him, talking without touching is strained and artificial. He is sharp with her; she protests; he denies; she withdraws. Now he is complaining that he cannot get any feedback at all about how to behave with her. The intensity of the battle initially masks the fact that it has become a long-standing ritual. If the therapist struggles with suggestions to them about how to modify their behavior, the ritual soon will come to include the thwarting of the therapist. Exploration usually will reveal that they are stuck not only because of power issues or problems with distance and closeness, but also because their legacies dictate that they cannot open themselves to a deeper commitment. Their recurring disagreement becomes a way of dramatizing where they are stuck. The sense of "emptiness" to which Fogarty (1979) and others have referred sometimes, at least, may serve to mask the excruciating pain of recognition that throughout one's life one has restrained those relational ventures that provide life with meaning.

1.11. Split Loyalty

A split between parents need not be intolerable for a child, unless the parents set up conflicting claims for the child's loyalty. If the child cannot move toward one without being accused of disloyalty by the other, the foundation of the child's trust is laid open to assault. This can become one of the deepest burdens of childhood. The child may resort to extremes in searching for substitutive ways to preserve his or her two-parent loyalty intact. One solution, which benefits no one, is for the child to turn cold toward both parents. If a child is forced to exclude one parent and devote itself entirely to the other, the substitutive payment to the excluded parent may come later in life when the grown child wihholds commitment from a spouse, saying, in effect, "I could not give anything to father so I repay him through my indifference to you."

In one situation, a husband came for help when his wife gave him a thirty-day deadline: Shape up or get out. His offenses included heavy drinking, long disappearances, and signs of involvement with another woman. His story was that his extramarital affair was a rescue mission, but every time he resumed it, he would abort the effort and leave his girlfriend stranded like his wife. He felt depressed, isolated, and worthless. His history was that his once-successful father had taken a spectacular plunge into alcoholism, highlighted by assaults on his wife. His descent did not stop because his wife heroically kept trying to arrange occasions, such as renting a vacation cottage, that would pull father back into the family. Each effort aborted, with an accretion of pain for the children. Father finally took off for good, with mother's curses literally ringing in the air as he left. Afterward, mother could not imagine her children giving their loyalty to anyone but her.

The son paid outward homage to the mother and made sporadic efforts to help her "get on her feet." At the same time he discharged his loyalty to his father by withdrawing emotionally from mother as well and paying only lip-service to being a dutiful son. Having withdrawn from his mother, he deserted his wife too; this was an invalid attempt at balancing the ledger with mother. Having made this payment, he felt free to undertake rescue missions to his girlfriend. He was actually astonished when he realized that neither his mother nor his girlfriend needed to be rescued at all. Meanwhile, it appeared that he had repeatedly crashed in the style that father had crashed. He was able to see that in his own collapse he was reaching out for father: "Look, Dad, I've been there too." But the father, who has rehabilitated and remarried, no longer needed such justification.

After a few sessions, the son was beginning to discover unexpected resources in his wife as well; it was no longer a disloyalty to either parent to do so.

The child's dilemma becomes deeper, of course, if one parent not only pulls the child away from the other, but also expects the child to break its ties to everyone in the spouse's family. The child then may be compelled to engage in many acts that he or she feels as betrayals of a basic commitment and for which compensation somehow will have to be paid. One way to pay is by failing to meet the expectations of the people who have tried to make their claim on the child an exclusive one. Or the child even may pursue the custodial family's goals so avidly as to make a mockery of them, for example, if my mother's family is coldly formal and my father's was warm and spontaneous, then I will become a very caricature of formality, but with a vengeance that takes its force from the invisible loyalty to father.

1.12. Invisible Loyalty

In the above illustrations, of course, none of the choices made contained any conscious intent to preserve loyalty to one parent or the other. The linkages that stem from common rootedness may be altogether covert. Invisible loyalty payments are often counterproductive to the self. Their most pernicious aspect is that, proceeding at an unconscious level, they are not subject to measurement; they may be infinite and endless. Invisible loyalty is not limited to cases in which a split has been imposed by parents on the child's loyalty base. For instance, a son who overtly rebels against a father may find covert ways of making loyalty payments. This may work to the son's detriment, as when the payment consists of dropping out of college at the same age that the father dropped out of college, or failing in business at just the point where the father failed.

1.13. The Revolving Slate

Loyalty and the lack of power leave children unable to deal directly with their parents on an equitable basis. The child who is abused or otherwise exploited cannot respond to the parent in kind, but the pattern of exploitation cannot be abruptly extinguished either. The pattern has been learned within the family. More important, it has become part of the family legacy, and so it continues. The dysfunctional solution is to bring in one or more substitutes who become engaged in the continuation of the pattern. (The spouse or child is the primary substitute, but the pattern also can be seen operating in relationships at work.) Having picked up momentum through two generations, the pattern is all the more likely to repeat itself in a third.

We can see how this revolving process gets under way in the case of split loyalty. Caught in the web of rootedness to the family, faced with the insoluble problem of how to give loyalty to a parent when neither parent can tolerate its being given to the other, the child can vindicate one parent only by somehow moving against the other. If mother says father is no good, one balances this by making out that neither is she any good. But such disloyalty impels a further balancing movement, usually against substitutive victims such as wife and children. Mother is exculpated if one can exclaim, "After all, *none* of you is any good." The stand-in victim, it seems, usually is impelled by his or her legacy to fit into the role, but this does not justify the aggressor. The series of substitutive steps taken to bring the ledger of loyalties into balance has no ethical validity.

Structurally, this pattern can be seen in terms of a series of interlocking triangles. Compelled by parent *A* to move against parent *B*, the child balances accounts by moving against parent *A* as well. This disloyalty in turn demands compensation, which is paid, for example, by bringing a spouse into the triangle with parent *A* and making the spouse suffer whatever parent *A* has suffered. The ramifications can be endless, including children as well as spouse. The grown child feels justified in his or her present behavior because it is a means, however invalid, of discharging the filial loyalty to parent *A*.

We refer to this revolving process as the "revolving slate" (Boszormeny-Nagy & Spark, 1973) and we submit that it is the chief factor in family and marital dysfunction (Boszormenyi-Nagy & Ulrich, 1981).

It is a common event in clinical practice to hear parents saying that they have tried not to repeat their parents' mistakes, yet it does not seem to be working out right. Or they observe with dismay that no matter how hard they try to avoid it, they are making the same mistakes their parents did. We suggest that the revolving slate is at work here. The abused child may struggle to avoid becoming the abusive parent. But if as parent his or her behavior is determined primarily by fear of being abusive, then the children may not get the controls they need and they in turn may become abusive. Thus the chain continues unbroken.

If an observer studies a family in terms of the positions of its members within triangles, without looking at the forces of legacy and loyalty that help to account for the shifts of alignment within the triangles, then key elements of therapeutic leverage may be ignored.

1.14. Interlocking Need Templates

In discussing the revolving slate, we referred to the stand-in victim whose own legacy seems to compel him or her to become engaged in the role. It seems uncanny at times how neatly the patterns of marital partners dovetail. The wife charges the husband with arrogant chauvinism, but it begins to appear that her investment in making this charge is even greater than his investment in living up to it. She had an overbearing father, against whom she learned to employ a wide repertoire of resistant behaviors. She continues the pattern with her husband; it fuels the flame of his arrogance. He thunders about her stupidity: she leaves the stove on, she lets house plants go dry. She drives the car without oil! The wife exultantly points out how he nags at her and the children, who get drawn into collusion with her against him. Each seems ready and eager to escalate the charges against the other. Boszormenyi-Nagy has referred to this acting out of mutually reinforcing patterns of legacy as "interlocking need templates" (1965). It is because of the mutuality of need for the dysfunctional patterns that each spouse so often will undermine any effort to bring about real change in the behavior of the other spouse.

1.15. Exploitation

We have referred to parents' exploitation of children and spouses' exploitation of each other as aspects of legacy and the revolving slate. The ingenuity of human beings in findings ways to exploit each other matches the proliferation of life forms in nature. Putting one's self on loan to be used as an object of exploitation by another may be a relatively benign part of life, provided the loan is temporary and the integrity of the self is not impaired. The patterns of exploitation to which we have occasion to refer tend to be of such a persistent nature that selves and relationships are warped by them.

One vivid instance of such persistent exploitation is in the relationship between modern professional life and family life. Children and spouses, for instance, may be continually drained of their resources of loyalty and caring to meet the insatiable needs of a father or mother who has opted for the pressures of career striving. Present society offers no clear and equitable guidelines for the upward-striving executive who wishes to balance his or her loyalties to self, family, and corporation. The strategy of advancement often is to look strong by making others look weak, so one must cover one's weakness. To most executives, it would be unimaginable to share their personal concerns with their colleagues, or to admit that they listened to their spouse. The emotional cost of maintaining such a posture of invulnerable strength can be enormous. This cost is passed on to the spouse and children, who are then left to struggle with the issues of balance that get overlooked at the executive level.

Our point concerning exploitation is not simply that it occurs but that its occurrence sets the processes of legacy and revolving slate in motion. The frustrated executive who hammers at his children to improve their school performance is setting up a substitutive chain: he is demanding the proof of prowess that has never been confirmed sufficiently in his own work. The invalid claim then may be passed on to the grandchildren, by which time its dysfunctional impact may have been multiplied several times over.

1.16. Parentification

When a person enters parenthood with needs that have not been met, he or she may expect the child to meet them; the child is expected to serve as surrogate parent. Sometimes the need is to combat loneliness or to have someone who can be depended upon. Sometimes it is to strike back for past unfairness. Through the child, the parent tries to make his or her self whole. The child may be kept from giving to others outside the family, and its own capacity for normal give and take may thereby be impaired. Often it is the child who is described as being "the best of the lot" who is the most heavily parentified. In a family full of symptoms, the symptom-free child may be the one whose prospects for normal growth are most at risk. In traditional "child guidance" work, this child was most likely to be overlooked. At the other extreme, the child with the heaviest symptoms might be serving in a scapegoat capacity as a kind of lightning rod to absorb all of the family dysfunction that could not be displaced anywhere else. This child too might be serving in a heavily parentified role. Its unwillingness to let go of the scapegoat role could result from its unconscious assessment of how necessary its own dysfunction was to meet its parents' needs and keep the family from splitting apart.

1.17. Stagnation

In the examples cited so far, a common element is the failure to deal with issues at the source. The constraints of legacy and loyalty, as well as the simple fact of being without power, may mean that a person cannot go back to the one who has done him or her an injustice in order to get redress for it. Then the tendency is to displace the blame, and the claim, on a third person who is more accessible but who is innocent except insofar as he or she permits the victimization or even works for it. The action appears to be taking place in the present, but this is in large measure an epiphenomenon. One party to the action is merely a triangled-in substitute. The real issue is with someone who is absent or even dead. As long as the blaming and claiming are directed at the wrong target, they are ethically invalid and nothing can get settled. The result may be lifetimes or even generations of stagnant patterns of relating.

These patterns cannot precisely be called "repetitive" because, as they persist in a family, they claim a spreading number of victims and their manifestations take various forms. We believe that this kind of "stuck" relating is a major aspect of what often has been called the homeostasis of the family. The "ritual disagreement" to which reference has been made is one instance of stuck relating.

A special case of stagnation is the situation where loyalty is ruptured, that is, when one member of a family simply breaks off all contact with the others. The issues that forced the break remain permanently unresolved, and all the persons who are direct parties to the break remain blocked in their efforts at true relief. When one spouse manages to force a complete break between the other spouse and the children, this may spare the children from conflict and abuse. In the long run, however, there is not much chance that anyone can benefit by making the break complete. The children may grow up feeding on the myth that one of their parents was a monster, a conviction that will undercut their own cohesive sense of self. They may grow up feeling that being deprived of a parent was the worst abuse of all or, if coached, they may suppress entirely the memory of the lost parent and then show a similar pattern of withdrawal toward their own spouse and children.

1.18. Exoneration

In discussing stagnation, our central point was that people fail to go to the source of their distress. As a child, one cannot face the parents on equal terms. Gradually, resentment compounds the problem. The parent or other who threw out the balance of fairness can be perceived as too powerful to challenge and too weak to be able to make amends. With the passage of time, the hope for new moves toward restoration of trust is gradually surrendered and stagnation ensues.

This, of course, is not always the case. Often enough, we find people who, as they mature, rebuild their relationship with their parents or at least are able to come to terms with their parents' limitations. These efforts can be characterized as "exoneration" of the parent. We submit that "exoneration" is one of the major aspects of movement toward mental health. If one has adopted the intention of working to exonerate the source of one's distress, this alone is an act of merit; it confers new entitlement.

The effort may progress along various fronts. The primary front, of course, is to seek to restore trustworthiness to the original relationship. This may have humble beginnings; it may mean a search for any kind of reconnection that can be made without reactivating the old conflicts in their old and futile forms. The married daughter may find that she can take her mother, who was once almost exclusively an object of hatred, on a shopping trip or invite her to come visit the grandchildren, with results that are meaningful for everyone. Yet the effort at suppression of old tensions may make the present contact seem superficial and lifeless. Really to bring the relationship alive, it may be necessary to face old issues in a new context. This could mean taking a stand. In the past, mother may have tried to dictate how her grandchildren should be handled. Daughter may have allowed it, fought with mother over it, or avoided mother. If the goal is exonerative, daughter will take a step beyond the old, "stuck" patterns and ask mother to face the problem with her: How can we both, appropriately, be together with these children? If mother responds, a move has been made to restore trustworthiness of relationship with her.

Sometimes the effort at exoneration may reach the level of confrontation. "I have always wondered why you found it necessary never to give me any approval. The things I did mattered to me; somehow they must have mattered to you. Did you have reasons for dealing with me that way?" The parent may be able to face the question and provide an answer that helps make sense of it.

Or the parent never may be able to respond. Freedom from the bonds of legacy comes not from succeeding in such efforts but from being willing to take the initiative in making them.

If it is too late—if the parent is dead, or unwilling over time to respond—then exoneration still can proceed on another front, one with which we are familiar in daily living. This has to do with the effort to understand the parents' behavior as being rooted in the parents' own families in ways of which they themselves could not be aware. It may take much amassing of fact and much forbearance before one can assemble a picture of a parent's life that will help to make sense of one's own. But the perspective on the past can be shifted. In one instance, a boy sensed throughout his childhood that his mother's life had been affected deeply by something that seemed to have been missing in his grandmother, whom he never had met. Later in life, studying family notes and letters, he pieced some of the picture of grandmother together. Her father had been, in effect, a refugee from Ireland and never ceased to suffer from a deep mix of homesickness and depression, made all the worse because he was an Englishman and thus twice displaced. Grandmother, the youngest of a large brood, herself had been displaced from Philadelphia to Oregon at a time when Oregon was very new to whites. She must have felt herself a refugee twice over. She never was able to give her daughter a sense of place. In such a perspective, the daughter's own restlessness and depression made sense. With this realization, the son felt a weight lifted. What had always seemed to be a bleakness intrinsic to himself and his mother now could be seen in the context of family history as the reaction to being displaced. If they had not handled it too well, perhaps he could do better.

The change of perspective can go to the core of how one perceives a relationship. In therapy or without therapy, one gradually may uncover hatred for a parent. If one simply accepts it as one of the facts of one's existence, that "I hate my parent," the result may be stagnation of relationships for at least three generations, for one's children inevitably will be drawn into this pattern of hatred. If one can push past the resentment and hurt to explore such questions as, "What could have been in their minds when they kept telling me I couldn't amount to much—what compelled them to do this?," the answers may not be altogether comforting, but at least the way is open to relieve the hate and to rework the sense of self in relation to family. A son finds that his incessantly critical father bore the brunt of support for his own mother and siblings, including one who was crippled; the grandfather had deserted them. The father's pain can be seen as the trigger for his criticism of his son; the son no longer need take it as a judgment of himself or a mandate for his future.

As such experiences as these unfold and one acquires the living sense of how the forces of legacy have converged within the family to work their impact on the present, one can discover simultaneously that one's predecessors were not altogether without redeeming virtues and that one is not without resources of one's own. Even when the facts come up showing that the parent indeed did suffer severe limitations and that one indeed was deprived as a result, the full understanding of this in its familial context relieves the deeply-felt personal need to go back and wrest forth a reckoning. Instead, if there is enough courage, one can test out whether, after all, one has the resources to make the future better than the past. This is loyalty in a deep sense. To enable someone to mobilize such courage may require an equal contribution of courage on the part of the therapist.

1.19. Multilaterality

Observance of the ethical dimension means consideration of how an action will affect the interests of others. For the therapist, as well as for the family member, this is a multilateral approach—that is, taking everyone's side of a question into account.

For a therapist trained in the psychodynamic approach, adoption of the multilateral approach requires a conscious shift in orientation and commitment. Imagine, if you will, a large transparency at the center of which is a point representing the patient. Scattered about the transparency are points representing significant others: family, friends, coworkers. Whenever the patient refers to any of these persons, a line is entered connecting the central point to one of the outer points. Occasionally a line is entered connecting two of the outer points with each other. But there is nothing systematic about the arrangement of lines. Even Erik Erikson, who actively has drawn attention to psychosocial factors, has not separated systematically family from nonfamily individuals in looking at their impact on the patient (1964, 1968). And the context of inquiry is the impact the others have had upon the patient. The therapist remains committed to the patient's subjective perception of self as center of the psychological universe.

Imagine, then, a second transparency placed over the first. It contains a systematic pattern of lines and symbols representing family relationships that are to be explored. Now the patient no longer is at the center. He or she becomes part of a complex pattern with many characteristics of its own, including the multigenerational chains of loyalty and legacy. We can now focus systematically and precisely on how the actions of the person in treatment will affect others as well as upon how he or she is affected by them.

The attitude of the therapist becomes one of "multidirectional partiality," that is, being partial in turn to all those whose interests are at stake (Boszormenyi-Nagy, 1966). Suppose, for example, that a couple with two children divorce. The husband remarries; his new wife brings a daughter of her own into the picture. The girl suffers from a debilitating illness that requires special considerations about diet and rest. The husband asks his former wife to shift the visitation schedule of his own children to lessen the impact on the sick child. The former wife insists that this is no concern of hers; she must consider her own needs first. The husband points out that under the present circumstances his relationship to his own children is being impaired. The ex-wife maintains that the quality of his relationship to the children is not her concern. A therapist concerned with the mental health of the ex-wife may support her contentions. A therapist committed to multidirectional partiality will first examine the possibility that the ex-wife after all does possess enough resources to face the issue with which she is confronted and to explore ways of resolving it. The therapist would see the issue as including the children's right to a good relationship to their father, the reciprocal advantages of their having good relationships within their stepfamily, and the mother's continuing accountability for doing whatever she realistically can to foster these relationships.

In raising the relational issues, the therapist would not see himself or herself as working against the basic interests of the former wife. The therapist would assume that in the long run her relationship to her children would be better served if she protected their access to both parents and that in the process she could develop a more adequate sense of self.

In a situation where a teenage son directs bitter and unforgiving rage toward his father, the therapist would inquire whether the adolescent is concerned about the impact on the mother and siblings.

These examples could lead to the inference that multilaterality is somewhere equated with advocacy of sacrifice or selflessness. This is not the case. We assume that the pursuit of genuine autonomy and the development of an adequate sense of self do not occur in a relational vacuum. The payment of one's relational debts as parent, spouse, or offspring is seen as a precondition of arriving at full selfhood and individual freedom.

We consider the commitment to multidirectional partiality to be an essential criterion of a contextual therapist. In the case cited above, the therapist may go as far as necessary in siding with the resentment and pain of the ex-wife, yet the therapist will be fully aware of a commitment to do whatever he or she can to help the ex-wife face her accountability as parent.

2. The Therapeutic Approach

2.1. Who Is Involved

We can now give more substance to our opening remarks about the terms *individual, marital,* and *family* therapy. When the therapist is committed to multidirectional partiality, the basic therapeutic orientation is the same whether one individual, a couple, or a family is present. The initial contact may be with someone presenting an individual complaint. It then may broaden to include spouse, children, parents, and so on. The presenting problem may be a marital dispute, but the therapist's recognition of the children's interests soon may lead to at least a temporary inclusion of the children. If the beginning contact is with the whole family, the need of one member for a private review of some concerns may emerge. In any event, the therapist perceives each individual not only as the center of a subjective universe, but also as part of a multigenerational pattern. The use of a genogram may prove even more effective with an individual than with a family because it provides guidance in speaking of and for the missing members. The distinction between *individual* and *family* therapy then becomes little more than a matter of who is available to participate in the work, given restrictions of time, distance, cost, and willingness.

When there is resistance to including, or even to talking about other family members, the therapist restates the multilateral contract: that within this approach to treatment, there is no way adequately to consider the interests of one family member without taking the others' interests into account as well.

Ideally, the initial contact is with all members of a nuclear family, but it is not always practical to insist on the ideal. The approach in any event is multidirectional. If a spouse refuses to work on a marital dispute, the therapist does whatever can be done to speak for the interests of the absent spouse. If, as is usually the case, the presenting problem involves two or more generations, the therapist works to become the advocate of those who are absent or dead. If a husband appears but says, "It's her life, I have nothing to do with it," the therapist addresses whatever factors have led the husband to distance himself.

As the example presented in the discussion of multilaterality suggests, the use of separate therapists for separate family members can work to the serious disadvantage of the multilateral effort unless these therapists are well coordinated in their outlook and in their grasp of what is going on. The approach does not require co-therapists, but the use of co-therapists usually will broaden and deepen the multidirectional partiality of the therapists' efforts.

2.2. Duration of Treatment

There is no fixed time limit for contextual therapy. One session may serve to help family members mobilize enough trust to face and handle a relational issue, such as the push of an adolescent toward autonomy. Years of treatment may be indicated when the impact of past on present has been especially severe. Under optimal circumstances, treatment will continue until the goals set by the family members with the active guidance of the therapist have been reached. In practice, the criterion a family uses in deciding to stop treatment may not be the relief of any specific symptom. It may be because of the confidence gained through trial actions and trial revision of attitude that there now is enough trustworthiness in the relationships for the family members to dare to venture on their own in dealing with symptomatic problems.

2.3. Applicability of the Contextual Approach

We do not regard the contextual approach as a specific methodology, but as a way of looking at and acting upon relational process. It generates methods of its own and also provides guidelines for the adoption of methods drawn from other sources. Accordingly, it is not limited by the nature of any particular patient population. Instead, its limits will depend upon the extent of its acceptance by mental health professionals and others charged with professional responsibility for human concerns, namely, judges, teachers, lawyers, physicians, clergy, and so forth.

2.4. The Goals of Contextual Therapy

The basic goal is to enable family members to take rejunctive action, that is, to make moves toward restoration of trustworthiness. This is worked at by helping the members of the family to bring to the surface and to face the issues that they have avoided facing out of fear that they could not afford the cost. A mother, for instance, may not be ready to face specific issues around her teenage son's use of the car because she unconsciously is afraid that her marriage cannot survive her son's growing up. A husband may avoid a wide spectrum of domestic issues because to surrender his chauvinism would be costly to his comfort, his narcissism, and his legacy. A husband and wife sidestep the issue of whether they have any relationship left by fretting endlessly about real or imagined rivals. A family continues living by worn-out prescriptions because they cannot face the cost of openly acknowledging to one another that the grandparent who laid down those prescriptions is dead and his time is over.

The movement is continually toward heightened awareness of multilaterality. A wife begins to recognize the impact on her marriage of continually denigrating her mother-in-law. The husband begins to realize that he cannot sit back while his mother and wife compete for him; he is accountable for engaging in the heavy work of deciding how much he owes to each and how to keep these accounts in balance. The interests of grandparents in children, and vice versa, are considered before steps are taken that exclude the older generation. The husband makes a greater effort to balance his work with his family life; the wife stops accusing him of making his work his "mistress." The issues of multilaterality involve not only triangular relationships but also whole family networks and even the junction of two family networks that takes place with a marriage.

2.5. The Relevance of Legacy to the Therapeutic Goal

In many situations, it becomes evident that the resistance to rejunctive effort comes from deeper sources than the family members' conflicts with each other. If the therapist conceptualizes in terms of triangles, it is important to know the forces that are keeping people stuck at one point or another of the triangle. It is not merely a task, for example, of helping the wife to recognize that her husband is not, after all, a monster; it is a task of helping her recognize that if she is to be loyal to her legacy, she feels compelled to make her husband look like a monster. Otherwise she will be disloyal to her father, whom she recalls as a monster. She makes an ethically invalid payment to father by acting as if her husband is even worse.

Or there is the husband who rejects all his wife's complaints because they make him look like an "evil person." Everybody knows he is really a good person, so his wife must be wrong. He turns out to be reflecting the legacy of a mother who became so terrified of the "badness" in her family of origin that she adopted a rigid posture toward her nuclear family: everything they do is good (and anything that does not fit this picture gets ignored). When his marriage exposes him to criticism, the son hears it as a multigenerational voice of doom: the facade of "goodness" is being threatened. His denials, of course, serve only to frustrate his wife.

The quickest way, and in some cases the only way to free people who are locked in combat often is to free them first from the past. We do not conceive of this simply in terms of freeing them from their conflicts with the people of the past. Instead, it is a matter of freeing them from the harmful effects of legacies in which both they and their parents were trapped. The recognition comes that they and their parents were not, after all, adversaries so much as they were common victims in a family drama of adverse legacy. This is one of the first steps toward multigenerational rejunction and liberation.

2.6. The Responsibility of Participants

The therapist is not there to "explicate" the family members to one another. Nothing will happen unless they are motivated to exert the effort to explore new approaches themselves. Once this effort is underway, the therapist may assist, as a resource person, by actively guiding the direction of inquiry. In the same spirit, the therapist may offer instruction, clarification, interpretation, or even confrontation, but only when people have shown that they are ready to use these materials to advance their own efforts.

Each participant is held accountable for his or her own position vis-à-vis the balance of relational accounts in the family. This is not a matter of the therapist's harshly demanding an accounting, of course. It is a matter of his or her persistently guiding people's attention back to the question of how they can play their part, pay their debts, and collect what is due them. The son says, "My father never opened up to me, but that's his life and his business." The therapist responds, "As a son, what might be your claim on your father? And if you have a claim, what could you do to make it?" When a daughter describes her mother's derogation of her, the therapist may at some point wish to explore what the daughter contributed to the problem. The goal is not to identify neurotic traits in the daughter; it is to explore how adaptations of new attitudes and actions might help to liberate the daughter from being stuck in her role as victim. It is sometimes astonishing how often it does not occur to people that they actually could do something.

2.7. The Therapist as Guide; Multidirectional Partiality

The contextual therapist will devote full attention, concern, and empathy to one family member, then to that person's adversary, and so on in a sequential process of "siding" with each family member. (This sequence does not have to be rigid, of course.) The therapist thus becomes advocate not only for all those who are present, but also for those who are absent for any reason, including death. As we have noted, the term "multidirectional partiality" refers to this process.

In the traditional psychodynamic approach to treatment, the therapist takes as a basic reference point the patient's own subjective perception of self as being at the center of the psychological universe (Kohut, 1977). This approach is reinforced by the therapist's own egocentricity. It is quite natural to adopt a protective stance toward the patient; indeed, the protective process begins with the use of the term *patient*. The offsetting effort to become equal advocate for all those others who are affected by the therapeutic process imposes a real demand on the therapist. It requires unlearning, relearning, and continual discipline. There is the temptation to collude with one family member against another. This is reinforced as one's own value judgments intrude. It is reinforced even more because the problems people bring with them are like the therapist's own problems and there is a pull toward the therapist's old nonsolutions. If one is to maintain the orientation we are describing, this means that one must keep a continual healing process going within one's self.

2.8. The Issues and the Dialogue

When a family or a couple enters treatment, the air soon may be full of recriminations. The therapist can be reasonably sure that all the things being said have been said hundreds of times before. One reason they are being said again is to probe whether the therapist will succumb to colluding with one or another party. As "ventilation" they are virtually worthless. They are addressed to postponement of solutions. They are worth the therapist's attention only insofar as they provide a quick initial assessment of how badly stuck people are.

The initial behavior may show something about power alignments and power shifts in the family. But in the contextual approach, application of power is seen as one sequel to the breakdown of trust in the family, and it is the root issue of trust we are concerned about.

As rapidly and firmly as possible, the therapist guides the participants toward focusing on one issue at a time. This may be difficult, for in most families there is a drift toward linking each issue with the next. Billy cannot have the car because he did not make his bed. He could not because his sister left her clothes all over it. She had to because mother made her empty out her closet to make space for cousin Jean. Now mother has to go to the station for cousin Jean, so mother is angry at Billy. And so on. The blaming is endlessly cycled; a clear target never emerges. It may take emphatic intervention by the therapist to get two or more family members to stay on one issue about which their adversary roles can be clearly identified. (It may be noted that the work of getting issues defined between adversaries also is a move toward detriangulation. If they must face each other, they cannot use a third person, or group, as a diversion.) The therapist invites each person in turn to give his or her side of the picture, while making it clear that the others are expected to listen. The focus is on making the complaint as concrete and specific as possible. In this process, the speaker may hear the flaws in his or her own case even while the listener is hearing the speaker's point of view clearly for the first time. Once a point of view has been stated, the therapist asks the other to respond, so that a balancing of adversary positions emerges. Simple as this process seems, it is the first step toward restoration of trust, and participants sometimes report their surprise at the effect it has on them.

The therapist gradually increases the pressure on each person to be accountable for making responsible statements and, in turn, be accountable for trying to explore and understand the point of view of the other.

The issue on which the therapist helps the participants focus at first may appear to be a very small one. The only requirement is that it can be brought into focus, usually between two people, sometimes with two or more family members on a side. It may be only a surface derivative of deeper issues in the family, for example, a wife's complaint about her husband's coming home too late to play with the children may mask her deeper concern about whether he cares for her. It probably will not be long before the exploration of surface matters reveals the underlying concerns and also indicates something of the impact of multigenerational issues on what is going on in the present. The speed with which the therapist moves from surface to depth will depend on both the therapist's and the family's readiness to deepen the context.

2.9. The Gradient of Change

As we have specified, the goal is to initiate action moving in the direction of trust. The intention to make a corrective effort is itself a step toward trust. Imagining how one would go about acting differently is a step. Wondering and trying to find out what accounts for the other person's behavior are steps. A phone call or a letter may be a step. A face-to-face conversation can be a major step if it helps resolve, or at least address, an issue. Within the family, new trial actions and new designs for action can provide leverage to break stuck patterns of relating. The target is not simply to get something done; it is to restore the hope and belief that things can get done. Such restorations may require very little time to effect or they may take years, depending on how badly trust has eroded.

If people remain stuck in mutually adversary roles, refusing to advance trust to each other, then it may become necessary to do some direct structural work within the family, for example, encouraging a wife to stand up for whatever entitlement she has earned and to take a more assertive role until her success in doing so can provide her and her husband with a new baseline for trust in the relationship, or until it has been demonstrated that no such gain is possible.

In the majority of situations, the goal is to improve functioning within a family unit that has not wholly stopped functioning. Occasionally, in connection with this task or as a separate venture, the goal is to restore a relationship that has been almost or wholly cut off, for example, between a married daughter and her mother. Here it is more likely that the therapist will have direct access to only one of the two. The rejunctive steps may have to be chosen with even greater care than in the case of the functioning family because the choices are so limited. What the daughter honestly can offer may not match up very well with what the mother chooses to accept. The daughter may wish to explore an old impasse; the mother may choose to let it stand. If together they are able to restore some common ground, this can be a move toward trust. If the daughter has made the utmost effort, consistent with reality, and still has made no progress, at least this provides her with some entitlement and some claim for freedom from the bonds of legacy.

The results of therapy may not be as great as people's initial expectations. The surrender of unrealistic expectations is itself a major step toward putting trust into the actuality of the relationship.

2.10. Siding

Multidirectional partiality means siding with people in turn. This is, of course, based on the conviction that each person has a legitimate interest in the proceedings. The opportunity is offered for each person to get past the stage of fruitless recrimination, to begin to define a point of view, and to make a serious statement. It may take time before people realize what is being asked of them and learn how to do it.

The therapist asks each person to be increasingly accountable, that is, to face the reality of his or her own part in what is happening as well as talking about what is happening to them. As this effort proceeds, it naturally runs into resistance. If someone has had an abusive parent and rigidly insists that his or her spouse is abusive, it may take a great deal of acknowledgement of later and earlier hurts before this person is ready to take a step toward a balanced perspective.

In any given exchange, the therapist must choose whether to go toward deeper siding or push for greater accountability. In one session, for instance, an adolsecent daughter was sobbing and complained that her father never treated her as a person. Her mother and brother had made similar complaints. The therapist asked the father, "What does your daughter's crying mean to you?" The father snapped, "When I think it's real, I'll respond to it." Wanting to protect the girl from the father's curtness, the therapist replied, "What makes you sure that you are entitled to ignore her now?" This was too much for the father, who lapsed into silence and permitted two years to go by before the next session. What the therapist had momentarily ignored was the father's own sense of isolation, whether self-induced or not, in the face of condemnation by the rest of the family. Further acknowledgement of his discomfort might have given him the extra measure of support he needed to begin to face what was happening between himself and his daughter.

Substantial acknowledgement of what has been endured may be necessary before a person is ready to rework a relationship in the direction of exoneration and reconnection. Pain and resentment may precede every step toward taking a fresh look at what did happen and what could happen. "Siding" is not, therefore, a matter of momentarily seeming to agree with someone. It is the art of helping people move through pain toward more accountable positions.

2.11. Mobilizing Accountability

In the contextual approach, the demand for accountability soon goes beyond the question of what one person may be doing to another. If it is a marital conflict, for example, the question very soon will be raised as to what effect the dispute is having on the children or other family members. Rather than deal with this by secondhand report, the therapist will push, if there are children, to have them included in treatment for at least long enough to see whether they too need help. When they are present, their expressions of concern for the parents' relationship may serve as a catalyst. The parents may begin to see their dispute in the context of what it is doing to their children. This touches the deepest level of ethical concern; it provides the most potent leverage for change. At the same time, if the parents are willing to acknowledge the child's concern for them and to reassure the child that they are working to make things better, this can be a first step toward deparentifying the overconcerned child and restoring structure to the family. In the contextual approach, ''marital'' issues are inseparable from the deeper issue of responsible parenting.

2.12. Loyalty Framing

In any contextual work, the underlying premise is that the therapist will encourage divisiveness only insofar as this will contribute to growth. Basic family loyalties will be respected. This is especially important when children are involved, because children have the heaviest investment in loyalty and their vulnerability is greatest. The therapist encourages the parents to carry the responsibility for talking to the child during the session, partly in order to relieve whatever fear they may have that the therapist is on the scene to rescue the child from them—an impression that puts the child into a loyalty bind. If the parents have a complaint about the child, the therapist not only will insist sooner or later that the parents offset this by some kind of positive assessment of the child, but also will ask for the child's comments on what he or she already is trying to do to make things work better. The negative images of parent for child and child for parent are not ignored or denied, but they are continually woven back into a context of movement toward trust.

2.13. The Task for the Therapist

In the effort to become a contextual therapist, it soon becomes clear that whatever prevented the therapist from taking a multilateral view in his or her own life is going to interfere. If, for instance, the therapist as a child was prohibited by one parent from giving loyalty to the other, the therapist will have to work at this issue in his or her life as a prelude to helping others. This does not mean that one must have experienced contextual therapy as such in order to become a contextual therapist. There are many ways in which the necessary preparation can be obtained. But its essential components will include an understanding of how intrapsychic variables operate to impede or facilitate the development of a multilateral point of view.

2.14. The Therapeutic Leverages

The contextual therapist is free to employ any responsible therapeutic method provided its manner of use is consistent with contextual premises. There is, moreover, no claim that the methods of contextual therapy are unique or exotic. On the contrary, their value derives from the fact that the basic contextual premises are addressed to what is universal in human nature. We can, nevertheless, review some of the basic therapeutic leverages that the contextual therapist employs.

Essential to all of them, of course, is the principle of multilaterality of point of view. For the therapist, this means active multidirectional partiality.

From the outset of treatment, the therapist presses for clear definition of conflictual issues, encourages each person to make serious statements of his or her position on these issues, and requires each individual to listen to the statements of the others. The participants are being asked to advance toward multipartiality of outlook. If there are no complications, this procedure alone may be all the treatment that is needed to help the family members get unstuck and go back to handling their own lives.

If, on the other hand, it appears that the participants are continuing to be stuck, the possibility will be explored that loyalty and legacy factors are impinging. (In considering the dynamics of legacy and loyalty, we do not overlook such dynamics as projective identification; we see these processes as mutually reinforcing one another.) If there are legacy aspects, then it will be necessary to focus therapeutic effort toward their source. In practice, this may mean shifting attention from a child or spouse to a parent or grandparent. If a person can overcome loyalty and legacy binds, then he or she will be freer to relate to child, spouse, or whomever has been pressed into service as a substitute victim.

In this process, the therapist will seek to mobilize the parenting responsibility of the participating adults, because it is a key therapeutic leverage. Any adult has parenting responsibilities to some extent, whether these involve children, aging parents, disabled relatives, or others. In the long run, no one is helped toward health by getting therapeutic permission to ignore this aspect of being a person. On the contrary, parental accountability provides leverage for facing other aspects of life, such as marital conflict.

In the process of dealing with legacy binds, the therapist also will work toward the exoneration of those who stand as sources, or as representatives of the original sources, of the legacy. Whether it includes the actual rebuilding of relationships or only the reworking of attitudes toward those who are no longer accessible to actual change, the process of exoneration offers liberation from invisible loyalties.

Exoneration is one of those processes through which people can build entitlement. Entitlement, in fact, can be derived from any act based on concern and addressed to the welfare of the other. Entitlement offers freedom from legacy and loyalty binds and also generates leverage for reworking the relationships of the present.

Where it exists, the claiming of entitlement is a significant strategy in movement toward health. This includes the ability to terminate overpayments. The courage required to take a stand may be the agent that initiates a new round of moves toward trust. At least it can interrupt the stagnation that comes from exploitation and absence of trust.

In all of these processes, healing is taking place through the continual effort at facing up to the entitlements of the other person, while defining one's own entitlements as well. This is a trust-breeding process. The ultimate goal is to build trustworthiness in the relationship. In this context, growth can take place, accompanied by affection and respect.

3. Converging Points of View

In keeping with its own basic premises, the contextual approach seeks to acknowledge and utilize all that is valuable and relevant in other therapeutic approaches. In this section, we will discuss some of the ways in which the contextual approach is congruent with those approaches.

3.1. Psychodynamic Aspects

We do not utilize transference as a therapeutic tool, but we recognize its persistence. Transference phenomena are ever-present, and the therapist must have some means of recognizing and dealing with them. A child, for example, almost invariably will transfer to the therapist some of the feelings and attitudes it holds toward its parents. Since these include loyalty, the mere presence of the therapist may tend to set up a loyalty conflict for the child. The therapist can act in such a way as to exacerbate or to relieve this conflict.

We can now gain new perspective on the concept of *repetition compulsion*. Repetitive behaviors indeed may be motivated in part by the need to master anxiety from old traumas. But a substantial part of the pressure for repetition of behavior may come from the revolving slate.

Affects also take on a different perspective in the contextual approach. Relief of pain or depression, for example, is not usually seen as the aim of treatment. Pain and depression are seen as signals of specific imbalances in relationships. The depth of pain provides a measure of the depth of perceived imbalance. The therapeutic task is either to bring the relationship toward balance or help the hurt person deal with the fact that such a balance cannot be accomplished. We do not see how valid relief from pain can be provided otherwise.

Those processes that have been identified as intrapsychic defenses can be seen as ways of sidestepping the facing of relational issues. Contextual therapy seeks to mobilize the resources that will help people to overcome these defensive efforts. For example, narcissistic withdrawal resulting from traumatic disappointment in parental figures may be relieved through the exoneration of the parents.

The development of a cohesive sense of self and the integration of ego functions may be seen in connection with being accountable for one's own part in events that affect others.

3.2. Transactional Aspects

The contextual approach has much in common with therapies that focus on the transactional dimension. Like other approaches, contextual therapy is concerned with communication and its impediments. We do not, however, tend to assume that failure of communication is at the core of relational problems. If people are not communicating, there is likely to be a reason why not. The withholding may be from fear; it may be a means of exercising power; or it even may be based on a realistic awareness that to blurt out what has been left unsaid will tear the relationship apart. Improving communication may be partly a matter of techniques, but we believe it essentially has to do with testing out possibilities for increasing trustworthiness in the relationship.

Concerning the communication of affect, we believe, of course, that openness of affect usually is desirable. But we do not set this up as an end goal of treatment. Likewise, we do not see catharsis as a therapeutic goal, although it may be a necessary stage in the movement toward health. We assume that affects have something to do with the state of the relational balance. It follows that modification of affect may require genuine shifts in the relational balance. To push for the expression of feelings without addressing the source of the feelings may be only to collude with one person's exploitation of another. The contextual therapist would not say, "Can you see that in spite of everything you love your grandmother?," but rather, "Can you find ways of understanding how your grandmother has behaved toward you, and can this lead to change?"

Accordingly, we do not encourage confrontation simply as a means to discharge feeling. We consider confrontation to be a measure for facing relational issues, to be used only when there is reason to hope that the encounter will help toward a solution.

Like other therapies, the contextual approach is concerned with structural aspects of the family. Overcloseness of a mother and child, for example, may be seen in some cases as parentification of the child. The mother's overutilization of the child may turn out to be the result of her being constrained by legacy factors from making an adequate commitment to her husband. The intrusion of a grandparent also may prove to have significant legacy aspects. We believe that restructuring moves are more likely to have a lasting effect if such factors as these are taken into account.

Concerning the geometry of triangles, the contextual approach does not turn on the concept of triangles, nor are its own therapeutic methods designed around that concept. It is safe to say, however, that our thrust toward facing the original source of relational difficulties instead of exploiting substitutes is consistent with the process of detriangulation.

4. A Model for Health Delivery

We stated earlier that contextual therapy eventually may provide a model for general health care delivery, a suggestion made recently by Lyman Wynne (1981).

At its worst, the medical model sees the patient as a passive recipient of the prescribed "treatment," whether this is medication, an operation, or whatever. This approach ignores the potential capacity of the patient and his or her family members to be partners in the restorative process; indeed, it begs the basic question of whether the patient wants to stay alive. Likewise, it fails to take into account the impact of the illness and of the treatment upon the patient's family, the members of which have considerable potential for helping or impeding progress. Of equal importance, it ignores the increasing body of evidence that the onset of various physical illnesses is correlated with psychological and relational stress. It also leaves out of account the crucial factors involved in the relationships of the professional health service providers to the patient and the family. Beyond these immediate concerns, there are, of course, large scale social questions of how medical treatment should be made available and to whom.

A contextual approach to physical medicine would seek to guarantee that the physician and other providers of health services would adopt a multilateral approach, seeing the onset of the illness, its course, and its treatment all in terms of how the providers, the patient, and the family members are affecting, and being affected by, one another's interests and concerns. This approach would help to generate new guidelines for prevention. Application of the appropriate resources at these points not only might bring substantial economies in health care delivery, but also help to restore trust in the physician–patient relationship.

On a broader scale, the same approach could be applied to issues of funding, priorities, coordination of health services, and others. As this effort progressed, the present relatively rigid boundaries between physical medicine and mental health services eventually might turn out to be as permeable as our present boundaries between "individual," "marital," and "family" therapy are.

5. References

Boszormenyi-Nagy, I. A theory of relationships: Experience and transaction. In I. Boszormenyi-Nagy & J. Framo (Eds.), *Intensive family therapy: Theoretical and practical aspects*. New York: Harper & Row, 1965.

Boszormenyi-Nagy, I. From family therapy to a psychology of relationships; fictions of the individual and fictions of the family. *Comprehensive Psychiatry*, 1966, *7*, 408–423.

Boszormenyi-Nagy, I., & Spark, G. *Invisible loyalties: Reciprocity in intergenerational family therapy*. New York: Harper & Row, 1973.

Boszormenyi-Nagy, I., & Ulrich, D. Contextual family therapy. In A. Gurman & D. Kniskern (Eds.), *Handbook of family therapy*. New York: Brunner/Mazel, 1981.

Erikson, E. *Insight and responsibility*. New York: Norton, 1964.

Erikson, E. *Identity, youth and crisis*. New York: Norton, 1968.

Fogarty, T. The therapy of hopelessness. *The Family*, 1979, *6*, 57–62.

Kohut, H. *The restoration of the self*. New York: International Universities Press, 1977.

Mahler, M. *The selected papers of Margaret S. Mahler* (Vol. 2). New York: Jason Aronson, 1979.

Wynne, L. Foreword. In A. Gurman & D. Kniskern (Eds.), *Handbook of family therapy*. New York: Brunner/Mazel, 1981.

11

Family Therapy as a Theory of Roles and Values

CHARLES P. BARNARD

In the January 1980 *AAMFT Newsletter,* Dr. Ben Ard provided the first of five interviews with what were called "seminal theorists in the field of marital & family therapy." Dr. Gerald Zuk was the first of these "seminal theorists" to be interviewed. As part of this interview, Dr. Zuk was asked: "This next question may be presumptuous, but if many years from now people look back on the work of Gerald Zuk in the field of marital and family therapy, what would you most like to be remembered for?" (Ard, 1980, p. 5). Dr. Zuk's answer identified six concepts, basic to his orientation, as what he regards as his most valuable contributions. He states that these concepts were derived from and "fundamentally grounded in observation in therapy" (Ard, 1980, p. 5). Although Zuk's ideas initially did emanate from his clinical experience, there is recent evidence from research documenting the presence and efficacy of most of his work (Garrigan & Bambrick, 1975, 1977a,b, 1979).

Referring to the scientific exploration of Zuk's ideas, it seems important to indicate that Zuk frequently has invited responses to his approach and encouraged research in the field of family therapy in general. He has stated:

> I am deeply concerned by efforts to picture the field as simply an art form. Without denying the importance of artistry, I believe there is an obligation to subject the various concepts and techniques that have emerged in the field to increasingly rigorous research, and that those found inadequate, deficient, or ineffective, should be discarded. . . . The ardent advocacy by members of "schools" has reached a point of diminished or zero returns, and credibility must now be established by hard-nosed evaluation. (Zuk, 1976, p. 300)

In this same article he identifies his approach, in outline form, in order

> to summarize the principles, et cetera, that appear to me to reflect more or less accurately my viewpoint in family therapy, thus offering the reader an opportunity to assess the consistencies

CHARLES P. BARNARD • School of Education and Human Services, University of Wisconsin-Stout, Menomonie, Wisconsin 54751.

> and inconsistencies therein, omissions (or erroneous commissions), validity of claims, and the capacity of the position to generate meaningful hypotheses. I hope in so doing to encourage other claimants (theorists) to duplicate my effort. (Zuk, 1976, p. 299)

To me, Zuk's request reflects the same integrity, as a person, that is found in the approach referred to as go-between therapy.

The six concepts Zuk referred to in his response were: (1) continuity values; (2) discontinuity values; (3) go-between role function; (4) side-taker role function; (5) celebrant role function; and, (6) pathogenic relating. These six concepts comprise the "basics" of family therapy from Zuk's point of view. Perhaps the provision of Zuk's definition of family therapy at this point also would facilitate understanding. He states: "It is the technique that explores and attempts to shift the balance of pathogenic relating among family members so that new forms of relating become possible" (Zuk, 1981b, p. 165). In *Family Therapy: A Triadic-Based Approach,* he further states that the shift from pathogenic relating evolves as a result "of a series of negotiations between therapist and family in which both parties vie for control" (Zuk, 1981b, p. 36), and the therapist judiciously applies the role functions of go-between, side taker, and celebrant.

These six concepts will comprise the basic format that this chapter will follow to provide an overview of Zuk's "Go-Between Therapy" (Zuk, 1966, 1971, 1975, 1981b). Although these concepts will constitute the "basic building blocks," the reader's attention also is called to the "mortar" that fastens them into the theoretical gestalt of go-between therapy.

1. Continuity and Discontinuity Values

Zuk's elaboration on the concept of varying types of values observed in family system operations is perhaps his most novel and significant single contribution. Although others have referred to characteristics of family operations that are operationally similar to values (rules in the case of Jackson, 1965, and loyalties in Boszormenyi-Nagy & Spark, 1973), Zuk's contributions are unique with respect to the degree of elaboration provided.

Zuk maintains that whenever there is conflict observed in the family, regardless of content, the clash between continuity and discontinuity values is extant. Prior to defining continuity and discontinuity, it seems appropriate first to identify Zuk's definition of value. He defines it as "an attitude, belief or way of evaluating events that typifies a person or group" (Zuk, 1978, p. 49). He believes, as do most of those who have attempted to be involved therapeutically with families, that there are three main intergroup conflicts that are observed and demonstrate basic value differences. These conflict groups are: (1) husband–wife, (2) parent–child, and (3) family–community. Upon reflection, it becomes obvious that the conflicts between these groups do not occur at random. Certainly the content of the disagreements can vary in numerous ways, but the values reflected seem more predictable. Wives, children, and families, in relation to husbands, parents, and community respectively, consistently will reflect what Zuk refers to as "continuity values" in contrast to the "discontinuity values."

Most recently, Zuk has defined continuity values as "the setting of a high value on emotional expressiveness, egalitarianism, humanitarianism, and holism" (Zuk, 1981b, p. 24). Discontinuity values he defines as "the setting of a high value on analytical thinking, on rules, regulations and codes, and on productivity, efficiency and individual achievement" (Zuk, 1981b, p. 25). We can add to discontinuity values the goodness of orderly procedures, discipline, law, and legal codes. Although individuals in a family will espouse one of these value systems more strongly at any given time, it must be remembered that both value systems have been, and will continue to be, important in human affairs. Along with the importance of the family therapist being aware of these basic classes of values, it is equally important that he or she respect each.

As with the family, we also can observe the implementation of these two basic value systems in political forms. A dictatorship would best be characterized as exemplifying discontinuity values, while a nation in a state of anarchy would best be characterized as operationalizing continuity values. Theoretically, a well functioning democracy would reflect acknowledgement and a well balanced implementation of both classes of values. Similarly, functional families would manifest acknowledgement and implementation of each of these value structures, while troubled families characteristically will present a chronic state of imbalance and rigidity regarding values. Trotzer has stated, "When an effective reciprocal balance between these two sets of values is not achieved, dysfunctional family patterns emerge which tend to interfere with both family growth and individual development. Thus most family problems revolve around a values conflict which creates tensions, anxiety, and disruption in the family" (1981, p. 49).

Zuk (1981a) presents a graphic portrayal of the consequence of a family's rigid adherence to a particular value system in the absence of the "reciprocal balance" to which Trotzer refers. In this article he provides a report of a family, referred to as the Ashbys, with which he was therapeutically involved for over 3½ years. Zuk notes that it is unusual for a family to be engaged for this period of time, but thinks it is important for attention to be devoted in the literature to "long-term cases," because they provide the best grounds for reliably and accurately assessing family processes and the effect of certain therapeutic interventions.

The Ashbys were a family consisting of mother, father, and three children. Each of the three children manifested psychiatric illnesses. Through presentation of clinical notes, Zuk illustrates how the parents had contributed to their children's difficulties by rigidly manifesting discontinuity values, with particular emphasis upon distance and coolness. He states:

> Although it is more or less normal for parents to espouse "discontinuity" values in the parent-child relationship, the Ashbys' emphasis on this set of values was excessive, and was the object of challenge or assault by their children, although each challenge was unique and related to special qualities in each. Each child challenged the climate of "discontinuity" established by the parents, and each challenge evoked pathogenic relating which led each to manifest symptoms of a mental illness. I am not suggesting that the particular parent-child atmosphere of conflict was the

Table 1. Categories of Contrasting Values Expressed in Family Interviews

	Values	
Categories	Continuity	Discontinuity
1. Affective/attitudinal	Empathic, sympathetic, "warm"	Distant, reserved, "cool"
2. Moral/ethical	Anticonformist, idealistic, egalitarian	Disciple of Law, order & codes, pragmatic, elitist
3. Cognitive/conceptual	Intuitive, holistic	Analytic, systematic
4. Tasks/goals	Nurturing, caretaking	Achieving, structuring

> only cause of the psychopathology, but rather that it was a significant and necessary contributor to the psychopathology, serving as it were as a trigger. I believe that children who feel deprived of the emotional intimacy (continuity values) that is the essence of the parent-child relationship, will react against the deprivation, seeking by so doing to restore it. (Zuk, 1981a, p. 20)

Table 1, (from Zuk, 1975, p. 29) illustrates the specifics of both continuity and discontinuity values. A brief examination of how the four categories of each value class is separated demonstrates that rigid adherence to either one or the other class likely would be counterproductive to individual and family development and functioning, as was illustrated in Zuk's portrayal of the Ashby family.

Zuk offers illustrations of how these contrasting classes of values are manifested in family operations in his article *Values and Family Therapy* (1978). He uses the three basic intergroup conflict categories identified earlier (husband–wife, parent–child, family–community) to facilitate this effort.

In husband–wife disagreements over child-rearing, it is generally the wife who accuses the husband of not being responsive and productive due to his "coolness," distance, reserve, and not caring (discontinuity). He typically responds by accusing the wife of being too sympathetic, a "victim of her emotions," and too "warm" (continuity). Although Zuk acknowledges that there are exceptions to every rule, he maintains that this example is a fairly typical one and illustrates the continuity–discontinuity division of values expressed on the affective/attitudinal axis (Table 1) between husband and wife.

In parent–child conflicts, the parents generally accuse the children of holding continuity values, while the children accuse the parents of espousing discontinuity values. Although the children accuse the parents of being too concerned with regulations, the parents accuse the children of being disobedient, rebellious, and anticonformist. In this we find the conflict joined along the moral/ethical dimension of the value system structure presented in Table 1.

In conflicts of the family–community level, the family generally is found holding to continuity values while the community is characterized as espousing the discontinuity values. An example would be the school or neighbors complaining to the family about a child. The parents/family are likely to defend their child by saying all children are not alike and allowances need to be made (continuity). Simultaneously, the school/neighbors maintain that good parents discipline their children and that certain rules and conduct of behavior must be maintained (discontinuity). The continuity–discontinuity dichotomy again is expressed along the ethical/moral dimension.

Although these examples characterize difficulties in the intergroup conflict categories most frequently encountered in family therapy, this value dichotomy can be applied to other elements of human relatedness as well. Table 2 (from Zuk, 1975, p. 30) illustrates contrasting values observed among conflicted groups, including those just described.

As one can see, those generally defined as less powerful, in relation to another, espouse continuity values, while the more powerful are found to reflect discontinuity values. In this observation, Zuk has identified a problem he discusses in two separate papers (1978, 1980). He believes that the mother assumes a central role with her children, while the father is peripheral. Keeping in mind that the mother most frequently espouses continuity values, while the husband manifests discontinuity values, he states:

> The tendency of children is to overlearn or over-identify with the values expressed by their mothers, with the result that they are poorly adapted to the values dominant in society which are primarily male values. . . . Because they are so identified with the values of their mothers

Table 2. Contrasting Values Expressed by Various Conflicted Parties in Family Interviews

Conflict between:	Values: Continuity	Discontinuity
1. Mates	Wife	Husband
2. Generations	Children	Parents
3a. Family and community	Family	Community
3b. Family and community: Race as a central factor	Black	White
3c. Family and community: Social class as a central factor	Lower class	Middle class
3d. Family and community: Politics as a central factor	Liberal	Conservative

("continuity" values), and because these values differ from those held by their fathers ("discontinuity" values) children, particularly males, are bound to have a difficult transition as they make their way into a society still dominated by male ("discontinuity") values. (Zuk, 1978, p. 52)

The polarization of continuity and discontinuity values between husbands and wives can be particularly problematic for children. Although this can be the case in the two-parent family, Zuk believes it to be of particular concern in the single-parent family:

> It (single parent family) is at higher risk than the so-called intact family because of the disproportionate emphasis, due to the absence of one parent (most often the husband-father), on a set of values which does not by itself satisfactorily prepare offspring for the workaday world. Both "continuity" and "discontinuity" values need to be effectively taught in the family, and it is my view that two parents do this better than one. (Zuk, 1980, p. 197)

Zuk has moved beyond identification of single adjustment problems people may experience secondary to the mix, or absence of the same, of continuity–discontinuity values they have integrated, into the realm of psychiatric illness. Table 3 (from Zuk, 1981b, p. 249) summarizes the connections he has formulated between various psychiatric illnesses and the continuity–discontinuity family value system structure.

At the "neurotic level," under continuity, the therapist will hear these people described as being impulsive, unable to control emotions, idealistic, naive, and manifesting such antisocial behaviors as drug use/abuse, runaway, and/or sexual promiscuity. As one can see, Zuk has characterized this as "delinquent behavior." Under discontinuity, on the neurotic level, he identifies the psychosomatic category. These are people who are described as almost "too good," "holding everything in," and being perfectionistic—

Table 3. Value Systems in Relation to Psychiatric Nosology

Psychiatric disorder	Values: Continuity	Discontinuity
1. Neurotic level	Delinquent behavior	Psychosomatic
2. Characterological level	Hysteric	Obsessive–compulsive
3. Psychotic level	Catatonic or hebephrenic	Paranoid

certainly an ample portrayal of someone with an overreliance upon the discontinuity position.

At the characterological level, the individual who is overly reliant upon the continuity position is referred to as the hysteric. This individual is described by self and/or others as too emotional, naive and immature, and either over- or underresponsive to those in his or her environment. At the opposite end of the continuum, we find the obsessive–compulsive who is overly demonstrative of the discontinuity position. This is the person who cannot tolerate disorder, dust, or dirt and may become very behaviorally ritualistic in order to avoid upset.

At the psychotic level, Zuk identifies the individual who will react to stress dramatically via either a catatonic or hebephrenic state as reflecting a heavy reliance upon the continuity system. They too frequently are identified as being naive, idealistic, easily influenced, and by other terms that fit the continuity system. On the discontinuity side, at the psychotic level, is the paranoid who has systematized his or her suspicions about persons or events into "tidy, delusional packages" which appear impenetrable. It is the extreme of the discontinuity system in the form of neatness, orderliness, hiding emotions, and maintaining interpersonal distance.

The reader should not extract the impression that individuals manifest solely either continuity or discontinuity values. It is not an either/or situation. It does seem apparent, however, that most individuals express continuity or discontinuity values along a dominant–recessive continuum. Trotzer has said:

> Each person has the capacity to portray either set of values but a tendency to express the dominant set as opposed to the recessive set. Each person has the capacity to resonate to both sets of values but the fact that one emerges as primary is due to the complex interaction of genetic heritage, societal and cultural norms, family orientation, and environmental circumstances. (Trotzer, 1981, p. 45)

Just as individuals to varying degrees manifest various ego defense mechanisms, so, too, do they attach themselves primarily to continuity or discontinuity values. It is likely that a combination of the same influences (genetic, societal, and familial) culminate in each of these phenomena occurring to the degree that they do.

The reader already may have detected a relation of the specifics characteristic of the continuity–discontinuity values to his or her own therapeutic method of operation. Zuk (1978, 1981b) has maintained that in implementing the role and functions of the family therapist it is virtually impossible to not be responding in accord with either the continuity or discontinuity position.

The three basic role functions that Zuk believes characterize the functioning of the family therapist are "go-between," "side taker," and "celebrant." Although each of these role functions will be elaborated upon later, they will be introduced here to illustrate the application of the value dichotomy in interactions between family therapist and family. Zuk has said, "In carrying out his role, the therapist is always expressing values of one sort or another, and I think it is helpful if he recognizes that these values are essentially of the two types considered at some length in this paper" (Zuk, 1978, p. 53). Table 4 (from Zuk, 1978, p. 53) will facilitate development of an understanding regarding when, and how, the family therapist projects continuity–discontinuity values while functioning in either of the three roles.

As therapists mediate or facilitate discussion within the family, set limits, and impose rules necessary for effective communication and therapy, they are operating in the role of go-between. As can be seen in Table 4, continuity values are expressed in the go-

Table 4. Values in Relation to the Therapist's Role

Role functions of therapist	Values	
	Continuity	Discontinuity
1. Go-between	Mediator, facilitator of communication	Sets limits, imposes rules or regulations on communication
2. Side-taker	Sides with wife against husband, children against parents, nuclear family against community	Sides with husband against wife, parents against children, community against family
3. Celebrant	Espouses mercy, compassion, forgiveness	Espouses justice, upholds law, codes, regulations

between role when mediating and facilitating discussion. Similarly, discontinuity values are manifested when the therapist, in the go-between role, sets limits and imposes rules or regulations necessary for effective communication.

In the role of side taker, as the term implies, the therapist aligns with one party or another for various reasons. If it is with wife against husband, children against parents, or family against community, continuity values usually are being espoused. If the therapist aligns with the opposite sides of the groups just identified, the therapist usually is espousing discontinuity values.

In the role of celebrant, the therapist certifies family events or happenings as important–unimportant or relevant–irrelevant and/or signifies and attaches other meanings to the same. When the therapist, in the role of celebrant, expresses mercy, compassion, and forgiveness, while encouraging the same of the family, continuity values are being espoused. When moral indignation and insistence upon justice and discipline regarding the event are expressed, the therapist is espousing discontinuity values.

As one can ascertain through analysis of these three role functions of go-between therapy and their relation to the continuity–discontinuity value scheme, the go-between therapist is always responsive, if not sensitive, to the values espoused in a particular family. This awareness on the part of the therapist naturally is important diagnostically (determining predominant values and connection to conflict in order to devise goals and interventions), but is of equal importance in evaluating the effectiveness of the therapeutic process. The Ashbys (the family Zuk provided an overview of his work with in his 1981a article) constitute a good example of this. They were a family with three children who manifested various psychiatirc illnesses and who Zuk portrayed as having parents who were rigidly overreliant upon the discontinuity system. The parents were described as cold, rigid, rational, and impersonal in their style. After observing this, one of his major goals became that of promoting the development of the contrasting continuity values within this family through his interventions as go-between, side taker, and celebrant. He states:

> In other words, the major goal of the therapist was to promote emotional expressiveness, warmth, and spontaneity, to encourage clear statements from family members of support and affection for each other, to be a sounding-board (as celebrant) of the succession of painful events that had beset the family, and serve as a clarion (again as celebrant) of a happier future in which parents and children would be more appropriately responsive to each other. (Zuk, 1981a, p. 20)

This seems to be an appropriate juncture at which to move into a more elaborate discussion of the three family therapist role functions Zuk has identified. It is through implementation of these three roles that families are helped to develop the more vital and reciprocal balance between the values just discussed and to displace other forms of pathogenic relating. Zuk defines the go-between process/therapy as the "therapist's application of leverage to displace pathogenic relating" (Zuk, 1975, p. 23). These three sources of leverage available to the therapist are described below.

2. Go-between Role

Zuk defines the role of go-between as the "member in family interviews who sets the rules for communicating" (1981b, p. 23). One can determine quickly that this particular role function is one that cuts across all the "schools" of family therapy. The reader can ascertain readily that many techniques easily could be categorized as the therapist fulfilling the go-between role. This is also a role function that seems inevitable for the therapist working with families. Zuk says:

> I think it is an unavoidable role. The therapist working with couples and families is continually engaged in being a go-between. The go-between role means that the therapist is engaged in three particular functions: setting the rules of communication, setting limits of communication, and facilitating communication. (Ard, 1980, p. 3)

Zuk offered a good example of establishing rules and limits for communication in an earlier paper. The following quote comes after his explanation of the situation when he had asked each family member to present his or her perception of a particular situation in order to clear up his confusion.

> The therapist then acted to establish his authority as the go-between by indicating that he would not allow interference in the telling of stories. He was thus introducing an unusual structure for the family: they were not used to letting each talk without frequent interruption, for one thing, and without efforts at intimidation, for another. (Zuk, 1971, p. 217)

Just as there are diverse interventions that could be categorized as belonging to the go-between role function, so too are there diverse styles of interacting within this role function. According to Zuk,

> the go-between can be very active, intrusive, and confronting, or inactive and passive. He may move into the role of go-between by the device of attacking two parties he hopes to make into principals; or he may move into the role by calmly pointing out a difference between two parties. On the other hand, he may become a go-between by refusing to take sides in a dispute that has erupted; or he may become one by presenting a new point of view in a dispute. (Zuk, 1981b, p. 147)

The style and timing of exercising leverage, via implementation of the go-between role, constitutes much of what is referred to as the "artistry" of the therapeutic process. Although the inexperienced therapist may implement the go-between role by insisting that a disagreeing couple engage in a shared meaning process to better insure understanding, the more experienced therapist may realize that the anger being expressed is valuable, albeit with sharp edges, and implement the go-between role by facilitating the exchange via presentation of a calm and disarming demeanor. Although both of these therapist behaviors would constitute implementation of the go-between role, the interventions appear very different to the outside observer. Zuk has said, "He [the therapist] may also exert therapeutic power by delaying or speeding up his arbitration [in role of go-between]'' (Zuk, 1981b, p. 147).

Just as the therapist can assume the role of go-between with various factions of a family, so too various family members may assume the go-between role to the detriment of the family's operation. Mothers in particular will cast themselves in this role. Zuk states:

> This is a common interaction in family therapy, observed frequently in mothers who wish to pit their husbands and children against each other so as to reserve for themselves a role of benevolent go-between. . . . In these rather commonly occurring clinical encounters, the mothers are employing go-between process to control relationships with both their children and husbands. In family therapy, they assume the role of go-between not only between husbands and children, but also between husbands and children, and therapist. . . . In reality, they may seriously undermine the therapist's efforts, for as go-between they are able to alter and rearrange his messages to the family. These mothers may actually be the strongest resisters of change in the family. (Zuk, 1981b, p. 150)

Although mothers will indeed assume the go-between role more often than fathers, this is not to say that fathers, or a child, may not assume the role as well. This may constitute one form of pathogenic relating (to be discussed later) which the therapist will need to change by exercising his own therapeutic leverage. Without intervention on the part of the therapist, it is likely he will become as inept, and neutered, as the rest of the family. ''Artistry,'' or therapeutic judgment, again must be exercised, for premature or obtuse intervention of a family member assuming the go-between role may result in their leaving treatment.

Just as there are those occasions when the therapist may need to move a family member out of a go-between role, there are others when the opposite move is most wise. As an example, the therapist may decide it is therapeutic to begin to promote a father assuming the role of go-between with his children, in contrast to his otherwise peripheral and uninvolved role. Naturally, sensitivity again must be exercised so as not to threaten mother's security which emanates from her long-standing status as go-between with her children. The therapist also may exercise the go-between role with the father by encouraging him to communicate, and otherwise demonstrate, his caring for the family members. This would exemplify encouraging the father to relate from the continuity value system as opposed to his more likely discontinuity value stance.

In exercising the role of go-between, the therapist must be cautious to be sure that the family does not trap him or her into too rigid a go-between role such as might occur by becoming the ''family judge.'' Barnard (1981a) has identified how this is a prominent danger in working with families that have an alcoholic member. The ''alcoholic family'' comes with a history of blaming and an obvious ''identified patient,'' expecting the therapist also now to ''fall into line.'' Zuk has said the following regarding those times when this entrapment may be occurring:

> As noted, family members will attempt to draw a therapist out of the role of go-between into the role of a principal or to trap him into being a certain kind of go-between. In the therapist's armamentorium are a number of devices to counter these efforts of the family. The therapist can simply refuse to intervene in a conflict in which he is pressed to take sides on the ground that this is not one of his proper functions. He can interpret or reflect on the conflict, thus sidestepping direct involvement. If he believes he is being trapped into the role of family judge, he may deny that he has any interest in judging or any authority to judge. If he believes the family is maneuvering to trap him out of the role of go-between, he may undermine their intent by changing the subject. (Zuk, 1981b, p. 157)

In concluding this discussion of the go-between role function, it seems important to underscore that this role is not synonymous with the go-between process/therapy. The go-between role is but one of three crucial roles fulfilled by the therapist utilizing the go-between process with families (the other two roles being the side taker and the celebrant) to exercise leverage such that the family might be dislodged from its more typical pathogenic form of relating. To maintain, or increase, his or her therapeutic leverage in this role, the therapist may employ such therapeutic gambits as confrontation, reflection, advice, denial, evasion, directing, clarifying, or blocking.

3. Side-Taking Role

The side-taking role function can be defined as follows:

> The side-taking role is just what it says: the therapist takes the side of one member in the family. The side taking may be momentary or for a longer period of time in a given session. Side-taking can be therapeutic because it disturbs a family's equilibrium. Side-taking is not necessarily anti-therapeutic or manipulative, although it may be. The family therapist cannot avoid side-taking. If a therapist believes that he/she is avoiding, chances are that the family will accuse the therapist of taking sides. The issue is not whether the therapist is going to take a side, but rather how the side-taking should occur. The issue is whether the side-taking is made in accordance with sound judgement. (Ard, 1980, p. 3)

As Zuk states above, this role is one that is unavoidable and one important consideration is whether or not the "side-taking is made in accordance with sound judgment." (Ard, 1980, p. 3) As he has indicated, the therapist must be aware of the family's state of equilibrium when engaging in side taking.

Whitaker (Barnard, 1981b) utilizes the analogy of the family operation to a chess game and indicates that the mother is analagous to the queen in that, particularly in the beginning stages of therapy, she needs to be protected or sided with. If the therapist precipitously sides against her, she might express her chagrin by utilizing her power to pull the family out of therapy. The therapist with sound judgment and sensitivity may realize that the more astute intervention, in light of the family's state of equilibrium and mother's role, is to side with the apparently overfunctional mother which results in her "changing her tune" for the first time.

An example of this would be the family with a mother, father, and two adolescent sons. The mother opens the session with an angry diatribe about the disobedience of the sons who appear to be overwhelmed by her attacks. Without knowing any more about the family, several alternative side-taking moves are available. One may be to take the mother's side, and amplify the deviation further (see Barnard & Corrales, 1979, chap. 6). This may result in her shifting and beginning to come to the assistance of her sons, who are being "attacked by this outsider." Indeed, this shift may be the leverage that is needed to change the rigid, pathogenic relating that has resulted in the family operation remaining stuck. Another may be judiciously to take the sons' side while continuing to engage mother, in an effort to facilitate the sons' feeling competent enough to involve themselves in more productive negotiations with their mother. In one sense of the word, this side-taking maneuver would be designed to lend the boys some ego strength so that they can cease their counterproductive, system maintaining, behaviors. Although these examples constitute only a few of the many side-taking interventions that may be generated, they may be sufficient to promote the readers awareness of the need for sound clinical judgment when adopting the side-taking role function.

Acknowledging the inevitability of side taking, the issue of countertransference becomes an important one. If the therapist finds himself or herself feeling particularly antagonistic toward a family member, resulting in consistent side taking against that member, it is important for the therapist to analyze his or her motives. At this time engaging a peer or supervisor in the role of consultant may be crucial not only to the therapist's development but also to the course of the therapy for the family. Without this issue being addressed, it is not unreasonable to assume that the family will terminate sessions as a result of their equilibrium being inordinately tilted by the therapist's excessive side taking. If this does not result in the family terminating therapy, it may result in intensifying the symptomatic behavior on the part of the person feeling excessively blamed. Along these lines Zuk has said:

> It is probably unwise for the therapist to give the message that he consistently sides with one member against others. It is advantageous for him to keep the family guessing as to whether he will engage in siding and what the tactics of his siding will be. The therapist must retain flexibility in the face of strenuous efforts by the family to get him to side predictably with one member or another, with the result that he becomes, in my opinion, a less effective therapeutic agent. (Zuk, 1971, p. 219–220)

To this point, the emphasis has been upon the therapist side taking with an individual. There also are times when it is appropriate to side take against the whole family. Zuk has written:

> It has been my experience that sometimes dramatic improvement may follow upon the therapist's notice of intention to terminate treatment because there has been no significant progress. . . . He chooses to employ this powerful confrontation because he is convinced that only by means of it can he undercut a powerful family resistance to change. (Zuk, 1971, p. 224)

Carl Whitaker (Barnard, 1981b) has referred to this action as the ''impotence ploy,'' while Palazolli and her colleagues (1978) have written of it as encouraging ''feeding of the enemy.'' All of the above have reported cases of dramatic change as a result of this intervention side taking against the entire family being judiciously employed. In using this type of side taking, the reader must be cautioned regarding assessment of his or her own motives in implementing this role function.

It seems that the particularly difficult family turns its strength (apparent resistance) against itself in responding to this side-taking action. Although the family appears to be stubbornly resisting being dislodged from its pathogenic relating, this move results in sudden and dramatic movement. ''It may be speculated here also that what has produced the change is actually the family's strenuous effort to prevent change; that is, a strenuous effort by the family to frustrate the therapist's avowed intention to withdraw from treatment'' (Zuk, 1971, p. 224).

4. Celebrant Role

> [The third role function is that of ''celebrant.'' Each year millions of people suffer a crisis or trauma, such as a death of a family member or friend, the running away of a child, the loss of a job, the loss of a marriage through divorce or separation. Those are the common accidents of life today.] When these accidents occur, families seek someone who can restore their confidence in life or in the meaning of life, and can give them a reason to continue to live. The family therapist today frequently occupies the role of celebrant. It is a very powerful role and can produce therapeutic change lasting for a short or for a long time. The role of celebrant can usually be held only for a short time. Once a family is restored to its sense of continuity and begins to pursue its regular living pattern, it will not want the therapist in that role any longer. The role of celebrant is

> in some respects too powerful, and families can tolerate a person in that role for only a short time. That's why all celebrations are relatively brief; they are too powerful. (Ard, 1980, p. 3)

This is the last role function to be identified by Zuk. It was defined in his 1975 book, *Process and Practice in Family Therapy.* In the mid-1960s he had introduced and discussed the roles of go-between and side taker. More recently others have begun to acknowledge how families may be in search of someone to fulfill the role of celebrant with them, that is, a therapist seen briefly, as opposed to longer term therapy. Whitaker (Barnard, 1981b) has stated his belief that perhaps family therapists have discounted prematurely the value of their "single session" families. He uses as an example the family that initiates therapy because of symptomatic behavior of an adolescent member. Upon completion of the first and only session, the father assertively states his expectations to the whole family. Along with these statements, he asserts that they will not be returning to therapy because "we'll handle our own affairs!" Indeed, the family does not return, as the single session with the family therapist in the role of celebrant has been sufficient for them to acknowledge that "things have gotten out of hand" and to move on to more constructive behaviors.

Although the family with the symptomatic youngster in crisis is an example of one type of family with which therapists frequently find themselves in the role of celebrant, the other is lower class families. Therapists should remember that "these are usually not long-term cases because, in the case of lower class families, while there is awe there is also a deep distrust of the therapist's expertise and an unwillingness to enter into a long-term relationship with an outsider who has superior education and sophistication" (Zuk, 1975, p. 24). These "short-term" families, while suspicious of therapists, will imbue them with a particular kind of power and authority only found in the role of celebrant. This power and authority, once attributed to the therapist, is what the family uses as a springboard from which to effect its own change.

Zuk has cautioned family therapists about deluding themselves into believing that families are eager about entering therapy. He believes that about one-third of all clients are comfortable sitting and talking about their difficulties, while the other two-thirds are not only not comfortable with therapy, but feel threatened by it. Because of this, he has said, "The majority of clients want something from us, want it in a hurry, want just certain things and not everything we have to offer. Many families are seen in times of crisis. Out of that experience came the notion of celebrant, a role that exists for a very short time, a powerful but short-time role" (Ard, 1980, p. 6). Zuk has indicated that there are others in society that fulfill a role similar to that of family therapist as celebrant, saying

> Rather like a judge, priest or civic official, he is often called on to officiate at or "celebrate" an event that has been deemed important by the family, such as a death or birth, a separation or reconciliation, a runaway or return from runaway of a family member, a hospitalization or release from hospitalization, a loss or recovery of a job. As celebrant the therapist confirms and signifies that the event did indeed occur. (Zuk, 1975, p. 13)

Although the therapist may be cast into and/or assume the role of celebrant for a single session, there is another possibility of which I have been acutely aware. As therapist it is all too easy, as it is for the family itself, to become preoccupied with pathology and lose sight of the "pockets of health" that Alberto Serrano refers to (Barnard, 1981b). I believe that it is important to help a family identify these pockets of health and to "celebrate" their existence and determine ways to further amplify them. A common example is that of taking time to "celebrate" with the family the decrease in bickering and tension that occurred between the current session and the previous one. As simple and obvious as this sounds, it occurs far too infrequently. It seems little wonder that families terminate therapy in light of each session apparently being designed solely to discuss more "gloom and despair."

Although the role of celebrant is one of the three identified by Zuk, hopefully the reader has developed the sense that the side-taker and go-between roles may be selected more intentionally by the therapist than that of celebrant. The therapist may be "assuming" the role of celebrant more as a result of the family's needs and desires than as a consequence of his or her own determination. In spite of this, the celebrant role should not be discounted as secondary to the others. Zuk has said,

> As celebrant the therapist should recognize that he may be in a very powerful therapeutic position, but that he is in the position for a brief time only, and that he does not so much introduce change in family members as "celebrate" the fact that a change has occurred or is about to occur. The members, in a sense, empower him to certify that something has happened or is about to happen that is important to them. (Zuk, 1975, p. 24)

5. Pathogenic Relating

Zuk has stated that pathogenic relating

> refers to formulations of the therapist about the distortions in patterns of relating among family members which may be important in a causal sense in producing symptoms in members. Silencing strategies are an example of pathogenic relating, as is scapegoating, which may also be a form of silencing strategy. Inappropriate labeling of a family member's behavior can constitute pathogenic relating, as can the promotion of inappropriate family myths. (Zuk, 1981b, p. 193)

Pathogenic relating is one of Zuk's basic concepts. It is a term that is generic in the sense that the goal of family therapy is to replace or dislodge the pathogenic relating noted. "The general goal of the therapist is to reduce pathogenic relating, or eliminate it, using those role functions described (earlier), while expressing differentially those values described (earlier). Pathogenic relating tends to erupt after an impasse in competing values, thus the therapist must also address the underlying values" (Zuk, 1976, p. 302). The three role functions and value schema discussed earlier constitute basic tools both for understanding and affecting change in the pathogenic relating found extant in the family according to Zuk's approach. In go-between therapy it is believed important for the therapist to assess the family's situation, identify the pathogenic relating present, and then to facilitate change through judicious utilization of the three therapeutic roles identified.

Zuk also is emphatic in pointing out that the therapist may become a constituent element in the family's pathogenic relating. For instance, the therapist may utilize excessive constraint in confronting a particular family member or excessively take sides with a particular member against another. In this regard, Zuk cautions therapists by saying:

> At the end of each interview, the second question the therapist should ask himself is, "what did they tell me that was new today?" The first is, "with whom or on what issue did they expect me to take sides?" In other words, information about the relationship of the therapist to family members takes precedence over other kinds of information. (Zuk, 1975, p. 16)

By continually addressing the relationship between himself and the family, the therapist is best able to ascertain to what degree, if any, he has become part of the family's pathogenic relating.

From Zuk's description at the outset of this section, the reader can determine that *pathogenic relating* is a broad term that can be used to describe a plethora of conditions and dynamics observed and/or reported in the family. As Zuk implies, the problems may be inappropriate labeling and scapegoating or other difficulties such as implementation of destructive silencing strategies, but the therapist can expect to find these problems consistently embedded within conflict surrounding the expression of continuity/discontinuity values in the family. Because of this, as the therapist formulates the assessment of the pathogenic relating present, the continuity/discontinuity value schema should be employed as the pervasive backdrop to the diagnosis.

The Ashby family (Zuk, 1981a), cited earlier, provides a good example of identifying the pathogenic relating in light of the underlying value disparity present. In his paper, where he describes the therapeutic process with the Ashbys, Zuk identifies various forms of pathogenic relating present, but characterizes the "basic" issue as that of a rigid reliance upon discontinuity values as formulating the basis of the family relationships.

As the elimination or reduction of pathogenic relating constitutes the major goal of family therapy, Zuk is realistic enough to realize that each family is not going to be "cured" at the termination point of therapy. As mentioned earlier, he believes that most families enter therapy because they want something specific from the therapist rather than all that he might be able to do for them. Certainly this idea of Zuk's is not unique, but rather is consonant with many other leading thinkers in the field of family therapy. Jerry Lewis and his colleagues (1976), established that even the most optimal families had their tensions, anxieties, and difficulties but differed from other families in their conflict resolution skills. Robert Beavers (1981) identifies how even these most optimal families will be seen in therapy at points of crisis (illness, death, unemployment, etc.). As Zuk has inferred, it is not unrealistic to expect that these families will benefit quickly from the therapist assuming the role function of celebrant and then move on about their own unassisted business of living. Whitaker (Barnard, 1981b) has stated his belief that the healthy, "self-actualizing" family is similar to the more dysfunctional with respect to tensions and problems, with the exceptions of the "wattage," or intensity of problems, and the time frame, in that their problems are more short-lived.

Zuk states that along with reduction and replacement of pathogenic relating, "the central aim of the therapist must be to return the family to functioning 'within normal limits' " (Zuk, 1975, p. 19). He then goes on to state that "within normal limits" for him does not mean an absence of frictions, rivalries, and competition between husband and wife or parents and children, of anxiety, guilt, and anger, nor does it mean that fair play is always present in the associations of family members. He then states: "'Within normal limits' means for me that those malevolent, intimidating, disruptive, inflammatory processes referred to as pathogenic relating are no longer observed by the therapist, or that they have been reduced, and that with reduction or elimination has come a noticeable improvement in family relations and/or individual functioning" (Zuk, 1975, p. 19). He concludes his discussion by saying that the therapist and the family need not stop at the point suggested above, but that realistically there are few families interested in proceeding beyond this point into more developmental or preventive work.

Although pathogenic relating can be multifaceted, Zuk has devoted particular attention to some specific types. One type he has attended to particularly is what he refers to as "silencing strategies." He defines them as "those interpersonal maneuvers designed to punish an individual for some transgression by isolating him in silence" (Zuk, 1981b, p. 102). Zuk, (1981b) has presented a number of descriptive statements and hypotheses about silencing strategies, some of which will be briefly presented at this point.

Zuk maintains that silencing strategies may be conducted primarily by either verbal or nonverbal means. Probably the most common verbal silencing mechanism is that of changing the subject. This certainly is a tactic, like others, that can be done crudely or with great subtlety. The therapist may put a sensitive question to a family member and find that member, or another, abruptly change the subject with, or without, such a note of urgency that the question is forgotten. On the nonverbal level, silencing mechanisms can take the form of laughing (Zuk, 1964), clearing the throat, coughing, yawning, changing one's posture, or a multitude of facial grimaces and contortions. Zuk (1981b) gives the example of a mother who, when criticized by her schizophrenic daughter, would grimace as though in pain. The mother's grimace would attract the daughter's attention and, "Observing this, the daughter broke off her comments and asked her mother what the matter was. The mother denied anything was the matter, but continued her facial expression of physical pain. The daughter halted her criticism, saying that now she couldn't remember what it was she had to say and perhaps it really wasn't justified after all" (Zuk, 1981b, p. 104).

Zuk cautions family therapists to be particularly sensitive to the silent family member. It is likely that this is a person with special significance for the family system. He has said of this person: "This is either the person who is powerful enough to get other family members to speak his thoughts and feelings for him, or the person who threatens to betray the system and agrees or is compelled to keep quiet" (Zuk, 1981b, p. 106).

Silencing strategies can be directed at an area of communication or at a person. Changing the subject is the primary silencing mechanism employed to "silence" a particular content area from being explored. The "silent treatment" is the silencing mechanism par excellence directed primarily at a person. "Scapegoating" an individual is a unique way of "silencing" not only that individual into only speaking a particular "language" (schizophrenia, juvenile delinquency, alcoholism, etc.), but also of molding others into "hearing" only what has been attributed to that individual emanating from them. Certainly this is tantamount to what Laing has identified as the "mystification process" (1965).

Zuk also has speculated that those who have been exposed to long-term silencing mechanisms are primarily candidates for employing them themselves. The silencing strategies employed by those who have been the victim of the same tactics may take the form of the "cold shoulder" or babbling (a type of meaningful sounding noncommunication).

6. Discussion

The reader familiar with Zuk's thinking is aware of both the tremendous quantity and quality of his work over the last two decades. He has been one of the most prolific writers in the field of family therapy as it has struggled through its early growing pains. In light of this, one of the most outstanding values of his work appears to be his ability to write at the "macrolevel" of family therapy (role functions, values, pathogenic relating), while effectively illustrating the microlevel (specific examples and interventions of the macro elements he identifies) with clear and concise case data.

For this reason, it appears to me that Zuk very adroitly provides the necessary cognitive map the family therapist needs in order to enhance therapeutic functioning, while leaving room for individual creativity and acknowledgement of personal style at the level of implementation.

One could take any of the techniques of various theorists in the field of family therapy and appropriately identify them as falling into one of the three role functions Zuk has presented. It also is possible to identify what any theorist claims he is attempting to change in the family system as pathogenic relating, and also probably to describe the issue in light of Zuk's continuity–discontinuity value paradigm. It is as though Zuk has painted with broad enough strokes to provide a structure for comprehending, while leaving room and freedom enough for the individual practitioner to provide the fine strokes or detail so that he or she can personalize it to a particular personality and style.

Along with Zuk's primary contributions, it seems appropriate to present briefly some of his ideas regarding the process of family therapy that have not yet been identified. Zuk believes that the focus of family therapy should be based in the present and that a focus on the past almost inevitably is destined to take on an individual focus and probably to become stalled. "For the same reason, the therapist usually rebuffs attempts to include in sessions discussions regarding family members who may not be present" (Zuk, 1981b, p. 38). As one might suspect, Zuk instructs the family that he wants all members currently living at home to be present for at least the first few sessions of therapy. He indicates that he would like the entire family present in order to avoid counterproductive discussion of members not present and that all members being present facilitates his making a more appropriate evaluation of whether or not the family will benefit from therapy. If he senses resistance in the form of family members being absent, or in other ways, he is quick to inform the family of his perception of their being involved in a game of "hide and seek" (Zuk, 1981b, p. 213), and that perhaps the family is really not in search of help, thus making termination a reasonable consideration.

As noted, Zuk expects the entire family to be present for the first three to five sessions. Beyond these initial sessions, his tendency is to not include children in sessions who are under the age of 10 unless they are the identified patient(s). If the youngster is the reason for initiating treatment he will include them for a longer period—10 to 15 sessions—but then again consider the advisability of their continuing in the direct treatment process. I believe that he provides a sound rationale for this action:

> The reason for my reluctance to include young children in more than the first few therapy sessions is not primarily that they should not be burdened by hearing confidences of the parents—although I believe that this is an issue too many family therapists pass over too lightly—but rather, that the loyalty of the children to the parents, especially the mother, is ordinarily so strong in children under 10 years of age that it is difficult to elicit conflict with the parents. Children of this age span ordinarily clam up tightly when examined about their relationship with their parents. Also, of course, the language they have available for the expression of conflict is still limited, and they tend to be very sensitive to and compliant with the many subtle silencing signals sent out by the parents. (Zuk, 1981b, p. 214)

Zuk believes that most family therapy is short-term in nature (six months or less), because most families either are not interested in or cannot tolerate the strain of a longer contact. In order to maximize the benefit from short-term contact, the therapist must focus on facilitating the development of the family engagement (commitment). Zuk believes that only a minority of families will engage themselves in a therapy process for longer than six months. He believes Jewish families are among those who are amenable to longer term contracts (Zuk, 1978), and describes a set of family values in Jews that he believes promotes engagement.

Zuk has identified four types of "contracts" families will make with therapists: (1) 1 to 6 interviews, for purposes of crisis resolution; (2) 10 to 15 sessions for the purpose of short-term therapy; (3) 25 to 30 interviews, which Zuk identifies as middle-range therapy; and (4) 40 or more interviews, described as long-term therapy. Zuk believes the goals of each of these contracts varies from tension reduction in the first type of contract to increased family solidarity and better acceptance of individual liberties and differences in the fourth type.

Within these various parameters there also are specific phases of family therapy that Zuk identifies. He believes that the first four or five sessions constitute the "engagement phase." The engagement of the family is important to the change process, and Zuk states that for many families the process of their being engaged is tantamount to change being effected. Beyond the engagement phase, he believes each issue subsequently presented by the family for exploration and negotiation constitutes a new phase of therapy. There is an engagement on successive issues, so to speak. The final phase of therapy, following the phases constituted by various issues being presented by the family beyond the engagement phase, is the termination point. The termination phase occurs when the therapist or family, either jointly or unilaterally, decides that a satisfactory goal either has been achieved or is unattainable in view of present circumstances.

Zuk also has identified some specific considerations regarding the successful engagement of families (Zuk, 1971). He has expressed his interest in deemphasizing to "non-talk" families the need for a long-term commitment. He believes this helps the family to feel less threatened and to maintain their engagement in the therapeutic process more easily. He also will arrange to schedule sessions with a greater interim period between them when he believes that these families otherwise may terminate prematurely. Another engagement technique is that of assuring families that he will not press to have secrets divulged. He also explains to families that he will respect signals that a topic is too sensitive to discuss. He believes that by providing families this reassurance, and freedom, it paradoxically promotes discussing issues they otherwise had the genuine intention of avoiding. Another engagement technique employed by Zuk is that of *not* providing the family an extensive rationale for why they are being seen as a unit. His concern is that a lengthy discourse on the rationale of family involvement will tend only to intensify the sense of guilt, and perhaps shame, that the family already is wrestling with. He believes the fact that the entire family has been asked into therapy is a sufficient contextual statement, without verbally relating the family functioning to the identified patient's behavior. He considers verbal rationales for family involvement particularly confusing and disconcerting to lower class families and likely to result in early termination.

7. Summary

Zuk can be characterized as a chronicler of the development of family therapy, and the reader can perceive from this chapter that he also has been a primary contributor and catalyst to the development of the field. In my role as a trainer of family therapists, I have found Zuk's contributions to be of immeasurable value and importance. Zuk's constructs provide the necessary cognitive map and orientation, yet permit the room for idiosyncratic expression that we all value. Although these ideas have proven valuable to me in my family therapy training capacity, they also have demonstrated their value to me in my practice with a multitude of presenting problems in both the inpatient and outpatient contexts. Although I may be accused of "side taking" with Zuk's approach, it seems important to acknowledge that rather than side taking, it was my intention to fulfill the role of "celebrant" in this effort. As Zuk states, the role of celebrant is designed to "certify and celebrate" important happenings (Zuk, 1981b, p. 24).

8. References

Ard, B. In focus: Gerald Zuk. *AAMFT Newsletter*, January 1980, pp. 1–6.

Barnard, C. P. *Families, alcholism and therapy*. Springfield, Ill.: Charles C. Thomas, 1981. (a)

Barnard, C. P. *Elements of family therapy: Drs. Carl Whitaker and Alberto Serrano*. (Videotapes and Monograph) Menomonie, Wisc.: University of Wisconsin-Stout, 1981. (b)

Barnard, C. P., & Corrales, R. G. *The theory and technique of family therapy*. Springfield, Ill.: Charles C. Thomas, 1979.

Beavers, W. R. A systems model of family for family therapists. *Journal of Marital and Family Therapy*, 1981, *7*, 299–307.

Boszormenyi-Nagy, I., & Spark, G. *Invisible loyalties*. New York: Harper & Row, 1973.

Carrigan, J. J., & Bambrick, A. F. Short-term family therapy with emotionally disturbed children. *Journal of Marriage and Family Counseling*, 1975, *1*, 379–385.

Carrigan, J. J., & Bambrick, A. F. Family therapy for disturbed children: Some experimental results in special education. *Journal of Marriage and Family Counseling*, 1977, *3*, 83–93. (a)

Carrigan, J. J., & Bambrick, A. F. Introducing novice therapists to "go-between" techniques of family therapy." *Family Process*, 1977, *16*, 237–246. (b)

Carrigan, J. J., & Bambrick, A. F. New findings in research on go-between process. *International Journal of Family Therapy*, 1979, *1*, 76–85.

Jackson, D. D. Family rules: Marital quid pro quo. *Archives of General Psychiatry*, 1965, *12*, 589–594.

Laing, R. D. Mystification, confusion and conflict. In I. Boszormenyi-Nagy & J. Framo (Eds.), *Intensive family therapy: Theoretical and practical aspects*. New York: Harper & Row, 1965.

Lewis, J., & Colleagues. *No single thread: Pyschological health in family systems*. New York: Brunner/Mazel, 1976.

Palazzoli, M. S., & Colleagues. *Paradox and counterparadox*. New York: Aronson, 1978.

Trotzer, J. P. The centrality of values in families and family therapy. *International Journal of Family Therapy*, 1981, *3*, 42–55.

Zuk, G. H. A further study of laughter in family therapy. *Family Process*, 1964, *3*, 77–89.

Zuk, G. H. The go-between process in family therapy. *Family Process*, 1966, *5*, 162–178.

Zuk, G. H. Family therapy. In Jay Haley (Ed.), *Changing families* New York: Grune & Stratton, 1971.

Zuk, G. H. *Process and practice in family therapy*. Haverford, Pa.: Psychiatry and Behavioral Science Books, 1975.

Zuk, G. H. Family therapy: Clinical hodgepodge or clinical science? *Journal of Marriage and Family Counseling*, 1976, *2*, 299–303.

Zuk, G. H. Values and family therapy. *Psychotherapy: Theory, research and practice*, 1978, *15*, 48–55.

Zuk, G. H. Value systems and psychopathology in family therapy. *International Journal of Family Therapy*, 1979, *1*, 133–151.

Zuk, G. H. Family therapy for the "truncated" nuclear family. *International Journal of Family Therapy*, 1980, 2, 183–199.

Zuk, G. H. Style of relating as pathogenic relating: A family case study. *International Journal of Family Therapy*, 1981, 3, 16–28. (a)

Zuk, G. H. *Family therapy: A triadic based approach* (Rev. ed.). New York: Human Sciences Press, 1981. (b)

12

Family Group Therapy

JOHN ELDERKIN BELL

My approach to family therapy emerged gradually after my beginnings in 1951 (Bell, 1961). To this day it continues to shift, though now in less dramatic ways. Starting without precedents I had the opportunity, without any input from other therapists, to devise a method that worked for me. Accordingly, the methods will not necessarily be functional for others whose personalities, family backgrounds, developmental experiences, and exposures to varieties of family therapy direct them to make their own different approaches to families.

The method I have developed is social-psychological, based on principles of small group therapy, but adapted to the constellations of the families and to their interrelations with me as therapist. This method contrasts with the intensely clinical approach taken by Ackerman (1958), Minuchin (1976), and others; with the intellectualized aggressive approach of the strategists (Palazzoli, Cecchin, Prator, & Boscolo, 1978; the MRI group—Watzlawick, Weakland, & Fisch, 1974; Weakland, Fisch, Watzlawick, & Bodin, 1974); or the historical, reconstructive methods of Bowen (1978) and his group.

I was very deeply indebted to a colleague, John Macmurray (1957, 1961), formerly professor of moral philosophy at the University of Edinburgh, with whom I taught a joint seminar in 1955, and whose point of view I largely adopted. What intrigued me was his philosophical analyses of such issues as the relation of thought and action, the separation of action from movement, the fundamental interpersonal or social nature of action, and derivatively, then, of experience, knowledge, and values. Thus, the word *action* has particular differentiation from *movement,* which occurs without social involvement. I now use *interaction* as a synonym for *action* in this sense, in order to avoid ambiguity, although the term *interaction* offends me because the *inter* is redundant, as is *communication,* which is subsumed within "action."

Foremost in my thinking is the *social* nature of man. The primary unit is social—persons in relation, persons in interaction. The individual as a person exists as an aspect of his or her social groups. The focus of the therapy is consistent with this position: "In the family treatment situation . . . we fight the tendency to give a primary and isolated significance to an individual who is in front of us" (Bell, 1964, p. 76). Because the nature

JOHN ELDERKIN BELL • 751 De Soto Drive, Palo Alto, California 94303.

of the family group is social and group oriented, that is family oriented, changes in the intrapsychic functioning of individual family members are seen as secondary aspects of the family action. Viewing the family as the problem, and not an identified individual as a patient, leads to primary therapeutic changes that occur as a family changes, and, derivatively, as an individual changes.

This group or social emphasis does not indicate that the individual is viewed as unimportant. The original presenting problem, frequently presented as existing in a child or adolescent, is never forgotten, though the problem may not be worked on in the therapy directly. With the family in focus as the "patient," the perplexing individual problems frequently disappear in behavior or by reinterpretation as the family becomes released from earlier strictures on action and thus more functional, current, and healthy.

Each individual of the family accordingly is extremely important to the effective operation of therapy. This is true of children, who commonly receive added initial help from me to become openly active in the therapy. Each individual is given equivalent opportunities to act yet remain an interdependent member of the family group.

Another major theoretical concept regarding the nature of the family is that the members engage in communicative acts, and the action of communication is effective in therapy when it is verbal as well as motoric. Coherent communication is so vital to family group therapy that I exclude preschool children and some of those in the early school grades because of insufficient verbal and conceptual development. Much family communication is by way of acts that have communicative as well as instrumental purposes among themselves. Such communication is nonverbal and/or symbolic and not comprehensible in its total meaning to outsiders. The task of clarifying communication is difficult when an individual is experiencing acute symptoms, since verbal communication then tends to become constricted, increasingly primitive, and nonverbal.

A final assumption is that persons are capable of change and that the family can change in the therapy. The changes in therapy may not always be as inclusive as I could visualize but the family can change nonetheless. The problem-solving abilities of the family are channeled within their own value system which I do not seek to modify in preconceived directions though those values change in accord with family expectations. The capability of the family to develop, maintain, change, and defend such value systems often is overlooked in individual therapy where change may occur in one individual and be stringently resisted by the family. The family's values motivate change toward new interactions but always compatible with these family values.

1. Concepts

Family group therapy does not contain unique terms. I am opposed on principle to using technical language if simple English will suffice as it usually does. This may make my ideas sound simple, but they are usually very precisely stated and often present translations from initial technically expressed formulations into more basic English. I always write with a thesaurus at hand to try to find the exact terms to express my intended meanings. I have not sought to become a leader of a cult, so have not had to depend on terms for in-group development and operation. Many people prefer to speak in such clichés, and some popularized terms in family therapy cater to this preference even though the terms often limit thought.

Many of the concepts in my theory are borrowed from the small group behavior literature, reflecting a theoretical bias. Two of these concepts especially merit discussion:

1. The first major concept is that of the family as a group. Four definitions of family were identified and discussed (Bell, 1962). These included the definition given to the family by a family-identified patient, often a child; the cultural definition, that is, the family as an institution; a corporate definition, reflecting the small group nature of the family; and, finally, a group bounded by community pressures, involving public, legal definition of the family. Family therapy is based primarily on the corporate definition.
2. The second major group is the therapy group. This consists of the therapist plus the family. This group forms for the sake of the therapy, exists during the therapy, and dissolves at the end. It is an artificial rather than a natural group, and its nature is much affected by the theories and practices of the therapist. The therapy group exists for changing the family in accord with the family's goals and with the therapist's interventions. The therapy group functions for one major purpose, to modify the behavior and relations within the family.

Later I began to acknowledge and use a third group, the family in the community. This concept extends back to the early 1960s. The stress on the family as group remains, but an emphasis also is placed on how that group interacts with other groups or systems in the community and on the impacts that such extrafamilial groups can have on the family.

2. Body of the Theory

One of the most pertinent questions a family therapy approach must attempt to answer is how family change occurs. I do not regard the concept of *change* as reducible to the simple definitions that most therapists reach for. As far as I can judge, change occurs through a complex multiplicity of causes in an immense variety of processes that are socio-, family-, and individual-syncratic. Rather than seeking simplification of theory at this stage of the therapy's development, I continue to struggle to identify and state descriptively what appear to be the behaviors and the contexts associated with observed changes. These appear to me to be so complex that I can only believe that we shall have to wait for grand theories, such as those in physics, to become possible. For the moment I am content with careful description of family behavior and that of myself as therapist. Large patterns gradually may become clearly visible.

One area of observable change is found within the family action. Changes in family action seem to occur through the nature of the therapist's relations with the family. As for my relations with the family, I do not join their group, but relate from outside the family. In this vein, I stated (Bell, 1963) that "toward this goal of keeping the boundaries around the family group as intact as possible, and toward strengthening them I try to avoid intruding myself into the family group" (p. 7). Wherever possible I approach an individual's problems as reflecting family problems, and help the family approach them from this perspective.

To respect and strengthen the family boundary, however, is sufficient to induce change. The typical frustration in a family is isolation, the separation of an individual from those to whom he or she should be nearest and most real (Bell, 1964). A primary means of altering the internal family functioning, that is the process of interaction, is through their communication. Specifically, covert communication patterns must be made overt and nonverbal patterns must be made verbal. The family's communication is a key to activation of interactional patterns and for that reason is a focus of therapy.

The theoretical progression of changes in the family's interactional patterns moves through the following sequence:

1. In all social groups and particularly the family, the interaction and communication are structured within certain operational limits that produce stereotyped patterns of reactions among family members. This results in the constriction of permissible behaviors.
2. Most older children and their parents have available to them potential or actual patterns of behavior beyond those they use in the family.
3. The therapist is a community figure in relation to whom family members may show behaviors that extend beyond those normally revealed in the family.
4. In response to the newly revealed patterns, the rest of the family members must revise their stereotypes about the family member, respond to him or her with new actions, and make new accommodations of their own behavior.
5. Having developed new models of interacting, supported by mutual commitment that they are better and should be continued, the family consolidates these new patterns. Thus the therapist, by encouraging interaction (and communication) among all the family members generates change in the functioning of the family. As new behaviors emerge, family members hear each other differently and accordingly come to view each other freshly and thus to respond to one another in new ways.

Because the therapist does not join the family, even temporaily, the family plus the therapist form a unique therapeutic group, similar in many respects to conventional ad hoc groups. In action seven stages of family therapy emerge: initiation, testing, struggling for power, settling on a common task, struggling toward task completion, achieving completion, and finally, separation. One of the most interesting of these stages theoretically is settling on a common task. As family members become freer in participation the diversity of goals becomes plain and the need for consensus essential. As the family determines the common task, it already is beginning to operate therapeutically. Further, focusing on their own task provides for the family (1) motivation for involvement of all the members and (2) specific information for evaluating therapeutic progress. Thus I see the improvement of process within family structure as the therapist's goal, although the selection and completion of the family's task is their responsibility.

Four stages of therapy develop during the course of therapy with most families that include children. These are the child-centered phase, the parent–child-centered phase, the spouse-centered phase, and the family-centered or termination phase. A family coming for therapy frequently presents a child-related symptom as the problem. Therapy begins where there is initial identification of a problem, but it seldom rests there. From the first session, emphasis is given to all interaction patterns and communication. As therapy progresses, different relations come into focus as the family members become increasingly free to show themselves in action, express negative emotions, admit relational difficulties, and strive for improved family functioning. In essence the family moves from an individual orientation, which often is maladaptive for all members, through a dyadic orientation, to a true group orientation in which individual needs can be met most effectively. This takes place in response to the consistent all-family orientation of the therapist. Thus the phases of therapy reflect a reorientation of the family in relation to itself (Bell, 1976).

3. Family Pathology

Pathology in an individual usually is approached as an indication of a deeper and more complex level of disturbance within the family group. All individual symptoms are not viewed as family related: some may be organic or in other ways physical, "but insofar as it is suitable to say that an individual's difficulties are created by or are a product of his or her family life, it is . . . just as appropriate to say that the family is disturbed" (Bell, 1975, p. 181). For this reason I appear to use the presenting symptom in an individual as a starting point for *family* interaction in therapy. Although I do not dismiss the presented symptom as unimportant, it may not and most probably will not become the focus of the therapy.

Family group therapy acknowledges the developing of a symptomatic "scapegoat" to cover some family disturbances. Pathological patterns in families often involve mutual projections of guilt and blame, frequently leading to a family member becoming a "patient." For me, however, that patient reflects a disturbance deeper within the family. I do not posit, however, that this individual necessarily is in any way inferior or weak or more troubled, only that he or she has been given the role of "patient" through the dynamics of family interaction (Bell, 1962).

Another characteristic of family disturbance is rigidified interaction among family members. Roles become static and inflexible, intensifying disturbing behaviors, reducing communication, and making it increasingly ineffective.

Family pathology is classified as either acute or chronic in terms of the symptoms presented. Acute symptoms often occur as family members enter new developmental stages that require changes in family interactions. Such symptoms show up in changes in communication patterns. Language commonly becomes more primitive and nonverbal, with increased incongruence between the verbal and nonverbal communications. Essentially this represents a regression to an earlier stage in family life, the employment of previously effective though no longer relevant patterns of interaction among family members.

If there are no resolutions of the crisis precipitating the acute symptoms, the pathological pattern will become entrenched and chronic. The symptoms, both in terms of interactions and individual behaviors, are perpetuated as roles. Chronicity is characterized by (1) a limitation or reduction in the range of methods of conflict resolution, (2) an increase in the use of simple sign language and primitive communication, (3) a reduction of intrapersonal and interpersonal awareness, and (4) insufficient or excessively radical changes in family values and traditional patterns of interaction. This overall rigidity is the focus of family group therapy at both the acute and the chronic stages. Flexibility in interactions among family members becomes a prime objective and a measure of therapeutic progress.

4. Therapist–Family Relations

As therapist I meet with the entire family at all sessions. I am so firm about this that I refuse to see a part of a family at any time. That sounds rigid—even to me—and it is. Any attempt by individual family members to meet separately with me is rejected flatly, for I regard the seeking of individual relations with me as a form of resistance to the treatment. For instance, if one or more family members cannot attend a session as a result of illness, a business obligation, or some other excuse, that session is postponed. Other therapists hold sessions with portions of the family, but from my perspective such a practice is not economical and tends to lengthen the course of treatment

I strive for a serious, businesslike atmosphere in the therapy. In order to maintain a working climate, the family and I sit at a table rather than lounging in easy chairs.

My approach to the family seeks to be friendly to all, especially at the beginning when solid working relations are being established. I do not join the family or assume the roles of persons therein, as others do (for example, Minuchin, 1976). My relations are most aptly described as those occurring between a task-oriented group leader and a group. Such relations encourage objectivity and diminish my need for a cotherapist.

5. Role of the Therapist

In my role as therapist, or group leader, two important principles guide my behavior: (1) I will work only with the entire family and (2) I am a facilitator of their new interactions. Within my role as group facilitator several key activities emerge:

1. I receive the referral, which may come from the family directly, from a social agency, the courts, a colleague, a school or college, a personnel officer, a mental health service, a physician, or others. I usually prefer to speak with a referral agent directly so I may explain some of my methods. Sometimes this deters an agent from making a referral; on other occasions it helps greatly by providing an orientation within which the agent may help to prepare the family for my work.
2. At the first meeting with the whole family, I have two aims: (*a*) to build a relation with the family that reduces somewhat their anxieties and gives practical orientation concerning the methods I will use; (*b*) to define how I shall conduct myself, by helping them to exchange their ideas about their problems and ways to change. I assist each person to participate to the full in assessing personal and family problems, to take part in solving them, to express their own reactions to each other and to the therapist, and to determine their readiness to terminate treatment.

Most commonly at least one person in the family begins with an account of difficulties with one or more family members, seldom with the family as a whole. Implicit is a message that the revision of one or more family members' behavior would solve their problems. I move the focus to the whole family immediately, but not abruptly. I may make a statement such as "I hear what you are saying, and I assume that when that problem is present there are problems in the whole family that are behind it. We will be exploring how the whole family can work together to so change that the problem can be diminished or removed, or so that what now seems a problem actually is found to be a useful, natural, and helpful way to function in your family." Although other outcomes are possible, these represent extremes within which the family may find new directions.

The shift to a family focus is not easy for many reasons. That is why I insist on full presence of the family members at all times. I go even further, to a refusal to speak with individual members apart from the family. Such a stance is not arbitrary. The speed of resolution of family problems depends on openness in communication and removal of *family* barriers to change. Absence from discussions provides powerful leverage to those who attend as well as to those who are absent. The leverage, however, is not in the direction of family problem resolution but against it. Absence represents a power grab for some family members and an escape from the family for others. To foster such power control or distancing works against the family as a unit and toward family destruction, or toward perpetuation of a family breakdown that has already occurred. What is more, it works against individual growth and freedom, which comes best from family sanctioned change rather than escape from the family.

For me, family therapy thus begins with the determination of who belongs to the family and their specification of who will be included in the treatment. Although it may seem arbitrary, I tell them that I will exclude from the topics that may be discussed any talk about family members beyond the agreed therapy group. This blocks an escape into one-sided presentations about family members who are not present that I would see as resistance to changes on the part of those making the presentations. It also accentuates the relevance of attendance and participation by those who are at hand. It defines, as well, my stance as a therapist, for it is a clear criterion of attendance that can be firmly applied. When a family makes an attempt to circumvent the rule, as most families do at some time, I refuse to see them with one or more persons absent. I close off for them an escape route from the requirement to examine the whole family and work through the problems all round. They cannot then continue to project problems onto a missing person or escape from pressures on themselves to change. In addition, this speeds up the therapy, which for me has been a consistent aim, though I suspect some others with whose work I am closely familiar have less concern about concluding therapy speedily.

I assume therapy process responsibility, but none directly for resolving symptom-producing intrafamilial conflicts. Resolution of family conflicts is the family's problem. They must work among themselves toward becoming released from painful former interactions and toward new functional interrelations. I am present to keep them at work but not to pattern the outcome.

Much of my attention is given to the family's interaction. I am watchful over the whole family at all times, insofar as possible. I do not center my gaze on an individual alone. My gaze keeps all persons in view to the greatest extent possible. This family-inclusive watching is a powerful therapeutic device. It keeps all persons engaged much of the time and allows my immediate intervention when someone appears to be dropping out. My interventions at such times may be nonverbal, for example, a more direct positioning of myself in relation to the person so that he or she senses the inclusion. If this is insufficient to keep a person in the group or bring him or her back into the family, then I make known the action that has taken place, describing the behavior that I have observed. I do not interpret what may be behind the behavior, for that is hypothetical and easy for a person or the family to ignore or attempt to refute. An open description of what I have seen permits each person to interpret the behavior as he or she chooses and thus to react in ways that bring about changed family interactions. This usually revises the action among all the family toward that person's reinclusion and often opens the way for that person to speak. What is said by the person if he or she does speak is especially powerful in deepening the whole communication within the family and breaking up a stereotyped old pattern of interaction. Problem behaviors are reduced, eliminated, or reinterpreted, as would be expected since the family is central in the precipitation of symptoms. This still leaves room for individuals to differ markedly in behavior, values, objectives, and functions, but within the positive valence of family endorsement.

6. Role of the Family

For the family two tasks form the center of their work. The first is to attend the sessions of treatment. If individuals are excluded, or if they absent themselves from a session, they threaten the group therapeutic process, the future integrity of the total family, and, most seriously, their own development toward adulthood and independence. Functional separation is thus a family group as well as an individual process. Absenteeism by protest precipitates or accentuates problems, as well, through its *public* acknowledgment of the incapacity of the parents to assert their functional adult and parental distinction from the child or children.

From my perspective, the family in therapy should include all members who have reached the age when they are able to conceive of the family as a functioning unit that includes the self, generally a level of conception reached during the early school years, around 7 or 8 years of age. On occasion younger children are included provided their presence does not generally disrupt the interaction of the rest. Children younger than 7, however, usually are unable to operate on a conception of the family as a unit within which they function as members rather than as separate individuals. An egocentric orientation from which they cannot be released until a certain level of intellectual development takes place, reduces their capacities to contribute positively to family problem solving, and often leads them to disrupt the progressing treatment.

The second major task for the family is to face the need to act with one another, rather than indirectly, as through speaking to and through the therapist. As an atmosphere of family trust in the therapist is established, the communication process increases through the family, promotes family discipline, and reduces the individual–to–therapist dimension. This represents, as well, growing assurance on the part of the family within which they can express hostility, resentment, private views, and expectations directly to other family members, as well as to the therapist, and gain release from inner pressures. As therapist I encourage this family-centered communication. I support the whole family in facing their open hostility through which such communications normally are initiated.

Although a stormy period of contention emerges, I maintain the family-centered perspective, facilitating the outpouring of negative feeling, supporting those who withdraw from it, and encouraging all family members to express openly to one another their reactions in the face of the hostility. The dominance of any speaker has to be countered by others who speak their reactions. This is done more by alerting the family to signs of restlessness or withdrawal of nonspeakers than by the therapist's suggestions. This more subtle approach does not challenge, but rather opens an opportunity if an individual is ready to seize it, and keeps alive for the family my continuing preoccupation within the total group rather than solely with the outpourings of a single speaker.

I liken my role to that of one who has been invited into a troupe of actors whose special drama form is improvisations. How each of the actors become a part of the troupe is an ancient story. They have been performing together for a long time and they are stale. They keep recycling their old routines and the excitement and freshness of earlier days has faded long ago. My job is to help them release themselves from the past and open up to the potentials that now are only latent among them. Obviously, I am not to join them as a performer. My task is to free them to discover fresh talents in one another and to so integrate these new potentials with old roles that the promise in each of them becomes a part of their total performance. Together they then can create new scripts for maximal use of the talents of each person in ways that are integrated into a comprehensive and exciting drama. Thus each actor feels a full partner in the performance and is liberated again to work with the others in developing fresh ideas as well as using the best of the old.

My role as a consultant is clarified. I first have to assure myself that the whole company is present. This does not mean that at some later time new actors cannot join the troupe, but for the moment, and for the quickest changes in their acting together, those who now belong have to be present. Further, each one has a role to play and this must be developed openly and fully.

To keep the company together and improvise drama, the roles must be integrated with those of others in mutually supporting ways. One person going on only to do his or her own thing can be as destructive to the whole drama as are boring, stereotyped, and frozen interactions. Together, they must call up from one another the unique capacities and qualities of each and put them into a framework that liberates rather than stifles each actor and facilitates the interaction of all the others. The performance as a whole must achieve an integration that satisfies and liberates each person.

This analogy brings out many of the characteristics of therapy as I conduct it. I note the following elements of my technical approach:

1. I am an outsider to the family. No matter how active, close, or functional I become for the family, I remain on the outside.
2. The basic performance is that of the family that is stuck in old, dying, or dead roles.
3. Their aim, as indicated by their coming for therapy, generally is to release one or more family members from roles that appear, at least to some, to be nonfunctional.
4. The whole family is implicated, but in a variety of ways.
5. The full capacities that are partly latent provide potentials for creative and functional transformations in persons and in the family as a whole.
6. Changes in persons are not sufficient to achieve the family potential but must be complemented by changes in the family as a whole.
7. The therapist creates a setting and supports the process of the family changing their interactions. The therapist does not direct the process, for the script and the performance would then be his or her creation, reducing the family's self-direction, sense of accomplishment, and unique integration.
8. The therapist strives to gain and maintain clarity about his or her functions in order to prevent a slipping into family roles and a disrupting of the family by joining it, though this can be done. If it does happen, then the family must suffer through an unnecessary and unproductive process of the therapist's final disengagement from the family group.

7. Reorientation of the Family

When the therapist and family have fulfilled their respective roles, dramatic changes in the family usually are observable. Effective working through of hostility opens new interaction and communication between the parents and children, among the siblings, and between the spouses. Concomitant behavioral changes accompany the development of renewed communication: (1) an increased fluency in the conversation, with everyone taking part; (2) an increase in active listening; (3) open discussion of roles required or permitted in the family; (4) increased understanding of the function of individual symptoms within the family; (5) shared responsibility for family problems, instead of the previous pattern of scapegoating one or more members; and (6) communication reflecting love and respect within the family, signifying a strengthening of the family bonds and boundaries.

The family, which prior to therapy may have been factious, begins to operate again or anew as a functioning unit. Old stereotypes, roles, and acts are challenged and through interactive processes the family members come to view themselves differently. When this reorientation is complete and the above goals and behaviors have been achieved to a functional degree, both family and therapist regard therapy as no longer needed, and termination is arranged.

In evaluation, it is recognized that this mode of therapy is not suitable for all therapists. It was, however, developed on the base of my own person, and is most operative for me.

8. Family Context Therapy

In my work of later years I have shifted much of my attention from the outpatient populations where family therapy originated and has been conducted most frequently. In 1963, at the suggestion of the director of the National Institute of Mental Health, for whom I was then working, I turned to the family situation of those who are hospitalized rather than receiving treatment on an outpatient basis. I was directed to examine primarily the possibilities of family therapy with such populations, and especially for those who are chronically ill with schizophrenia. Little was being done with family therapy among such populations; many persons remained hospitalized rather than receiving treatment on an outpatient basis. Typically, in fact, the patients were ostracized by family and community.

The disparity between the success of family therapy in the community and in the hospital suggested that patients in the latter setting were unsuitable for family therapy, had not been offered sufficient family therapy, or needed some alternative forms of family involvement, treatment, and relations. Few models were available; none were particularly successful; and the psychiatric community generally was skeptical about the prospects for family treatment of such hospitalized patients, though some successes with schizophrenics treated on an outpatient basis were reported.

In my scouting around I came across a report of a family-oriented mental hospital in India (Kohlmeyer & Fernandes, 1963) and it was proposed by the director of the National Institute of Mental Health (NIMH) that I visit and report on this hospital. In view of the expense I volunteered to find out if other hospitals in India or elsewhere abroad involved the families of patients and discovered that the practice was widespread (in about two-thirds of the nations of the world), but never had been studied and systematically reported. Accordingly, I was commissioned by NIMH to investigate this practice on a wide scale, and in 1964–65 visited about 150 hospitals in Africa and Asia to observe and report on the family activities (Bell, 1970). Not only did the family involvement in these hospitals intrigue me, it suggested possible ways by which families could remain integrated with their members who were hospitalized.

This study turned my attention to efforts to integrate families more effectively into mental hospitals, general hospitals, and other institutions. From the technical point of view, hospitals in the Western world obviously are advanced in comparison to most hospitals in the developing countries. From a social perspective, however, only in most recent years has systematic hospital attention been given to the involvement of families, although in earlier times families were included more actively in hospitals. It is a matter of pride to me that I have been a part of the effort to change the family culture from the earlier days of a new movement toward family inclusion in hospitals. The roots of the recent changes in the Western world were planted over 50 years ago with the attention given to children in English hospitals by Sir James Spence (1946), and later by Bowlby (1949, 1952) and Robertson (1958, 1963) among others. By the 1950s, when family therapy was just beginning, an international movement toward parental involvement with children in hospitals was well in progress. Only token attention was given, however, to the families of adult patients, although their permission to visit has a long history.

The investment of staff time in planning and developing programs for the families of patients has reached many hospitals and is being developed in orderly ways. I count my own work in the developing countries, and in application of the principles and practices discovered there, as a major contribution to family well-being in relation to institutional care.

To take the observations in hospitals in the developing countries and attempt to apply their precedents directly here would generally be foolhardy. Family structures and hospital conditions there do not match our conditions here, although some hospitals, particularly the teaching hospitals at universities and some of the large urban hospitals abroad, would fit equally well into the Western world. It was, however, most often in unlikely places—a small clinic far out in the bush in Africa, an overcrowded mental hospital in tents in India, a ward for the tubercular on the slopes of Kilimanjaro, a family self-help ward for premature babies in South Africa—that some of the most telling lessons about family involvement were realized (Bell, 1970). I initiated an effort to import some of these practices.

A mental transformation of the lessons from these hospitals was required before the development of derivative applications in the West was possible. The principle characterizing the observed example was extracted and then used as the base for devising applications pertaining to our hospitals.

The sequence of experiments was as follows:

1. The first experiment grew out of observations of various kinds of living arrangements for families at hospitals, all the way from allowing them to share the patient's space to sleeping on a cot in a tent or living in a hostel, as in the Harari Hospital in Salisbury, Zimbabwe, where a former but no longer used nurses' residence was converted into living quarters for families. In the first workshop based on the African-Asian observation, I showed a slide of this residence and the idea was caught by one of the participants, the director of the Children's Hospital at Stanford. He was just beginning to determine prospective uses for a recently vacated nurses' residence on the grounds. The idea of a center for the families of patients caught his imagination and he began to develop the concept. It was applied first in the former nurses' residence, but ultimately grew into the Ronald McDonald Residence, the forerunner of an extensive chain of such facilities built or now being constructed in various parts of the country.

2. The second development involved the construction of a home-like experimental unit at the Stanford Medical School and Hospital (Sasano, Shepard, Bell, Davies, Hansen, & Sanford, 1977). This unit was organized to provide family training prior to discharge of a newly handicapped patient and for education of students toward a family orientation rather than an exclusive patient-centered training. A hospital patient and his or her family moved into the constructed home three days prior to discharge, and care of the patient was turned over to the family. Medical staff of all necessary kinds served as consultants and teachers for the family, rather than providing direct services. This project, which ran for seven years, had a major impact on the concern of the hospital for families

at the time of transition from the hospital back to the community. Its example has spread arious forms to other hospitals across the nation.

This represents modification of only one phase of hospitalization, treatment, and care. It is beyond emergency care at the time of the first shock of illness, a time when families are critically involved, but so centered on the patient's problems and the securing of the earliest and most direct service for him or her that family considerations are to a major extent set aside or thrust upon others. Soon, however, issues of family as well as patient reconstitution begin to assert themselves, often in the basic elements of actual physical survival: food, heat, transportation, sanitation, and so on. There is a long history of provision of support services for families during this immediate crisis period—much of it on an informal basis. In large urban centers where families may be more isolated, a variety of support networks by both professional and lay persons is present and proliferating. Most of these services may be regarded as in the area of family interventions and therapy.

3. A small home for severely disabled veterans was founded on a new principle of placement learned in a rehabilitation village in Northern Thailand (Bell, McDonough, & Toepfer, 1976). A rented home was secured and patients were selected on the following bases: (*a*) None had families available to help in community placement. (*b*) All had severe enough illnesses or disabilities that they were hospitalized full time and had no prospects other than to remain in a hospital for the rest of their days. (*c*) Each patient had to have a different diagnosis than any of the others. (*d*) The handicaps of each patient had to be compensated by assets available elsewhere in the group.

The selection of the patients for the home was difficult. All were hospitalized at the Palo Alto Veterans Administration (VA) Hospital. Medical staff were reluctant to release some of them from the hospital. Skeptics were certain that the absence of live-in staff would lead to failure of the living arrangements and require rehospitalization of patients who would then be in worse shape.

But the principles behind the project proved generally sound, although a patient or two had to return to the hospital and was replaced by others. Some moved on from the home into other community settings of their own choice.

This project represented family treatment of a new kind: construction of a "family" to provide a self-help social setting in the community for the care of severely disabled hospital patients who were virtually completely isolated from their families of origin, although the effect of community living for some of the patients led to restoration of ties with families of origin, as though living in the community rather than in the hospital was a mark of normalcy in place of pathology.

4. My moving in 1973 into a hospital setting full time allowed my developing, supporting, or extending a whole range of new programs, services, and philosophies of family–hospital integration. I worked collaboratively with staffs who were being helped to envision wider roles for families in the hospital. Through this I gained a broader vision of the practical and therapeutic goals that could be reached through the involvement of families. Having been given a mandate to concern myself with the family–hospital relations and the freedom to initiate or facilitate new programs and activities in these directions, I was able to move on many fronts.

Some of the projects that were initiated were as follows:

1. Educational efforts with staffs of various units to widen their perspectives on the place of families in the hospital and some of the potential developments in family involve-

ment that could be initiated. For example, the reconstitution of family ties with long hospitalized, mostly elderly patients was facilitated through the simple device of family open-house days on wards, where families were invited to provide a favorite dessert of the patient or of the family. Since such open houses were rare, the staff, even the dietician, were willing to look the other way as a patient on a restricted diet sampled the family treats in a trade of social values for nutrition. A family therapist might ask if this is "treatment." The question would be irrelevant to the patient who had not seen his family for five years and at last was reunited with them for an afternoon and perhaps, as happened with some, gradually reintegrated into the family.

2. Rewriting of the protocol for staff that governs visiting at the hospital. The basic memorandum, issued every three years, had become more and more protective of staff and had gained a negative tone about family visiting, emphasizing all the restrictions that the hospital was imposing—limits on days and hours of visiting, prerogatives of staff in preventing various "intrusions" on hospital routines, protections for the staff, and so on. Such memoranda might seem innocuous to a casual reviewer, but in use they become the basis for limits and controls that often are instituted to take care of a single case and then applied widely to the detriment of larger populations. Is it family "therapy" to engineer the rewriting of such protocols to emphasize the positive benefits of family? in a classic sense, no; in an extended framework, emphatically yes.

3. In former years the Veterans Administration hospitals have not always lent themselves easily to community rehabilitation of patients. Many factors, including the priority standards for admission and the financial benefits from service-connected hospitalization, may account for this. These hospitals have been directing their efforts increasingly to the prevention of long-term hospitalization. I have been a part of the planning and consultation staff for such care programs. This has allowed me to direct staff attention especially to the resources in families for continuing care of persons who earlier might have been hospitalized for long periods and thus become integrated into the hospital community. Consultation to staff in the Palo Alto Hospital Nursing Care facility and in the Senior Day Care Center has facilitated their developing programs of day care and extended but yet time-limited respite for families of patients who in earlier days would have been fully hospitalized indefinitely. Similarly, within the same unit, the development of an hospice allows family members to maintain responsibilities for and lively communication with patients and staff during the days or months of a terminal illness. The family part goes much beyond visiting and enters direct care, formerly the province of nursing staff who now assume consulting and supporting roles for both family and patient as well as providing care that is beyond family capacities.

The growth of family involvement and concern in the VA in the past decade has been dramatic, and the momentum of the Regional Blind Rehabilitation and the Spinal Cord Injury Centers has brought family members to the hospital for orientation to treatment, instruction about the changes produced through treatment, and effective planning for placement and rehabilitation. Now units of service throughout the whole hospital are modifying their programs to include families.

Impetus has been given to these developments by a national effort whereby 104 new positions were created in 1977 to promote family therapy and personnel were placed in these positions throughout the total system of VA hospitals and clinics.

One of these positions at the Palo Alto VA Hospital was assigned to a team of professionals devoting themselves to followup of psychiatric inpatients for six weeks after they had returned to their homes. As consultant to the program I gained rich insights into the practical complexities that face patients returning to the community and the need to have staff to mobilize helping resources there to tide the family over the multiple domestic and community crises during this period, as restabilization of the patient, family, and community is being sought and developed.

Ultimately my family efforts alone and in collaboration with others led to my constructing a new paradigm for family therapy, to which I have given the name *Family Context Therapy*. The basic aim is to "modify the family *environment* so as to solve family problems and promote beneficial family growth" (Bell, 1978, p. 111). Rather than treating the family directly, the family context therapist becomes involved with changing the environment of the family toward the target of improved family functioning. Such interventions may range all the way from improving circumstances for one patient whereby the family is drawn closer, to managing or assisting the reprogramming of central components of a total institution in order to facilitate and improve family relations.

The last 31 years of my professional life have been devoted primarily to the invention and promotion of new family developments. These activities range from working with a single family in therapy to modifying total institutions for family orientation and operations. In my semiretirement hopefully my health and energies will permit me to continue in the invention and extension of such professional efforts. If not, the momentum developed through my work and that of an array of colleagues whom I have taught, counseled with, consulted to, and challenged, will promote further the health and well-faring of families and of the family as an ever changing institution.

9. References

Ackerman, N. W. *Psychodynamics of family life: Diagnosis and treatment of family relationships.* New York: Basic Books, 1958.

Bell J. E. Family group therapy: A method for the psychological treatment of older children, adolescents, and their parents. *Public Health Monograph No. 64.* Washington, D.C.: United States Government Printing Office, 1961.

Bell, J. E. Family group therapy: A new treatment method for children. *American Psychologist,* 1953, 515T, *Family Process,* 1967, *6,* 254–263.

Bell, J. E. Recent advances in family group therapy. *Journal of Child Psychology and Psychiatry,* 1962, *3,* 1–15.

Bell, J. E. A theoretical position for family group therapy. *Family Process,* 1963, *2,* 1–14.

Bell, J. E. The family group therapist: An agent of change. *International Journal of Group Psychotherapy,* 1964, *14,* 72–83.

Bell, J. E. *The family in the hospital: Lessons from developing countries.* Washington, D.C.: U.S. Government Printing Office, 1970.

Bell, J. E. *Family therapy.* New York: Jason Aronson, 1975.

Bell, J. E. A theoretical framework for family group therapy. In P. J. Guerin (Ed.), *Family Therapy.* New York: Gardner Press, 1976.

Bell, J. E. Family context therapy: A model for family change. *Journal of Marriage and Family Counseling,* 1978, *4,* 111–126.

Bell, J. E. Veterans—their families. In F. Kaslow & R. I. Ridenour (Eds.), *The military family.* New York: Guilford Press, 1983.

Bell, J. E., McDonough, J. M., & Toepfer, H. Achieving community living by preplanned interdependence. *Psychosocial Rehabilitation Journal,* 1976, *1*(1), 7–18.

Bowen, M. *Family therapy in clinical practice.* New York: Jason Aronson, 1978.

Bowlby, J. The study and reduction of group tensions in the family. *Human Relations,* 1949, *2,* 123–128.

Bowlby, J. *Maternal care and mental health* (2nd ed.). Geneva, Switzerland: World Health Organization Monograph No. 2, 1952.

Kohlmeyer, W. A., & Fernandes, X. Psychiatry in India: Family approach in the treatment of mental disorders. *American Journal of Psychiatry,* 1963, *119,* 1033–1037.

Macmurray, J. *The self as agent.* New York: Harper, 1957.

Macmurray, J. *Persons in relation.* New York: Harper, 1961.

Minuchin, S. *Families and family therapy.* Cambridge: Harvard University Press, 1976.

Palazzoli, M. S., Cecchin, G., Prator, G., & Boscolo, L. *Paradox and counterparadox.* New York: Jason Aronson, 1978.

Robertson, J. *Young children in hospitals.* New York: Basic Books, 1958.

Robertson, J. *Hospitals and children: A parent's eye view.* New York: International University Press, 1963.

Sasano, E. M., Shepard, K. F., Bell, J. E., Davies, N. H., Hansen, E. M., & Sanford, T. L. The family in physical therapy. *Physical Therapy,* 1977, *57*(2), 153–159.

Spence, J. C. *The purpose of the family: A guide to the care of children.* London: Epworth Press, 1946.

Watzlawick, P., Weakland, J., & Fisch, R. *Change: Principles of problem formation and problem resolution.* New York: Norton, 1974.

Weakland, J., Fisch, R., Watzlawick, P., & Bodin, A. Brief therapy: Focused problem resolution. *Family Process,* 1974, *13,* 141–168.

13

Behavioral Marital Therapy

GAYLA MARGOLIN

The emergence of behavioral marital therapy, approximately 13 years ago, drew attention primarily for the innovative and distinctive treatment procedures that were introduced. Similar to other theoretical perspectives, behavior therapy originally was applied to a variety of individual problems. Only later, in response to what was perceived as the needs of clients, was it deemed a viable treatment option for marital problems. What behavior marital therapy offered in its early stages of development was a set of orderly, step-by-step procedures for intervening into the complicated, and difficult-to-treat world of marital conflict. Behavior marital therapy's promise for the future was an even more precise technology in which there would be treatment "modules" matched to specific target problems. Although welcomed by some for its precise, systematic, and time-limited technology, this approach was attacked by others for being overly rational, task-oriented, and narrow in focus.

Within the mixed reviews to behavior marital therapy there was a misleading tendency to equate behavioral marital therapy with specific procedures. What distinguishes the behavioral model from other marriage therapies is not its procedures *per se* but its commitment to an integration between clinical and research endeavors (Jacobson & Margolin, 1979; Vincent, 1980). Behavior marital therapy is best described as a method of inquiry, both for analyzing clinical problems and for designing intervention techniques. Clinical observations, whether systematic or serendipitous, prompt theoretical refinements and additional empirical study. Through continued empirical investigation, clinical procedures undergo considerable change over time. A self-corrective process thus ensues from this constant interplay between clinical and research endeavors.

The clinical–empirical integration has important practical implications. First, the interventions themselves are derived from experimentally based principles, primarily from operant learning principles, social exchange principles, and cognitive psychology. Second, there is a strong emphasis on the empirical evaluation and validation of therapeu-

GAYLA MARGOLIN • Department of Psychology—SGM 923, University of Southern California, Los Angeles, California 90089–1061.

tic procedures. Clinical innovation, at least in part, is data based. Third, the behavioral marital therapist uses experimentally based procedures with each couple to understand their behavior and to monitor the effects of the intervention. In other words, there is a detailed evaluation before therapy begins to determine what internal and external influences control the couple's presenting problems. Then, as therapy progresses, there is a continuous monitoring of target problems to ferret out successful from unsuccessful treatment procedures.

The identity of behavioral marital therapy as an empirical approach is inexorably linked to its theoretical underpinnings, namely, the innovative blending of operant learning principles (Skinner, 1963) and social exchange theory (Thibaut & Kelley, 1959). From the operant model comes the perspective that important determinants of behavior are found in the external environment. Thus, the understanding of marital problems requires a careful analysis of behavior–environment relationships to identify antecedent stimuli and consequences that control marital behaviors. What social exchange theory contributes is a model for analyzing how ongoing behavioral exchanges influence long-range outcomes of relationships. Based on the assumption that spouses' behaviors and attitudes incur reward and cost values, relationship satisfaction in marriage can be understood in terms of long-term appraisals of reward/cost ratios. As such, the improvement of unsatisfying marriages rests with identifying potentially rewarding events that are missing and displeasing events that are occurring in excess (Jacobson, 1981a).

These principles initially were applied to distressed marital relationships in the pioneering work of Liberman (1970), Rappaport and Harrell (1972), and Stuart (1969). The early behavior change experiments conducted by these therapists had couples collect data on their own problem behaviors to discover stimuli that set the occasion for undesirable behaviors and consequences that maintained those behaviors. Data on target behaviors also were used to monitor the progress and success of each intervention and, most importantly, to assess the need for changing the treatment course if progress were not satisfactory (Rappaport & Harrell, 1972). The primary treatment component at this early stage of behavioral marital therapy was teaching spouses to use reinforcement principles to produce an environment that was supportive of desirable relationship behavior. It was assumed that having both spouses working simultaneously in this direction would result in a reciprocally rewarding interaction.

In rapid succession to this initial wave of studies came the highly influential work of the marital research team at Oregon (Patterson & Hops, 1972; Patterson, Hops, & Weiss, 1974; Patterson, Weiss, & Hops, 1976; Weiss, Hops, & Patterson, 1973). These researchers proposed and found supporting evidence for the social exchange concept of reciprocity, that is, that over time spouses reward and punish each other at equal rates (Birchler, 1973; Wills, Weiss, & Patterson, 1974). They also found evidence that marital distress was accompanied by lower schedules of reinforcement and higher levels of aversive stimuli (Birchler, Weiss, & Vincent, 1975; Vincent, Weiss, & Birchler, 1975). A further contribution of this group was the hypothesis that marital distress was a function of faulty behavior change operations or what they termed the "coercion process." Coercion occurs when one partner gains compliance or behavior change through actions such as threats, guilt, or abuse or through passive strategies such as withdrawal or the withholding of rewards. In such a process, one person is reinforced for behaving unpleasantly while the other is reinforced for complying. Over time the aversiveness intensifies and there even may be a shift in roles. The unfortunate net result is a general reduction in positive consequences, a reduced frequency in enjoyable social interchanges, and general marital dissatisfaction. The intervention that followed from this formulation had, as one of its major goals, the acquisition of problem-solving skills to be used in the constructive negotiation of behavior change. More generally, the innovative work of the Oregon group led to a multidimensional approach for assessing marital relationships, including self-report questionnaires, the daily monitoring of pleasing and displeasing events, and the direct observation of problem-solving discussions. The treatment program that was used in conjunction with these assessment procedures involved training to discriminate pleasing and displeasing exchanges, operationalizing requests for change, and negotiating contracts for behavior changes (Weiss *et al.*, 1973).

By the late 1970s and early 1980s, the pioneering stage of behavior marital therapy had been replaced by a period of replication, refinement, and rapproachment. Controlled, between-group designs have been conducted to replicate the earlier uncontrolled case studies and to attempt to identify treatment components responsible for change (e.g., Harrell & Guerney, 1976; Jacobson, 1977a, 1978b; Liberman, Levine, Wheeler, Sanders, & Wallace, 1976). Theoretically speaking, recent developments have been characterized by efforts to integrate social learning views with those derived from other theoretical perspectives. From systems theory has come appreciation for the interdependence in the behavior of marital partners, for the cohesiveness of the marital system, and for therapeutic interventions that "prescribe the symptom" and reframe the problem. Although the social learning approach always has looked upon cognitions as mediators of behavior, increasing attention also is being paid to the role of cognitions in marital dysfunction, that is, unrealistic expectations about marriage, faulty attributions about relationship problems, and negatively skewed perceptual filters that affect how spouses process relationship information (Doherty, 1981a,b; Epstein, 1982; Jacobson, in press; Margolin, Christensen, & Weiss, 1975; Margolin & Weiss, 1978b).

In view of these recent developments, behavioral marital therapy is best thought of as a treatment model in transition (Gurman, 1980). Just as there is no one application of systems theory or psychodynamic theory, there is no singular approach to behavioral marital therapy. This has become exceedingly clear by the differences found among the three separate books on behavioral marital therapy published in the past few years (Jacobson & Margolin, 1979; Liberman, Wheeler, deVisser, Kuehnel, & Kuehnel, 1980; Stuart, 1980).

This chapter has been written to highlight the major principles and applications of behavioral marital therapy and to evaluate how well behavioral marital therapy fulfills its mission as an empirical approach. We turn first to a social learning theory explanation of marital distress. This is followed by a relatively detailed description of procedures for assessing and treating marital problems. The chapter concludes with a brief look at research examining the effectiveness of behavioral marital therapy.

1. Concomitants of Marital Distress

Identifying concomitants of marital distress ultimately comes down to the question of what contributes to spouses' subjective feelings of unhappiness and discontent with their marriage. This basic question certainly is not unique to any one theoretical perspective, but choices about which factors are to be explored definitely vary according to theoretical assumptions about marital distress. The way behavior marital therapists respond to this question reveals an orientation toward interpersonal as opposed to intrapsychic phenomena. Based on the assumption that it is impossible to understand the behavior of one partner independently of the other, the behavioral marital approach explores characteristics of interactions that occur between two marital partners and environmental influences that affect those interactions. Although not ruling out the importance of individual characteristics that each spouse brings to the relationship system, these factors receive attention primarily for their impact on the interaction as opposed to being important variables in their own right.

According to this perspective, the understanding of marital relationships comes from a detailed exploration of the discriminative and reinforcing stimuli that spouses provide for one another and the extent to which such stimuli have either a pleasing or a displeasing effect. Looking first at couples' day-to-day behavioral exchanges, we find that distressed, compared to nondistressed, couples exchange lower rates of pleasing behaviors and higher rates of displeasing behaviors (Birchler *et al.*, 1975; Margolin, 1981b). It also has been discovered that the subjective impact of behavioral events differs for distressed and nondistressed couples. The most consistent finding in this regard is that the occurrence of displeasing behaviors has a stronger negative influence on satisfaction ratings of distressed than nondistressed couples (Jacobson, Waldron, & Moore, 1980; Margolin, 1981b). Thus, distressed couples engage in more negative exchanges and also are more emotionally responsive to such interactions.

Similar findings emanate from analyses of couples' communication in the context of problem-solving discussions. Here again, distressed, relative to nondistressed, couples emit higher rates of punitive unhelpful communications and lower rates of socially reinforcing and task-oriented problem-solving communications (Billings, 1979; Gottman, 1980; Gottman, Markman, & Notarius, 1977; Margolin & Wampold, 1981; Vincent *et al.*, 1975; Vincent, Friedman, Nugent, & Messerly, 1979).

More important, however, is the way that spouses constantly influence one another toward a mutual pattern of rewarding or punishing exchanges. Interactions between spouses reveal a lawfulness or predictability in the way that spouses influence and control one another's behavior. That is, the probability that a rewarding behavior will be emitted is linked to whether a rewarding behavior has just been received. Likewise, a punishing behavior is more likely to occur given that a punishing behavior has been received. This particular phenomenon of marital interaction, namely, for there to be an immediate balancing between spouses in their exchange of positive (or negative) behaviors, has been called reciprocity (Gottman, 1979; Patterson & Reid, 1970). As concomitants of marital distress, we find that reciprocity of negative behavior is more characteristic of distressed than of nondistressed couples (Billings, 1979; Gottman, Notarius, Markman, Bank, Yoppi, & Rubin, 1976; Gottman *et al.*, 1977; Margolin & Wampold, 1981). In other words, distressed spouses are more immediately reactive to negative behavior and demonstrate a tendency to "pay back" all insults and injuries. Reciprocity of positive exchanges, in contrast, is equally characteristic of distressed and nondistressed couples.

Empirical demonstrations of the association between overt behavioral transactions and marital satisfaction have provided an important foundation for behavioral marital therapy and have led to specific intervention strategies, such as behavior exchange procedures, communication training, and problem solving. However, full understanding of these connections requires knowledge of how the spouses themselves interpret the transactions. It is hypothesized that marital satisfaction reflects, in part, spouses' estimations of positive versus negative outcomes from the behavioral transactions. Specifically, spouses are presumed to sum the overall benefits and costs in their marriage and compare this sum to their anticipated cost–benefit ratio and to their expected ratios from alternative relationships (Homans, 1961; Thibaut & Kelley, 1959). These comparisons help to explain the stability of a relationship as well as satisfaction with the relationship.

Introducing questions of how spouses interpret behavioral transactions enters cognitive variables into the model of marital distress. Indeed, recent experimental evidence strongly supports the necessity for examining the attributions and perceptions that spouses impose on their own and the partners' behavior. Data from Gottman and his colleagues (Gottman *et al.*, 1976) indicate that distressed spouses receive messages from the partner more negatively than the partner intended the message to be sent. Nondistressed spouses, in contrast, demonstrate more agreement between how the message was intended and how it actually was received. A follow-up study by Notarius, Vanzetti, and Smith (1981) introduced still another dimension—expectations of how the partner would receive a communication. In accordance with their hypothesis, these investigators found that distressed, compared to nondistressed, couples predicted that the partner would respond more negatively than was, in fact, the actual response. A longitudinal study along the same vein by Markman (1979) perhaps provides the most intriguing findings regarding perceptual measures. Markman found that the way spouses rated the impact of one another's communication was predictive of relationship satisfaction at a 30-month follow-up, thereby demonstrating the first etiological relationship between perceptions of communication and the development of marital distress.

There are, in addition, other cognitive variables presumed to be related to marital distress that have only preliminary or no direct empirical support. It is expected, for example, that distressed, compared to nondistressed, spouses: (a) subscribe to more unrealistic expectations about relationships (Eidelson & Epstein, 1981); (b) attribute more blame to the partner (Doherty, 1981a); (c) have low efficacy expectations about their ability to resolve problems (Doherty, 1981b; Weiss, 1980); and (d) engage in negative tracking, that is, sustaining an acute awareness of undesirable relationship events while being relatively oblivious to positive events. In view of the obvious importance of these cognitive variables, cognitive restructuring and reattributional procedures are becoming more common in behavior marital therapy.

The behavioral and cognitive factors discussed thus far illustrate two important features about the behavioral marital approach to marital distress. First, whether the evidence is experimentally or clinically derived, significant advances in our understanding of marital distress come from comparisons between distressed and nondistressed couples. These comparisons, better known as the "match-to-normal" approach, have provided important leads in the formulation of therapeutic interventions. Yet the approach also has an important drawback: As Gurman and Klein (in press) caution, relying upon nondistressed couples as a basis of comparison simply may reinforce a traditional view of marriage. A second important consideration in the research cited thus far (with the exception of Markman, 1979) is that we have no way of sorting out whether differences between the two groups are antecedents or outcomes of marital distress. All that is known about the processes described here (e.g., positive to negative ratios of behavioral exchange, negative reciprocity, and cognitive misperceptions) is that they are current manifestations of marital distress. The ultimate objective from a preventative perspective is to identify precursors to marital distress. Behavior marital therapists offer a number of ideas that will be discussed below about possible precursors, but these remain speculative in the absence of adequate data.

The presumed antecedents of marital distress that have received most attention in the behavioral marital literature are relationship skills deficits, particularly skills related to conflict resolution. Given the inevitability of conflict in a long-term relationship, couples are distinguished not by the presence or absence of conflict but by the way they respond to it (Jacobson & Margolin, 1979). Couples skilled in handling conflict deal directly and openly with conflictual issues, using problem-solving and behavior change skills to prevent the accumulation of unresolved problems and lingering resentments. Less skilled couples, who either attempt to ignore conflict or who repeatedly analyze but never act on the problem, are likely to experience a cumulative build-up of unexpressed problems that, over time, becomes insurmountable. The less skilled couples also may resort to coercive tactics to bring about change in the partner's behavior. Deficits in problem-solving skills thus play havoc with relationships in two ways: Each new problem-solving attempt creates additional immediate resentment and there is an ever-increasing build-up of unresolved issues.

There also are other skills deficits associated with marital dissatisfaction. Skills related to expressing and receiving emotion-laden material influence the way intimacy is experienced in the relationship. Similarly, skills related to maintaining an enjoyable sexual relationship are important to spouses' overall relationship satisfaction. Various instrumental skills also are necessary, including child-rearing abilities, and household and financial management. Granted, spouses' budgetary skills rarely are the source of a couple's initial attraction. Yet, repeated mismanagement of financial matters can create a desperate marital situation. Skills training, whether for parenting, communication, financial management, or other purposes, is an important component of behavior marital therapy.

However, what at first glance might appear to be a skills deficit instead may be a problem in stimulus control, that is, a deficiency in conditions that set the stage for certain interactions. A couple's communication problems, for example, may not be a skills deficit but a reaction to important conditions regarding the way their lives are structured. For example, if the wife works all day while the husband works at night, communication problems simply may reflect the fact that each spouse makes important decisions without ever consulting the other. Time schedules are a particularly important stimulus condition since they affect spouses' availability for shared activities. Other stimulus conditions worth considering include the amount of privacy afforded in a couple's living quarters, presence of extended family, the predictability of family finances from month to month, and so on. Stimulus control interventions involve altering stimulus conditions so that they are as favorable as possible for a desired outcome.

A slightly different but equally powerful type of stimulus control comes from the rules that govern relationships. Whether the rules are explicit or implicit, relationships are characterized by a complex set of assumptions, such as how labor and responsibilities are divided, what are acceptable sexual activities, how leisure time is planned, when are appropriate times for displays of affection, and who handles the finances. Relationship discord is likely if spouses function under discrepant sets of rules or if the rule structure contains significant gaps necessitating ad hoc decisions (Jacobson & Margolin, 1979).

Another possible precursor to marital distress concerns spouses' reinforcing capabilities for one another. This is not usually an issue in the early stages of a relationship since partners are caught up in the excitement and novelty of a new relationship. However, for some couples there is a process of reinforcement erosion (Jacobson & Margolin, 1979) or a gradual deterioration in spouses' capacities to gratify one another, primarily due to habituation. Spouses who rely on restricted types of rewarding interactions may find that the relationship has become increasingly routinized and dull. Since this is a subtle and gradual process, spouses themselves often are perplexed about the source of their dissatisfaction and question the very basis of their relationship. Couples who effectively counter this satiation process find ways to expand their repertoires of reinforcing interactions by varying their recreational activities, developing and sharing new interests, and learning to communicate in a more intimate manner. Similar strategies must be instigated with couples who suffer satiation with their current relationship reinforcers.

Despite the heavy emphasis in behavioral marital therapy on environmental characteristics of behavior, recognition also is given to spouses' individual differences that lead to relationship difficulties. Marital compatibility can be affected significantly by differences in spouses' preferences for intimacy (versus independence), their liking for intellectually stimulating activities, their varying energy levels, and so on. Whether these individual differences stem from each partner's individual learning history, physiological factors, or cognitive abilities, they play a fundamental role in spouses' attraction for one another as well as their dissatisfaction with one another.

It must be noted that relationships continually are undergoing change. They change from within as they pass through various development stages, such as the birth of a child (Vincent, Cook, & Brady, 1981). These changes obviously require considerable accommodation, including new rules about the distribution of responsibility, previously untapped parenting skills, and adjustment to the new stimulus condition of having less time together as a couple. Relationships also can be changed by outside factors, including health factors and imbalanced career progress, or even larger sociopolitical considerations, such as disadvantageous economic conditions and the women's movement (Jacobson, 1981a). Understanding a particular relationship system requires drawing connections among these various factors; that is, identifying which characteristics of a couple's behavioral exchange, which environment variables, and which individual factors affect marital satisfaction. Below we examine how the behavioral marital therapist addresses those questions.

2. Assessment

The basic objectives of behavioral marital assessment include (a) identifying behaviors in need of change as well as variables that control those behaviors, (b) formulating an appropriate treatment plan, and then (c) evaluating the effectiveness of that plan. For most behaviorists, and particularly for those studying intimacy, the definition of behavior goes beyond overt motor activity and includes cognitive/verbal activities as well as affective/physiological reactions (Nelson & Hayes, 1979). How behaviors are selected to be the target of assessment jointly reflects priorities of the couple and the therapist. Specific complaints that spouses present as the source of their marital stress, for example, lack of affection or too many arguments, constitute one type of assessment target. A careful evaluation of these responses takes the form of a functional analysis to describe accurately the behavior and to identify environmental conditions that elicit and maintain those behaviors. Assessment targets also include relationship processes that the couple does not identify as problematic but that reflect the therapist's formulation of marital distress. That is, there are procedures that examine couples' rewarding and punishing behavioral exchanges in the natural environment, their skill deficits, particularly in the area of conflict resolution, and the ways that they appraise and evaluate the relationship.

In behavioral marital therapy, assessment provides the indispensible link between blanket formulations about what accounts for marital distress and individually designed intervention strategies for a specific couple. Since behavioral marital therapy is grounded in the assumption that therapy is to be tailor-made for each couple, pretreatment assessment holds the key to what ultimately is decided upon as the treatment plan. Rather than presume similar characteristics of distress in all couples seeking therapy, pretreatment assessment data point out differences between distressed couples and direct attention to exigencies that are unique to the individual couple and thus serve as the basis for individualizing treatment plans.

As Gurman (1978) observed, behavioral marital assessment tends to be more formalized than traditional types of assessment. Stemming from its identity as an empirical approach, behavioral marital therapy has made standardized assessment a priority. Typically, the first two or three therapy sessions are primarily, although not exclusively, devoted to assessment. Within that time period, there are structured and unstructured assessment procedures that take place in the therapy sessions in addition to assessment tasks that the couple carries out at home. It is important to note, however, that assessment is not simply a stage preceding the instigation of intervention procedures. The continuation of data collection throughout the duration of therapy makes it possible to infer what aspects of the treatment have been effective.

The task of evaluating the effectiveness of marital therapy is, of course, made difficult by the fact that there is no ultimate measure of relationship success. There are, on the contrary, countless models of what constitutes a successful relationship. Thus, marital assessment cannot presume that there is one criterion response for the construct of marital satisfaction, nor one set of behaviors representing marital distress. The assessment of marital therapy is further complicated by the fact that the two partners rarely have the same goals for therapy; in fact, it is often the case that spouses' separate sets of goals conflict with one another (Margolin, 1982). Inasmuch as couples enter marital therapy with a wide variety of objectives and goals, some of which represent individual as opposed to relationship improvement, the therapist cannot be too closely tied to a singular set of standards for treatment efficacy.

A particular strength of behavioral marital assessment is its multidimensionality. Although limited to the context of relationship improvement, behavioral marital assessment spans a wide variety of behaviors, cognitions, and feelings. Furthermore, the multidimensional approach strives to integrate demands that are unique to each couple with the behavioral marital therapist's formulation of marital distress. This integration has produced four major assessment strategies: the direct sampling of communication, spouse-monitoring of daily interactions, self-report questionnaires, and interview procedures. In the remaining portions of this section, these four strategies will be described briefly in terms of what they contribute to our understanding of couples and to our specification of treatment plans. More comprehensive information about individual assessment procedures can be found in the recent reviews on behavioral marital assessment (cf. Jacob, 1976; Jacobson, Ellwood, & Dallas, 1981; Margolin, 1983; Margolin & Jacobson, 1981; Weiss & Margolin, 1977).

2.1. Direct Sampling of Communication

The direct sampling of behaviors of interest through observational procedures is a hallmark of behavioral assessment. In the general field of behavioral assessment, direct observations of behaviors are obtained by trained observers, by significant others, or by clients observing themselves in either a naturalistic or a controlled setting. In marital assessment, the opportunities for observation by outsiders or by trained observers are relatively limited since marital interactions of importance tend to occur infrequently and unpredictably and to be intimate and private (Bellack, 1979; Margolin & Jacobson, 1981; Patterson *et al.,* 1976). For the most part, the direct sampling of behavior has been confined to what can be observed in the therapy setting. Particular attention has been paid to how spouses handle themselves during sample problem-solving discussions. In addition to objective observations by outsiders, what has taken on tremendous importance in behavioral marital assessment is participant observation, in which spouses observe themselves and one another. Participant observation refers, on the one hand, to immediate observations made during an ongoing interactional sample, for example, during a problem-solving discussion. Participant observation also has been used to obtain a more generalized accounting of spouses' behaviors over wide-ranging activities that occur during the course of an entire day.

2.1.1. Outsiders' Observations of Problem-solving Discussions

The rationale for directly observing samples of couples' problem-solving skills has theoretical as well as methodological origins. As indicated previously, social learning theory identifies deficits in problem-solving skills as an important precursor to marital distress. Methodologically, the direct sampling of problem-solving discussions through observational techniques is deemed preferable to relying on spouses' retrospective, and most likely distorted impressions of how they discuss problems. The assessment procedure standardly used for obtaining communication samples is for spouses to spend approximately 10 minutes in uninterrupted discussion about a conflictual issue of their choosing. Specific instructions for this discussion range from the vague injunction "Discuss this topic" to the more deliberate "Discuss this topic as you would discuss it at home" or "Work toward resolution of this conflict." Audiotaping, or preferably videotaping, allows for detailed observations at a later time. Although this assessment task typically has been conducted in the therapy setting, audiotapes also can be made at home, which, according to Gottman (1980), may prove to be a more realistic sample of couples' interactions.

Observations of brief communication samples are, of course, plagued by problems of reactivity (e.g., Is the couple's behavior influenced by the fact that they are being observed or by the demand characteristics associated with beginning or ending therapy?) and questions of generalizability (e.g., Are the samples of behavior representative of what might occur under naturalistic conditions?). Despite these constraints, useful information emerges about how the couple defines a problem, whether they offer specific solutions, and, if so, how the suggestions are received and how affect is expressed. These discussions also offer important information about repetitive communication patterns, for example, what does one partner do that serves as an antecedent for constructive versus destructive problem solving by the other?

When used as a treatment outcome measure or for other empirical purposes, data from these discussions are quantified through complex coding systems. The two predominant systems that have been developed are the Marital Interaction Coding System (Hops, Wills, Patterson, & Weiss, 1972) and the Couples' Interaction Coding System (Gottman, 1979). In both of these systems, observers are trained to code in as objective a manner as possible. The Hops *et al.* (1972) system contains 30 behavioral categories spanning verbal (e.g., problem solution, criticism) and nonverbal behaviors (e.g., smile/laugh, not tracking). In Gottman's system, each behavioral unit is assigned one of eight content codes (e.g., disagreement, problem information) and one of three affect codes (positive, negative, or neutral). The principal value of these coding systems comes from their representation of the ongoing sequential patterning of behavior. The systems not only provide information on how often specific behaviors occur. They also are used to determine whether specific patterns, such as negative reciprocity, are present.

Whether there is a formal examination of problem solving through structured coding systems or an informal examination through careful listening, information from these discussions bears directly on the therapist's treatment plan. Occasionally it becomes obvious that the spouses display adequate conflict resolution skills, which obviate the need for problem-solving training in therapy. The more likely outcome, however, is that the discussion helps to pinpoint specific strengths in the couple's problem-solving attempts, for example, creative solutions or a good sense of humor, as well as their particular problems, for instance, vague problem definitions, inaccurate listening skills, and a limited view of options.

2.1.2. Participant Observation of Problem-solving Discussions

When analyzing patterns of how one behavior leads to another which leads to a third behavior and so on, spouses' interpretations of each action may be viewed as the essential link between behaviors. Is it the behavior *per se* that is problematic or is the interpretation of the behavior distorted? What complicates this analysis are the multiple levels of cognitive processing that occur simultaneously. For each action, there is a sender and receiver, each of whom has a perception of that behavior, as well as a metaperspective perception, that is, "how I see you seeing me."

Assessing spouses' ongoing perceptions of their interactions is a relatively new dimension in behavioral marital assessment but one that is growing in importance. The primary thrust thus far has been for spouses to rate, at frequent intervals, their reactions to each communication along a five-point scale from supernegative to superpositive. This procedure was pioneered by Gottman and his colleagues who had spouses rate both the impact of messages received and the intent of messages sent. Used primarily for research purposes, these procedures have shown that perceptions of communication deficits, as measured through impact ratings, are associated with the development and maintenance of marital distress (Gottman *et al.*, 1976; Markman, 1979). In an interesting alternative to the procedures described above, which require interval ratings, Knudson, Sommers, and Golding (1980) periodically would interrupt the videotape playback of an interaction and have spouses independently discuss their ongoing impressions. Both the Gottman *et al.* (1976) and Knudson *et al.* procedures elicit information that is unavailable to outside observers by assessing the attributions and personalized meanings that spouses assign to their interactions. These procedures, when used clinically, help spouses to become careful observers of their own behaviors and to operationalize what they find helpful in problem discussions (Margolin & Weiss, 1978a).

2.2. Spouse Monitoring of Daily Interactions

Having spouses become careful observers of critical incidents in their everyday interaction is essential to the behavioral aims of: (a) modifying couples' behavioral exchange; (b) understanding environmental influences of couple behavior; and (c) identifying links between cognitions, behavior, and affect. To a certain extent this type of monitoring goes on in all forms of marital therapy. What is unique to behavioral marital assessment is the use of systematic procedures for monitoring and recording observations at regular intervals. The questions explored by spouse monitoring instruments reflect an assumption of circular causality between internal and external processes: How do the events that comprise spouses' daily interactions affect their impressions about their relationship? Or, alternatively, how do overall appraisals about a relationship influence the way spouses behave in the relationship?

Of the major procedures for collecting data in the home, the Spouse Observation Checklist (SOC) (Patterson, 1976; Weiss, 1978) is used most frequently and has the most supporting data. Working from the assumption that marital relationships are comprised of instrumental behaviors, expressive–affectionate behaviors, and companionship events, the marital research group in Oregon devised a 400-item listing of representative pleasing and displeasing behaviors that span 12 separate categories, including companionship, affection, sex, communication, consideration, coupling activities, household management, finances, parenting, employment, personal habits, and independence. Spouses independently read through the entire checklist each night before retiring and place a check mark indicating which events occurred during the previous 24 hours. Spouses also indicate their satisfaction with the relationship for that day by using a 1-9 rating scale, ranging from totally dissatisfied to totally satisfied.

The SOC has proven to be an invaluable tool for the marital therapist. Its most obvious use is to provide information on overall frequencies of pleasing and displeasing events across many domains of interaction. From this, the therapist readily can perceive the absence of certain desirable behaviors and the presence of undesirable behaviors. In addition to sheer frequencies of behavior, the SOC also can be used to examine what types of behaviors positively or negatively affect marital satisfaction. That is, SOC data are a good basis for formulating hypotheses about what specific behaviors, either through their presence or absence, are associated with fluctuations in spouses' daily satisfaction ratings. Careful inspection of SOC data for associations between behavior and satisfaction ratings helps to identify important intervention targets, that is, targets that are likely to affect satisfaction, and points out how each partner could be more effective in pleasing one another. Demonstrations of an association between behavior and satisfaction also show spouses just how much control they have in the relationship, providing evidence to counter their feelings of futility and lack of efficacy. Finally, the SOC also can be used to monitor the ongoing progress of therapy since, by continually checking SOC recordings throughout the treatment period, the therapist can observe change in areas targeted for intervention (Jacobson, 1981a).

Although the SOC evaluates seemingly mundane dimensions of marital interaction, there is substantial empirical evidence for the validity of this type of detailed analysis of relationship behaviors. Comparisons between distressed and nondistressed couples, for example, indicate that distressed couples report fewer pleasing and more displeasing behaviors. Please: displease ratios are approximately 4:1 for distressed and 12:1 to 30:1 for nondistressed couples (Birchler *et al.*, 1975; Margolin, 1981b). The data further demonstrate that there is an association between spouses' behavioral exchanges as recorded on the SOC and their impressions of marital satisfaction (Jacobson *et al.*, 1980; Margolin, 1981b; Wills *et al.*, 1974). As one would expect, there is a positive correlation between pleasing behaviors and daily satisfactions and a negative association between displeasing behaviors and satisfaction. Additionally, it has been found that the significance of specific content categories (e.g., sex, companionship, household activities) varies according to gender and level of marital adjustment.

In contrast to the SOC which strives for breadth of information, other self-monitoring procedures have the spouses observe and record specific types of interactions. The Interactional Record (Peterson, 1977, 1979; Protzner, King, & Christensen, 1981), for example, has spouses independently identify the most important interaction that occurred each day. They are to describe (a) the conditions under which the exchange took place, including setting and feelings; (b) how the interaction started; and (c) what happened from start to finish. These records then are coded in terms of affect ("I hate you") and construal ("I think it was your fault that our bank account is overdrawn") and expectations that each partner held in regard to the subsequent response of the other. Another procedure, the Marital Satisfaction Time Lines (Williams, 1979), has spouses rate time segments as positive, neutral, or unpleasant and then report on the most and least pleasant behaviors that occurred during the morning, afternoon, or evening.

In addition to these structured procedures, a self-monitoring format can be devised to assess almost any individualized complaint that a couple presents. What one strives for with these procedures is to learn how the specific complaint fluctuates over time and to discover what factors account for the fluctuations. As Margolin and Weinstein (1983) suggest, a couple who complain of feeling emotionally distant can be instructed to examine this feeling by rating emotional closeness versus distance at given intervals during the day and by monitoring the situational variables that seem pertinent to each rating. Factors that consistently influence feelings of closeness versus distance will emerge and then can be taken into account when engineering an intervention to enhance emotional closeness.

2.3. Self-Report Questionnaires

Despite the emphasis on direct observation in behavioral assessment, self-report questionnaires still play an important role in the assessment of marital dysfunction. The questionnaires are used to evaluate global, relatively stable dimensions of marital adjustment that do not reflect moment-to-moment or daily fluctuations. Since these measurements are well validated and have already established norms, they offer a quick, inexpensive way of comparing couples to one another or comparing the same couple across time. On the negative side, these instruments are limited in what they contribute to the actual planning of an intervention as well as by their susceptibility to demand characteristics and social desirability factors.

The two most widely used instruments to measure global marital satisfaction are the Marital Adjustment Scale (Locke & Wallace, 1959) and the more recent Dyadic Adjustment Scale (Spanier, 1976). Reliability and validity studies have indicated that these two instruments are internally consistent and accurate discriminators between satisfied and dissatisfied couples. Based on their psychometric properties and the fact that they are accepted measures of the general construct of marital adjustment, these instruments are popular choices as screening measurements, as treatment outcome measurements, and as criterion measures for examining the validity of other instruments (Margolin & Jacobson, 1981). Other self-report instruments include the Areas of Change Questionnaire (Weiss *et al.*, 1973) which asks couples to indicate which of 34 behaviors they would like to see changed as well as how much change is desired and the direction of that change; the Marital Status Inventory (Weiss & Cerreto, 1975), a Guttman scaling of steps toward divorce; and the Marital Pre-Counseling Inventory (Stuart & Stuart, 1972), a comprehensive instrument to measure behavior change goals, resources for change, and the degree of mutual understanding between spouses.

2.4. Interview

The interview serves several important functions in behavioral marital assessment. It is an excellent opportunity to observe how the spouses interact, that is, how they present their problems to the therapist and how they relate to one another. Does one take the lead? How do they handle disagreements? How much warmth do they express toward one another? The intake interview also may be used to probe actively the spouses' interaction with the objective of evaluating the range and flexibility of their response repertoire, for example, assessing their verbal facility, their self-awareness, and their responsiveness to therapeutic directives.

In addition to what it offers as an observational device, the interview also is an opportunity for gathering information that is not obtained elsewhere. Despite the extensive array of assessment instruments in the behavioral marital therapist's armamentarium, a number of questions important to our understanding of marital adjustment remain virtually untapped. A priority for behavioral marital assessment, for example, is the identification of relationship strengths. Strengths in communication processes are evident from observing problem-solving samples and strengths in certain other relationship domains are notable in the SOC data. However, it is equally important to find out what the spouses themselves perceive as relationship as well as personal strengths, which is a question that is overlooked in structured assessment procedures. Second, further clarification generally is needed to understand global relationship patterns. To understand the common attack–withdrawal pattern, for example, requires knowing what provokes each stage of the cycle, how each partner contributes to the escalation and deescalation of conflict, and how the cycle eventually abates. Third, it is important to assess what precipitated the couple's decision to enter therapy: Was there a crisis? Had they been in therapy previously? What do they expect to achieve through therapy? Is therapy the last effort before ending the marriage or has the decision to end the marriage already been made? (Weiss & Birchler, 1978). Fourth, the developmental history of the relationship is necessary in order to identify historical antecedents of the current distress (Jacobson & Margolin, 1979). What has the couple done to accommodate to transitions from one development stage to another? What factors initially attracted the partners to one another? Fifth, what are the rules or expectations that govern the relationship (Birchler & Spinks, 1980; Weiss, 1978)? To what degree do spouses agree on these rules? Finally, what changes have occurred in spouses' lives outside of the relationship that make the marriage more or less attractive (Thibaut & Kelley, 1959)? Has either spouse experienced recent changes in employment, health, or in relationships with family or friends?

Although behavioral marital therapists generally hold off structured interventions until pretreatment assessment has been completed, initial interviews do serve important treatment as well as assessment functions. As Jacobson and Margolin (1979) assert, "the most desirable goal of an initial interview is not to gather assessment information but rather to set the stage for therapeutic change by building positive expectancies and trust in the couple, and by actually providing them with some benefits" (p. 51). Whatever therapeutic tone is set in that initial interview can have tremendous impact on what is to come. When the first session is structured as a forum for constructive as opposed to blaming interactions, couples leave it feeling they have benefited. This, then, is likely to reduce their fears about therapy and to create positive expectancies about continuing in therapy. It also is likely to increase couples' compliance with the other, more structured data collection procedures. It is hypothesized that characteristics of enthusiasm, confidence, and control are essential to the therapist in establishing a constructive therapeutic atmosphere and for generating cooperative, optimistic reactions in the couple (Jacobson & Margolin, 1979). Thus, in addition to demonstrating sensitivity to the couple's pain, the therapist must be able to keep the session focused, retain a sense of humor, and communicate confidence in his or her ability to be of help to the couple.

The two- to three-week period of evaluation concludes with an interpretive meeting during which findings from the assessment data and an overview of the treatment are presented. The therapist delineates both the strengths and the problems of the relationship, suggesting possible antecedents for the latter. A treatment plan that follows directly from the summarization of problems is proposed and discussed (Jacobson & Margolin, 1979). This session also is time for the therapist to express optimism about the outcome of marital therapy, while simultaneously conveying the message that hard work by the couple is the key to successful outcomes.

3. Treatment

Speaking globally, there are two general goals of behavior marital therapy: to increase the couple's experience of intimacy and to disrupt the negative, destructive patterns associated with recurrent conflicts. The development of problems in each of these broad domains certainly is not independent: Destructive patterns of anger, for example, are likely to detract from feelings of intimacy. Yet, it cannot be presumed that an intervention directed to one or the other of these goals necessarily generalizes to the other. As Weiss (1978) so cogently summarized, "The reduction in rate of aversive behaviors merely reduces dissatisfaction but does not in itself add to satisfaction. If all annoyances fell to zero rate/hour, one would be quiescent but not necessarily satisfied; soporific drugs might accomplish the same end" (p. 199). Likewise, although helping couples to experience feelings of closeness and to enjoy each other's company is, in itself, a significant therapeutic gain, this step may have no bearing on unresolved disagreements. If anything, the unresolved conflicts simply will wear away at the renewed feelings of intimacy. Thus, couples presenting both types of problems require therapy that takes each objective into account.

In order to accomplish either of the broadly stated objectives the therapist must choose a level at which to intervene. In the early days of behavioral marital therapy, that decision was quite easy; the intervention would be directed to overt behavioral transactions based on the assumption that changes in perceptual processes automatically would follow. Although overt behaviors remain the primary target of intervention, it is recognized at this point that interventions sometimes are better directed to cognitions (Birchler & Spinks, 1980; Doherty, 1981b; Epstein, 1982; Margolin & Weiss, 1978b; Weiss, 1980) and to affective processes (Margolin & Weinstein, 1983).

3.1. Increasing Intimacy and Positive Interaction

Aside from cases in which negative interaction patterns between spouses are too dangerous or devastating to ignore even temporarily, an increase in positive interaction often proves to be an effective opening step in behavioral marital therapy. This step is a powerful attention-getter. Focusing for so long on what is wrong with the marriage, the couple generally approaches therapy assuming it is a time to labor in earnest on serious problems. Strategies to increase intimacy are designed instead to put the couple in touch with good things that can occur in the marriage by challenging them to experiment with more positive sorts of interaction. As an unexpected opening step, this strategy tends to jar spouses out of entrenched positions and to set the stage for the more difficult issues that lie ahead.

When enacting such strategies, the therapist's objective is to improve the overall emotional tone of the marriage rather than to resolve any one specific problem. Such a decision comes from having a good grasp of what the specific problems entail but determining that, for the moment, attention to the couple's overall emotional well-being supercedes the resolution of a particular conflict area. This message translates to the couple that the hard work of relationship improvement also can be a time for playfulness, imagination, and humor. Thus, the key therapeutic atmosphere for implementing this message is what Tiesmann (1979) describes as "serious playfulness," in that the serious responsibility of effecting change at times incorporates dimensions that may be frivolous or illogical.

The common denominator of interventions to increase intimacy is that they require spouses to engage in activities at home between sessions. As Jacobson concludes (1981b), "The ultimate goal is that spouses are actively involved in a sustained effort to improve the relationship. Rather than having the therapist decide what each spouse should do, it matters only that they do something to improve the relationship—particularly during the early stages of therapy" (p. 10). The activity chosen generally is directed to discovering new ways to increase spouses' reinforcing capabilities for one another. The dimensions along which intervention strategies vary is the extent to which the therapist actually determines what specific steps will occur as opposed to leaving the final decisions to the spouses.

A frequently adopted strategy (Jacobson, 1981a,b; Jacobson, Berley, Newport, Elwood, & Phelps, in press; Jacobson & Margolin, 1979) is having spouses be behavior analysts in regard to their own relationship by expanding upon the assessment task in which they use the SOC to track daily satisfaction ratings and daily frequencies of pleases and displeases. This intervention requires spouses to study the partner's checklist to learn which of their own behaviors has a functional impact on the other's subjective satisfaction. In other words, the spouses are to attempt to identify characteristics of their own behavior that differentiate whether the partner is relatively satisfied or dissatisfied with the day. These observations, once discussed in the therapy session, are then put to a direct test. Actually increasing the frequency of actions each spouse believes to impact positively on the partner should result in increased satisfaction for the partner, as measured by satisfaction ratings on the SOC. Jacobson maintains that the success of this intervention depends upon spouses having maximum degrees of freedom in choosing what to increase. By determining for themselves what to increase spouses are not forced to concede to the partner's demand. This increases the likelihood of the assignment being carried out and reduces the potential for devaluating attributions, for example, "She did it because just because I asked her to" (Jacobson, in press). In making these assignments, the therapist will find that some spouses can be encouraged to put forth the necessary efforts in the spirit of collaboration. For others, it is more effective to issue a competitive challenge, saying, for example, "We find in our work with couples that they often lose touch with how to make each other happy. They think they know what the other person wants, but it turns out that they are wrong. Let's see if you can do it'' (Jacobson, 1981, p. 570). The goal, in either case, is to get each partner to prove how much she or he knows about making the other happy.

Weiss *et al.* (1973), Stuart (1980), and Margolin and Weinstein (1983) instigate similar interventions with their respective ''love days,'' ''caring days,'' and ''consideration'' interventions, which are prespecified times for spouses to increase the number of pleasing actions that they emit. In Stuart's technique, spouses identify for one another, in the form of requests, specific small behaviors that they would like to receive. Spouses then commit themselves to a certain number of requests per day. Weiss's procedure calls for dramatic increases of pleasing actions, that is, doubling one's usual rate on a certain day during the week. Margolin and Weinstein's procedure asks spouses to show consideration at least once a day and to keep a record of these actions.

Each of the procedures discussed thus far falls under the rubric of behavior exchange techniques and is designed to foster a more favorable exchange of pleasing behaviors. In such techniques, relationship enhancement comes about by having spouses engage in either affectionate gestures, for example, back rubs or leaving notes for one another, or instrumental activities, such as stacking up the newspapers or filling the car with gasoline. For successful implementation of the procedures, it is recommended that the actions be highly specific and that they avoid the key conflictual relationship issues. A secondary benefit of the procedures is that spouses learn the importance of making requests to one another rather than presuming that the partner simply can intuit what is wanted. In learning to express requests in a precise and direct manner, spouses often find that vague injunctions such as ''Give me more attention'' translate into a request as specific and simple as ''Ask me how my day went.'' The more narrowly defined request is, of course, easier for the recipient to accept and increases the likelihood that, if implemented, it will fulfill the desired objective.

In contrast to behavior exchange strategies, which have spouses doing activities for one another, other strategies employed by behavior marital therapists have spouses engage in mutually rewarding experiences to enhance their experience of intimacy. These interventions include any experience that heightens spouses' shared affective experience. The objective of these interventions is to supply situational variables that lessen the emotional distance that is reported by distressed couples and thereby overcome problems of reinforcement erosion.

A primary intervention to increase couples' feelings of closeness involves evoking or reevoking core symbols, which are events, places, rituals, or objects that have special meaning in terms of the couple's relationship (Stuart, 1975). These symbols help the spouses get in touch with each other in ways that may have been buried under layers of hostility and discouragement (Liberman *et al.*, 1980). Examples of core symbols include the ritual of reserving Friday nights for each other, wearing special articles of clothing or going to favorite places, celebrating anniversary dinners, or resurrecting long-time private jokes. Whatever the core symbol may be, its importance lies in its mutual and special meaning for the couple.

When couples lack core symbols or have little desire to resurrect old core symbols, the therapist then must help the couple develop new core symbols. Developing mutually enjoyable recreational activities is one way for spouses to come to view each other as discriminative stimuli for pleasure, for example, going dancing on a Saturday night, taking a class in photography together, or learning to play tennis. Undergoing an emotionally moving experience together, such as viewing and discussing an emotion-evoking film, is another way to help spouses discover new sensitivities in one another. Key factors linked to the success of these interventions include seeing that they involve novelty, perhaps even risk taking, and carefully avoid all core conflict areas.

Implementation of these strategies requires strong commitment to their importance on the part of the therapist. Although not denying the reality of the couple's pain, the therapist must strive to minimize negative tracking in order to help the couple focus on positive aspects of the marriage. In the therapy sessions the therapist makes sure that positive aspects of the week, for example, days with high daily satisfaction ratings, receive at least as much attention as low-rated days. Even when faced with a relationship crisis, the therapist still must debrief how the couple handled their homework assignment to increase intimacy, rather than be sidetracked solely to what went wrong that week. In making each assignment, the therapist relentlessly must point out the seriousness of implementing the task and apply the "antisabotage" techniques of Birchler and Spinks (1980), that is, anticipating reasons why they may not carry through on the task and discussing how sabotage behavior will be identified and dealt with. Additionally, it is important that the therapist enthusiastically reinforce positive outcomes and, likewise, that the spouses give credit to one another for making changes. Toward this end, it is helpful for the therapist to build in specific steps so that the spouses themselves focus on what went right during the week and communicate these observations to one another. "Appreciation notes" (Jacobson & Margolin, 1979; Margolin & Weinstein, 1983) is one such procedure whereby spouses inform each other, through the daily exchange of written messages, what they have welcomed and enjoyed in the partner's behavior.

It should be noted that many of the clinical steps outlined here involve cognitive as well as behavioral interventions. Promoting the collaborative spirit that is essential to taking any of these steps toward greater intimacy comes primarily from cognitive restructuring procedures, that is, introducing a focus that implies reciprocal causality and mutual responsibility (Jacobson & Margolin, 1979; Margolin *et al.*, 1975). Toward the same objective, reframing is widely used to point out how being upset with one another actually is a sign of strong affiliative bonds. Why else would spouses' sense of well-being be so dramatically affected by the other person if they did not care greatly about that person (Weiss, 1980)? Secondly, spouses' attributions about requested changes are carefully explored (Epstein, 1982; Jacobson, in press; Jacobson & Margolin, 1979), with particular emphasis placed on the distinction between "intention" and "actions." This attributional "analysis" is designed to interrupt spouses' automatic inferences of malevolent motivation. When further action is required, alternative explanations for undesirable behaviors (other than bad intentions) are given with the aim of lessening the emotional intensity attached to certain behaviors and easing the resistance to making requested changes (Jacobson, in press). Finally, if the procedures to increase intimacy are received positively, this is interpreted as a sign of spouses' commitment to relationship improvement. This attribution is particularly crucial in encouraging continued efforts during the upcoming, still more difficult stages of therapy.

3.2. Disrupting Negative Patterns

Relationship patterns occur on several different levels, ranging from moment-to-moment interactions to patterns that repeatedly unfold over weeks, months, or even years. Problem-solving discussions portray important facets of the moment-to-moment interactions. Molar relationship patterns, which are more difficult to assess, similarly prove to be the source of repeated relationship upheaval. Consider, for example, the familiar pattern in which one spouse's withdrawal elicits resentment and conflict, which triggers efforts toward heightened intimacy, but then, once again, gives way to the withdrawal and a repetition of the entire cycle. Whatever the time span, the focus on patterns makes sequences of interaction the primary point of interest, that is, how one spouse's behavior affects the other spouse, which affects the first spouse and so on. In disrupting negative patterns, it does not suffice simply to decrease the frequency of negative behavior or, alternatively, to increase the frequency of positive behavior. Instead, "distressed couples must learn to treat negative behavior as a discriminative stimulus for positive behavior and, thereby, interrupt the chain of negative reciprocity. That is, negative behavior must become a cue for some strategy which will circumvent the tendency to reciprocate" (Jacobson & Moore, 1981, p. 198).

Communication training (e.g., Birchler, 1979; Guerney, 1977; O'Leary & Turkewitz, 1978; Rappaport, 1976; Weiss, 1978; Weiss & Birchler, 1978) and problem-solving training (Jacobson, 1977b; Jacobson & Margolin, 1979), both of which are designed to alter moment-to-moment interaction patterns, receive a great deal of emphasis in behavior marital therapy. Communication training, a component found in most forms of marital therapy refers to (a) accurate and empathetic listening skills, (b) the expression and reception of feelings, and (c) conflict resolution. Problem-solving training, which sometimes is subsumed under the general category of communication training (e.g., O'Leary & Turkewitz, 1978), teaches couples how to communicate in order to facilitate the resolution of conflict. The emphasis on teaching couples strategies for the effective resolution of conflict reflects the overriding objective that couples apply these skills rather than coercive tactics to bring about future relationship change.

Behavior therapy is set apart from other therapies that offer communication training by its systematic approach to teaching skills. By applying principles of learning, such as operationalizing behavior, shaping, and social reinforcement, the behavior therapist teaches a process of enhanced communication for negotiating change agreements. Jacobson (1977c, 1981a) divides the training procedure into three components: instructions, feedback, and behavioral rehearsal. Instructions refer to the way that the therapist actually imparts information about what is necessary for effective communication. Believing couples must understand the general principles underlying a new skill as well as clearly envision how that new skill will be enacted, the behavioral marital therapist generally uses more than one vehicle for instruction. Description of the new skill usually is presented verbally or through written materials (cf. the problem-solving manual contained in Jacobson & Margolin, 1979). Illustrations of the new skill are offered through role-played demonstrations in which the therapist takes the place of one of the spouses. Once the skills are presented, the spouses repeatedly practice these new behaviors until they achieve competency. As with most behavioral rehearsal, the couple works up to skills of greater complexity and problems of greater proportion after first achieving competency on simpler tasks. Feedback is, of course, essential to progress in the behavioral rehearsal. Using shaping as the underlying principle for feedback, the behavioral marital therapist reinforces successive approximations to the ultimately desired response. That is, the therapist continually refines the spouses' behaviors by giving frequent and detailed feedback describing ways that their behaviors approached (and did not approach) the desired response. Thus, the training involves a constant interplay among the three components of instruction, rehearsal, and feedback. Instruction is presented; the couple rehearses a particular skill, usually imperfectly at first; feedback and possibly further instruction is used to refine the spouses' responses; the practice is repeated; and so forth.

Communication training, as it relates to the expression of affect, follows this general format. Instruction on how to make clear affective statements and how to be an empathic listener are presented, after which the spouses rehearse each role, with the therapist frequently interrupting to give specific and descriptive feedback. Once the couple becomes competent in their speaker–listener roles on nonrelationship issues, they then move on to more important relationship issues.

Training in feeling expression plays a less central role in behavior marital therapy, compared to other marital therapies, but nonetheless is important. It was recognized at an early point that acceptance and recognition of feelings were necessary before a couple could turn to the more rational demands of problem solving (Weiss, 1978; Weiss *et al.*, 1973). That is, expressiveness and listening skills were seen as a way to dissipate the emotions that interfered with the structured task of problem solving. More recently, expressive skills have been stressed for other functions as well. As summarized by Margolin and Weinstein (1983), both positive and negative feeling expression affords partners access to one another's subjective reality and offers important feedback regarding the impact of one's behavior on the partner. This information can be very useful in short-circuiting negative communication patterns.

Problem-solving skills, the aspect of communication training that has received the most attention in behavioral marital therapy, directly circumvents negative interaction patterns on several levels. Problem solving provides a mechanism to discuss conflictual issues that avoids rapidly escalating patterns of blame, withholding, coercion, and the like. The skills also provide a mechanism to cope actively with the problem so that it does not become a sore point in the marriage, festering and growing in importance due to spouses' unability to reach resolution. Most importantly, problem solving is taught with the hope that the skills will help couples cope, on their own, with conflicts that are unanticipated during the time of therapy but arise at a later date.

The most clearly defined guidelines for problem solving are presented by Jacobson and Margolin (1979), who separate the problem definition stage from the problem solution stage. In developing clear, well defined problem statements, spouses are to:

1. Always begin with something positive when stating the problem.
2. Use specific behaviors to describe what is bothersome rather than derogatory labels or overgeneralizations.
3. Make connections between those specific behaviors and feelings that arise in response to them.
4. Admit one's own role in the development of the problem.
5. Be brief and maintain a current or future focus, that is, do not list all previous incidents of the problem, analyze causes, or ask "why" questions.

When deciding what action is in order to solve the problem, spouses are to:

6. Focus on solutions by brainstorming as many solutions as possible.
7. Focus on mutuality and compromise by considering solutions that involve change by both partners.
8. Offer to change something in one's own behavior.

9. Accept, for a beginning, a change less than the ideal solution.
10. Discuss the advantages and disadvantages of each suggestion before reaching agreement.
11. Prepare a final change agreement that is spelled out in clear, descriptive behavioral terms, that is recorded in writing, and that includes cues reminding each partner of changes she or he has agreed to make.

There are, in addition, the following general guidelines for problem solving:

12. Develop an agenda for each problem-solving discussion.
13. Discuss only one problem at a time, that is, be aware of sidetracking.
14. Do not make inferences; talk about only what you can observe.
15. Paraphrase what the partner has said and check out perceptions to what was said before responding to the statement.

To follow these rules, spouses must adopt a collaborative attitude in which problems are viewed as mutual. This attitude, although difficult at first, is reinforced repeatedly when spouses learn that each time a problem is solved, the relationship improves. So crucial is this attitude that problem solving cannot continue in its absence. When couples are more interested in fighting than in collaborating, the problem-solving session should be terminated since it is unlikely that reasonable agreements will be reached under these circumstances.

The final stage of problem solving is a written change agreement or a contract (Weiss *et al.*, 1973; Weiss, Birchler, & Vincent, 1974). Although contracts have had a variety of meanings in behavioral marital therapy and come in a variety of forms, they essentially are written agreements specifying behaviors to be changed. It is strongly urged that agreements be put in writing so that: (a) there is no need to rely on memory to recall the conditions of the agreement; (b) the contract can act as a cue, reminding spouses to carry out the agreement; and (c) the written format (requiring signatures and perhaps a witness) underscores the significance of the agreement (Jacobson & Margolin, 1979). Originally, it was recommended that contracts specify contingencies; that is, by specifying environmental reinforcers, there would be a greater likelihood that the change would occur and that "who goes first" problems would be circumvented. These contingencies sometimes came in the form of the other spouse engaging in his or her requested behavior (i.e., Sarah agrees to put the children to bed each evening and Sam agrees to give Sarah a backrub each evening). At other times contingencies were independent of the other person, for example, Sarah earns a half-day on Saturday totally free from family responsibilities if she puts the children to bed each evening. The empirical literature does not support the efficacy of one type of contingency over the other, nor the necessity of contingencies *per se* (Jacobson, 1978b). Clinical experience, however, shows that couples tend to have strong preferences about the inclusion versus exclusion of contingencies, and this should be explored with couples when preparing change agreements.

Finally, it should be noted that the cognitive aspects of problem solving are receiving increasing attention. Rather than simply accepting each request for change and automatically applying a problem-solving approach, therapists are finding it necessary to explore the meaning of the requested behavior and the expectations surrounding that request (Epstein, 1982; Jacobson, in press; Jacobson & Margolin, 1979). Jacobson (in press), for instance, provides the example of a husband who defined the problem of his wife going to bed earlier than he did. Since he retired at 2:00 A.M., her compliance with his request would have meant that she would have to limit her sleeping to five hours per night. Upon further exploration, it became clear that he considered her bedtime hour an attempt to avoid sex and intimacy, an obviously unwarranted interpretation. By uncovering the husband's unrealistic and irrational expectations, the therapist opened up two new avenues for therapy: modification of the husband's expectations and further exploration and possible intervention into the area of sex. As can be seen in this example, cognitive procedures based on the models of Beck (1976), Ellis (1962), and Meichenbaum (1977) can be integrated with behavioral marital therapy to expose and challenge the irrational and dysfunctional cognitions that may underlie specific behavioral complaints.

Although communication and problem-solving skills provide alternatives to couples' frequent reliance on coercion to bring about relationship change, couples also may be entrenched in other, equally destructive and self-perpetuating cycles. Weiss (1980), for example, describes an alternating pattern of fighting, reconciliation, fighting, and so forth that may not be evident to the therapist until several repeating cycles have elapsed. The danger inherent in this roller-coaster pattern of anger is that the couple may come to rely on fighting (or making up from the fighting) as the stimulus for intimacy. Margolin (1981a) describes how issues of jealousy and trust are another common dimension in self-perpetuating cycles: Reactions to jealousy, such as guilt-producing maneuvers, demands, or excessive scrutiny, are immediately reinforcing in that they may terminate the jealousy-provoking situation. In the long run, however, they breed more suspiciousness, resentment, and frustration. Similar to the anger patterns, these cycles are particularly devastating because what initially appears to be a corrective reaction repeatedly is followed by renewed disappointment.

The treatment objective in dealing with anger is to teach couples to disrupt hostile, negative chains. Negative feelings are not to be suppressed altogether but are to be expressed and dealt with in a manner that does not simply evoke a reciprocally negative reaction. Recommendations in behavioral marital therapy for expressing and responding to negative emotions include the following guidelines (Jacobson & Margolin, 1979; Liberman *et al.*, 1980; O'Leary & Turkewitz, 1978): (a) Use feeling statements, not threats or labels: (b) Express the feelings verbally but do not demonstrate them nonverbally: (c) Take responsibility for the feelings, saying, for example, "I feel . . ." (d) Use affect–behavior statements that connect a particular feeling to a specific behavioral cause. These recommendations, although useful for coping with the inevitable conflict that occurs in any long-term intimate relationship, are insufficient for severe problems with anger. Margolin (1979) recommends the following, more definitive steps for couples who are abusive in their anger expression: (a) Establish a ground rule that physical abuse is unacceptable and be prepared to carry out that ground rule: (b) Identify cues that elicit and maintain the destructive expression of anger: (c) Teach the spouses to use early signs of anger as discriminitive cues for coping, that is, for taking steps antagonistic to destructive displays of anger: (d) Develop a plan of action to interrupt the conflict pattern, for example, temporary disengagement from contact with a plan to reunite later: (e) Modify faulty cognitions, including unrealistic expectations and assumptions that inhibit clear communication of dissatisfaction.

Several investigators (Epstein, 1982; Jacobson, in press; Novaco, 1979) have suggested that cognitive self-control strategies may be a way to halt cognitive-behavioral-affective cycles that culminate in destructive expression of anger. Epstein (1982, p. 23), for example, suggests that spouses learn to identify impulsive responses (e.g., "I am interrupting my partner") and task-interfering cognitions (e.g., "I am thinking about how my partner's ideas are incorrect) and to respond instead with self-instructional statements (e.g., "Stay calm. Listen carefully to my partner and try to understand how she/he views things. Do not respond with my ideas until I have communicated understanding of my partner's views to him/her."). This self-instruction initially can be practiced individually or in role playing with the therapist, and then rehearsed with both spouses together. Further suggestions from Jacobson (in press) indicate that self-instructional strategies can be built into problem-solving training by having spouses instruct themselves to focus on collaborative efforts rather than drift into adversarial positions.

The therapeutic objectives for negative cycles regarding jealousy and mistrust are to refocus attention from one person's infidelity or the other person's jealousy and to disrupt the entire interactional pattern that surrounds this issue (Margolin, 1981a; Tiesmann, 1979; Watzlawick, Weakland, & Fisch, 1974). Reframing is an important initial treatment step to relieve resentment by altering perceptions of specific behaviors, for example, viewing jealousy as an indication of caring and devotion as opposed to possessiveness or insecurity. Then, more direct steps are taken that require the couple to approach the jealousy-provoking situation while simultaneously engaging in actions that defuse rather than escalate the jealousy cycle. That is, the couple is offered ways to cope with rather than to avoid the threatened situation, thereby learning that the discomfort of the situation, although certainly unpleasant, can be endured and perhaps eventually overcome. Margolin (1981a) presents the following example of a plan to break out of a jealous cycle surrounding the wife's work as a cocktail waitress. On nights that the wife worked, the husband typically greeted her arrival home with a barrage of accusations and anger. As part of the plan to disrupt this pattern: (a) the husband was to dispense temporarily with his "rules" that she could not drink on the job and could not go to parties with co-workers; (b) the wife was given an opportunity to demonstrate how she actually handled men's advances by role playing these situations in the session and by jotting down notes throughout an evening at work about every man who made a pass at her; and (c) the wife was to reassure that husband that she cared for him, even in her absence, by leaving notes around the house and by calling him on breaks.

As demonstrated in these examples, it is of primary importance in altering negative patterns that the problem not be construed as one person's behavior, that is, one spouse's anger or jealousy. Rather, the entire cycle is construed as the problem, including both spouses' covert and overt reactions at each stage as the pattern unfolds. Based on a thorough assessment, the therapist and couple together can learn what perpetuates and exacerbates these patterns. Then, decisions can be made about whether disrupting this pattern best can be accomplished by training in feeling expression, listening skills, problem-solving skills, self-control procedures, cognitive restructuring procedures, or, most likely, some combination of these various components.

Presenting intervention plans to disrupt negative cycles requires an active, directive therapist who has captured the clients' attention and trust (Jacobson & Margolin, 1979). Therapeutic instructions, for the most part, are quite direct; the therapist not only prompts interactional changes but teaches the couple how to solve their own problems in the future. This is not to say, however, that instructions always are direct. Paradoxical interventions have been employed by behavioral marital therapists to bring home a particular message (Jacobson & Margolin, 1979), to get spouses to react out of character and to overcome cognitive belief barriers (Weiss, 1980), and to help the therapist gain control of and/or modify a maladaptive behavior (Birchler & Spinks, 1980). In most instances, however, these indirect procedures are an intermediary step to the more direct cognitive or behavior modification procedures.

4. Empirical Support for Behavioral Marital Therapy

How well does behavioral marital therapy live up to its mission as an integrated clinical and empirical approach? As indicated previously, the empirical endeavors of behavioral marital therapy are exhibited in at least three distinct ways. First, there is the empirical exploration of principles underlying behavior marital therapy and, more specifically, of factors that differentiate distressed and nondistressed couples. The current behavior marital literature shows a burgeoning of research in the past few years attempting to explain the etiology and maintenance of marital problems from a social learning perspective (e.g., Barnett & Nietzel, 1979; Billings, 1979; Christensen, Sullaway, & King, 1983; Gottman, 1979, 1980; Haynes, Follingstad, & Sullivan, 1979; Jacobson & Moore, 1980; Jacobson *et al.*, 1980; Margolin, 1981b; Margolin & Wampold, 1981; Markman, 1979, 1981). These recent data have begun to serve as the basis for some reformulation in behavioral marital therapy. Jacobson and Moore (1981), for example, point out that the common behavioral practice of training distressed couples to use contingencies more effectively may be ill-advised; distressed couples, compared to nondistressed couples, already rely more heavily on contingency control. As an alternative suggestion, they recommend inducing high rates of noncontingent positive behavior.

A second type of integration between clinical and empirical endeavors occurs when treating each individual couple. Experimentally based procedures are used to understand each couple's behavior and to monitor their progress in therapy. Although it is tempting to suggest that all behavioral marital therapists are busy collecting and analyzing their data as the basis for upcoming clinical decisions, this, of course, cannot be presumed. The plethora of data-based case studies in behavioral marital therapy indicate at least that some clinicians are applying this model. However, the overall extent to which behavioral marital therapists actually rely on data for information about the effectiveness of any one procedure or about their overall efficacy with a couple is unknown.

The third and perhaps most pertinent type of research evidence for this particular review concerns the investigation of treatment outcome. This research has been examined in detail in a variety of sources (Greer & D'Zurilla, 1975; Gurman & Kniskern, 1978a, 1978b; Jacobson, 1978a, 1979b; Jacobson & Margolin, 1979; Jacobson & Martin, 1976), and thus is briefly summarized here.

Series of uncontrolled case studies have shown behavioral marital therapy to be associated with a variety of positive changes in couples' behavior and in their perceptions of marital satisfaction (Azrin, Naster, & Jones, 1973; Patterson *et al.*, 1976; Stuart, 1969; Weiss *et al.*, 1973). Controlled and comparative investigations also have shown that multifaceted programs of behavioral marital therapy are an effective treatment for marital problems; however, the extent of the treatment effects vary considerably among studies. The strongest data come from a pair of studies by Jacobson (1977a, 1978b), who found behavioral marital therapy to be superior to a no-treatment control as well as to a nonspecific control group on both observational and self-report measures. Similarly, positive findings were reported by Tsoi-Hoshmand (1976). Her results, however, are difficult to interpret due to methodological flaws. Comparing behavior exchange procedures, combined behavioral and nonbehavioral communication training, and a no-treatment control, O'Leary and Turkewitz (1981) found more ambiguous results. Both treatment groups improved significantly more than the control group on self-report measurements but not on behavioral measures. In addition, there were no overall differences between the two treatment groups.

Two studies examining group-administered behavioral marital therapy also provide mixed results. Liberman *et al.* (1976) compared behavioral marital therapy to an "interaction–insight" approach. Observational measures favored the behavioral group, although both groups improved substantially on the self-report measures. Similarly, Harrell and Guerney's (1976) study, which employed a group format but with nondistressed couples, compared a combination of communication training and contracting to a no-treatment control. Here, once again, the behavioral group showed greater improvement on the communication task but not on subjective reports of marital satisfaction. In interpreting these studies, plus the O'Leary and Turkewitz (1981) study, there is no obvious way to reconcile the inconsistencies across different measures.

Other studies have been designed to identify the essential ingredients of behavioral marital therapy. Jacobson (1978b), for example, contrasted two types of contracting procedures, that is, "good faith" versus "quid pro quo" contracts, but found no differences in their effectiveness. More recently, Jacobson and Anderson (1980) conducted an analogue study comparing problem-solving training through instruction only, videotaped feedback and instruction, behavioral rehearsal and instruction, and all three components. The complete treatment package including instruction, feedback, and the opportunity to rehearse produced greater change than any other condition. In a similar vein, Baucom (1982) assigned distressed couples to problem-solving/communication training plus contracting, problem-solving/communication training only, contracting alone, or a wait-list condition. The total treatment group that received all active therapeutic ingredients was the only condition to show significant improvement on all behavioral and self-report measures. The three behavioral conditions, however, did not differ significantly on any measure at posttreatment. A similar finding, that the total treatment package is superior to any of its component parts, also received support from Margolin and Weiss (1978b) in an analogue study that compared a strictly behavioral intervention, a behavioral-cognitive intervention (which included cognitive-restructuring procedures), and a nondirective control condition. Although negative behaviors dropped in all three conditions, couples in the behavioral-cognitive group, compared to the other two groups, showed more positive changes in terms of positive communication behaviors and self-reported marital satisfaction.

These studies are but a beginning. Further attention currently is being directed to specific treatment components as well as to a variety of treatment parameters, that is, the conditions under which therapy is offered. For example, Baucom and his associates (Baucom, 1981; Mehlman, Baucom, & Anderson, 1981) are comparing: (*a*) immediate versus delayed treatment and the use of a single therapist versus cotherapists and (b) cognitive-behavioral versus behavioral-only interventions. Jacobson (1979a) is midway through a study that compares three treatment formats (behavior exchange, problem-solving training, and a combination of behavior exchange and problem solving). Studies also are underway to apply behavioral marital therapy to select populations, for example, male alcoholics and their wives (O'Farrell & Cutter, 1981) and families with both marital and child problems (Margolin & Christensen, in press). These new directions will delineate further which aspects of a behavioral approach are effective under what conditions and with what types of couples.

Overall conclusions about the status of outcome research in behavioral marital therapy reflect a promising but cautious tone. Gurman and Kniskern's (1978b) overall computation of therapeutic effectiveness for behavioral marital therapy results in a 64% success rate, indicating that behavioral marital therapy may not be any more effective (nor any less effective) than other marital therapy approaches. At this stage of the empirical enterprise, our assumptions about how to intervene clinically certainly surpass what has been demonstrated empirically. Perhaps behavioral marital therapists never will obtain sufficient empirical data to support their broadening applications and their increasingly more intricate procedures. It is likely, however, that behavioral marital therapy will continue to devote time and energy toward that objective, and, in the process, will develop a rich empirical basis that will be responsible, at least in part, for theoretical and clinical refinements.

5. Conclusions

This chapter has presented an overview of behavior marital therapy, an approach, according to Gurman (1978), that "offers the most recent important perspective on marital dysfunction and treatment" (pp. 479–480). Although recognized primarily for specific procedures, such as problem solving and contracting, behavioral marital therapy is distinguished mostly for its commitment to the scientific process. The extensive use of formalized assessment procedures, both for formulating a treatment strategy and for evaluating the efficacy of treatment, attests to this clinical-empirical perspective. Originally grounded in operant learning principles and social exchange principles, the social learning approach currently reflects an effort to integrate alternative conceptual approaches, particularly cognitive and systems perspectives. As forecast by the theoretical evolution that has occurred thus far, any number of experimentally based principles that can be applied to marital problems may be incorporated over time into the behavioral marital therapy approach.

Although behavior marital therapy's overall therapeutic objectives of increasing intimacy and disrupting negative patterns are not particularly unique, what sets this approach apart from others is how the objectives are accomplished. Spouses themselves become behavior analysts of their relationship, identifying specific actions and events that affect the way they think and feel about the marriage. Specific skills deficits, particularly in relation to communication and problem solving, are remedied through precise instruction, behavioral rehearsal, and detailed feedback. Faulty relationship cycles are identified and altered through training in new behaviors, cognitive restructuring, and modification of the stimulus conditions that set the stage for such patterns. Implementation of each intervention strategy involves a stepwise progression introducing the intervention in the therapy session, practicing new behaviors at home, and then tracking and formally acknowledging all signs of progress. The research on behavioral marital therapy, although suggestive of its overall efficacy, has not yet directly examined many of the variables deemed most important by behavioral marital therapists nor assessed the newer directions in behavior marital therapy. With further exploration of these important dimensions, some of which already is underway, behavior marital therapy is certain to continue undergoing considerable revision and refinement.

6. References

Azrin, N. H., Naster, B. J., & Jones, R. Reciprocity counseling: A rapid learning-based procedure for marital counseling. *Behavior Research and Therapy*, 1973, *11*, 365–382.

Barnett, L. R., & Nietzel, M. T. Relationship of instrumental and affectional behaviors and self-esteem to marital satisfaction in distressed and nondistressed couples. *Journal of Consulting and Clinical Psychology*, 1979, *47*, 946–157.

Baucom, D. H. *Cognitive behavioral strategies in the treatment of marital discord.* Paper presented at the meeting of the Association for the Advancement of Behavior Therapy, Toronto, November 1981.

Baucom, D. H. A comparison of behavioral contracting and problem-solving/communication training in behavioral marital therapy. *Behavior Therapy*, 1982, *13*, 162–174.

Beck, A. T. *Cognitive therapy and the emotional disorders.* New York: International Universities Press, 1976.

Bellack, A. S. A critical appraisal of strategies for assessing social skill. *Behavioral Assessment*, 1979, *1*, 157–176.

Billings, A. Conflict resolution in distressed and nondistressed married couples. *Journal of Consulting and Clinical Psychology*, 1979, *47*, 368–376.

Birchler, G. R. Differential patterns of instrumental affiliative behavior as a function of degree of marital distress and level of intimacy (Doctoral dissertation, University of Oregon, 1972). *Dissertation Abstracts International*, 1973, *33*, 14499B–4500B. (University Microfilms No. 73–7865, 102).

Birchler, G. R. Communication skills in married couples. In A. S. Bellack & M. Hersen (Eds.), *Research and practice in social skills training.* New York: Plenum, 1979.

Birchler, G. R., & Spinks, S. H. Behavioral systems marital and family therapy integration and clinical application. *American Journal of Family Therapy*, 1980, *8*, 6–28.

Birchler, G. R., Weiss, R. L., & Vincent, J. P. Multimethod analysis of social reinforcement exchange between maritally distressed and nondistressed spouse and stranger dyads. *Journal of Personality and Social Psychology*, 1975, *31*, 349–360.

Christensen, A., Sullaway, M., & King, C. E. Systematic error in behavioral reports of dyadic interaction: Egocentric bias and content effects. *Behavioral Assessment*, 1983, *5*, 131–142.

Doherty, W. J. Cognitive processes in intimate conflict: I. Extending attribution theory. *American Journal of Family Therapy*, 1981, *9*(1), 3–12. (a)

Doherty, W. J. Cognitive processes in intimate conflict: II. Efficacy and learned helplessness. *American Journal of Family Therapy*, 1981, *9*(2), 35–44. (b)

Eidelson, R. J., & Epstein, N. *Cognition and marital maladjustment: Development of a measure of unrealistic relationship beliefs.* Paper presented at the meeting of the Association for the Advancement of Behavior Therapy, Toronto, 1981.

Ellis, A. *Reason and emotion in psychotherapy.* New York: Lyle-Stuart, 1962.

Epstein, N. Cognitive therapy with couples. *American Journal of Family Therapy*, 1982, *10*(1), 5–16.

Gottman, J. M. *Marital interaction: Experimental investigations.* New York: Academic, 1979.

Gottman, J. M. Consistency of nonverbal affect and affect reciprocity in marital interaction. *Journal of Consulting and Clinical Psychology*, 1980, *48*, 711–717.

Gottman, J. M., Notarius, C., Markman, H., Bank, S., Yoppi, B., & Rubin, M. E. Behavior exchange theory and marital decision making. *Journal of Personality and Social Psychology*, 1976, *34*, 14–23.

Gottman, J. M., Markman, H., & Notarius, C. The topography of marital conflict: A sequential analysis of verbal and nonverbal behavior. *Journal of Marriage and the Family*, 1977, *39*, 461–477.

Greer, S. E., & D'Zurilla, T. Behavioral approaches to marital discord and conflict. *Journal of Marriage and Family Counseling*, 1975, *1*, 299–315.

Guerney, B. G. *Relationship enhancement.* San Francisco: Jossey-Bass, 1977.

Gurman, A. S. Contemporary marital therapies: A critique and comparative analysis of psychoanalytic, behavioral and systems theory approaches. In T. J. Paolino & B. S. McCrady (Eds.), *Marriage and marital therapy.* New York: Brunner/Mazel, 1978.

Gurman, A. S. Behavioral marriage therapy in the 1980's: The challenge of integration. *The American Journal of Family Therapy*, 1980, *8*(2), 86–95.

Gurman, A. S., & Klein, M. H. Women and behavioral marriage and family therapy; An unconscious male bias? In E. A. Blechman (Ed.), *Contemporary issues in behavior modification with women.* New York: Guilford Press, in press.

Gurman, A. S., & Kniskern, D. P. Behavioral marriage therapy: II. Empirical perspective. *Family Process*, 1978, *17*, 129–148. (a)

Gurman, A. S., & Kniskern, D. P. Research on marital and family therapy: Progress, perspective, and prospect.

In S. L. Garfield & A. E. Bergin (Eds.), *Handbook of psychotherapy and behavior change: An empirical analysis* (2nd ed.). New York: Wiley, 1978. (b)

Harrell, J., & Guerney, B. Training married couples in conflict negotiation skills. In D. H. L. Olson (Ed.), *Treating relationships.* Lake Mills, Iowa: Graphic, 1976.

Haynes, S. N., Follingstad, D. R., & Sullivan, J. C. Assessment of marital satisfaction and interaction. *Journal of Consulting and Clinical Psychology,* 1979, *47,* 789–791.

Homans, G. C. *Social behavior: Its elementary forms.* New York: Harcourt Brace, 1961.

Hops, H., Wills, T. A., Patterson, G. R., & Weiss, R. L. *Marital interaction coding system.* Eugene, Oregon: University of Oregon and Oregon Research Institute, 1972.

Jacob, T. Assessment of marital dysfunction. In M. Hersen & A. S. Bellack (Eds.), *Behavioral assessment: A practical handbook.* New York: Pergamon, 1976.

Jacobson, N. S. Problem-solving and contingency contracting in the treatment of marital discord. *Journal of Consulting and Clinical Psychology,* 1977, *45,* 92–100. (a)

Jacobson, N. S. Training couples to solve their marital problems: A behavioral approach to relationship discord. Part I: Problem-solving skills. *International Journal of Family Counseling,* 1977, *5*(1), 22–31. (b)

Jacobson, N. S. Training couples to solve their marital problems: A behavioral approach to relationship discord. Part II: Intervention strategies. *International Journal of Family Counseling,* 1977, *5*(2), 20–28. (c)

Jacobson, N. S. A review of the research on the effectiveness of marital therapy. In T. J. Paolino & B. S. McCrady (Eds.), *Marriage and marital therapy: Psychoanalytic, behavioral, and systems theory perspectives.* New York: Brunner/Mazel, 1978. (a)

Jacobson, N. S. Specific and nonspecific factors in the effectiveness of a behavioral approach to the treatment of marital discord. *Journal of Consulting and Clinical Psychology,* 1978, *46,* 442–452. (b)

Jacobson, N. S. *Behavior marital therapy: Comparing formats and modalities.* Unpublished manuscript. University of Washington, 1979. (a)

Jacobson, N. S. Behavioral treatments for marital discord: A critical appraisal. In M. Heisen, R. M. Eisler, & P. M. Miller (Eds.), *Progress in behavior modification.* New York: Academic Press, 1979. (b)

Jacobson, N. S. Behavioral marital therapy. In A. S. Gurman & D. P. Kniskern (Eds.), *Handbook of family therapy.* New York: Brunner/Mazel, 1981. (a)

Jacobson, N. S. Marital problems. In J. L. Shelton & R. L. Levy (Eds.), *Behavior assignments and treatment compliance: A handbook of clinical strategies.* Champaign, Ill.: Research Press, 1981. (b)

Jacobson, N. S. The modification of cognitive processes in behavioral marital therapy: Integrating cognitive and behavioral intervention strategies. In N. S. Jacobson & K. Hahlweg (Eds.), *Marital interaction: Analysis and modification.* New York: Guilford Press, in press.

Jacobson, N. S., & Anderson, E. A. The effects of behavior rehearsal and feedback on the acquisition of problem-solving skills in distressed and nondistressed couples. *Behavior Research and Therapy,* 1980, *18,* 25–36.

Jacobson, N. S., & Margolin, G. *Marital therapy: Strategies based on social learning and behavior exchange principles.* New York: Brunner/Mazel, 1979.

Jacobson, N. S., & Martin, B. Behavioral marriage therapy. *Psychological Bulletin,* 1976, *83,* 540–556.

Jacobson, N. S., & Moore, D. Spouses as observers of the events in their relationship. *Journal of Consulting and Clinical Psychology,* 1980, *48,* 696–703.

Jacobson, N. S., & Moore, D. Behavior exchange theory of marriage: Reconnaissance and reconsideration. In J. P. Vincent (Ed.), *Advances in family intervention, assessment, and theory: A research annual* (Vol. 2). Greenwich, Conn.: JAI Press, 1981.

Jacobson, N. S., Waldron, H., & Moore, D. Toward a behavioral profile of marital distress. *Journal of Consulting and Clinical Psychology,* 1980, *48,* 696–703.

Jacobson, N. S., Berley, R., Newport, K., Elwood, R., & Phelps, C. Failure in behavioral marital therapy. In S. Coleman (Ed.), *Failure in family therapy.* New York: Guilford Press, in press.

Jacobson, N. S., Ellwood, R., & Dallas, M. The behavioral assessment of marital dysfunction. In D. H. Barlow (Ed.), *Behavioral assessment of adult disorders.* New York: Guilford Press, 1981. (a)

Knudson, R. M., Sommers, A. A., & Golding, S. L. Interpersonal perception and mode of resolution in marital conflict. *Journal of Personality and Social Psychology,* 1980, *38,* 751–763.

Liberman, R. P. Behavioral approaches to family and couple therapy. *American Journal of Orthopsychiatry,* 1970, *40,* 106–118.

Liberman, R. P., Levine, J., Wheeler, E., Sanders, N., & Wallace, C. Experimental evaluation of marital group therapy: Behavioral vs. interaction-insight formats. *Acta Psychiatrica Scandinavica,* Supplement, 1976.

Liberman, R. P., Wheeler, E. G., deVisser, L. A., Kuehnel, J., & Kuehnel, T. *Handbook of marital therapy.* New York: Plenum Press, 1980.

Locke, H. J., & Wallace, K. M. Short-term marital adjustment and prediction tests: Their reliability and validity. *Journal of Marriage and Family Living*, 1959, *21*, 251–255.

Margolin, G. Conjoint marital therapy to enhance anger management and reduce spouse abuse. *American Journal of Family Therapy*, 1979, *7*, 13–23.

Margolin, G. A behavioral-systems approach to the treatment of marital jealousy. *Clinical Psychology Review*, 1981, *1*, 469–487. (a)

Margolin, G. Behavior exchange in distressed and nondistressed marriages: A family cycle perspective. *Behavior Therapy*, 1981, *12*, 329–343. (b)

Margolin, G. Ethical and legal considerations in marital and family therapy. *American Psychologist*, 1982, *37*, 788–801.

Margolin, G. An interactional model for the assessment of marital relationships. *Behavioral Assessment*, 1983, *5*, 105–129.

Margolin, G., & Christensen, A. Treatment of multiproblem families: Specific and general effects of marital and family therapy. In L. A. Hamerlynck (Ed.), *Essentials of behavioral treatments for families*, in press.

Margolin, G., & Jacobson, N. S. The assessment of marital dysfunction. In M. Hersen & A. S. Bellack (Eds.), *Behavioral assessment: A practical handbook*. New York: Pergamon, 1981.

Margolin, G., & Wampold, B. E. A sequential analysis of conflict and accord in distressed and nondistressed marital pairs. *Journal of Consulting and Clinical Psychology*, 1981, *46*, 1476–1486.

Margolin, G., & Weinstein, C. D. The role of affect in behavioral marital therapy. In M. L. Aronson & L. R. Wolberg (Eds.), *Group and family therapy 1982: An overview*. New York: Brunner/Mazel, 1983.

Margolin, G., & Weiss, R. L. Communication training and assessment: A case of behavioral marital enrichment. *Behavior Therapy*, 1978, *9*, 508–520. (a)

Margolin, G., & Weiss, R. L. A comparative evaluation of therapeutic components associated with behavioral marital treatment. *Journal of Consulting and Clinical Psychology*, 1978, *46*, 1476–1486. (b)

Margolin, G., Christensen, A., & Weiss, R. L. Contracts, cognition, and change: A behavioral approach to marital therapy. *The Counseling Psychologist*, 1975, *5*, 15–26.

Markman, H. J. Application of a behavioral model of marriage in predicting relationship satisfaction of couples planning marriage. *Journal of Consulting and Clinical Psychology*, 1979, *47*, 743–749.

Markman, H. J. Prediction of marital distress: A 5-year follow-up. *Journal of Consulting and Clinical Psychology*, 1981, *49*, 760–762.

Mehlman, S. K., Baucom, D. H., & Anderson, D. *The relative effectiveness of cotherapists versus single therapists and immediate treatment versus delayed treatment in a behavioral marital therapy outcome study*. Paper presented at the meeting of the Association for the Advancement of Behavior Therapy, Toronto, November 1981.

Meichenbaum, D. *Cognitive-behavior modification: An integrative approach*. New York: Plenum Press, 1977.

Nelson, R. O., & Hayes, S. C. Some current dimensions of behavioral assessment. *Behavioral Assessment*, 1979, *1*, 1–16.

Notarius, C. I., Vanzetti, N. A., & Smith, R. J. *Assessing expectations and outcomes in marital interaction*. Paper presented at the meeting of the Association for the Advancement of Behavior Therapy, Toronto, November 1981.

Novaco, R. W. The cognitive regulation of anger and stress. In P. Kendall & S. Hollon (Eds.), *Cognitive-behavioral interventions: Theory, research, and procedures*. New York: Academic Press, 1979.

O'Farrell, T., & Cutter, H. S. G. *Evaluating behavioral marital therapy for alcoholics: Procedures and preliminary results*. Paper presented at the Banff International Conference, Banff, March 1981.

O'Leary, K. D., & Turkewitz, H. Marital therapy from a behavioral perspective. In T. J. Paolino & B. S. McCrady (Eds.), *Marriage and marital therapy: Psychoanalytic, behavioral and systems theory perspectives*. New York: Brunner/Mazel, 1978.

O'Leary, K. D., & Turkewitz, H. A comparative outcome study of behavioral marital therapy and communication therapy. *Journal of Marital and Family Therapy*, 1981, *7*, 159–170.

Patterson, G. R. Some procedures for assessing changes in marital interaction patterns. *Oregon Research Institute Bulletin*, 1976, *16*(7).

Patterson, G. R., & Hops, H. Coercion, a game for two: Intervention techniques for marital conflict. In R. E. Ulrich & P. Mountjoy (Eds.), *The experimental analysis of social behavior*. New York: Appleton-Century-Crofts, 1972.

Patterson, G. R., & Reid, J. B. Reciprocity and coercion: Two facets of social systems. In C. Neuringer & J. L. Michael (Eds.), *Behavior modification in clinical psychology*. New York: Appleton-Century-Crofts, 1970.

Patterson, G. R., Hops, H., & Weiss, R. L. A social learning approach to reducing rates of marital conflict. In

R. Stuart, R. Liberman, & S. Wilder (Eds.), *Advances in behavior therapy.* New York: Academic Press, 1974.

Patterson, G. R., Weiss, R. L., & Hops, H. Training of marital skills: Some problems and concepts. In H. Leitenberg (Ed.), *Handbook of behavior modification.* New York: Appleton-Century-Crofts, 1976.

Peterson, D. R. A plan for studying interpersonal behavior. In D. Magnusson & N. Endler (Eds.), *Personality at the crossroads: Current issues in interactional psychology.* New York: Wiley, 1977.

Peterson, D. R. Assessing interpersonal relationships by means of interaction records. *Behavioral Assessment,* 1979, *1,* 221–236.

Protzner, M., King, C., & Christensen, A. *Naturalistic interaction of married couples: A descriptive analysis.* Paper presented at the WPA meeting, Los Angeles, 1981.

Rappaport, A. F. Conjugal relationship enhancement program. In D. H. L. Olson (Ed.), *Treating relationships.* Lake Mills, Iowa: Graphic, 1976.

Rappaport, A. F., & Harrell, J. A behavioral exchange model for marital counseling. *The Family Coordinator,* 1972, *22,* 203–212.

Skinner, B. F. Operant behavior. *American Psychologist,* 1963, *18,* 503–515.

Spanier, G. B. Measuring dyadic adjustment: New scales for assessing the quality of marriage and similar dyads. *Journal of Marriage and the Family,* 1976, *38,* 15–28.

Stuart, R. B. Operant interpersonal treatment for marital discord. *Journal of Consulting and Clinical Psychology,* 1969, *33,* 675–682.

Stuart, R. B. Behavioral remedies for marital ills: A guide to the use of operant–interpersonal techniques. In A. S. Gurman & D. G. Rice (Eds.), *Couples in conflict: New directions in marital therapy.* New York: Aronson, 1975.

Stuart, R. B. *Helping couples change: A social learning approach to marital therapy.* New York: Guilford, 1980.

Stuart, R. B., & Stuart, F. *Marital Pre-Counseling Inventory.* Champaign, Ill.: Research Press, 1972.

Thibaut, J. W., & Kelley, H. H. *The social psychology of groups.* New York: Wiley, 1959.

Tiesmann, M. W. Jealousy: Systematic problem solving therapy with couples. *Family Process,* 1979, *18,* 151–160.

Tsoi-Hoshmand, L. Marital therapy: An integrative behavioral-learning model. *Journal of Marriage and Family Counseling,* 1976, *2,* 179–191.

Vincent, J. P. The empirical–clinical study of families: Social learning theory as a point of departure. In J. P. Vincent (Ed.), *Advances in family intervention, assessment, and theory.* Greenwich, Conn.: JAI Press, 1980.

Vincent, J. P., Weiss, R. L., & Birchler, G. R. A behavioral analysis of problem solving in distressed and nondistressed married and stranger dyads. *Behavior Therapy,* 1975, *6,* 475–487.

Vincent, J. P., Friedman, L. C., Nugent, J., & Messerly, L. Demand characteristics in observations of marital interaction. *Journal of Consulting and Clinical Psychology,* 1979, *47,* 557–566.

Vincent, J. P., Cook, N. I., & Brady, C. P. The emerging family: Integration of a developmental perspective and social learning theory. In J. P. Vincent (Ed.), *Advances in family intervention, assessment, and theory: A research annual.* Greenwich, Conn.: JAI Press, 1981.

Watzlawick, P., Weakland, J., & Fisch, R. *Change: Principles of problem formation and problem resolution.* New York: Norton, 1974.

Weiss, R. L. The conceptualization of marriage from a behavioral perspective. In T. J. Paolino & B. S. McCrady (Eds.), *Marriage and marital therapy: Psychoanalytic, behavioral and systems theory perspectives.* New York: Brunner/Mazel, 1978.

Weiss, R. L. Strategic behavioral marital therapy: Toward a model for assessment and intervention. In J. P. Vincent (Ed.), *Advances in family intervention, assessment, and theory: An annual compilation of research* (Vol. 1). Greenwich, Conn.: JAI Press, 1980.

Weiss, R. L., & Birchler, G. R. Adults with marital dysfunction. In M. Hersen and A. S. Bellack (Eds.), *Behavior therapy in the psychiatric setting.* Baltimore: Williams & Williams, 1978.

Weiss, R. L., & Cerreto, M. *Marital status inventory.* Unpublished manuscript, University of Oregon, 1975.

Weiss, R. L., & Margolin, G. Marital conflict and accord. In A. R. Ciminero, K. S. Calhoun, & H. E. Adams (Eds.), *Handbook for behavioral assessment.* New York: Wiley, 1977.

Weiss, R. L., Hops, H., & Patterson, G. R. A framework for conceptualizing marital conflict, a technology for altering it, some data for evaluating it. In L. A. Hamerlynck, L. C. Handy, & E. J. Mash (Eds.), *Behavior change: Methodology, concepts, and practice.* Champaign, Ill.: Research Press, 1973.

Weiss, R. L., Birchler, G. R., & Vincent, J. P. Contractual models for negotiation training in marital dyads. *Journal of Marriage and the Family*, 1974, *36*, 321–330.

Williams, A. M. The quantity and quality of marital interaction related to marital satisfaction: A behavioral analysis. *Journal of Applied Behavior Analysis*, 1979, *12*, 665–678.

Wills, T. A., Weiss, R. L., & Patterson, G. R. A behavioral analysis of the determinants of marital satisfaction. *Journal of Consulting and Clinical Psychology*, 1974, *42*, 802–811.

14

Network Therapy

JODIE KLIMAN AND DAVID W. TRIMBLE

Family therapy demonstrates the need for conceptualizing and treating emotional difficulties contextually. It looks beyond the individual to the family as the system of concern. Ackerman's (1970) "interpersonal unconscious of the family group," Minuchin's (1974) of the "extra-cerebral mind," and Palazzoli, Cecchin, Prata, and Boscolo's (1978) of the "family in schizophrenic transaction" all have helped us to understand that there is a dialectical relationship between intrapsychic and social experience. In such a relationship, intrapsychic and interpersonal or social processes reflect and influence each other; each is an ever changing creation of and counterpoint to the other. Human consciousness is a dynamic interplay between these two processes.

Unfortunately, this systemic approach restricts itself to the family itself. Families and their members too often are viewed as if they were independent of the other, larger, social systems to which they relate (Kovel, 1980). Although some family therapists may incorporate school, work, or welfare concerns into the course of treatment (Minuchin, 1974) or help family members with their relations to extended family (Bowen, 1978), there has been little systematic attention to the relationships between extrafamilial ties and difficulties that are manifested in the family.

Families are no more independent of the social systems in which they are embedded than individuals are independent of their families. This chapter explores how networks of relationships with kin, friends, and other social ties can be considered and utilized systematically in the treatment of emotional distress. Dysfunctional family dynamics and interactional structures associated with individual psychological distress can be harnessed and modified toward the well-being of families; so can the dysfunctional dynamics and structures that characterize the social networks of families and individuals in distress.[1]

[1]Minuchin and Fishman describe hierarchies of systemic organization, e.g., the individual, family, extended family, and community, utilizing Koestler's concept of the *holon*, in which every level of organization is simultaneously its own whole and part of a larger system. As such, it "exerts competitive energy for autonomy and self-preservation as a whole. It also carries integrative energy as a part. . . . Part and whole contain each other in a continuing, and ongoing process of communication and interrelationship" (Minuchin & Fishman, 1981, p. 13).

JODIE KLIMAN • New England Center for the Study of the Family, Newton, Massachusetts 02159.
DAVID W. TRIMBLE • North Shore Professional Associates, Lynn, Massachusetts 01901.

This chapter is concerned with social networks' involvement in the development and maintenance of psychological well-being and distress (Sussman, 1970) and with techniques for therapeutic intervention into networks. Before beginning, we wish to emphasize that a complete analysis of the origins and phenomenology of psychological experience cannot stop at the level of the social network. The network is one organizing level of psychological experience and social arrangements, intermediate between family life and the workings of overarching social, economic, political, and cultural structures. It is not the only intermediate level, and the investigation of network relations alone cannot illuminate all aspects of the dialectical relationship between social and psychological phenomena.[2] Society is more than an aggregate of interconnected networks. The focus of the present work, the social network, is a mediating structure that is relatively accessible to clinical investigation and intervention.

Psychological experience reflects the dynamic tension between an active self, which is as social as it is biological at the very core, and a society that creates, shapes, and satisfies partially and frustrates partially, and which itself is changed by the psychological and material needs and desires of human beings (Fenichel, 1938; Marcuse, 1955). There is a profound and dynamic interpenetration of psychological self and the structures and arrangements of society. This interpenetration is manifested and experienced differently in different kinds of societies and for different relationships of individual to the social order (e.g., based on class or gender position).

We believe that the key to understanding the relationship between individual (and family) psychology and organization of society lies in an ever deeper and more critical investigation of the interplay between depth psychology and social arrangements and how they reflect, modify, and reproduce each other.

Such work is beyond the scope of the present effort. However, the psychological experiences and social arrangements examined in the context of social networks provide a window into both psychological and social dynamics. The network is an active and changing medium through which the social order makes its indelible mark on individual consciousness and activity and through which the changing experience of individuals, families, and other small groups ramify out to larger society. Social networks are where people live much of their lives. As such, they are fertile ground for psychological—and social—understanding and intervention.

1. Social Network Defined

Although we will be using the network concept within a clinical discussion, a definition of social networks requires mention of the concept's origins in anthropological and sociological network analysis. Barnes (1954) first used the term *social network* to describe a matrix of relationships between persons and groups of persons that can be diagrammed as a set of points. Some points are connected by lines, which indicate interaction between people. He distinguished between "unbounded networks," interconnected and endlessly ramifying sets of relationships, and "bounded," "personal," or "ego-centric" networks, which consist of all the people one individual knows and of all the links among those people. The latter definition is of interest here. Barnes excluded

[2]Other structures mediating individual psychology and the social order are the work place, school, the mass media, and religious institutions. Social arrangements based on different positions of class, gender, and race are mediating structures that are fundamental to the continuing development of individual psychology and society.

formal ties, such as those to the workplace, from his definition of networks; other network analysts, and these authors, do not.

Personal networks are variously defined in the literature (Barnes, 1954; Boissevain, 1968; Boissevain & Mitchell, 1973; Bott, 1957; Wellman, 1980), but all network analysts point to a set of relationships, actual or potential, between an individual and the people in that individual's immediate social context, as well as the relationships among those people. The social network mediates between the individual (or family) and society. Interaction with this complex reticulum of ties contributes to the development of one's sense of psychological self. It also contributes to one's sense of belonging, loneliness, and the constraints, limitations, privileges, and deprivations characterizing one's relationship to society.

Boissevain (1968) describes membership in an individual's network as falling into six concentric zones of decreasing intimacy and increasing inclusiveness. These zones are: (1) *the personal cell,* which includes the index person's household and one to three closest relatives and friends; (2) *the intimate zone A,* whose members are relatives and friends with whom the index maintains close and active ties; (3) *the intimate zone B,* whose members are friends and relatives with whom the index maintains more passive ties but who still are considered important; (4) *the effective zone,* including all those people with whom the index has ongoing affective or instrumental relationships of any kind; (5) *the nominal zone,* which is comprised of people the index knows slightly or once knew, which shades off into; (6) *the extended zone,* an amorphous collection of the acquaintances of people who know the index, that is, people to whom index could gain access if necessary. Membership in these six zones is dynamic. In industrialized and mobile society, there is considerable movement of people across network zones. Brief reflection about the reader's own network points to the flux in membership and in the intimacy and closeness of network ties that an individual's network can experience over relatively short spans of time.

Personal networks consist of an individual's family, other household members, kin, friends, neighbors, work associates, classmates, social acquaintances, fellow members of church or temple, voluntary associations, unions, and the like, as well as people such as neighborhood bartenders, baby-sitters, storekeepers, and so on. These personal relations constitute the *primary sector* of the network. The *secondary sector* of the network comprises more formalized relationships with representatives of social institutions: personnel of schools, health and mental health facilities, social service agencies, clergy, landlords, police, the courts, and others.

There is no clear dividing line between the primary and secondary sectors of the network. A priest, employer, teacher, or bookie could fall into one sector or the other, depending on the nature and complexity of ties to the index. Most people have strongest emotional ties to the members of their primary sector, but the secondary sector has a powerful—if not necessarily obvious—effect on personal life. Chronic psychiatric patients and other marginal members of society frequently have their most significant, frequent, and reliable contacts with members of the secondary sectors of their networks. Network therapy necessarily involves intervention into both the primary and secondary sectors.

Clinical definitions of networks are simple and based on pragmatics of therapeutic practice. Speck and Attneave (1973), the first network therapists, loosely refer to social networks as those people an index individual or family considers to be significant in their lives. Their use of the term is roughly equivalent to Boissevain's (1968) inner four network zones. For a relatively well functioning person, the effective zone of the network may number well over 100 people (of course, the combined network of a family would be larger still). A psychiatric patient who has been instituionalized for years may have no more than a handful of people in his or her effective zone. Although not all the members of the effective zone necessarily attend a full-scale network assembly, Speck and Attneave (1973) tend to use *network* and *participants in network assembly* interchangeably. We prefer not to gloss the two definitions, since network members who do not attend network assemblies (recently estranged lovers or spouses, the sister who is no longer on speaking terms with the patient, and crucial inpatient treatment team members, for instance) are often vital to the shape of an individual's network and to the effectiveness of intervention into that network.

Some epidemiologists define networks still more narrowly. Many of the epidemiologists addressing stress, social connectedness, health, and mental health use the network concept to mean those close personal relationships that provide social and emotional support (Dean & Lin, 1977; Liem & Liem, 1978). This use of the term is problematic, since not all personal ties are supportive (indeed, some can be quite destructive) and not all supportive relationships are personal. Unless otherwise specified, we will rely on an anthropological definition of networks, with emphasis on Boissevain's (1968) inner four zones.

1.1. Clinical Applications of the Network Concept: An Introduction

Network therapy involves any psychotherapeutic intervention that focuses on the social network of an individual, family, or larger group in distress. A variety of network therapy techniques, ranging from the ambitious and dramatic full-scale network assembly in which dozens of people are assembled to private coaching of individuals or families to make changes in their network relations, will be discussed elsewhere in this chapter. For the moment, the question is: What does the network concept bring to clinical practice?

The answer, we believe, lies in an expanded understanding of psychological dysfunction. Family therapy practice demonstrates that what otherwise might be labeled as individual psychopathology often can be treated effectively as a simultaneous reflection of, comment upon, attempt to maintain, and criticism of increasingly dysfunctional patterns of interactional sequences, structures, and rules. While one (or more) family member serves as the identified patient, the whole family shares a commitment to maintain and uphold the very family dysfunction that the identified patient's behavior symbolizes. The behaviors, perceptions, and level of functioning of every family member can be understood within the framework of the system in which he or she is embedded. The system and its members maintain each other.[3]

It is important not to assume a linear causality here. Palazzoli and her colleagues (1978), among others, posit an alternative, circular, causality in which every behavior influences and is influenced by all other behaviors that constitute the "game" of the family system. We do not suggest that any given arrangement of family relations *causes* symptomatic behavior in family members, or that any given abnormality in a member *causes* a dysfunctional family system. A truly systematic view would incorporate a

[3]All systems and their members maintain each other. There is nothing inherently problematic about that fact, except when rigidification occurs, for instance with families who have trouble accommodating to developmental change. Homeostasis is as vital to the survival of any system as is the capacity to change.

multivariate and dialectical understanding in which family history, social structure, biological factors (e.g., a genetic vulnerability to schizophrenia or manic depression), individual experience and the relationship between family members and the outside world all influence each other in an ongoing and changing manner.[4]

The same systemic model can be applied to social networks. A distressed family expresses the dysfunctionality of the network in which it is embedded. Simultaneously, the network patterns itself around the discomfiting behaviors or stances of the index family. Here, as with individual families, it is best to avoid seeking causal relations. Epidemiological evidence is inconclusive at best on the sequential ordering, for instance, of the onset of psychosis and network interactional patterns. Despite this uncertainty as to causality (which probably reflects a nonlinear reality as much as it does the underdeveloped state of the art), clinical experience demonstrates that intervention into the networks of families in distress can bring clinical relief to those families and improved coping skills for their networks (Curtis, 1974; J. Garrison, 1974; Speck & Attneave, 1973; Speck & Rueveni, 1969; Trimble, 1980, 1981; Trimble & Kliman, 1981).

The brief case description that follows[5] exemplifies the relationship between network transactions and family dysfunction. By the time George Jones, the oldest of five children, was 13, his delinquent activities already had involved his family with the police, courts, juvenile services, and foster care. His mother, Cynthia, single after several divorces, and the juvenile authorities had been unsuccessful in containing the boy's defiance and stealing. Mother and son were locked into an unhappy cycle in which Cynthia's feelings of incompetence and her negative expectations of male behavior were intensified by George's unchecked antisocial behavior, which in turn was heightened by Cynthia's helpless and angry stance, and so on, through escalating sequential spirals. By the time the family entered treatment, Cynthia not only was desperate about her inability to control George, but also worried about her second child, Deborah, who had begun to drink and to stay out too late.

Over the course of several months, the family was seen conjointly and George participated in individual and group therapy. No positive changes were made, but a number of significant dynamics concerning the family's relationship to its network began to emerge. The repeating sequence in which Cynthia presented herself as an incompetent and helpless authority and George complementarily presented himself as uncontrollable was maintained not only by the family, but also through the network's reinforcing participation in and mediation of the mother–son relationship.

Cynthia blamed her son's behavior on a group of older friends who frequently set him up as the "fall guy" in their delinquent escapades. In particular, she blamed Sally, an adult who once had been Cynthia's friend and neighbor. Cynthia, along with a number of other parents and juvenile workers, believed that Sally actively encouraged the youngsters' antisocial behavior. It appeared that Sally saw these activities as constituting a justifiable protest against their families and against society in general. The peer group, with the sanction of Sally, provided George with enough support to withstand the attempts of his family and the authorities to return him to his predelinquent ways. This group not only sanctioned George's otherwise unacceptable behavior, but also provided him with an

[4]Beels's (1978) introduction to a special issue on networks and schizophrenia in the *Schizophrenia Bulletin* discusses some of the multiple and interactive variables involved in the course of schizophrenia.
[5]This case is presented in more depth in Trimble (1981).

alternative context for feelings of belonging and loyalty. Since he no longer experienced his family as a primary reference group, his behavior did not present him with sufficient loyalty conflict and ambivalence to draw him effectively into treatment.

Cynthia agreed to a full-scale network assembly when George was sent to a court-ordered foster care placement but kept running back to his mother and friends. Attending the assembly were: George, Cynthia, Deborah, Cynthia's mother and brother, eight of her friends, Sally, five young friends of George, Deborah and Sally, George's foster parents, and three workers from the foster care agency. The purpose of the network assembly was to modify the toxic dynamics and structure of the network so as to allow for effective work with the index family.

In the first of the Jones's two network assemblies, the polarization between Sally and the other adults was rapid and intense. Sally was harshly criticized for her contributions to the adolescents' delinquency and to their parents' suffering. She seemed distressed to hear about Cynthia's misery, but maintained a defiant stance, drawing on the support of her young friends. George continued in his angry and evasive behavior and the adults continued to feel helpless.

During the second assembly, the network's collective depression in the face of this impasse was profund. In order to break through the group's frustration and depression and activate the network, the network conductor seated George in the middle of the room, across from an empty chair. Network members then were asked to sit facing George, one at a time, and "speak from your heart." Placed in one-to-one contact with George in an atmosphere of emotional intensity and in the presence of others, network members found themselves expressing great sadness and nurturant compassion toward him, rather than the anger they had felt only moments earlier. George appeared confused about how to respond to this show of adult caring, while the group shared its mounting distress at its inability to help a boy who was only 14.

Breakthrough was achieved when Sally, moved by the level of caring expressed by the previously antagonistic network, confronted George for refusing to help himself despite the collective concern of the people in his life. She publicly withdrew her support for his delinquent activities and for his rejection of his network's care for him, stunning him with this dramatic shift in her position. George was left without adult sanction for his rebellious behavior as Sally moved into an alliance, however strained, with the other adults in the network to monitor George's activities. She was able to use her influence with George's friends to convince them to stop drawing the younger boy into their criminal acts.

A systemic approach to this problem that stopped at the boundaries of the family system would have failed to address the ways in which dysfunctional family patterns relate to the workings of larger systems. George's disobedience and delinquency and his mother's ineffective attempts at exerting authority must be considered in the context of network members' collusion in maintaining the family impasse. It also should be considered in the context of the economic and social forces in which juvenile delinquency is an expression of social discontent as well as of individual dynamics.

2. Network Therapy Strategies

The practice of network therapy can be divided into five domains: network coaching, partial network assembly, full-scale network assembly, community network therapy, and network construction. The role of the therapist varies across domains. Working with an individual or family, one acts as a coach or advisor on network relations. When the unit of intervention is a partial assembly (a group of 5 to 20 interrelated people who are not all of the same household), the therapist acts as a mediator and arbitrator. The therapist who assembles full-scale network assemblies of 20 to over 80 people takes the position of shaman or tribal healer. Community mental health strategies require that the network therapist take a community organizer role. Network construction, in which the therapist helps clients to build healthy new network structures, employs strategies from the four other domains and from techniques of group psychotherapy.

2.1. Network Therapy with Individuals and Families[6]

Coaching a family on the conduct of relationships within their network often provides the path of least resistance to achieving constructive changes in the family's relational context. Families frequently are reluctant to bring significant network members into direct contact with their therapists and the participation of nonrelatives in psychotherapy may conflict with agency policy. Even when such obstacles are present, the therapist may conclude that coaching the family is the most efficient means of achieving the desired systemic change. Network therapy with a family is analogous to Bowen's (1978) systemic family therapy in which work with one motivated family member can produce relational changes beneficial to the family system of the individual client.

The first step in coaching is to introduce the family to the social network concept, through helping family members develop detailed descriptions of their personal networks and teaching some basic principles about the relationships between networks and mental health. The combined family network (i.e., the combined networks of all the family members) is then examined critically concerning both its contributions to the family's difficulties and its strengths and the access it provides to helping resources. Finally, family and therapist develop strategies for changing network patterns, and/or making better use of the network to meet family needs.

This final stage differs according to level of the family's ability to cooperate with treatment. A straightforward counseling approach, which provides the family with direct advice, is effective with cooperative family members on issues that do not arouse irrational opposition. Indirect approaches are necessary when dealing with homeostatic impasse. Instead of suggesting a specific course of action for the family to take with a problematic sector of their network, the therapist might instead propose that the family invite everyone in their network to attend a full-scale assembly, fully expecting the family to declare such a meeting impossible. By examining the family fantasies about what would happen at a network assembly and exploring family beliefs about why certain key network memebers could or should never attend, the therapist helps the family members to develop new perspectives on their network problems and to imagine potential solutions. Frequently, the therapist's graceful surrender of the network assembly proposal following such an exploration results in the family significantly changing their transactions with their network. Some families may have strong investments in maintaining maladaptive network relationships, which in turn maintain rigid and dysfunctional relational patterns within the family. In such cases, the network therapist may turn to paradoxical strategies, for example, positively connoting the family's network and intrafamilial behavior and prescribing that the family continue or intensify their network transactions.

[6]Although we discuss primarily the coaching of families, this approach also can be used with individual clients.

There are several techniques for ''mapping'' the personal networks that can be used in the first step of coaching. The work of Attneave (1975), Todd (1980), and Pattison (1975) is particularly helpful. Attneave's (1975) complex and emotionally evocative ''network map'' is a printed instrument enabling family members to list and characterize all their significant relationships. Network ties are organized spatially in a diagram representing degree of closeness, relational strain, membership in kinship and nonkinship groups, and patterns of interrelationship among network members. Attneave's map requires judging degree of closeness and difficulty for each relationship. Observing families' efforts to deal with these stressful tasks provides a great deal of clinically useful information.

Todd's (1980) network diagram method has a more flexible format and does not require a printed form. It tends to focus on the conflict-free, practical dimensions of the network, and is less likely to evoke conflictual material. Todd's method is most useful when the clinician is looking for network strengths and resources rather than difficulties.

Pattison's Psychosocial Kinship Inventory (Pattison, 1975) was developed for research purposes. In addition to identifying significant network members and the relations among them, it requires clients to evaluate their relationships along such dimensions as positive versus negative attitudes, strength of attitudes, degree of emotional support, frequency of contact, and so forth. These are rated in both directions: client to network member and vice versa. Although Pattison's method provides rich material, it does not provide for a network diagram. It is therefore difficult for the therapist and family to develop a shared image of the family's network.

Describing the network leads into definitions of network strengths, weaknesses, and problems. The therapist draws on clinical experience, epidemiological research, and social network analysis to help the family understand the network's bearing on the problems that have brought them into therapy. What follows illustrates the use of this information in clinical practice.

Network size shows a well established relationship to mental health (this relationship is discussed in more detail elsewhere in this chapter). If family members report fewer than 25 people with whom each interacts regularly, the therapist can discuss strategies for enlarging network size. Examination of the reasons for small network size can reveal information concerning some of the behavioral and/or social structural origins of a family's difficulties.

Other network attributes have more complicated relationships with personal problems. Network density, or the extent to which network members know each other, is one such attribute. Networks that are more or less dense each have their own advantages and disadvantages. Dense networks have strong potentials for intimacy, support, and normative consensus. At the same time, they restrict individual autonomy, expression, and access to relationships beyond their relatively rigid boundaries. Less interconnected networks provide greater freedom at the cost of shared values and a sense of belonging. Variation in network density interacts with individual and family pathology and with cultural, ethnic, and class differences.

For example, a young woman, Carol, complains of depression, which appears related to frustrated efforts to develop autonomy. Examination of the problem in its network context reveals that her social field is limited to a very tight-knit, kinship-based network whose members share a rigid and restrictive definition of acceptable behavior. She cannot tolerate the powerful group sanctions against any move toward independence and has no alternative sources of social support. Such a client might be coached to form additional relationships in new contexts (work, voluntary associations, church, recreational activity, etc.). These new sectors in Carol's network would form few cross-ties to the original tight-knit sector. They could provide support for new kinds of social behavior and buffer against the conformity pressures of the original group. If it appears to be too difficult for the client to develop ties on her own, the therapist might use a network construction strategy, such as a transitional group.

The enmeshed family (Minuchin, 1974) tends to maintain a fairly small combined family network. Most network members have relationships with each member of the family and with almost every other member of the network. The majority of the network are kin to the family and to each other. These tiny, dense networks tend to develop idiosyncratic values and perceptions, further isolating them from the rest of the world. Ideally, the network coach would encourage each family member to form new relationships that would not overlap with those of other family members. Family loyalties are so strong in such systems that a more practicable first step would involve the whole family joining a large, cohesive group. This will dilute enmeshed family ties somewhat, making it possible to expand the networks of individual members further.

In contrast to the very dense network of isolated, enmeshed families, the networks of socially isolated individuals are composed primarily of nonfamily relations, with few or no ties among them. A client from such a sparse network may complain of anomie, loneliness, and confusion about personal identity. In disengaged families (Minuchin, 1974), each family member relates to an independent personal network that overlaps minimally with the networks of the others. The combined network of such a family is structurally similar to the personal network of the isolated individual in its sparseness and family members are likely to suffer loneliness and uncertainty. The therapist can try to increase density by helping the individual to acquaint separate friends with each other or by having family members introduce their friends to each other. Alternatively, individual or family clients may be encouraged to join a new and relatively dense group, such as a church congregation or voluntary association.

Assessment of network resources is as important to network coaching as is the diagnosis of network pathology, particularly in crisis situations. In cases where a client is expressing suicidal ideation, for instance, a thorough knowledge of the client's patterns of interaction with others helps the therapist assess the actual risks. Generally, the more a client is able to confide in others and the more that others are supportive in response, the less the risk of self-destructive behavior. It is important to know the position and relative influence of network members who insist that the client survive and of those members who are giving the client "don't exist" messages. How likely is a client to suffer dysfunctional pressures from a densely knit cluster of relationships in his or her network? The answer may depend on the number and accessibility of network members who are not connected with the problematic cluster. The more "outsiders" to the problem cluster in the client's network, the greater the protection against the cluster's harmful effects.

2.2. Partial Network Assembly

Coaching a family or individual is not always sufficient to create healing network transformations. It may be necessary to recruit network members to participate in group meetings or to provide more concrete help in the construction of new, supportive network relationships. Because the group methods often are used for purposes of network construction, they will be discussed first.

Auerswald (1971), Curtis (1974), and J. Garrison (1976) have described techniques of partial network assembly designed for groups of 3 to 20 members. All emphasize rational problem solving within a systemic frame of reference. Auerswald and Curtis invite troublesome network members in an effort to change dysfunctional relationships. In contrast, Garrison invites only those who are seen as having positive contributions to make. He allows clients to exclude potential participants.

J. Garrison (1974) describes partial network assembly in most detail. The therapist, or "convenor," acts as a mediator in a negotiation session, helping parties to rise above emotion, recognize common interests around which they can cooperate, and agree upon a course of action. When therapist and client agree to convene a partial assembly, they draw up a list of network members who have the most positive influence on the current problem and who are likely to cooperate in finding solutions. The partial assembly may be convened for such problems as adolescent delinquent behavior, preparation for discharge from a residential facility, family crisis following injury or illness of a family member, and difficulties in service integration with a "multiple family problem." It is particularly indicated when there is a need to coordinate the efforts of several service workers.

The first phase of the meeting involves greeting arrivals and socializing over refreshments. The convenor calls the group together and asks them to share their definitions of the problem by eliciting a "laundry list of complaints." Each complaint is written down and is not to be repeated. The convenor helps participants phrase their grievances in terms of observable behavior. For example, a complaint about a 16-year-old's irresponsibility is rephrased as, "he stays out late and never calls when he knows he will be late."

The "laundry list" phase serves to discharge accumulated frustration and resentment in the network in a controlled fashion. The convenor acts as an objective nonjudgmental arbitrator, channeling expressions of sentiment into factual statements. Network members receive support for expressing their angry feelings and are assured by the convenor's businesslike attention to the list that expressions of anger will not get out of hand. The convenor's rational, instrumental response to group anger stands in dramatic contrast to the full-scale network assembly conductor's approach to group polarization, which is discussed later.

Once the list is competed, the convenor helps members to transform complaints into consensual goals for group actions. For instance, the network of the boy who stayed out late may set a goal that he come home on time and always call when he knows he will be late. Considerable negotiation skill is required to help people reverse negative expectations and to reach consensus on goals derived from their grievances. The convenor seeks attainable goals for changing the problem situation.

The convenor then helps the network establish its own model for problem solving and decison making. Some networks may follow the strong leadership of one or two key activists. Others may require that each issue be discussed by all members until consensus is achieved. Every partial network assembly develops its own unique group process for planning and attaining goals. At the conclusion of the meeting, each task is assigned to specific group members who agree to carry out their assignments. The group arranges to reassemble in one or two weeks in order to review progress and, if necessary, make new plans.

In industrial society, access to power and resources often is mediated through secondary relationships. Because it gathers those actors with most influence in a problem situation, the partial network assembly often includes a substantial proportion of secondary relationships. When several agencies are involved in helping an individual or family, problems develop around defining their respective spheres of authority.

Serious problems may develop in the social matrix of the "multiple problem family," which often has antagonized or exhausted most of the potentially helpful people with whom they have primary ties. Supportive primary ties have been replaced over time by secondary ties to service workers. Each household member may relate to several different agencies that are trying to help, often in contradictory ways.[7] Role constraints, organizational boundaries, and territoriality often prevent or restrict communication among agencies and service workers. Under these circumstances, secondary relationships may be drawn unwittingly into the fray, just as the primary relationships have been before them. At the same time, families and their intimates are sucked into the dysfunctional systems that already exist within and between the agencies. Two preexisting systems, the primary sector of the network and the matrix of social agencies, are inducted into each other's dysfunctional patterns. Agencies are rendered ineffectual and family conflicts are displaced onto the secondary sector of the network. This displacement reduces stress and emotional intensity within the family, making their situation more bearable and stabilizing dysfunctional interactional patterns. Network intervention into such an "ecological system disorder" (Auerswald, 1968) helps members of the secondary sector attain objectivity and detachment and to retreat from territorial, rescuing, and competitive behavior. Agreements about specific task assignments at a partial network assembly help reduce territorial conflict among agencies and to ensure improved interagency communication.

Revitalization of primary relationships is particularly important in network therapy. Dysfunctional relations between family and the primary network sector perpetuate family disturbance. Primary ties have the advantage, however, of freedom from the institutional constraints which make secondary relationships inflexible and unresponsive. At their best, primary relations operate around the clock, cover a multitude of functions, and adapt readily to the specific demands of situations that make each client's case unique. A partial network assembly can effectively rebalance primary and secondary relations within a network.

A meeting convened for a young woman having difficulties making plans for leaving a psychiatric halfway house illustrates the process of partial network assembly. Marilyn's mother and sister, two of her mother's friends, and her friend Julie (a former resident of the halfway house) represented Marilyn's primary ties; the secondary ties included her individual therapist and the halfway house director.

The laundry list revealed problems in the relationship between mother and daughter. Marilyn complained that her semi-invalided mother pressured her to get a job, but also to provide the housekeeping the mother herself could not manage. Mother complained that Marilyn would not talk with her; Marilyn complained that her mother would not listen. Marilyn had to take care of her mother; she claimed her sister would not help. Sister, in turn, complained of feeling excluded from the family. Marilyn complained that her mother would not cooperate in getting medical care.

The halfway house director complained that Marilyn was not keeping her contract

[7]This situation is more common among those families who do not have the material resources to stay clear of public agencies. When a middle-class wife is too depressed to work and her son has been caught shoplifting, the family may quietly enter private family therapy. When a marginally employed mother is too depressed to work and her son has been caught shoplifting, mental health centers, welfare and Medicaid social workers, family court, school psychologists, etc., all may enter the scene.

with the house; she was violating rules and was risking expulsion from the house. The therapist, in obvious disagreement with the director, complained that he pushed Marilyn too much. The director countered by complaining that instead of attending her rehabilitation program, Marilyn was spending her days at her mother's house.

After these complaints were aired and recorded, the convenor helped the group agree upon these goals: Marilyn would attend her scheduled programs. The halfway house contract would be renegotiated. Marilyn's mother would get care for her leg. Communication and cooperation between mother and daughter would be improved.

The group's decision making involved strong leadership by mother's friend and the halfway house director. Marilyn was willing to attend the day program because her sister and her mother's friends agreed to take over daytime responsibilities for her mother. The director agreed to extend Marilyn's stay at the house in exchange for her compliance with rules and serious work toward her transition out of the house. The therapist agreed to monitor Marilyn's compliance with the contract. Julie suggested that Marilyn could live with her when she left the halfway house. Marilyn's mother accepted the director's help with getting health and household care. Mother and daughter agreed to restrict their phone calls and visits to a schedule that would be monitored by their entire network. Sister and friends pledged to increase their involvement with mother. After some discussion, mother and daughter agreed to begin family therapy.

Because of the expense, inconvenience, and potential embarrassment involved in bringing together the significant people in a family's life, the partial network assembly is reserved for situations where conventional therapies prove insufficient. The partial assembly can be used more readily than the full-scale assembly, which involves a much larger number of participants and therapists. A major limitation of the partial network assembly is its requirement that network members participate in rational problem solving. This approach assumes that everyone shares common interests, when in fact there are often very real contradictions among network members. Also, it often is not possible to engage group members in rational discourse about the emotion laden issues in a problem situation. When the assumptions of group rationality and common interest cannot be met, a partial network assembly can get out of hand. Partial assemblies are contraindicated when it is likely that emotions will run too high, network members cannot work rationally in a group, or that the most significant network members will not reconcile their differences. Under such circumstances, if the problem is severe enough, it may be time to consider a full-scale network assembly.

2.3. Full-Scale Network Assembly

The full-scale family network assembly was the first network therapy technique reported in the literature (Speck, 1967, Speck & Attneave, 1973). It is the most dramatic and ambitious approach to clinical work with social networks. A conductor, with a team of three to five clinicians, leads a series of one to five gatherings to which everyone who has significant relationships with the index family members is invited. The assembly is generally attended by 30 to over 80 people. Objectives for a full-scale assembly include mobilization of supportive and healing resources within the network, restructuring patterns of relationships (e.g., loosening pathological binds and tightening supportive bonds and assisting the activists in the network to become more effective leaders and helpers).

Network assemblies are especially applicable to crisis situations, such as an acute psychotic break that otherwise would lead to a psychiatric hospitalization unacceptable to the family, serious and recurrent suicide attempts, or the threatened removal of a child from his or her family. Other situations may involve enduring pain or steady deterioration, as in chronic mental illness, incorrigible juvenile delinquency, or alcoholism. Particularly for these long-standing, debilitating problems, the full-scale assembly can restore and strengthen the "burnt-out" members of the client's support system.

The therapist presents the possibility of a full-scale assembly to the client in as detailed a manner as possible. Once the family agrees to a full-scale assembly, the therapist helps them draw up a list of all their significant relations. This list often includes people who are not in frequent contact, who are geographically distant, or who have negative or ambivalent relationships with the family. One family member sometimes is unwilling to invite an important person to the assembly. The therapist can turn to other family members or close friends to do the inviting if this exclusion appears to have a homeostatic function.

Full-scale assemblies describe a predictable, spiraling sequence of six stages of group process. These stages are: (1) retribalization, (2) polarization, (3) mobilization, (4) depression, (5) breakthrough, (6) exhaustion/elation (Attneave & Speck, 1974; Rueveni, 1979; Speck & Attneave, 1973). Knowledge of the spiral model guides the team in conducting the meeting. The team "reads" the group process during the meeting, determining the stage in which the assembly is functioning and whether to shift from one stage to the next or to let the sequence unfold on its own. Each stage of the spiral sequence requires its own specific group leadership techniques.

Retribalization begins with the family's first calls to the network and the activation of communication channels among network members in response to receiving the invitations to the assembly. It bonds the group together, providing members with a powerful sense of belonging. At the beginning of the assembly itself, the conductor often uses nonverbal exercises, such as leading the group in jumping, whooping and hollering, and dancing in a circle. Team members, dispersed throughout the group, facilitate by joining in and encouraging others to join in as well. Out of breath, the participants gather in a circle with their arms about each other, swaying back and forth. The conductor may direct members of the troubled family to select a song for the group to sing. The emotionally evocative retribalization ritual is used to begin subsequent meetings or for helping transcend temporary impasse in later stages. Although vigorous exertion and song are most effective, retribalization also can be achieved through a simple ceremony in which each network member announces his or her name and relationship to the family.

Once retribalization has been established, the *polarization* phase begins. The team's task during this stage is to surface as many conflicts as possible. Unlike the partial assembly convenor (J. Garrison, 1976), the network therapy team actively draws out and intensifies group conflict. They interrupt and redirect the participants so that the group does not settle on a single complaint or an individual scapegoat. Polarization involves the emergence and dialectical interaction of the many conflictual positions in the network. The information and high level of energy generated in this process can help the group transcend the obstacles that previously have constrained them.

When polarization is difficult to achieve, differences can be brought into the open by having vocal network members form a circle in the middle of the room and discuss the problem without allowing interruption from the rest of the group. Others are allowed to speak only if they join the circle. When polarization is intense, but undirected and counterproductive, it can be structured by forming two concentric circles, each of which represents an opposing camp within the network. Dialogue between the two circles only occurs after each circle has had the opportunity to express its collective opinion without interruption. These techniques both draw out and direct existing conflict in the network. Conflict may be drawn along generational lines, between two sides of a family, between primary and secondary sectors of the network, and so forth.

The polarization stage is marked by an intensification of group energy, which had begun to build during retribalization. Angry feelings can build to extraordinary levels of intensity, yet network members rarely leave the field; nor do they appear harmed by angry confrontations. The size of the group and the long-time relationships among many members create a protected setting for otherwise risky confrontations. Although some participants seize upon the invitation to vent their negative feelings, the conductor can rely on implicit and explicit group sanctions for preventing vindictive, violent, or wilfully destructive behavior during polarization.

Transition into the *mobilization* stage begins when a small group of activists emerges from the network. Visibly frustrated at the inconclusiveness and apparently nonproductive friction of polarization, these activists start making specific proposals for action. Under their leadership, the group energy level continues to rise and the tone of the meeting shifts from anger to hope. It often happens spontaneously that the network activists emerge and the network shifts into mobilization. Conductor and team then can step back and allow the mobilization process to run its course with only occasional facilitative interventions. In some cases, the mobilization stage does not unfold unassisted and the group remains stuck in polarization. The conductor must then move the group into mobilization, cutting off unproductive arguments, exhorting the network to come up with plans of action, and only allowing participants with constructive proposals to speak.

The optimism and excitement of the mobilization stage are contagious. The network experiences a surplus of creative solutions and energy for carrying out network plans. Network members may find it hard to remember why the problem seemed so difficult in the first place.

Depression begins as the network encounters obstacles to their efforts. Family members (and other intimates) resist the well-meaning plans laid for them. Enthusiastically developed strategies suddenly seem impossible in the face of the network's homeostatic pulls. The activists begin to falter and the group energy plummets. Depression is intensified when participants confront the severity of the problems around which the network assembled. The team's task at this stage is to help the network endure this painful but necessary collective experience. It often is necessary to hold the unwilling network in this stage and to conduct network healing around issues of unresolved mourning, denial of loss, feelings of impotence, and other shared pain.

A number of exercises can be used to facilitate the network's working through its collective depression. Rueveni (1979) suggests making a severely suicidal network member the focus of a "mock funeral." The potential suicide is laid on the floor and covered with a sheet. Network members kneel one by one at his or her side, expressing their feelings as if to a dead body. This ritual can bring the network's depressive helplessness (which passively permits suicide) to an intolerable point, so that the group is jolted into refusing to allow suicide as an option.[8] Such emotionally evocative ceremonies can surface previously unmourned family loss, which has been both signaled and obscured by

[8]It may be that the mock funeral ritual also reduces vengeful motives for the potential suicide. He or she has an opportunity to act out fantasies of "getting even" without loss of life.

the suicide attempts. Working through the original loss reduces the powerful systemic demand for the suicidal behavior.

The team is fairly active in bringing the depression to a focus, with ceremonies such as the "mock funeral" and "speaking from the heart," described in the accounts of the Jones (cf. pp. 281–282) and Duquesne (cf. pp. 299–300) assemblies, which promote group support through retribalization at the same time that they evoke expressions of unhappy feelings. As network members discover that group support can make their helpless and hopeless feelings tolerable, they share in expression of their despair. They then can reexamine their original plans realistically, without the collective denial of difficulties and complexities that adheres to the planning during the mobilization stage.

Transition to the *breakthrough* stage occurs quite rapidly once the network has adequately confronted its real despair. This next stage is marked by a lifting of group spirits and a sense of renewed hope. Team members now challenge and encourage the activists to do something about the network's predicament. The network begins to set realistic goals, to develop new and creative problem-solving strategies, and to contract with individual members to carry out tasks. At this stage, the team may divide the network into small "committees." Committees often are gathered around each member of the troubled family and charged with meeting goals established for him or her in the assembly. Alternatively, committees may form around specific tasks, such as finding a job or apartment. Because earlier stages have reduced the irrational and homeostatic obstacles to productive network activity, this stage somewhat resembles the partial network assembly process described by J. Garrison (1976).

The breakthrough stage is followed by *exhaustion/elation*. Some members of the network experience a profound sense of fatigue after the group's work has been done for the evening. This exhaustion is quite distinct from the low-energy state of depression. Other participants are exuberant over the network's accomplishments. Once the group reaches this stage, the team can leave the meeting, which often continues informally into the night. With the six-stage sequence completed, the group naturally spirals up into a new retribalization, drifting into small clusters for informal conversation. Retribalization initiates a new network sequence, this time at a higher level of group development.

The spiral sequence occurs predictably at each assembly, although different stages of the spiral dominant different meetings, and later sequences are more highly evolved. The sequence also occurs between network assemblies, both for network members and for the network therapy team.

The role of conductor is as shamanistic as it is psychotherapeutic (Speck & Attneave, 1973). The term *conductor* has two meanings here. The conductor leads the assembly as an orchestra leader might direct an orchestra. He or she is also a channel that conducts network energies and experiences, much as metal conducts heat or electricity. As a conductor in the second sense, the network therapist cannot (and should not) avoid submitting to the powerful demands for emotional fusion with the retribalized group. Acting as a shaman or tribal healer, the conductor accepts this fusion and spends much of the assembly in altered states of awareness, tapping into the powerful unconscious currents of the network. The conductor's acts and utterances become vehicles for generating the network's unique symbols, symbols that guide the assembly as they help and heal.

Shamanism requires that the conductor act from unconscious and preconscious centers of the self. In order to ensure consistently sound therapeutic work, the conductor must rely on the discriminating judgment of the team, whose members are less fused with the group unconscious. Strong ties develop rapidly among team members (if they do not already exist) as the conductor and team guide each other through the manifest and hidden "worlds" that converge in the full-scale assembly.

The conductor's altered state limits certain capacities while it sharpens and strengthens others. Conductors often experience "tunnel vision" in the midst of the hubbub and confusion of full-scale assemblies. The assembly generates more information and emotional stimulation than the conductor can assimilate at the moment of intervening in network process. Team members are essential to provide a reasonably rational, consensual comprehension of a complex group situation in which much of the essential communication takes the form of whispers and gestures among people who are clustered throughout a crowded room.

Team analysis of the spiral sequence process of the network is crucial to maintaining clinical judgment and effectiveness over the course of a full-scale assembly. The team's own group process involves more than the necessary exchange of perceptions and strategies regarding the assembled network's process. The team and conductor experience a self-conscious spiral evolution as they apply their understanding of the spiral sequence model to the dynamics of their own small group. When the network's group process appears undecipherable at certain critical moments, the team's analysis of its own experience usually provides a reliable guide for appropriate intervention into the larger group.

The team's own spiral sequence is often one step ahead of the network's sequence. Knowing this is particularly helpful for managing the depression phases in assemblies. Alerted to their own depressive process, the team members can prepare themselves for the emergence of this difficult interlude in the larger group. While network activists are still leading the group through mobilization, the team and conductor have time to turn to each other for comfort as they simultaneously rediscover the severity of network problems and their own capacity for sustaining painful emotions through group support. Without this self-conscious team process, conductor and team are liable to act out their own defenses against depression through their network interventions. The team's meetings before, between, and following network assemblies also help to make sense of what emerges in the network.

Psychotherapeutic teams have capacities for imagination and creativity that are well suited to the most demanding of clinical challenges (Palazzoli *et al.*, 1978). These faculties are particularly important in full-scale assemblies, in which floods of information and excitation require the constant invention and modulation of strategies. As team members repeatedly shift their frames of reference, they discover solutions that organize the proliferating alternatives generated by the assembly.

2.4. Network Construction

At times the therapist may conclude that a family's network is too small or that the family (or individual) is trapped in a web of pathogenic network forces that the therapist does not expect to be able to treat successfully. Under these circumstances, the client(s) can be helped to build new networks through coaching techniques, "networking,"[9] or mutual support group therapy.

[9]The practice of networking (Miles, 1978; Parker, 1977) involves developing, maintaining, and utilizing relatively informal network ties organized around specific needs or interests (e.g., teachers interested in sharing information about limited educational resources or new teaching techniques). The network therapist can help family members locate appropriate informal interest networks.

One way to construct networks of unrelated individuals is through the establishment of psychotherapeutic mutual support groups. Trimble (1980) describes such a group in which members were encouraged to rely on each other's support around the clock not only during formal meeting times. Child care, crisis intervention, emotional nurturance, information, and material resources were exchanged among members of this constructed network. Anything exchanged within such a network is subject to group discussion. Group membership provides a relatively protected context in which to learn less dysfunctional strategies for managing personal relationships. Many clients devote themselves exclusively to relations within the constructed network at first, which enables them to withdraw from the toxic webs of their own personal networks and to gain perspective on their network problems. This "transitional network" sustains its members and offers them new ways to relate to others so that members eventually can form their own personal networks which will support future health and growth.

The mutually supportive relationships characteristic of constructed networks often emerge spontaneously in multiple family therapy groups (Laqueur, 1972), which include designated patients and family members. Multiple family groups provide isolated and enmeshed families with new network ties that dilute family binds and offer alternative ways of interacting. Groups set up for the mutual support of the relatives of psychiatric patients (Atwood, 1978) provide similar opportunities for network construction. Day hospitals and halfway houses can serve similar functions.

2.5. Community Network Therapy

Comprehension of the elusive, invisible structures of relationships that ramify among people and groups is essential to effective network therapy. The more fully one understands the social context of clinical problems, the more certain one can be of network therapy techniques. The network perspective requires that the network therapist understand his or her own network of personal and professional ties in the community where he or she practices. This understanding provides a "window" through which to apprehend the social structures and dynamics of the community.[10]

The practice of community network therapy involves the use of many interacting networks within a community. Some networks are client-centered and others are defined by group or professional membership (mental health agencies, youth gangs, church congregations, etc.). The community network therapist develops a position in the community from which to navigate the existing pathways within and between networks, construct new linkages, and generate new patterns in this ever changing social field. Such practice, especially as it involves dealing with service workers, provides one with access to many community groups. Establishing marginal memberships in many groups, the community network therapist becomes a broker and mediator of information and resources among groups and is in a good position to engage in "networking" for clients. In this process, the network therapist initiates many new linkages among previously unconnected workers and agencies. These ties often are informal and based on shared interests. As such they are well adapted to "networking" among service workers as well.

Community network therapy is particularly applicable when the therapist works in

[10]The view through the window of the therapist's own network can be narrow and misleading, however. Communities are more complicated than mere "networks of networks." In addition, one cannot know everyone in the community, and forming certain ties excludes the possibility of developing others.

one community, primarily with a single clinical population, for example, chronic psychiatric patients or dying people and their families. Careful cultivation of ties with the primary and secondary sectors of client-centered networks puts the therapist in a good position to understand and influence local agency practice and to facilitate future clients' effective integration into existing contexts.

Community network therapy is especially effective with the networks of chronic psychiatric patients (the development of such a practice is described in detail in Trimble & Kliman, 1981). Family members in schizophrenic transaction, who have difficulties managing relationships, frequently must rely on secondary ties with service workers from a number of different agencies. At the same time, serious differences often exist among agencies, between clients and agencies, or between agencies and intimates. The community network therapist can draw on his or her multiple memberships to mediate among agencies and between the primary and secondary sectors of clients' networks.

When the community network therapist utilizes the full-scale network assembly, the emergent difficulties between the primary and secondary network sectors, and within each sector, often are expressed through polarization against the conductor. The conductor comes to represent all the service workers for members of the primary sector and all other service workers for the competing members of the secondary sector. When the entire assembled network polarizes against the conductor, their shared temporary antagonism toward a single target can facilitate new levels of cooperation. Families and service workers both tend to feel helpless and hopeless in their relations with and advocacy for chronic patients. Their united polarization against the conductor is welcomed by the network therapy team and the energy it generates is channeled into constructive action. Through this process, both primary and secondary sectors can experience some measure of control and competence.

It is not always possible to resolve differences between the primary and secondary sectors or between competing agencies. It sometimes happens that differences in the secondary sector of the network are exposed in the course of community network therapy but prove to be irreconcilable. Under these circumstances, instead of serving as a vehicle for empowering the network, polarization against the conductor rigidifies into scapegoating of the network therapist. The community network therapist's local recognition can turn into notoriety, making it difficult for him or her to facilitate interagency cooperation around the target population within the community.

3. Advantages of the Network Approach

The family is a small and relatively homogeneous social system. Its members share a unique history. Their identities, personality structures, ideologies, and transactional styles are intertwined with each other's, historically and evermore. In our society, the family unit is a veritable crucible of the most intense and emotionally significant of human bonds, providing the earliest and most enduring experiences of nurturance and authority, of satisfaction and frustration of desire.

These characteristics contribute to a powerful loyalty to the familial homeostasis even when individual members are painfully at odds with each other. This loyalty, while essential to the family's survival, can rigidify into resistance to change when families who are confronted with new and developing circumstances are unable to expand their transactional repertoires and grow in response to those changes. The same holds true for intense nonfamilial relationships.

The network is a larger, more heterogeneous, and less densely interwoven system, which shares its experience of history less intimately and collectively than does the family.[11] Network members' relations with family members are shaped by individuals' differing personal experiences, circumstances, and beliefs. The network is diverse and flexible in its membership and in the kinds of ties that exist among members. This diversity allows the network to sustain a wider range of individual behaviors and roles than a single family can tolerate. The therapist intervening in a network is therefore more likely to find allies who can help foster and maintain therapeutic change than if he or she were working alone with an index family. Although psychologically less salient than the family itself, the network is important enough to the family that changes in the network or between the network and the family can lead to changes within the family. At the same time, the ties between the family and the network are weaker than those within the family itself, and network members are likely to be less invested in the familial homeostasis. That is not to say that they have no such investment; witness the homeostatic responses of relatives and friends to spouses who begin to discuss the possibility of divorce.

3.1. The Power of Crisis

Times of crisis provide the clinician with particularly valuable opportunities to reframe and restructure dysfunctional interpersonal systems and to foster changes in individual beliefs and perceptions about their relationships. Any system that is thrown into crisis and unknown experience first attempts to fall back on familiar strategies for managing stress. When old strategies prove unsuccessful, flexible systems begin to experiment with alternative approaches, thereby adding to their repertoires. More rigid systems keep returning to their accustomed patterns, despite obvious failure. The therapist often can break through this self-defeating attempt to maintain sameness by reframing family members' behavior (Palazzoli *et al.*, 1978) or through using therapeutic authority to restructure interactions (Minuchin & Fishman, 1981). When a family system is too rigidified to permit change from within, or when the network contributes to the family's rigidity and perceived helplessness, a network intervention may be appropriate.

Our work with the McShane family network illustrates how networks can be used to promote constructive change in times of crisis. Alice McShane, a 32-year-old unmarried woman diagnosed as borderline psychotic and alcoholic, had been temporarily judged incompetent to care for her children by the local protective services agency. Nine-year-old Lynnette had been shuttled among the homes of several foster parents and of her maternal grandparents for several years. Her 2-year-old half-sister Susan had spent most of her life with foster parents who hoped to adopt her.

The authors were called in by one of the many agencies involved with the McShanes, just six weeks before the courts were to make a final determination of custody. Alice, drinking heavily and threatened with eviction because of her raucous drinking parties, wanted "another chance" to live with Lynnette (who acted parentally toward her) but could not decide about whether to allow Susan to be adopted by her psychological parents. Alice's divorced parents half-heartedly supported Lynnette's return, but explicitly refused to sanction the return of Susan, who reminded them of her addict father. Alice's sister,

[11]Some networks, however, are extremely tight-knit and intimate in historical and present relationships and as such share a carefully enforced normative code and a collective belief system that is not open to challenge. Some networks of recent immigrants have such characteristics.

Molly, and Sharon, Alice's adolescent lodger, argued angrily against Lynnette's return. Alice's drinking buddies cheered on her maternal spirit and offered to include the youngsters in their partying. The plethora of social workers were aghast, anxiously reminding Alice of her past neglectfulness and irresponsibility and threatening legal action to rescue the children. Lynnette said she wanted to come home so that she and Mommy could take care of each other. Susan became tearful when separated from her foster parents.

With the future of two children and their various caretakers in the balance, it was only possible to hold one full-scale network assembly, as the authors and the network were in different states. The assembly was held to facilitate the decision-making process concerning the permanent placement of the two little girls, a decision ultimately to be made by the courts. One author was the conductor; the team consisted of the other author and the two social workers who had asked us to consult. The network members who attended were: Alice, her parents and their spouses, her sister and brother-in-law, Lynnette, Lynnette's present foster mother and two previous foster mothers, Susan's foster parents, (Susan was not present), and their two best friends, a former parent aide, Susan's estranged father, Alice's lover, Alice's landlady, several angry neighbors, several drinking buddies, Alice's boarder, Lynnette's teacher, and eight representatives of five social agencies involved with the family, including Alice's individual therapist.

The network assembly began with a sense of despair. Advocates for the children were convinced that Alice could not care adequately for the girls, but that Lynnette and possibly Susan would be returned to her anyway. Alice and Lynnette were profoundly ambivalent about living together, but could express only the positive side of their ambivalence. They did so more belligerently as service workers and relatives argued against their reunion. Susan's foster parents were frightened that they would lose the child to a "crazy lady" or to a string of foster homes if she were not immediately freed for adoption. Alice's drinking buddies exuberantly supported her efforts to bring her children into her home without altering her hard-drinking, partying way of life.

Polarization in the meeting was intense, alternating with depression. A deadlock that prevented constructive decisions centered on the network's erroneously dichotomized perceptions of Alice. The implicit network ideology, in effect, was: If you care about Alice, then you must wholeheartedly support her right to live with her children; if you criticize or question her ability to mother, then you reject her as a person. The network fell into two opposing camps of staunch believers. One camp accused the other of rejecting Alice, while the other accused the first of gross irresponsibility toward dependent children. Only Alice and Lynnette appeared unsure of what they believed. Everyone felt angry and hopeless, including the network therapy team.

Breakthrough finally was achieved much as it was for the Jones family network. When depressive anger became so intense that some network members no longer could tolerate staying, Alice and Lynnette were seated next to each other in the middle of the room. Network members were asked to speak from the heart to one or both of them. Facing both dependent and needy people at once, network members were forced to respond to the conflicting dependency needs of both mother and daughter and to acknowledge their confusion in the face of such complexity. The simplistic dichotomy no longer was tenable. After several false starts in which a number of people mistakenly assumed that it was decided that Lynnette would move in with Alice, "speaking from the heart" gave expression to network members' own sadness. It also provided mother and daughter an important opportunity to express their love and longing for each other, along with an acknowledgment of the limitations of their relationship.

Receiving a new, more unified message from the network, Alice was able to accept love and support without being overwhelmed by internal and external expectations she could not meet. For the first time, she was blocked from using network splits to externalize the splitting-off that characterized her intrapsychic and interpersonal relations. She no longer could use her drinking buddies' unqualified support to rail against her relatives, her therapist, and the service workers. Seeing that her mother was receiving support and nurturance from the adults, Lynnette was able to begin to relinquish her parental role and to express her desire to "visit Mommy on Saturdays."

The network ended with Alice letting go of her symbolic hold on Susan and agreeing to her adoption. She was less ready to release Lynnette, whom she had mothered for three years, but was willing to acknowledge her present inability to care consistently for her. Arrangements were made to keep mother and daughter in touch and the protective services agency agreed to recommend that the coming legal decision be made on a temporary basis. Alice's parents and sister, greatly relieved that she would not be taking the girls home, committed themselves to providing more emotional and material support to Alice.

3.2. Treatment Impasse

Family therapists have at their disposal a variety of effective strategies for dealing with the grim collective determination of many families to rid themselves of troublesome symptoms without making any changes in their family systems (Haley, 1976; Minuchin & Fishman, 1981; Palazzoli *et al.*, 1978; Papp, 1980). Network therapy is not necessary when breakthrough can be achieved through systemic techniques within family treatment. It is sometimes the case, however, that changes are not possible within the family holon so long as family members' various relationships in extrafamilial holons remain unchanged.

A clear example of network collusion in maintaining dysfunctional family transactions was provided in our discussion of the Jones family network, in which the ineffectual mother–delinquent son sequences were perpetuated through mother and son's extra familial experiences with network members. The son's delinquency and premature moves out of tbe family were encouraged, while the mother's authority was undermined by her son's older friends. Under these circumstances, it was virtually impossible to help the family find new interactional strategies without activating the network's cooperation.

Network intervention also can be helpful in breaking through treatment impasse when the family is underinvolved (rather than destructively involved) with its network. Deeply enmeshed families in schizophrenic transaction often have minimal contact with other people. An isolated family often functions almost as if it were a closed system, so that the family's decreasingly effective coping strategies become ever more deeply entrenched. The psychological quicksand in which such a family is immersed is liable to suck in a family therapist, rendering him or her as powerless to change within the therapeutic system as is the family. It is rarely possible to pull oneself out of a pit of quicksand and the therapist would be wise not to count on the family for assistance. The family therapist sinking waist deep in the family quicksand would do well to cry out for the network's help; a chain of people can effect a rescue over treacherous and shifting terrain. If it is impossible to renew or strengthen enough network ties, the therapist can help the family construct a network.

3.3. Shared Problem-Solving

Because networks are larger than families, they offer more possibilities for creative problem solving and more resources for carrying out plans. An individual family can be overwhelmed, for instance, by the task of helping a recently released psychiatric patient to find a job or apartment. A group of 40, however, may well be able to come up with information about apartments or new ideas and concrete opportunities for employment. Middle-class and wealthy networks may be able to provide direct employment in addition to job-hunting suggestions. Members of poor and working-class networks may set up exchanges of services, for instance, lodging in return for childcare. The network often can supply more muscle in getting the designated patient to follow through on plans, and to prevent sabotage from within the family than can the therapist. Network members can provide short-term concrete assistance during crises, circumventing the need for hospitalization, foster care, or recourse to the courts. An entire network can be mobilized to share responsibility for around-the-clock suicide watches, with far less exhaustion, burnout, and risk of communicating "don't exist" messages than can despairing families. Relatives or family friends of a severely acting-out adolescent may take him or her temporarily into their home when the family can see no alternative but court-ordered placement. These adults may be better equipped to demand the young person's respect and cooperation at such a time, perhaps even insisting on esteem-building responsibilities within the household.

Network members also are in a position to offer assistance with child care and housework, loans of money or car, advocacy with social agencies, companionship, information, and advice (for which families might otherwise turn to impersonal and beleaguered social agencies). Some of these offers can be made unilaterally; often they are most beneficial when offered on a reciprocal basis so that a family in need can experience themselves as helpers as well as helped.

3.4. Changing Dysfunctional Family and Network Patterns

The very intensity of emotional ties that characterizes the family can be either the strength or the undoing of a family in severe distress. At its most extreme, this intensity is manifested in families in schizophrenic transaction (Palazzoli *et al.*, 1978), who can neither tolerate living with each other nor the thought of living without each other, and who cannot discover the means to express, let alone resolve, their dilemma. Such circumstances breed despair. The despair of these families often is communicated as a hopeless, angry challenge to any who would try to make their lives better.

Such challenges can lead to two outcomes. First, they drive away many people who otherwise might engage in helping or reciprocal (mutually helpful) relationships with family members. As the family's predicament worsens and their presentation of themselves become more unpleasant to witness, ties to network members are lost or impoverished. The range of available relationships narrows. Generally, it is easier to get rid of friends and co-workers than relatives or social workers. An increasingly circumscribed set of accessible behaviors and roles accompanies the narrowing social range. The family who interacts less, in a narrower range of relationships, turns in on itself and develops increasingly rigid and stereotypic transactional sequences and styles.

The second outcome of the impossible challenge is less obvious. Some people do not give up and desert when they meet such a challenge. Palazzoli and her colleagues (1978) demonstrate how powerfully these challenges can induct the dedicated (and ambitious) therapist into the family's self-destructive dance. Offers of help toward change are distorted into help in perpetuating the dance. The family's endlessly repeating cycle of protest against and desperate attempts to maintain their deteriorating system attracts and then exhausts not only therapists, but others as well. Those relatives, acquaintances, co-workers, social service institutions, and social service workers who maintain ties with families in schizophrenic transaction all enter into increasingly stereotyped patterns in their doings with (and about) the family. Even as they try to support, advise, blame, comfort, and threaten family members, they unwittingly join the family's efforts to "perfect" the constricted steps of the family's unhappy dance. In doing so, they implicitly sanction and promote the very dysfunction they protest and deplore.

Network members are not passively seduced into the family's destructive dance, however; they participate in its creation. The dance is choreographed over years of interaction within the family and between the family and the network. It takes form in relation to the structure, circumstances, and requirements of the network and the quality of family members' interactions with each other and with individual network members (indeed, with society as a whole). The dance manifests the interpenetration of interacting individual psyches, the family system, the network system, and the forces, structures, and institutions of society. All of those elements influence, and are influenced by, the dance.

The therapist can do relatively little within the confines of clinical practice to alter the distorting impact of society. Clinical changes are possible, however, through the network, which mediates between individual and family psychology and society. For instance, the identified patient and one parent in severely disturbed families frequently are profoundly fused, while other family members collude in their own exclusion, appearing to escape the suffocating closeness of the dyad. Family therapists can not always effect the "appropriate" changes in which the parents (in two-parent families) are given back to each other and the designated patient returns to the sibling subsystem (Minuchin, 1974). They find that the apparently disengaged family members and the enmeshed family members want little to do with each other. The fusion seems impenetrable and everybody (all the individuals and the enmeshed twosome) remains profoundly lonely.[12]

Exploration of network dynamics in such cases is likely to reveal that the network, as well as the family, colludes in this state of affairs. Network members argue that "he only listens to his mother anyway," or that "they're both so impossible, they deserve each other," or that "no one can help you but family, so it's good that she and her mother are so close." These rationalizations and the homeostatic needs they serve can not always be changed within many families, but can be challenged effectively in the less entrenched system of the network.

In the Duquesne family (described in more detail in Trimble & Kliman, 1981), the father's physical disability exempted him from responsibility toward his only child, Janet. The mother, enraged at her sick husband, devoted most of her energy to her institutionalized daughter, while still managing to maintain a surprisingly high level of community ties. The 28-year-old daughter kept her mother angrily engaged with her through floridly psychotic and exaggeratedly dependent behavior, thereby saving her father from desertion or strangulation. Despite the fact that Janet had lived in residences and hospitals for a decade, neither mother nor daughter made a move without the other.

The Duquesnes' entire network ostensibly had been kept ignorant of Janet's psychiatric career; her parents had informed friends and relatives that she had moved out of state. When a full-scale assembly was convened before Janet's release, however, it became

[12]Occasionally, a "well sibling" manages to escape this collective loneliness, most often by effecting an early escape from home and establishing a new network not based on kinship ties. Some of these "well siblings" are able to avoid replicating their original situations in their new lives; others are not.

apparent that most had known about Janet's hospitalization but had colluded in keeping the "secret." After a couple of network assemblies, the network's negative view of the mother–daughter fusion emerged.

The network's initial handling of the issue of fusion was homeostatic in nature. Some members blamed mother for being overprotective, others criticized Janet for acting like a baby. No one held the father or any other network member responsible for the present state of affairs. None of these positions held any possibility for change. During the third assembly, the network conductor set up a kinetic sculpture in which mother and daughter were instructed to hold onto each other for dear life and members of the network were instructed to tear them away from each other. Not surprisingly, the network failed in their task. A team member huddled briefly with a few network members, instructing them to draw the two women apart by inviting them, warmly and firmly, to engage in separate activities with the members. The group was surprised to discover that this tactic was far more effective than force.

Assimilating the metaphor of the exercise, the network began dealing with the family in new ways. One couple invited the parents to join them for their first weekend away from home without Janet in many years. The invitation was acceptable for two reasons. First, the couple did not have to spend the weekend alone together (an unpleasant idea, considering the state of their marriage), since each spouse had a friend for the weekend. Second, several network members agreed to keep Janet occupied for the weekend, so that she could not sabotage the trip. Thus, activation of each family member's extrafamilial ties reduced the fusion between mother and daughter, simultaneously easing marital tension.

3.5. Changing Network Size and Structure

A number of epidemiological studies suggest a relationship between network size on the one hand and psychopathology and prognosis on the other. These findings have significant implications for clinical work. Pattison, De Francisco, Wood, Frazier, and Crowder (1975) found that "normal" individuals related to 20 to 30 people in the intimate zones of their networks and that these relationships generally were rated positively. Neurotic individuals in the study could count only 10 to 12 people in their intimate networks (some of whom were physically distant or even deceased), including people with whom they had negatively or ambivalently rated relationships. Pattison found that psychotic individuals related to tiny intimate networks of 4 or 5 people, most of whom were immediate family. Their relationships uniformly were ambivalent. Pattison did not examine the network beyond the intimate zone.

Other authors, using different network measures (often extending beyond the intimate zone) also report a decrease in network size associated with increasingly severe psychopathology. Cohen and Sokolovsky (1978), in a study of schizophrenic and nonpsychotic residents of a single-room occupancy hotel, found that even actively psychotic schizophrenic residents averaged network ties to 10.3 people. Schizophrenics without residual symptoms had networks averaging 14.8 people. Nonpsychotic residents (most of whom were alcoholic or indigent) had networks averaging 22.5 people. Tolsdorf (1976) and Hammer (1978) found that schizophrenics and nonschizophrenics did not vary in number of ties to kinfolk, but that the non-kin segments of schizophrenics' networks were considerably smaller. Garrison, in her study of schizophrenic and nonschizophrenic migrant Puerto Rican women in the Bronx, found that relatively well functioning schizophrenics relied more on non-kin ties than on family. The most disturbed women maintained very few, overdependent relations with kin who were not of the same generation, and with virtually no one else except service workers (V. Garrison, 1978).

There appear to be relationships not only between network size and severity of diagnosis but also between network size and course of illness. Sokolovsky, Cohen, Berger, and Geiger (1978) found that expatients who relate to larger, more highly interconnected (dense) extrafamilial networks are hospitalized less frequently. Strauss and Carpenter (1977) report that the patient's degree of social connectedness with friends prior to psychotic break is one of three most powerful prognostic predictors. Brown, Birley, and Wing (1972) found that, for schizophrenics living with family, the *relatives'* degree of social connectedness is a predictor of rehospitalization rates for the patient; patients whose relatives had more ties had lower rates of rehospitalization. Leff reports that schizophrenics are less likely to be rehospitalized when they do not live with family. Schizophrenics who do live with family do significantly better when both patient and relatives spend sizable portions of time out of the home, in independent social interactions (Leff, 1981; Faughn & Leff, 1976).

Density, or the extent to which network members are interconnected, also is related to the course and outcome of schizophrenia. Cohen and Sokolovsky found that schizophrenics without residual symptoms had denser networks than schizophrenics who were actively psychotic, and that nonschizophrenics had even more densely connected networks. They also reported that, of the schizophrenics without residual symptoms, those with denser (and larger) non-kin network sectors were able to stay out of the hospital for longer periods of time.

Tolsdorf's (1976) and Hammer, Makiesky-Barrow, and Gutwirth's (1978) studies of the smaller nonkin sectors of schizophrenics' networks suggest that the nonintimate zones of schizophrenics' networks are less dense than those of normal and neurotic individuals. Hammer indicates that schizophrenics' networks show fewer clusters of non-kin members, and fewer cross-ties among those clusters. Unsupported ties (relationships with network members who do not know each other) frequently are lost during hospitalization, further decreasing network size for chronically or periodically hospitalized people. Finally, she suggests that many of the people in schizophrenics' networks themselves have sparsely populated networks; thus a source of new network ties is lost (Hammer, 1978).

Although we do not know of related epidemiological evidence, at this writing, our clinical experience suggests that a number of other clinical populations present variations in network density. We find that borderline psychotic patients (who tend to split off intrapsychic and interpersonal relationships) often have networks that are larger than those of psychotics, but which are fragmented, consisting of a high proportion of unsupported and fragile relationships. In contrast, abusing families tend to have smaller, but very dense networks consisting of people with similar and overlapping networks of their own (Kaplan, Salzinger, Pelcovitz, Samit, Krieger, Artemyeff, & Ganeles, 1981).

Another significant variable involves directionality of social ties between the index person and network members. Toldsdorf (1976), Sokolovsky *et al.* (1978), and Hammer *et al.* (1978) all report that, in comparison with others, schizophrenics have fewer ties that are reciprocal, that is, in which help and definition of the relationship are bilateral. Schizophrenics also have fewer relationships in which they are helpful to others, and more in which they are dependent on the help of others. In a related finding, schizophrenics were shown to have a smaller proportion of multiplex relationships (ties with more than one dimension, e.g., friends who are also co-workers or neighbors) than nonschizophrenics. Uniplex relationships tend to be more fragile and less enduring than multiplex ties. Cohen and Sokolovsky (1978) found that schizophrenics who did not have residual symptoms had more success in avoiding hospitalization when they had more multiplex ties.

To summarize without suggesting a causal direction, the more severe psychological disturbances are epidemiologically associated with greater social isolation of the index patient, and frequently of that person's intimates as well. More disturbed people tend to have less densely interconnected networks with a higher proportion of unsupported ties outside the intimate zone.[13] Finally, the more severely disturbed the individual, the fewer reciprocal or helpful (rather than dependent) relations, and the fewer multiplex ties he or she is likely to have.

These findings have significant clinical implications. All of the network variables just described interact with family and individual variables. For instance, there is considerable evidence that social connectedness (or "social supports," a related concept in psychiatric epidemiology) buffers people against the psychological and physical consequences of stress (Dean & Lin, 1977; Dohrenwend & Dohrenwend, 1974; Liem & Liem, 1978; Lin *et al.*, 1979; Mitchell & Trickett, 1980). Schizophrenics and their families are particularly vulnerable to stress; they are less able to manage stress effectively and they are more likely to create stressful situations than most people. Yet the very people who most need the buffering that networks afford have the smallest and least effective social networks.

Network underpopulation also interacts with schizophrenics' characteristic problems with initiating social contacts and carrying on reciprocal relationships (Beels, 1978). Small networks reduce the number of opportunities to engage in beneficial interactions and difficulties in engaging in such behavior can lead to reduction of network size, and so on, in circular fashion. Sparse family networks often are associated with high indices of expressed emotion in which family members' hostile and critical communications toward the index patient are unmodulated by extrafamilial opportunities to complain or by extrafamilial supports of various kinds (Brown *et al.*, 1972; Vaughn & Leff, 1976).

Many of the problems of underpopulated networks of severely disturbed families (and more highly functioning families in acute distress) can be ameliorated, if not completely corrected, in the course of network therapy. Effective network size can be increased through network construction and coaching. Dormant ties can be reactivated, particularly when other network members can influence the people whose relationships with the index family are broken or deteriorated. Some dormant ties, previously toxic, can be neutralized through therapeutic intervention and careful monitoring by concerned network members.

We have noted that psychotic and borderline patients and their families tend to have a high proportion of unsupported ties in their networks. Unsupported ties (which are not problematic when they constitute a low proportion of the network) often are lost during periods of hospitalization. Many of these losses may be explained by the fact that network members do not communicate with each other and therefore may not know the index patient's whereabouts or how to reach him or her. Some network members may not

[13]Cultural differences must be considered here. For instance, an Italian working-class immigrant who is schizophrenic may have a denser network than a middle-class and well-functioning Yankee, but a far less dense network than his normal Italian neighbor.

initiate renewed contact on their own, but would do so if encouraged by others. Increasing network density can help hospitalized patients to maintain needed social connections. Sometimes it is even possible to prevent hospitalization when network members are in touch with each other and can communicate and act on concerns, for instance about signs of decompensation.

For patients with borderline personalities, their many unsupported ties and the intrapsychic splitting off of internal objects seem to reflect each other. The many people who are drawn into isolated relationships with borderlines come to represent split-off part-objects, and as such are played against each other. Many of these relationships end when the index patient rejects the friend, relative, or therapist who has come to represent an unacceptable internal object, or when the other person is pushed into doing the rejecting. A network history is likely to show disastrously broken relationships with now-detested or idealized former friends, lovers, work associates, therapists, and estranged relatives, as well as some active relationships that are in serious trouble. Sometimes such a network includes several therapists, each unaware that the others exist and each prescribing different medications.

One such network was assembled when Roberta White made a serious suicide attempt with medications collected from four different mental health clinics. Roberta, the divorced mother of two children with sickle-cell anemia, had succeeded in alienating her parents and sisters, her estranged lover, and most of her local friends. She kept her more distant and friendlier relatives and her assortment of therapists ignorant of most of what was going on in her life. Her remaining friends did not know each other. At the assembly, everyone who had been closely involved with Roberta for any length of time was angry, frustrated, and frightened by her and upset with each other. New friends and distant relatives could not understand how the others could be so rejecting of this charming woman.

During the full-scale assembly, however, network members who previously had been set up against each other began to exchange stories about Roberta that revealed her triangulation of her network. As Roberta's self-destructive and alienating manipulations became increasingly apparent, network members began developing a "united front" to undercut her maneuvers so that they could support her without feeling exhausted or abused. As relatives recognized that Roberta might succeed in dying before her ailing children, they were able to take explicit and cooperative responsibility for the care and upbringing of the two frightened children in the event that their mother's suicide could not be prevented.

3.6. Interdependence and Shared Responsibility

Mainstream American culture holds that individuals are entirely responsible for their own fates. Success and failure, contentment and misery, all are seen as individual accomplishments. The sufferer is responsible for his or her own suffering either through direct action or through failure to protect against victimization by another. (Here an additional target of blame emerges. If the individual sufferer has been victimized, then the victimizer usually is seen as the parents, particularly the mother.) There is little room in such a view for the social aspects of human suffering.

Not all Americans hold this view, of course. Some ethnic American subcultures continue to integrate personal experience more closely with community life. In such cultures, interdependence is valued over individuality and blame for suffering is more likely to be placed on the failure to uphold community norms than on failing to care for oneself.

Although any treatment requires some measure of respect for individual responsibility, a comprehensive clinical approach recognizes the network's deep involvement in the psychological and social well-being of its members. Through the process of retribalization,[14] network therapy makes networks—who usually do not experience themselves as social collectivities and whose members often are unaware of their mutual impact—conscious of their responsibilities for each other, and of their collective potential for constructive action. Retribalization helps take the onus of badness or madness off the individual or family. Distress, neediness, confusion, anxiety, anger, loneliness, and helplessness are deprivatized, reducing shame in the sufferer(s) and embarrassment among the network members. A sense of shared responsibility begins to undermine the individualistic beliefs that have contributed to the isolation and despair of the network, family, and individual. This transformation of beliefs about responsibility for emotional suffering has positive consequences for the future mental health of members of the network and for relations in the personal network of each member, as well as for the immediate psychotherapeutic task.

3.7. The Network Effect

When Speck and Attneave (1973) began experimenting with social network therapy, they discovered that not only did the index family demonstrate clinical gains in the course of treatment, but that other network members began to do better as well. An aunt and uncle who reach out to a family in distress begin to address their own marital difficulties in new and more effective ways. A neighbor's generous offer to help an overwhelmed single parent with childcare is also an opportunity for the neighbor, who has been feeling depressed and useless since her children went to school, to regain self-esteem by helping another.

This "network effect" (Speck & Attneave, 1973) can be understood in a number of ways. The networks in which dysfunctional families are embedded often show dysfunctional interactional patterns as well. An intervention that helps network members find new ways to interact with the index family can ripple out to influence their relationships with each other and with their own personal networks. Not only specific interventions concerning network interactions, but the very experience of participating in the powerful group process of the full-scale assembly, has an impact on individual and collective psychology.

Another aspect of the network effect involves network members' relationship to stress. Even "healthy" network members are subjected to considerable stress because of their ties to disturbed members or clusters of the network. As the healing process of network therapy continues and stress is better modulated within the network, individual stress levels decline and tolerance for stressful experience improves.

The network effect also occurs when network interventions are made into the networks of relatively healthy people who are in severe situational crisis. Such crises as death, angry divorce, a fire in an apartment building, or natural disaster can have pro-

[14]Although the term *retribalization* has unfortunate overtones of nostalgia for an unrecapturable and romanticized tribal past, it does place important emphasis on the collective power of the network experience made conscious.

found effects on entire networks (J. Kliman, Kern, & Kliman, 1982). Nine-year-old Tanya James and her family came into treatment after Tanya had been slightly injured when her best friend, Ruth, drowned in an ice skating accident. Tanya had begun taking on Ruth's mannerisms, spending her afternoons at the neighboring home of Ruth's family, and insisting on being called by her friend's name. Meetings with the James family revealed that the bereaved family was contributing to Tanya's efforts to replace her dead friend. Tanya's parents had not interfered, since they hoped that their daughter might be a comfort to their grieving neighbors and since they were painfully aware that the dead child could have been their own. The two families lived in a tightknit neighborhood and their children attended the same school. The accident had been witnessed by several neighborhood children.

The tragedy that brought a single family into treatment had affected the lives of an entire neighborhood, dozens of schoolmates and their teachers, and the friends and extended families of two households. A network therapy intervention with a primary goal of helping the two families find a more adaptive way to mourn also provided a very large group of people (the overlapping networks of the two families) the opportunity to mourn collectively.

Such work has preventive as well as reparative consequences. Every loss recalls earlier losses and provides an opportunity for further working through of those losses. In addition, when one experiences the death of someone who was not very close, a "psychological immunization" (G. Kliman, 1968) takes place. This immunization helps prepare one for the eventuality of more personally significant future losses. In the case described, young neighbors and classmates were helped to utilize the tragic, but somewhat removed, experience of Ruth's death for developing their abilities to cope with the eventual deaths of intimates.

Another preventive benefit of the network effect involves network members' heightened sense of social belonging. This greater (or renewed) awareness of connectedness is related to network members' participation in a collective problem-solving process and the demonstration of caring in a large group. The recognition that mutual support is possible even when conflict and anger are expressed openly can ramify into network members' developing relationships with each other and with members of their own personal networks. Finally, witnessing and participating in an entire network's mobilization to meet the needs of one individual or family help participants to feel safe about expressing their own needs and about asking and receiving help.

3.8. Empowering the Network

Most people turn to the mental health industry when they feel that something they ought to be able to control has gotten out of hand. When serious psychological symptoms are involved, people often feel helpless and mystified. Something has gone mysteriously and terribly wrong and relief seems attainable only through the ministerings of experts trained in the secret workings of the human mind. Popular culture informs the troubled that psychological distress is the result of their own inadequacy or that the blame for serious symptoms lies with a history of poor parenting. Troubled individuals and families thus enter therapeutic relationships bearing a burden of guilt for being bad, incompetent, or both.

Interactions with many psychiatric facilities and therapists perpetuate these feelings of guilt and incompetence. Families often are blamed for their own distress by the very people who try to help them. The very act of hospitalization communicates to the family that they are unable to care for their own, or even that they are destructive to one another. By demonstrating their relative ability as caretakers, mental health workers unwittingly reinforce family members' feelings of incompetence—and perpetuate a self-defeating strategy for managing family problems.

Under these circumstances, the designated patient is thrown into conflict: how can he or she allow strangers to be more helpful than family? Family members, who genuinely may wish for improvement, nevertheless find it hard to tolerate others' success where they have failed. "Resistance" to therapy, which often is a show of family loyalty as much as it is a show of family stuckness, proves to therapists how "sick" or "bad" these families are and how much more help they need. This unfortunate cycle can go on for years.

After years of relinquishing their potential for competence and control over their unhappy lives to mental health and other service workers, families are bound to feel as angry as they do helpless. Their anger most often is turned inward, expressed in continuing family conflict, passive resistant dealings with agencies, and ever deteriorating self-esteem among family members.

The equilibrium of this chronic system is upset when the entire system is brought into therapy. The network therapists challenge people who feel resentful and helpless (toward each other and toward the agencies) to do what the therapists and institutions have been unable to do: to change a situation that has become intolerable. This reversal in expectations about who is responsible (as opposed to blameworthy) confuses everybody. Initially, the network fights the reversal; after all, who are the doctors? The group process of the full-scale assembly is powerful, however. Polarization that begins as an intragroup conflict can develop into an energizing polarization against the network therapy conductor, as a representative of mental health and other social service agencies. A well handled polarization against the conductor can draw the network into angrily proving that they can manage their problems more effectively than the paid professionals have been doing for years.

It sometimes happens that when network members begin to take back power and responsibility, they make choices contrary to the beliefs of therapists and institutions. This conflict is particularly likely to emerge when the network's culture differs from that of the professionals. The responsible network therapist must respect the directions the network chooses for itself, if he or she is to facilitate the empowerment of the network. This respect takes the form of accepting the network's decisions and resisting the temptation (and institutional pressures) to wrest back control when network actions run counter to therapeutic beliefs.

Networks can take power and responsibility for members' well-being in a number of ways. Network members may insist upon getting a recently deinstitutionalized person out of his parents' home before the concerned therapist thinks it is wise. They may be far more controlling, and even bullying, in their maneuvers to get an unemployed young man back to work than the therapist finds acceptable. They may hold rituals with an espiritista[15] to rid a schizophrenic of the spirits possessing her. They may organize tenants' associations or lobbying efforts to prevent the curtailment of needed local services (Trimble & Kliman, 1981). These network-initiated activities sharpen network members' awareness of their collective ability, strength, and potential for change within their network and in larger social contexts.

[15]A spiritual medium in a number of Hispanic cultures.

3.9. Coordination of the Secondary Sector

Families confronting a multitude of problems over a long period of time often end up relating to a large number of social institutions, each of which has a different definition, plan of action, and set of constraints for the family. It is all too common to encounter a family in which father and daughter see individual therapists, son meets regularly with his probation officer, and mother gets tranquilizers from the doctor she sees for hypertension. The therapist who is called in when mother makes a suicide attempt is liable to be overwhelmed by the complexity of competing institutional ties. Therapeutic effectiveness is undermined by the contradictory messages emanating from so many directions. The secondary sector's response to the family's disorganization leads to still more disorganization.

In a full-scale or partial network assembly, service workers who previously had access only to isolated elements of their clients' situations can see a more complete picture and recognize their part in maintaining the family's difficulties. Those helpers and gatekeepers who are inclined to be cooperative can begin to form collaborative ties based on a shared new understanding of the problem at hand. Competition and territoriality among agencies and their workers can be reduced at such meetings. Once collaborative ties are developed in the course of network therapy for one family, service workers can continue to cooperate with each other on behalf of other clients as well. More is involved, however, than the good will and understanding of individual service workers. The workers are subject to the regulations and constraints of the institutions that employ them, and the network therapist is less likely to succeed in restructuring institutional relationships than personal relationships.

4. Class, Ethnicity, and Gender

In the preceding sections, we have examined network dynamics and structures as they relate to psychological dysfunction. A thorough clinical understanding of network relations is not possible without addressing such mediating factors as class, race, ethnicity, and gender. People apprehend their social world, and their relationships to that world, through the lenses these mediators provide.

Relationships of class, race, and ethnicity profoundly influence the ways households are established and organized, as well as the interactions between households within networks. These relationships also inform expectations and perceptions of family, kin, friends, workplace, neighborhood, and social institutions such as schools, churches, and clinics. Across class, race, and ethnic lines, gender differences are associated with different relationships to networks. This variation can be explained in part by men and women's differential participation (and psychological preparation for that participation) in the workplace, the domestic sphere, kinship ties, and contact with institutions involved with children and family life.

Both the degree of urbanization in a network's locale and the geographical mobility of its members also influence network relations. All the variables mentioned above interact with each other. The respective networks of an urban poor black woman, an economically marginal male farmer of Swedish stock, a middle-class suburban Jewish man, a working-class Italian-American in the city, a recent female immigrant from the Dominican Republic, and a male WASP multimillionaire with homes in both city and countryside will be markedly different, irrespective of disturbance.

The economic situation of a household and the network to which it relates influences transactions and expectations within the network. In networks whose members are impoverished or working poor, it generally is necessary for related households to pool their severely limited resources (money, child care, food, appliances, living space, etc.) if everyone is to survive. Network members understand that when emergencies arise, relatives and close friends are obliged to provide each other with whatever assistance they can muster. Intimates are expected to give what they can and take what they need. Declining to help or to accept what is offered is met with strong negative sanctions which can go so far as exclusion from the network. Household boundaries are fluid, with money, clothes, food, and child care rotating as needed among intimates. Although men contribute significantly to this pooling, it is women who tend to initiate and monitor resource pooling (Rapp, 1978; Stack, 1974).

This kind of network arrangement is adaptive in that basic survival is ensured for people who might not be able to manage independently. It is disadvantageous in that getting ahead is impossible within such a structure. One can accumulate resources and break out of poverty only by leaving a network that insists upon sharing whatever is not essential to one's own survival; yet to leave such a network without already having adequate resources is perilous both psychologically and financially (Stack, 1974).

Relatives and close friends may move in with each other, temporarily or permanently, in times of difficulty. It is not infrequent to find children who are raised for months, years, or lifetimes by relatives or "fictive kin" (friends who are "taken" as kin, with all the obligations of kinship) while maintaining close ties with natural parents. Even more children live in one household, while relatives in other households are involved actively in rearing and supporting them.

Such network arrangements have important ramifications for the therapist. Conflictual relationships with the aunt or grandmother who raised an individual may be more significant to the work of therapy than those with natural parents. Children grow up with the advantage of multiple nurturant relationships with adults, but also with a greater number of triangulated relationships.

Privacy and independence are impossible when people are obliged to help each other meet survival needs. Network members are more likely to complain of others' intrusiveness, or of the burdens of obligations to relations, than of loneliness or isolation. Everyone knows whose welfare check did not come, who just bought a car or lost a job, whose mother is sick, who came into some money, and who needs help with the kids while she sees her new lover. This lack of privacy is a decided advantage for the therapist proposing network therapy; friends and relatives already know much of what is going on.

Families of the middle class and stable working class, in contrast, have much more clearly defined household boundaries. Sharing economic resources, if it occurs at all, is restricted to the households of immediate relatives (most often parents and their grown children) and then it takes the form of gifts and loans rather than of the rotation of resources. When in need, members of individual households are more likely to turn to institutions or paid service providers—banks, baby-sitters, private duty nurses, car rentals, and so forth—than to friends or relatives (Rapp, 1978). Although grandparents, aunts, and uncles may baby-sit, children rarely live outside their natural families except under such extreme circumstances as the death or prolonged hospitalization of a parent.

This kind of network arrangement is associated with a high value on privacy and self-reliance. With some ethnic variations, information about finances tends to go no farther than immediate relatives, and emotional difficulties are shared only with intimates. Network members are more likely to complain about loneliness than lack of privacy. Network therapy is less easily accepted in these networks, except under the direst of situations.

We can say less about the networks of the very wealthy, perhaps because they value—and can maintain—privacy much more than others. Rapp (1978) speculates that, like the poor, the very rich also share financial resources, but only among close kin, and then in order to augment surplus income. Because privacy is of the greatest significance, it is unlikely that a ruling-class network would consent to being assembled for psychotherapeutic purposes.

Class variations in network structure and belief systems interact with variables of race and ethnicity (which are treated together here). Ethnic differences in normative relationships with immediate family, kin, and non-kin are associated with varying transactional styles and different patterns of dysfunction. Different groups hold divergent normative expectations of behavior concerning privacy/openness, emotional reserve/ expressiveness, dependence/independence/interdependence, individualism/group cohesion, individual freedom/normative consensus. They also vary with respect to what constitutes proper relations between the generations, between the genders, between kin and non-kin, and between households. The sanctions imposed for deviating from network norms also differ among ethnic groups (McGoldrick & Pearce, 1982).

A detailed discussion of ethnic variations is not possible here. (McGoldrick and Pearce, 1982, provide a helpful clinical examination of ethnic variables in family relations, with some attention to the network.) A few generalizations suggesting ethnic differences in network relations and receptivity to network therapy are possible, at the risk of painting too narrow a picture with strokes too broad. Only a few groups are mentioned, and without adequate attention to intragroup class differences or relative recency of immigration.

Working with a network composed, for example, of first-generation Italian-Americans is markedly different from working with a network whose members are mostly Connecticut Yankees. Italian networks generally place tremendous value on emotional and geographical closeness to kinfolk (especially among women), loyalty to family and neighborhood, and emotional expressiveness. Moves toward independence from the network are liable to be met with powerful negative sanctions. Men and women tend to have separate but closely related networks; women interact with relatives and female neighbors, while men interact with relatives, male neighbors, and male co-workers. Trust is reserved for the extended family. Italian networks may be receptive to network intervention so long as it is limited to kinfolk, and perhaps the priest and godparents (Antonioli, 1981).

Greek networks are structured rather like Italian networks, but are less likely to accept the suggestion of network therapy because of the competitive, symmetrical struggles among kinfolk (Welts, 1981). Hispanic assemblies tend to be more inclusive than Italian networks, with such fictive kin as comadres and compadres, a few close friends, and possibly an espiritista as well as a priest. It is not uncommon that when networks of Hispanic families are assembled, relatives fly in from their home countries in order to attend.

WASP networks are likely to espouse the values of self-reliance, privacy, individual achievement, and emotional reserve. Family bonds do not require frequent contact, and family feeling may not extend beyond parents, siblings, spouse, and children (McGill & Pearce, 1982). Negative sanctions are more probable when an individual fails to attain independence than when he or she acts on beliefs that are at odds with majority network opinion. Privacy is foremost; people may not discuss troubles even with immediate family. This emphasis on privacy and self-reliance makes network assembly difficult, although it is possible if the index family is desperate enough to air its dirty laundry. Network coaching and construction, which do not necessitate self-disclosure, frequently are more acceptable solutions. Such approaches also are advisable for ethnic groups with similar values (e.g., Germans and Scandinavians) and for other ethnic groups whose families have been here long enough to acculturate to British-American values.

Extended families in Jewish networks tend to be less close-knit than in Italian networks, but Jews value independence and privacy less than WASPs. Family and kinship bonds are strong, but emotional closeness is stressed over geographical proximity. Family loyalty is expressed through frequent communication and sharing emotional states (to an extent WASPs might consider intrusive). Adherence to consensually defined norms is not particularly stressed, except in the networks of religious Jews. Religious and first-generation Americans tend to trust only kinfolk and the rabbi to know family business. More assimilated Jews would be more willing to welcome friends and co-workers to network assemblies. Family relations are a favorite topic of conversation, so assembling people to talk about relationships is a familiar idea. This attitude provides an interesting contrast to that of Polish networks, which would be willing to assemble in order to make plans for changing a difficult situation, but not to talk about relationships or feelings.

Because blacks in this country are disproportionately poor and working class, discussing black networks separately from class issues is problematic. The networks of most American blacks are structurally similar to these described for poor and working-poor people. Interdependence is highly valued; privacy and individualism are regarded as threats to the common interests of network members. Intimate ties exist between friends who take "fictive kinship" relations (Stack, 1974). Information about network members passes freely throughout the group. These patterns hold less true for middle-class and upwardly mobile blacks, whose individual advancement is antithetical to the collective values of the poor. Middle-class blacks are more likely to espouse such "mainstream" values as independence and self-reliance.

Any examination of ethnicity and race requires analysis of class difference. Certain network characteristics are determined primarily by network members' relations to the economy. At the same time, transactional styles, values, and world views are influenced greatly by racial and ethnic experience, regardless of economic position.

The influence of gender difference on network relations cuts across class and ethnic lines. It is pervasive to the point of invisibility. The nature and loci of men's and women's social relations are divergent. In our society, women are seen, first and foremost, as belonging to the domestic sphere; whatever paid work or other involvements they may have are "extra." Men belong, first and foremost, to the work world; they travel as families' ambassadors between home and outside world.

Women are largely responsible for keeping the culture (passing its practices on to children) and maintaining kinship ties. Their unpaid domestic labor keeps households going and frees men to engage in paid work (Rapp, 1978). Women generally maintain this position even when they work outside the home. Network ties for the housewife in poor and working-class networks focus on the immediate family, relatives, female neighbors, and children's friends. Middle-class housewives relate to their husbands' colleagues as well, and may develop ties through voluntary associations and activities. The working wife and mother of either class relates to co-workers, but is likely to have little time for socializing with them because of household responsibilities. Single women's social relations may resemble men's more except among those ethnic groups (e.g., Puerto Ricans or Italians) that closely monitor the activities of unattached women. In contrast, men's social ties focus largely on the work world. Among the working class, men's social ties to relatives and male neighbors are significant, but less so than for women. Men's extrafamilial social involvements generally are more positively sanctioned than women's.

Because men and women relate primarily to distinct parts of their networks, they are differentially vulnerable to stress in network relations. A man who underfunctions on the job is more likely than a woman to attract widespread concern and resentment in his network. If he is too depressed at home to do anything but drink beer in front of the television, no one outside his family even may notice. When a woman cannot carry out her domestic functions, her entire network may respond, while doing poorly at work attracts only the attention of those co-workers directly affected by her behavior. These differences are associated with patterns of network dysfunction. A man's unemployment may provoke a network crisis, while the impending marriage of the last child at home may precipitate a crisis for the network assembled around a woman's suicidal depression.

Issues of power and control are central to gender relations in families, networks, and society. Men and women have differential access to power and differential interests in maintaining existing social arrangements. Their respective socialization to and perceptions of gender relations reflect and shape their struggles for ascendency, although these struggles often are perceived as the result of individual conflicts rather than underlying conflicts based on gender.

Gender-related conflicts invariably emerge in network assemblies (and in any therapy, for that matter), in many guises and with many variations. When the network conductor and team members are aware of their own positions in the political dynamics of gender relations, they can facilitate a critical understanding of these conflicts within the network. The plight, for instance, of the suicidally depressed housewife can be redefined dramatically. The problem that originally was understood as resulting from the individual frailty of a woman experiencing the "empty nest syndrome" is reframed as a reflection of gender arrangements that render women without children at home useless and dependent. At this moment of redefinition, the network therapist can turn to women in the group who would gladly help mobilize the client through consciousness raising.

5. Conclusions

In the 15 years or so since its inception, the field of network therapy has advanced rapidly in developing psychotherapeutic and preventive strategies. Progress in social network research, particularly with schizophrenic populations, has stimulated conceptual and technical invention in clinical practice and holds promise for outcome studies in the future. Despite these encouraging beginnings, however, practicing network therapists still are few and far between.

Some of the obstacles to a more widespread use of network therapy among psychotherapists include the challenge it presents to conventions of confidentiality, the issues of interagency "turf" struggles it can provoke, difficulties concerning billing procedures, and the extraordinary demands it places on the therapist. Other obstacles involve the therapist's own fears about managing so large a group as a network assembly and about relinquishing control to the assembled group. Nevertheless, practitioners find network therapy techniques to be effective in dealing with a variety of situations and populations, in breaking through treatment impasses that have been otherwise unresponsive, and in the preventive strengthening of the "at risk" members of dysfunctional networks.

This chapter has provided more than a discussion of network therapy techniques. It has offered a perspective that encompasses systems larger than the family alone. A network perspective, integrated into the daily work of family therapists, enriches our work.

6. References

Ackerman, N. Family interviewing: The study process. In N. Ackerman (Ed.), *Family therapy in transition.* Boston: Little, Brown, 1970.

Antonioli, L. Personal communication, March 29, 1981.

Attneave, C. Family network map, 1975. Available from the author at 5206 Ivanhoe Place, N.E., Seattle, Wash. 98105.

Attneave, C., & Speck, R. The temporal cycle of retribalization. In A. Jacobs & W. Spradlin (Eds.), *The group as the agent of change.* New York: Behavior Books, 1974.

Atwood, N. Group support for the families of the mentally ill. *Schizophrenia Bulletin,* 1978, *4*(3), 415–425.

Auerswald, E. Interdisciplinary versus ecological approach. *Family Process,* 1968, *7,* 212–215.

Auerswald, E. Families, change, and the ecological perspective. *Family Process,* 1971, *10,* 263–280.

Barnes, J. Class and committees in a Norwegian island parish. *Human Relations,* 1954, *7,* 39–58.

Beels, C. C. Social networks, the family, and the schizophrenic patient. *Schizophrenia Bulletin,* 1978, *4,* 512–521.

Boissevain, J. The place of non-groups in the social sciences. *Man,* 1968, *3,* 542–556.

Boissevain, J., & Mitchell, J. (Eds.). *Network analysis: Studies in human interaction.* The Hague: Mouton, 1973.

Bott, E. *Family and social network: Roles, norms, and external relationships in ordinary urban families.* London: Tavistock, 1957.

Bowen, M. *Family therapy in clinical practice.* New York: Jason Aronson, 1978.

Brown, G., Birley, J., & Wing, J. The influence of the family in schizophrenic disorders: A replication. *British Journal of Psychiatry,* 1972, *121,* 241–258.

Cobb, J., & Sennett, R. *Hidden injuries of class.* New York: Vintage, 1973.

Cohen, C., & Sokolovsky, J. *Schizophrenia Bulletin,* 1978, *4,* 546–560.

Curtis, W. R. Team problem-solving in a social network. *Psychiatric Annals,* 1974, *4,* 11–27.

Dean, A., & Lin, N. The stress-buffering role of social support: Problems and prospects for systematic investigation. *Journal of Nervous and Mental Disease,* 1977, *165,* 403–417.

Dohrenwend, B. P., & Dohrenwend, B. S. (Eds.). *Stressful life events: Their nature and effects.* New York: Wiley, 1974.

Fenichel, O. The drive to amass wealth. *Psychoanalytic Quarterly,* 1938, *7,* 69–95.

Garrison, J. Network techniques: Case studies in the screening-linking-planning conference. *Family Process,* 1974, *13,* 337–353.

Garrison, J. Network methods for clinical problems. In E. M. Pattison (Chair), *Clinical group methods for larger social systems.* Symposium presented at the meeting of the American Group Psychotherapy Association, Boston, February 1976.

Garrison, V. Support systems of schizophrenic and nonschizophrenic Puerto Rican migrant women in New York City. *Schizophrenia Bulletin,* 1978, *4,* 561–596.

Haley, J. *Problem-solving therapy.* San Francisco: Jossey-Bass, 1976.

Hammer, M. Influence of small social networks as factors on mental hospital admission. *Human Organization,* 1963–1964, *22,* 243–251.

Hammer, M., Makiesky-Barrow, S., & Gutwirth, L. Social networks and schizophrenia. *Schizophrenia Bulletin,* 1978, *4,* 522–545.

Kaplan, S., Salzinger, S., Pelcovitz, D., Samit, C., Krieger, R., Artemyeff, C., & Ganeles, D. *Psychopathology, stress, and social network research instruments in the treatment of families of maltreated children.* Paper presented at the meeting of the American Orthopsychiatric Association, New York, April 1981.

Keller, S. Psychotherapy with Polish-Americans. In M. McGoldrick, J. Pearce, & J. Giordano (Eds.), *Ethnicity and family therapy*. New York: Guilford Press, 1982.

Kliman, G. *Psychological emergencies of childhood.* New York: Grune & Stratton, 1968.

Kliman, J., with Kern, R., & Kliman, A. Natural and human-made disasters: Some therapeutic and epidemiological implications for crisis intervention. In U. Rueveni, R. Speck, & J. L. Speck (Eds.), *Interventions: Healing human systems.* New York: Human Sciences Press, 1982.

Laqueur, H. P. Mechanisms of change in multiple family therapy. In C. Sager & H. Kaplan (Eds.), *Progress in group and family therapy.* New York: Brunner/Mazel, 1972.

Leff, J. Presentation at workshop at the meeting, *Schizophrenia—New Approaches to the Family,* Columbia University, New York, April 1981.

Liem, R., & Liem, J. Social class and mental illness reconsidered: The role of economic stress and social support. *Journal of Health and Social Behavior,* 1978, *19,* 139–158.

Lin, N., Simeone, R., Ensel, W., & Kuo, W. Social support, stressful life events, and illness: A model and an empirical test. *Journal of Health and Social Behavior,* 1979, *20,* 108–119.

Marcuse, H. *Eros and civilization.* Boston: Beacon Press, 1955.

McGill, D., & Pearce, J. Family therapy with British-Americans (WASPS). In M. McGoldrick, J. Pearce, & J. Giordano (Eds.), *Ethnicity and family therapy.* New York: Guilford Press, (1982).

McGoldrick, M., Pearce, J., & Giordano, J. (Eds.). *Ethnicity and family therapy.* New York Guilford Press, (1982).

Miles, M. *On "networking."* Unpublished manuscript, National Institute for Education, 1978.

Minuchin, S. *Families and family therapy.* Cambridge: Harvard University Press, 1974.

Minuchin, S., & Fishman, H.C. *Family therapy techniques.* Cambridge: Harvard University Press, 1981.

Mitchell, R., & Trickett, E. Task force report: Social network as mediator of social support. *Community Mental Health Journal,* 1980, *16,* 27–34.

Palazolli, M., Cecchin, G., Prata, G., & Boscolo, L. *Paradox and counterparadox.* New York: Jason Aronson, 1978.

Papp, P. The Greek chorus. *Family Process,* 1980, *19,* 45–57.

Parker, L. A. Networks for innovation and problem-solving and their use for improving education: A comparative overview. Unpublished manuscript, 1977. (Available from the author at Center on Technology and Society, P.O. Box 38–206, Cambridge, Mass. 02138)

Pattison, E. M. *Psychosocial network inventory.* Unpublished manuscript, 1975. (Available from the author at Department of Psychiatry and Health, Medical College of Georgia, Augusta, Ga. 30904)

Pattison, E. M., DeFrancisco, D., Wood, P., Frazier, H., & Crowder, J. A psychosocial kinship model for family therapy. *American Journal of Psychiatry,* 1975, *132,* 1246–1251.

Rapp, R. Family and class in contemporary America: Notes toward an understanding of ideology. *Science and Society,* 1978, *42,* 278–300.

Rubin, L. *Worlds of pain: Life in the working class family.* New York: Basic Books, 1977.

Rueveni, U., & Speck, R. Using encounter group techniques in the treatment of the social network of the schizophrenic. *International Journal of Group Psychotherapy,* 1969, *19,* 495–500.

Rueveni, U. *Networking families in crisis.* New York: Human Sciences, 1979.

Sokolovsky, J., Cohen, C., Berger, D., and Geiger, J. Personal networks of ex-mental patients in a Manhattan SRO hotel. *Human Organization,* 1978, *37,* 5–15.

Speck, R. Psychotherapy of the social network of a schizophrenic family. *Family Process,* 1967, *7,* 208–214.

Speck, R., & Attneave, C. *Family networks.* New York: Pantheon, 1973.

Speck, R., & Rueveni, U. Network therapy: A developing concept. *Family Process,* 1969, *8,* 182–191.

Stack, C. *All our kin: Strategies for survival in a black community.* New York: Harper Colophon, 1974.

Strauss, J., & Carpenter, W. Prediction of outcome in schizophrenia. *Archives of General Psychiatry,* 1977, *34,* 159–163.

Sussman, M. The urban kin network in the formulation of family theory. In R. Hill and R. Konig (Eds.), *Families in East and West.* Paris: Mouton, 1970.

Todd, D. *Social networks, psychosocial adaptation, and preventive/developmental intervention: The support development workshop.* Paper presented at the meeting of the American Psychological Association, Montreal, September 1980.

Tolsdorf, C. Social networks, support and coping: An exploratory study. *Family Process,* 1976, *15,* 407–418.

Trimble, D. A guide to the network therapies. *Connections,* 1980, *3*(2), 9–22.

Trimble, D. Social network intervention with antisocial adolescents. *International Journal of Family Therapy,* 1981, *3,* 268–274.

Trimble, D., & Kliman, J. Community network therapy: Mobilizing the networks of chronic patients for return to the community. *International Journal of Family Psychiatry,* 1981, *2,* 269–289.

Vaughn, C., & Leff, J. The influence of family and social factors on the course of psychiatric illness: A comparison of schizophrenic and depressed neurotic patients. *British Journal of Psychiatry,* 1976, *129,* 125–137.

Wellman, B. *A guide to network analysis.* Toronto: Structural Analysis Programme, Department of Sociology, University of Toronto, 1980.

Welts, E. Personal communication, September 10, 1981.

15

Multiple Family Group Therapy

A MODEL FOR ALL FAMILIES

PAULA HOLLINS GRITZER AND HELEN S. OKUN

Multiple Family Group Therapy (MFGT) is a combination of family and group psychotherapy in which several families meet simultaneously at agreed upon intervals with therapists present. In this marriage between two recognized and established treatment modalities, the therapists fill an important role as creators, catalysts, and organizers. The special MFGT structure is one in which adults meet with children, families with other families, and members of one generation with those of another generation. The therapist's selection criteria can include families whose system structures are similar (homogenous), families whose system structures are different (heterogenous), families that are intact or single parent, and families that are intergenerational or nuclear. Through the application of a family systems approach within a group therapy format, the therapeutic process is accelerated and enriched.

The underlying assumption for choosing MFGT rather than individual family therapy is that systemic and individual growth can be promoted more fully when outsiders other than the therapists are included in the family treatment. The inclusion of the outside world in the form of other families fosters an unpredictable and complex group process that

Paula Hollins Gritzer and Helen S. Okun are both social workers formerly employed by the Jewish Family Service (now the Jewish Board of Family and Children's Services—J.B.F.C.S.) in Brooklyn, New York. Ms. Gritzer was a family and group therapist at J. F. S. from 1971 to 1975, and a supervisor from 1975 to 1980. During this time she co-led numerous multiple family therapy groups and wrote about that experience with another senior staff member, Florence Bass. Any references in this chapter to the co-therapists leading MFGT are references to Gritzer and Bass.

Helen S. Okun was Assistant Borough Director of the Brooklyn Jewish Family Service (J.B.F.C.S.) from 1973 to 1981. In her capacity as Assistant Borough Director she was closely involved in the group program developed during that period. All references in this chapter to the authors refer to Gritzer and Okun.

PAULA HOLLINS GRITZER and HELEN S. OKUN • 243 President Street, Brooklyn, New York 11231.

cannot occur in any other therapeutic settings. It is inherent in MFGT, irrespective of specific definitions, that circumstances and events within the group create a milieu that does not exist in other therapies. The group members create, re-create, and demonstrate universal family dilemmas, crises, problems, pathology, and environments existing in all people; for in all of us there are parts of the external others. This can be a recognizable personality trait, a means of dealing with others, or a similar family life situation.

Current conceptualization and actual practice of MFGT covers the entire spectrum of theoretical bases, therapeutic styles, and structural variables. For some practitioners the group constitutes 45 people from 10 family units, meeting once a month for a total of 12 sessions. For others, the MFT group would consist of 20 individuals from four families meeting weekly in a closed group for one year. In one setting MFGT may be a preparation for psychotherapy while in another setting it is the actual treatment. Some therapists maximize and capitalize upon group process, others basically dispense with it. Some practitioners refer to couples' groups as MFGT while others define MFGT as groups consisting of identified patient plus parents. In any MFGT setting, the number of therapists, foci, style, goals, patient population, and format can vary. This broadly defined spectrum poses difficulty in trying to write about the modality.

In this chapter we have attempted to include some overview of the MFGT field but have placed a heavier emphasis on our own experience. Our family therapy experience is based on a psychodynamic understanding of the individual within the family and a systems approach to the family. We have not applied the recent purely structural approaches to our MFGT work. Our group and family experience relies on a use and understanding of process.

In our review of the literature we found a diversity of principles and methodology related to MFGT. Therefore the statements that we present related to the literature are our own assumptions and distillations of commonalities or differences. We have chosen to draw largely from the writings of Laqueur (1964, 1968, 1976), McFarlane (in press), and Strelnick (1977). We recognize that articles by Bowen (1976), Leichter (1962), Leichter and Schulman (1968, 1974), and others contain significant well developed models and theories for MFGT.

Reflecting the variability of the field, authors have conceptualized MFGT in different ways. Laqueur (1976) describes MFGT as uniquely allowing in the outside world in the form of several random families entering into the therapeutic relationship. Strelnick (1977), in noting the range of settings in which MFGT has been used, mentions the open and closed models. The former includes extended family members and significant social others. The latter family group membership includes the patient and significant adult others, that is, spouse or parents. The MFGT programs described by Laqueur and McFarlane are an outgrowth of planning for the needs of seriously ill patients in an inpatient psychiatric or aftercare setting.

Our use of the term MFGT refers to a group in which several families are present, including well siblings, led by two therapists. We form groups that are heterogenous, that is, single parent plus intact families with a range of presenting problems and system types. We emphasize the need for at least three screening sessions that must be well structured and focused. Goals described in the MFGT literature are focused on behavioral change of family members in relation to each other in order to bring about family system reorganization (Laqueur, 1976; McFarlane, in press). The primary goals of MFGT as we conceive it are the healing of dysfunctional aspects of the individual (intrapsychic) *and* the shifting of family systems.

1. Statement of Purpose

The overview discussions on MFGT in the literature draw largely on information from in-patient settings. We think a more comprehensive description of MFGT is required to incorporate into the literature the experience with the out-client[1] population. We will therefore give added emphasis to the out-client experience in an effort to contribute new writings to the literature. We will provide a brief history of MFGT and some discussion of the evolution of this form of treatment in both hospital and out-client settings. We will draw selectively on and summarize those ideas and concepts from the existing literature that are particularly relevant to our focus. We will provide a model and a structure for working with families on an out-client basis in the hope that a ''blueprint'' for comprehending the whole will encourage more practitioners to report and expand its use.

2. Brief History

Philip Laqueur is credited with beginning MFGT in the early 1950s in a New York psychiatric hospital. He and his staff held community ward meetings on weekends but had difficulty containing the patients because they would leave the group meetings to visit with family members. The groups also were interrupted by the queries of family members about the ward meetings. According to McFarlane (in press) a decision was reached to have a parents' meeting at the same time as the community meeting. Laqueur recognized that some patients preferred attending the parents' group and acted more appropriately when there. He then combined the two groups and the results were incredibly positive. From that time to the present MFGT usage has grown and the literature cites numerous examples of such groups. Laqueur (1964, 1968, 1976) evolved his own theoretical constructs for understanding and leading MFGT, and others have followed, amplifying and expanding what he began.

There are reports in the literature of MFT group programs for patients suffering from cancer (Spiegel & Yalon, 1978; Wellisch, Mosher, & Van Scoy, 1978) and substance abuse (St. Luke's, 1980); however, it is rare in hospitals that families and patients are brought together in the MFGT format. Although a literature relating to family therapy has been prolific and has produced divergent schools of thought, the literature related to MFGT has experienced a limited expansion, staying almost exclusively in the arena where it began, that is, within the inpatient psychiatric hospital.

The literature indicates that MFGT practice and theory derive from varied theoretical approaches, therapeutic styles, and structural factors. However, the application of MFGT to types of problems has been largely delimited to the psychiatric inpatient populations. Although expert consensus attests to MFGT efficacy with this population, we believe that the practical and theoretical utilization of MFGT can be improved by incorporating the out-client experience more fully into the literature.

In addition to the literature addressed to MFGT use in specific settings, a number of authors have contributed useful overviews of MFGT that draw together the varied MFGT applications in an attempt to unify concept and theory in the field (Laqueur, 1976; McFarlane, (in press); Strelnick, 1977). These overviews are written largely from data collected in serious-illness settings, thus reflecting a narrower use of MFGT. They do not

[1]We are using this term to differentiate between MFGT inpatient and MFGT for families involved in psychotherapy outside of medical–psychiatric settings.

broaden the existing conceptualizations to include the out-client realm. Leichter and Schulman (1972, 1974, Schulman, 1976) are major contributors of articles based on out-client populations. Their early premises, derived from MFGT work together, constitute an excellent beginning theoretical framework with MFGT out-clients. Their thread has not been picked up, however, and the resulting gap in the literature presents an anomaly. The very success of MFGT with serious psychiatric illness has prompted speculation about its unexplored potentialities with the less seriously afflicted populations in out-client settings. Nevertheless, the hopes for MFGT with these populations remain largely unexplored or, if explored, undocumented.

3. Homogeneity and the Evolution of MFGT in Hospitals

The literature describes various settings where serious psychiatric illness is treated within the context of an MFGT format. The settings in which serious psychiatric illness is treated are most often public and private hospitals. In either structure there are families represented from all socioeconomic, ethnic, and age groups. The life stages of the identified patients in hospital MFT groups range from early childhood to late middle age.[2]The psychiatric illness is a life-style altering or threatening one, whose management and aftercare ideally require the involvement of family members on behalf of the patient. To this end, involvement of the nuclear family is vital, and MFGT lends itself to the accomplishment of goals that affect more than one person, generally the entire nuclear family of the identified patient.

It is understandable, then, that the psychiatric hospital structure constitutes a natural host setting in which MFGT was first conceived and from which it has since developed. It can be prudent and expedient to bring together families who are all experiencing the same life crisis. It makes sense that MFGT formed on the basis of similar life crises be open-ended, so that families at later stages of the same crisis can offer hope and help to those just beginning the process. Since all groups are formed on the basis of some unifying commonality, the illness theme occurring in hospitals and drug addiction centers provides a natural raison d'être for bringing families together in MFGT. The greater use of MFGT with the inpatient population may have to do with the relative ease of beginning programs in those settings. The more extensive reporting of hospital related MFGT in the literature also may be related to academic connections of large teaching hospitals and publishing to aid career mobility.

Within the various hospital settings there are a variety of opinions about the degree of homogeneity or heterogeneity in selecting the MFGT. Against a setting of hospitalized or ambulent patients, Laqueur recommends that family group membership be as random as possible in socioeconomic, ethnic, religious, and age characteristics, so that the group work can be on basic human behavior problems (Laqueur, 1976). This preference presents a minor contradiction since all families considered for MFGT by him had a hospitalized member suffering from what was likely to be the same diagnostic syndrome as other identified patients. Therefore, although Laqueur recommends diversity of religion, age, socioeconomic standing, and so forth, the circumstances in which families were chosen were markedly similar in that they all had a psychiatrically hospitalized member. Regardless of statements recommending the desirability of a heterogenous group composition, the MFT groups in hospital settings are by one major definition largely homogenous.

[2]The literature reflects an absence of work in MFGT on behalf of more senior patients.

McFarlane describes MFGT as helpful with more isolated and fragile families and deems it advisable that MFGT be comprised of like family types and like disorders, lest one set of concerns submerge others (McFarlane, in press). Skynner states that "the membership must be sufficiently evenly matched to insure that no one member or subgroup can dominate the whole" (Skynner, 1976, p. 250). We have found that the shifting dominance of various subgroups within MFGT can be utilized. The dominance struggle is inherent in any group situation and can be capitalized upon in MFGT to make explicit themes of power, control, and their opposites.

Hospital programs offering MFGT are on the upswing, spurred both by the natural setting factors listed above and by the favorable published literature reporting positive outcomes of existing groups. The MFGT modality provides a more cohesive, effective, and supportive treatment milieu for the identified patients and their families. In hospitals, MFGT additionally offsets a degree of the usual fragmentation that is part of the bureaucratic structure. For instance, psychiatrists and social workers frequently treat members of the same family, but do not necessarily confer with sufficient regularity about progress, goals, prognosis, and so forth. The coleadership arrangement of MFGT promotes regular communication between professionals and offers a forum in which family members can clarify questions, distorted information, and fears. Social isolation and fragmented communication are common factors in many families whose members are admitted to inpatient psychiatric wards (McFarlane, in press). The MFGT format in hospitals lessens the miscommunications that are inherent in the bureaucracy while at the same time minimizing fragmented and distorted family communication factors through the involvement of several families meeting together in a supportive environment. The MFT groups also are cost efficient in hospitals in that several families can be seen at one time.

On the other hand, we can see impediments to beginning MFGT programs in hospitals. Many professionals are involved in the medical/psychiatric service units from which families are drawn for MFGT, thereby presenting the possibility of different treatment recommendations based on different philosophies and orientations. The choice of families for MFGT often is structured according to ward assignment. The hospital structure is such that in these wards there are different chiefs for each service and the operation and philosophy of each ward can vary greatly. For instance, the head of a psychiatric hospital division may have a different practice orientation from other professionals on the ward, thereby ruling against a modality such as MFGT.

The length of an MFGT hospital group or any family's membership in the group is frequently time-limited due to the trend toward shorter term hospitalization. This time factor will affect the focus of the group and rule out certain psychotherapeutic goals, such as the working through of many intrapsychic conflicts. One hospital professional told us that because of the hospital dictates of group brevity, MFGT is considered as preparation of families for therapy rather than a treatment in and of itself. Practitioners utilizing briefer therapies that emphasize behavior modification and structural techniques could posit that even within a shorter time frame, treatment would be effective utilizing their methodology. Regardless of methodology, a group's short time in the hospital does influence therapists to seek further homogeneity since sufficient time does not exist to work through issues of dramatic difference.

The stringent demands of accreditation and fiscal accountability already have had an impact on the structure and extent of MFGT program development in hospitals. Bureaucratic requirements may alter the course that MFGT will take in all large treatment facilities. MFGT was begun in the hospital setting and has largely perpetuated itself in that same milieu. The MFGT practice is richer because of the available literature, but the unanswered questions as to why the evolution of MFGT has not gone beyond that setting remain unclear. One must be aware, however, that within the hospital milieu MFGT as the sole treatment of choice rarely if ever exists. There is almost always the ongoing individual psychotherapy for the identified patient; often the dispensing and supervision of medication; and sometimes the involvement of parents or spouse in separate individual auxiliary sessions. When discussing the efficacy of MFGT in the psychiatric hospital setting, there are other major treatment applications existing and impacting on the identified patient, and often the family, simultaneously. Any conclusion about MFGT efficacy in hospitals must take this into account.

4. Out-Client MFGT: A Choice between Homogenous and Heterogenous Groups

In the hospital setting there is generally a crisis that has removed one member from the existing family system and placed that person in an institution at a point of maximal psychiatric distress. In an out-client family clinic setting or private practice the family also makes application during a time of crisis. By definition, however, the crisis is different. Societally there is usually a greater stigmatic association to psychiatric hospitalization than to other life crises, for example, child abuse or divorce. Although no person can be objective in the comparison of pain, in that it is a highly subjective variable, there remains a distinction between psychiatric hospitalization and other major life crises, perhaps because the illness itself is disorganizing and frequently irrational. Nonetheless, the choice for MFGT in the out-client setting has broader client selection potential and the group model can be homogenous or heterogenous.

There are two basic philosophical or conceptual points operant in making this choice. Homogenous groups are stronger on such themes as identification, support, and shared realities, and they soften the impact of facing issues of difference. Therapists choosing homogenous groups have a less conflictual bonding or cohesion process in the group but ultimately have to work harder to reach deeper levels of difference and conflict. The heterogenous group has built-in counterforces that highlight difference from the beginning and make group cohesion and bonding more of a struggle to achieve. For example, issues of competition are highlighted by greater diversity of social class, presenting problems, traumatic life events, and so forth. The difficult therapeutic task with heterogenous groups is to help members see beyond their differences and acknowledge the universality of their human situation. Heterogeneity requires a longer therapeutic time frame to work through issues of dramatic difference, while homogeneity lends itself to therapeutic work bound by briefer time constraints. The time constraints of the out-client setting often are expansive as compared to those in hospitals, thereby permitting more time to work with families making application.[3]

The organization of MFGT in the out-client setting is substantially different from MFGT organized in a hospital setting. The out-client group selection criteria can be arrived at with greater flexibility on the therapists' part because the therapists are selecting from a client population who most often voluntarily have applied for service. The potential family group members are not a captive audience in the same way that a family is

[3]For example, private practitioners and agencies are less bound by the constraints of insurance reimbursement than are hospitals.

captive to an institution. Because the degree of pathology is frequently less severe in the out-client sector, many therapists leading out-client groups put families together with different diagnostic considerations and variable social class and ethnic backgrounds.[4] In fact, it could be postulated that to limit a group according to family system type, individual diagnosis, or socioeconomic standing gives a counterproductive skew to the group. In contrast, heterogenous selection of families provides a therapeutic opportunity for the family unit to expand their experience of and behavior in the world. If, for example, a homogenous MFT group has three different families with mother–child mergers, it is more difficult for any one mother or child to see the debilitating effect of the closeness. On the other hand, if only one family has mother–child merger as a presenting problem, it is likely that there will be more rapid and accurate feedback about the pathological pairing and its debilitating impact.

In summary, there are two ways to organize out-client MFGT. The first is to select heterogenous groups with less specific family similarities, so that the unifying link is the existential reality of living in society as a sharing family. In the heterogenous groups, the universality of life's experience is more the common theme once the group is underway, although specific identifications occur in great numbers whether the family perceives a problem in itself or in one of its members. The unifying factor in the heterogenous out-client group is that *we are a family in the world.*

A second choice is to organize the group along homogenous lines, for example, learning disabled child–family groups or divorced family groups. The unifying themes of similarity enhance the cohesive working of such a group. The diagnostically homogenous MFGT in hospitals, substance abuse facilities, or out-client agencies brings families together around shared life crises. They may be in varying stages within the crisis process. Families can say to each other, "oh, yes, we know exactly what you are going through." There is comfort in that shared experience and the therapist is no longer alone with a family who feels strongly that the therapist cannot really understand. To some extent either choice is influenced by therapist preferences.

There are difficulties in beginning MFGT programs in all psychotherapeutic settings. It remains unclear whether hospital settings have more factors in their favor and therefore can do more to establish MFGT or whether in the final analysis the possible deterrents for out client group development have little to do with the dearth of related literature. In Washington, D.C., there are many private practitioners leading MFGT. Perhaps the concentration of systems oriented therapists in that area of the country has as much to do with MFGT usage as anything else. Certainly, the systems orientation is more compatible with MFGT than is psychoanalytically oriented psychotherapy.

4.1. Developing MFGT in Out-Client Settings

The implementation of out-client MFGT includes both easy access to families and great challenge. On the positive side there are broad selection possibilities for a diversity of family types and presenting problems in an agency or private practice. The limited evening hours, at a premium everywhere, could be used to see several families in a one and one-half hour time period. However, a variety of factors can mitigate against MFGT

[4]As mentioned earlier, much of the hospital literature indicates agreement that only like-diagnosed patients should be in groups with each other. There is a consistently strong emphasis on homogeneity.

expansion on an out-client basis. Therein lies the need for energetic, enthusiastic therapists.

In order to develop MFGT programs, family agencies have to be involved philosophically and practically in family and group work. The agency must employ staff already well trained in family and group therapy or offer ongoing training programs. The cost of training, supervision, and planning time has to be calculated to insure that cost factors do not outweigh the budgetary realities. There has to be existing available space and two compatible trained therapists.[5] Fee sharing within the private practice setting between the MFGT co-therapy team could pose a concern. Some private practitioners believe that they would not have the expertise to lead MFGT without agency backup and resources. Most important, there must be a strong commitment on the part of the therapists to undertake the responsibility.

Those who lead MFGT in the out-client setting know that the members of those groups are accessible to systemic and individual change in a flexible and exciting way. Our intent in exploring inpatient versus out-client MFGT is not to polarize the two but rather to interest the professional community in developing further and reporting MFGT use with the out-client population. To rephrase E. James Anthony (1975) with a similar "what if" question, what if Laqueur had begun MFGT because his experience with families seen in private practice led him to believe that putting them together in groups might be beneficial? Perhaps the position that MFGT occupies today in the world of treatment and the frequency of reported out-client usage would be quite different.

4.2. Screening: Philosophy to Practice

The specific criteria applied when screening families for MFGT are as diverse as are the types of MFT groups. The criteria for acceptance into a group can be as vague as taking any family willing to attend regular group meetings, or as specific as seeking a family with a certain presenting problem where children and parents fall into some acceptable category of age and economic standing. The pattern over the past 20 years has been to give increasing importance to the screening process. McFarlane describes as many as four or five sessions to prepare families for the group, reduce anxiety, and build a trusting alliance (McFarlane, in press). Leichter and Schulman discuss the screening process on an out-client basis as consisting of three or four sessions where the co-therapists try to obtain a beginning grasp of the family system and see if the family can be engaged as a family group (Leichter & Shulman, 1972). We found that the methods for choosing group members varied from a brief factual explanation of the group to a multiple session differential process. For instance, the staff at one large teaching hospital told us, "privately people shop around for therapists, but once they reach the hospital they do not look further. We tell the family what we have and then offer or recommend it. That is in essence our screening process" (Personal communication).

In screening for MFGT there are variations in the number of participants and number of sessions. More than four or five sessions might reinforce too strongly the individual family treatment format and ultimately mitigate against the family's ability to integrate into the group setting. A more prolonged screening period also could increase the expected beginning anxiety before offering the real group experience. A briefer screening experience does not permit the time for a thorough structure to be set and a process to

[5]There is consensus that two therapists are desirable, even necessary, due to the group's complexity.

evolve. When the use of group process is considered to be indispensable by the therapists, then the screening interviews are the beginning of a portion of that process. There are, however, several family therapy approaches where a process with the family in preparation for the group is secondary to the therapists' treatment plan. These methodologies involving certain behavioral or structural techniques would require a different format for MFGT—perhaps along the lines that Bowen utilizes where the therapist works with each family in turn and group process has lesser importance. The model that we are describing does utilize group process fully.

The interviews with the family unit begin a reciprocal experience between family members and the co-therapy pair. The co-therapy pair connect to the family members individually and as a unit. The family unit and its members begin a relationship with the therapists as individuals and as a team. In the course of the screening process therapists come to relative agreement about many issues, for example (1) the family system and its function and design; (2) the individuals and their roles within the family; (3) the individual behavior patterns of each member; (4) the way in which life stage and role blend to influence the whole; (5) whether or not the family is motivated to change; (6) whether or not the family is compatible with them as a therapeutic duo; (7) the extent of the family units' ability to recognize the functional and dysfunctional aspects of their way of interacting; and (8) goals that are mutually agreed upon. A tentative diagnostic assessment of each member and of the family system then is made. Special attention is paid to the nature of the existing pathology in order to determine what is manageable and appropriate for the family, for the setting, and for the therapeutic pair. A plan for intervening in the family system is agreed upon. For example:

> The Greene family consisted of mother (48), father (50), Jennifer (18), Naomi (15), and Gail (12). Jennifer called the agency on her own behalf but was immediately receptive to involving all family members when this was suggested by the intake worker. In the first screening session, the parents initially focused all dissatisfaction around Jennifer, who earlier had made an unsuccessful attempt to live independently. The therapists used the three screening sessions to elicit from the family their perception of the problem and to prescribe agreed upon treatment for the group.
>
> The theme of the first screening session was each person's unhappiness related to feelings of deprivation. There was serious somatization for each parent as a result of this. At the end of the first screening session the therapists knew that all members believed they had been understood by the therapists on the issue of each person's deficit.
>
> The second session focused on communications and behaviors that perpetuated the lack of gratification and the various dyads and triangulations that complemented this. For instance, Mr. Greene was then unemployed. The therapists identified that in Mrs. Greene's own family of origin she felt neglected and unappreciated. In her marriage to Mr. Greene these feelings were reactivated. Her withdrawal from making needs explicitly known and her close alliance with Gail made it difficult for needs to be gratified within the marriage. This and other aspects of the family's structure were discussed. The particular triangle involving Mrs. Greene's closeness to Gail as a wedge in shutting out Mr. Greene was underscored. Jennifer's role in distracting from the marital discord was another aspect of the family system. Naomi ran a third variety of interference between the two parents. The lack of marital gratification became a primary issue.
>
> By the third screening session the therapists had clarified each individual's unmet needs, each person's strengths, and the general family system and what it served to

perpetuate that was growth inhibiting. Goals for each person were agreed upon and the effect that the individual changes would bring about were predicted. Therapists offered feedback about the system and the family agreed to work on specific issues within the group. Although much input was offered directly to the family during the screening, there were obviously individual and systemic matters that the therapists did not include in their discussions with the family.

Just as individual psychotherapists vary in their preference or nonpreference for certain types of clients, so do co-therapy pairs complement each other in their range of preference and nonpreference. Some co-therapists will include a 5-year-old child in MFGT while other pairs will not. Some pairs can tolerate seriously acting-out families while other pairs can not tolerate any in such a group. Sometimes conflict arises within the pairing as to whether or not a certain family can be in a group because one therapist says no and the other insists yes. These differences must be successfully resolved before the family in question can join the group. Often the therapists' complementarity is a factor aiding group cohesion.

There are variable rules for inclusion or exclusion of families in MFGT. To a great extent selection of families is influenced by the setting, by the therapists' treatment philosophies, and by idiosyncratic variables regarding the therapeutic pair. Our own guidelines for out-client group family selections, presented here, are the outgrowth of 10 years of work in a family agency setting. If the co-therapy pair understand the family dynamics, if they like the family, and if they believe that the family is amenable to change, then the family can be put in an MFGT program. That is the most broad and simple qualifier. There are some exclusions which include the following: severely acting-out or violent families, impulse disorders in family members who cannot sit still for one and one-half hours or attend regularly, or families in which the revelation or disclosure of unknown secrets would be problematic for the family or for the group. We recognize that for each of these exclusion guides there can be exceptions.

When the co-therapy pair have a variety of families from whom to choose, the second desirable and unifying consideration is some comparable age range of children. We try to select children who share a range such as older teens, younger teens, latency age, and so forth. This will not insure that family life stage or parents' ages will be comparable, however, or that the ages of children represented will be confined to an absolute range. We additionally will not put more than one seriously disturbed family system into a group. Leader preference varies, of course, and we have known colleagues who put groups together with several seriously disturbed families, the selection choice determined by the population they served. Those therapists were comfortable with the choice.

The screening experience helps the family evaluate how well they believe the therapists understand what they are presenting. The family experiences the leadership styles of the therapists and can assess their interventions and feedback. Basic trust begins to evolve on the part of the family toward the therapists. The family members have to hear and agree with the therapists's plan so that there is relative concurrence about why they are entering the group and the goals they want to attain. The family unit and its membership must have some concept about what they would like to shift as a system and as individuals.

Potential MFGT families referred for screening can be selected from new applicants to a service, undercare case loads of other therapists, or from the case loads of either co-therapist. We have found little or no appreciable difference between therapeutically experienced and novice families once the therapy is underway. There is no difference in their progress in the group, the accuracy of their contributions in sessions, or in their ability to sustain and integrate new learning and change. Although there is no difference in old versus new clients, there are major transferential issues stemming from the source of the referral.

If the family is selected directly from intake or from a waiting list, they are new to the co-therapy pair; thus, all begin from a similar vantage point of newness. If the family is referred by a colleague who is terminating with them, there are competitive implications of the old therapist versus the new and possible covert themes about the setting in which the client will be most helped. If either co-therapist refers families currently seen by them individually, this referred family can occupy a favored position in that therapist's eyes. Conversely, if the therapist referred the family out of exasperation and/or desperation, the family can become the symbolic unfavored or rejected child. Regardless of the source, important transferential material regarding parental favoritism or sibling rivalry is often stimulated.

In groups where remarried families are members, parallels can emerge with regard to the stepparent phenomenon. There can be a residue of systemic splits that occur. The dynamics that emerge are similar to the "my children," "your children," and "our children" issues in remarried families. From the beginning screening sessions the co-therapy pair must be acutely sensitive to positive and negative countertransferences. We recommend that this transferential and countertransferential material be anticipated and acknowledged in the screening process, as well as utilized within the group as rivalries and favoritism become more pronounced.

Any and all expectations emanating from the co-therapists during the screening are very powerful for the group. For instance, the therapists may be very firm that families enter the treatment contract as a unit, while within the group they will promote responsibility on an individual level for attendance and participation. This concept emphasizes the unification of the whole system while encouraging autonomy in each member. Thus, the therapist might say that any family member needing to be absent from a session call on his or her own behalf and that other family members attend the session in question. Therefore, the therapists would later question a parent calling on behalf of a child or an entire family absenting themselves due to one person's unavailability. The expectation that each person will be responsible for "self" can initially be foreign and alien to the mode of functioning of many members. Maintaining this expectation in the group over time ultimately helps break forcefully into disabling family alliances or mergers. It is important to state these expectations directly in screening sessions and again at the group's inception. Therapists must insist that all family members whom the therapists and the family consider vital participate in the MFT group. This permits the inclusion in the group of single parent families, families with children away at college, extended families, and significant nonrelated persons. Families do not have to be intact and single parent families mixed into intact family groups work quite well.

In the time between the screening sessions the therapists can observe how the family is utilizing input from them and by what method the family synthesizes and integrates information about themselves. The interval between the sessions also allows the therapists to plan strategically for shifts in the family system. Areas of difference or disagreement between the co-therapists must be acknowledged by the therapists as not posing impediments to the greater purpose of the group. Goals that can be striven toward and attained begin to be identified. Feedback is offered to the family about the feasibility of accomplishing mutually stated goals of therapists and family members so that ultimately family and therapists can arrive at an agreed upon contract. Because the screening occurs in an out-client setting, captive audience factors are eliminated and each party has the more attainable option of looking elsewhere if not satisfied; that is, therapists can look elsewhere for other families as group members and families can choose other therapists and therapies. When therapists convey a genuine excitement about MFGT and a belief in its benefits for a particular family, it is rare to have a family decline the invitation to participate.

When the therapists are able to make good connections to the family members, concur with them about goals for the family system and the individuals within, offer a plan, and anticipate potential trouble spots, then the group process has much of its content cut out for it. The therapists can weave together past therapeutic and family knowledge with present process in the group and with the family. It is admittedly an awesome task for the therapists but also an act of respect and confidence in the families' capacity to be self-determining and to change.

5. Fee Structure

The literature did not give any data on fee charges for the groups. An informal review of some hospitals' present structure indicated fee charges at minimum costs (under $10), and only a few on a sliding scale. At the Jewish Family Service in New York City (now the Jewish Board of Family and Children's Services), clients in MFGT were charged for MFT group sessions. This was consistent with the view that MFGT was unique and that families were getting something quite special. It was not unusual for a family to pay a maximum fee for MFGT.

Where Medicaid costs are involved, there are definite restrictions related to reimbursement based on frequency of patient contacts. The implications for arranging sessions with fee collection in mind first and family need second are distressing. Oddly enough, even in situations where MFGT is valued highly, fees set (if at all) generally are lower.

6. Co-therapy: Philosophy and Structure

Having discussed a format for screening families, we now will make some comments about the co-therapeutic relationship in this type of group. The rationale for co-therapy includes the complexity of the group, the quantitative and qualitative interactions, and the necessity to observe these with accuracy and perceptivity. MacLennan cites the most common and desirable qualities of group therapists as perceptiveness, warmth, understanding, empathy, self-awareness, and the capacity to be accepted as a leader (MacLennan, 1975). She lists some of the different leadership styles that are advantageous, such as: the leader as resource person, clarifier, benevolent authority, stimulator of emotional confrontations, and so forth (MacLennan, 1975). We agree that the above qualities are positive ones for group leaders and that the styles of leadership described all can be incorporated into the co-leadership of MFGT. All agree that consistent and honest communications between therapists are necessary.

McGee and Schuman describe the senior–junior co-therapy relationship utilized for training purposes (McGee, 1974). MacLennan distinguishes co-therapists from observers (MacLennan, 1965). She offers the rationale for two leaders: assumption of different roles and combining resources for mutual support and training reasons. Frequently these reasons result (or the pairing results) in a hierarchical division of labor. All literature reviewed on co-therapy reaches general agreement that the pairing compounds the transference reaction and countertransferential phenomena, or that it adds further to the complexity of that reaction (McGee, 1980; McGee & Schuman, 1970). As reported in the literature, the styles of group leadership and schools of thought vary. There is general agreement on the importance of more than one therapist as MFGT leaders. McFarlane recommends two therapists as the minimum for all but the most seasoned clinicians (McFarlane, in press). He also recommends that both sexes and the racial composition of the group be represented. The practical and pragmatic feasibility of achieving a heterosexual ethnically balanced match is a dilemma in many situations. The unattainability of this match, however, need not be a deterrent to a creative co-therapy pair. The co-therapeutic pairing must be based on complementarity and some equivalent, although not necessarily similar training. Practitioners from varied backgrounds can work together (psychiatric nurses, family therapists, group specialists) so long as there is mutual respect.

We have found that age and sex of the therapists are not crucial because whatever is idiosyncratic to the pairing will evoke the group members' transferential response. This basically means that the therapists' awareness and understanding of issues that might emerge and their handling of the issues when they do become manifest is most important. The optimal arrangement is thought to be a male/female pairing, but given that this can often be difficult or impossible, we will make some points about same-sex therapists.

It is likely that two female therapists of comparable age and temperament would be perceived according to the needs of each individual group member. Often several members of a group will agree that one therapist is aggressive–negative while the other is perceived as passive–benign. This is true regardless of the therapists' age, sex, style, and personality, but it is noteworthy in the MFGT context when part of the group perceives one way, and the other part of the group reverses the same perception applying it to the same therapist. The therapists' encouragement of discussions in the group about the split allegiances produces useful material related to the obvious parallels in the lives of individuals and their perceptions of significant-authority others.

The co-therapy model provides an opportunity to draw upon parallel analogies between the co-therapist and the parental dyad. Unlike couple's or adolescent's groups, both parents and children are present to comment upon and hear how these parallels are drawn. As the symbolic figureheads of a large group "family," the therapists are in the mainstream of much transferential material. With so many issues arising out of the group process and the interaction of the various family systems, the co-therapists frequently can represent at least two points of view. As with the parental figures, what is acceptable to one therapist or parent is not necessarily acceptable to the other. These differences often can be shared in front of the group[6] and can serve as a model for conflict resolution. In a similar vein, the two leaders provide different personalities with whom group members can identify. Any set of two people working together with mutual respect and without destructive elements therefore has to serve as a positive model for the group regardless of the specific content and style. Openness and trust between the co-therapy pair serve as a model for openness and trust in the group. The time spent before and after each session either recording the session or discussing what happened and planning for the next time can become an ongoing vehicle for examining and reexamining the co-therapeutic rela-

[6]Of course, not all issues are appropriate to discuss before the group so that the pair have to be in relative agreement about what can be open and what needs to remain private. Here, too, the parallels to parenting are strong.

tionship. It would not be possible to lead a successful group without a high degree of collaboration that begins long before the actual screening starts and ends long after the group itself has terminated. Like a marriage that works, the relationship requires care, fine tuning, and input from significant outsiders in order to endure in the most effective way.

7. Supervision and Training

The literature contains several references to supervision and training for MFGT co-therapists. Institutional settings frequently have group observers who sit in on sessions and learn through observation. In the senior–junior hierarchy one co-leader is the "real" therapist while the other is a beginning learner (MacLennan, 1965). In some settings for training purposes the senior group leader is fixed, whereas the junior partner changes during the life of the group (MacLennan, 1965, McGee, 1974).

Many settings continue to have one identified supervisor who has the responsibility for overseeing the work of a co-therapy team. We believe it is optimal to have MFGT in settings where group supervision is available and, more specifically, groups of co-therapy pairs. Between 1972 and 1975, Elsa Leichter, Director of Group Training at the former Jewish Family Service in New York City, supervised and led a co-therapy pairs group comprised of six to eight pairs of co-therapists all leading MFT groups. In essence, this couples group for therapists was the vehicle for learning. The parallel processes that grew out of this group supervision were an ideal model for teaching and learning MFGT. Where this arrangement is not possible, it is effective to have a general supervision group for all therapists of groups with one or two MFGT pairings participating.

8. The Unique Features of MFGT

There is agreement throughout all of the literature on MFGT that the modality itself has unique features not found in other therapies. A number of authors have conceptualized their understanding of what these features are and on that topic there is no real consensus. Each writer uses a different organizational approach.

Laqueur describes the unique aspects of MFGT as "mechanisms of change" and uses systems theory concepts to specify the particular phenomena (Laqueur, 1976). Laqueur lists the following 10 mechanisms: (1) delineation of the field of interaction; (2) breaking the intrafamilial code; (3) competition; (4) amplification and modulation of signals; (5) learning through trial and error; (6) learning by analogy; (7) learning through identification; (8) the use of models; (9) creating a focus of excitation; and (10) use of families as co-therapists. We will restate his definition of the "delineation of the field of interaction." About number one he writes, "The therapist tries to see the total field of interaction between sub-systems (patient, family) and supra system (the total social environment), and makes the participants in the group aware of the importance for sickness and health of this changing surrounding field" (pp. 412–414).

McFarlane (in press) refers to the unique aspects of MFGT as "therapeutic mechanisms" and lists nine specifics. They are: (1) modulated disenmeshment; (2) rapid resocialization; (3) stigmatic reversal; (4) indirect restructuring; (5) interfamily competition; (6) interfamily support and confrontation; (7) positive feedback stabilization; (8) tertiary prevention; and (9) medication maintenance. His descriptive language, like Laqueur's, follows the historical process of the group. We will give his definition of "modulated disenmeshment" to give some idea of his frame of reference. About modulated disenmeshment in MFGT he says, "It uniquely allows gradual, regulable reduction in family enmeshment simultaneously and interdependently with the creation of new interactional and relational bonds with members of other families. At the same time the family bonds are preserved and validated."

Leichter and Schulman refer to several unique aspects of MFGT as "dynamics and process phenomena (Leichter & Schulman, 1968)." We are in agreement with Strelnick that the "dynamics of mechanisms of change at work in any group are still a matter of debate" (Wellish, *et al.*, 1978). A formal, professional language unique to families does not yet adequately exist. Strelnick adds, "The vocabulary for family interaction and therapy has not reached the same sophistication or proliferation as vocabularies for other forms of treatment" (p. 319). In fact, Bowen (1976) states that:

> It is inaccurate to refer to the entire concept of psychotherapy; but there is no accurate and acceptable word to replace it. As we move more into systems thinking, we will have to find new terms to describe what we are doing, for conventional terms simply no longer apply. (p. 403)

The evolution of language for family therapists has not yet reached a new refined consensus. Thus, in MFGT we have several authors, including ourselves, struggling to find a language to apply.

We have evolved our own way of viewing and categorizing the unique aspects of MFGT and will elaborate on them. First, there is the introduction of the outside world into the therapeutic setting. Laqueur mentions this outside world concept in an early publication (Laqueur, 1968). The introduction of the outside world into the treatment setting always exists in the person of the therapist. It is additionally introduced in groups of unrelated individuals and in couples groups. In MFGT one expands the diversity of the group "universe" by having complete family units, thereby rounding out the global composition. Family units of ethnic, educational, and economic diversity are brought together.

In many ways MFGT is analagous to an urban center such as New York City and can be the comparable melting pot for the therapeutic experience. The "outside world" factor also can be an impetus for change in that family units can see that other families have problems too. In a protective setting group members can experience positive and negative competition which aids the refinement of their life survival skills. They can test out their private convictions about themselves and their fantasies about others. Laqueur refers to the impact of the outside world as partly "learning by analogy" (Laqueur, 1968). McFarlane brings it in with "interfamily support and confrontation." We would say that the introduction of the world into the therapeutic situation is a contributing factor in all of these unique aspects.

It is different to witness family struggles than to hear or fantasize about them. By putting families together in MFGT, all communications made in the group become public. This heightens the degree of exposure for each group member and for each family unit. The exposure to other families in the outside world is more powerful than the exposure to an individual therapist. It can have either positive or negative impact, leading to supportive input, or, on the other hand, to negative vulnerability. Most important in the public nature of the group is the opportunity to correct distortions. It becomes more difficult to hide inappropriate behavior between family members and to convince others outside of the family to join in this. In a large group with a variety of people and perspectives, someone usually can speak for what is more real or objective.

Additionally, substitutes for missing family members can be found outside the family unit among group members. In this vein MFGT provides an opportunity for "re-peopling" families where there are absent members. For example, a child from one family can be adopted by another family as a "subling," or substitute sibling. Since all of the above features derive from the introduction of the outside world, none of the variables would be attainable without the external others in MFGT.

The second special factor is the possibility for relationships to develop that one might avoid in one's everyday life, or which simply would not be available to cultivate. Although this is true for all groups, the age disparity in MFGT allows for a broader range of possibilities to emerge. For example, in a specific MFT group, the Blue family membership included a twice divorced mother with two teenage daughters. All three Blue women had a negative and conflicted stance in regard to men, primarily evident in the abusive types of males they chose and then rejected. In the group they were more able to work on resolution of their conflict, given a face to face experience with three outside male heads of households. This opportunity for a variety of men to be present in the family's treatment could not have existed in any other form of therapy. In individual family therapy, the therapists' appraisal of how the women were progressing outside could only be inferred. In MFGT it can be witnessed and the process toward resolution is sped up.

The third feature has to do with modification *of* and changes *in* diverse norms and values. Families can observe vast differences in functioning, expectation, and production in each other. The exposure to difference in all of these spheres can encourage change by stimulating redefinition of the system interaction, role functioning, individual behavior, and attitudinal stances. Laqueur takes this factor into account in his "breaking the intra-familial code," "competition," and "learning through trial and error." It is partially incorporated in McFarlane's "modulated disenmeshment," "indirect restructuring," and "inter-familial competition." It is touched upon in what Leichter and Schulman call "differentiation of families in the group," "spontaneous insights," and "well sibling shifts." For example, parents from different families who have similar conflict situations with children or with each other can observe first hand what is growth inhibiting in the "outsider's" situation. They can evaluate this behavior in others and apply by analogy those aspects relevant to their own situation. Families hearing other families discuss how to handle similar situations are exposed to value and norm differences they might not otherwise experience. With the development of interfamily mutual respect it is possible for defenses to become less rigid as one family absorbs a new perspective about a previously nonnegotiable subject.

Fourth, in grouping families together for a therapeutic purpose, we encourage the creation of a large symbolic family with co-leaders as therapists and role models. Within the new structure we superimpose our own guidelines which are purposefully different than those norms and guidelines existent in the operational life of the family as they come to us. All of the therapists' interventions, structures, and expectations, overt or covert, create a new "group ego." Family systems and the individuals within can experiment with new behaviors and new ways of communicating. Different family norms and patterns can be tested and tried under the protective group ego umbrella in an arena different from the existing expectations and norms of each family unit and each individual member. In the Blue family, for example, the intense overidentification of the mother and 18-year-old daughter was viewed by them as positive and desirable, "just like sisters." Although we acknowledged some positives about the pairing within the group, we also stated a different opinion, which was that their particular closeness was growth inhibiting and served to keep away any anger or issues of difference. This anger was present but could not emerge.

Initially mother and daughter joined to project their rage onto the therapists, but eventually the group process made it acceptable for the mother's and daughter's anger with each other to surface. An arena existed for the newly surfaced anger and the experience was advantageous in disrupting the intense joining of the two. The group ego, being different, permitted and encouraged different behavior from them, and they received positive feedback whenever the new behavior was overt.

The group ego also provides room for any group member to demonstrate leadership qualities that are inhibited or unknown in the nuclear family system. One man, Mr. Greene, always had been viewed by his family and friends as a ne'er-do-well, and he thought of himself in a similar vein. In the group the leaders made special efforts to give recognition to his input, and this was reinforced regularly by others. By the time the group ended he had emerged as an important contributor, completely overturning the view that he and all members of his family previously held. His family members witnessed the respect others offered him and began to see him in a new light. In both of these examples, the different group ego provided an arena in which the group members could try out new behaviors and roles. This is true for all individuals in all groups. The major difference in MFGT is that family members and outsiders witness these changes.

The fifth special feature of MFGT in the way that we conceive it is that an egalitarian environment is created where equality of all on many levels crosses generational lines not possible in other forms of therapy (Leichter, 1969). We attempt to make equality operant among group members without denying the essential authority of the parenting role or the ultimate responsibility for control on the part of the group leaders (Leichter & Schulman, 1968). By putting everyone on a first-name basis, for instance, there is a leveling of all to a quasisibling position which highlights competition and, when constructively used, can promote additional motivation for growth. We believe that the contribution of any group member can be equally or more important than the input of the therapists (Leichler & Schulman, 1968). Many times in the course of a group, a child can connect to an adult in another family in a way that no adult could do. By making the importance of each member overt, we build in equality of each person as central, diminishing the world-hierarchical view that some people are more important than others by virtue of their life role or status. This also neutralizes the strong hierarchy in families without tampering with the essential power structure. Parents remain parents. In MFGT one thus has the possibilities for the child in each adult to be freed and the burgeoning adult in each child to link up to adult others in supportive and growthful ways.

The sixth special feature of MFGT is the likelihood that in a group of such diversity old feelings and experiences will be activated through material produced in other individuals or families. In all group therapies past life experiences are aroused in this way. The difference for MFGT is that as areas of resistance are broken into in one family, similar processes are stimulated in other family units that might not be responsive to the interventions of individual family therapy. For example, the revelations of one couple's domestic crisis brought forth similar material from another couple who had been strongly invested in denial of their marital conflict while in individual family therapy. Or in a sculpting exercise with the Greene family, a 45-year-old woman in the group cried profusely as she watched Jennifer and listened to her. Jennifer sculpted her family situation as she perceived it, dramatizing the marital discord and inevitable separation that she feared, that is, the pushing apart of her parents and their disconnectedness from each other. The exercise itself stirred up for the other woman, Mrs. Red, recollections of her own parent's separation and the pain associated with it for her, which she had never shared aloud before. In addition to relieving Mrs. Red of a long held burden, Mrs. Red provided warm feedback for Jennifer Greene and an alliance was formed between them. This interaction could be referred to as transference, or as positive identification, or just as human universal understanding. Whatever one labels it, the bonding of one outsider to another across generational lines and before one's own family can occur only in the MFGT setting. Life situations are reactivated *in vivo* with the entire cast present in the form of real and symbolic others. This provides an opportunity for an experiential reworking and reintegration of critical moments with those significant real or symbolic individuals present.

The seventh area of specialness, and we believe the most potent feature of MFGT, is the possibility for endless transferences and alliances. The multiple age, sex, and role differences offer possibilities for identifications, projective material, and extensions of self to develop. Perhaps these could be called "poly-transferences." A child first may get angry with another child's parents before being encouraged to tackle his own. One husband might see in someone else's wife those qualities that he abhors in his own wife. The anger can emerge first in terms of the "other." In the area of positive transferences there is room on all levels for attachments to develop. The wide range of group members representing people from all walks and ages in life makes possible the discovery of substitute relationships, perhaps the opportunity for simultaneous poly-transference. Group members can find people to substitute for people absent in families through death or departure. In this respect MFGT can re-people families where absences, literal or figurative, are existent. A variety of techniques are employed to make the arena of love and conflict live. Also, the therapists are repositories for diversified transferential material, although this is diluted somewhat from other group experiences due to the available others in the group.

In summary, family units often have a stake in perpetuating mores, systems of behavior and interaction, and role functioning as they have existed through time. The powerful difference in the structure of MFGT is that the group ego has to provide room for a multiplicity of family life-styles, attitudes, and communication patterns to emerge and shift. In essence, the arena of MFGT is really a live theatre where families enact their life realities before participant observers. Individual family members and family units can be witnessed interacting within the family system as well as before others. The "theatre" of MFGT is in many ways a microcosm of the world. As our former colleague, Gerda Schulman, pointed out (Schulman, 1976), MFGT is an environment "in which bridges can be built from individual to individual, from family to family, and from subgroup to subgroup." Unlike other treatment modalities, there is the potential for narrowing the distance between generations and the possibility for altering divergent attitudes, norms, and role functions.

9. Structure, Time, and Process

In an effort to give form to an otherwise confusing and complex therapeutic modality, we will first break the group's entirety into three major components. These interactional components are time, content, and process, a trio of shifting and interwoven forces simultaneously in motion. Although recognizing that there is a blurring of those boundaries, we will nonetheless attempt to isolate them. In this way we can continue to understand the parts of MFGT as a means for understanding the whole. Figure 1 shows how we envision the group. First is the suprastructure whose major components include:

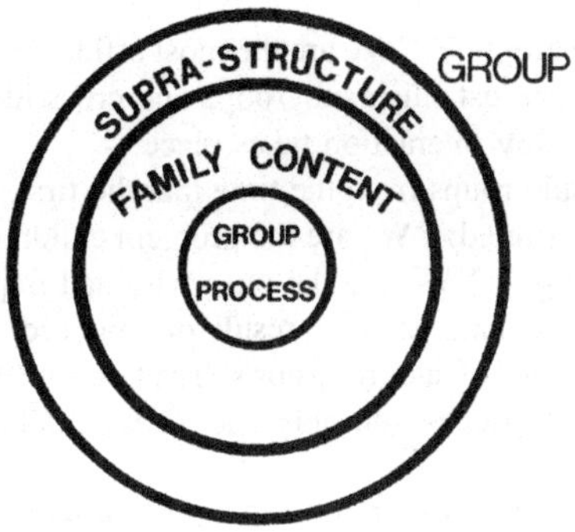

Figure 1

(1) number of therapists, (2) length of each group session, (3) whether group follows an open or closed model, (4) length of group over months or years, (5) which family members are included, (6) therapeutic model and methods of intervention, (7) rules and guidelines for all, (8) imposed and inherent structures. These are the major suprastructure factors giving form and boundaries to the group.

When the leaders select an imposed time limit, as we do, it follows that a group will have three clear stages or phases: a beginning, a middle, and an end. Each of these has an inherent process in terms of the kinds of arising issues. These stages are part of the group's suprastructure.

The second major component of MFGT is the family data gathered and understood during the screening process. This data give the group concrete content. The family data include: (1) family composition, (2) presenting problem, (3) system type, (4) family life stage, (5) roles of each member, (6) family relationships with each other and with therapists, and so forth. Many of these factors were discussed in the section on screening.

The third component, that is, group process, evolves as a direct result of the first two. This process is woven of all spoken and acted-out transactions, communications, agreements, alliances, differences, and so forth, between and among group members. In order to lead MFGT successfully, the therapist always needs to be aware of these three major components so that each event in the group's life can be understood within the context of the whole.

Some component parts of MFGT have not been discussed in previous sections. We will examine them in the following sections.

9.1. Inherent and Imposed Structure

As in any group therapy situation, there are two kinds of structure, one inherent in the group at its inception and one that the therapists impose once the group has begun. The inherent structure remains fixed for the group while the imposed structure becomes part of the process. The MFT groups exist with a variety of inherent structures around which, in spite of which, and with which the therapists must work; for example, the subsystems of women, problem children, husbands, family units, co-therapy pairs, and so forth. These are the most obvious subsystems existing at the group's inception and members can almost look around the room and categorize: "We are the children," "We are the mothers,'' ''We are the parents,'' ''We are the most affluent looking,'' and so forth. This kind of visual sizing up can establish subgroups and cross identification patterns before any words are spoken or any interaction takes place.

The emergence of subgroups from the time that the first words are spoken relates to what cannot be seen or assumed: ''We are the problem children,'' ''We are the ones who have difficulty functioning,'' ''We are the ones who had impoverished parenting,'' for example. These subgroups emerge as a result of imposed interventions that fuel the process. In this way a variety of subgroups or subsystems develop. The therapists need to keep this in mind as the process unfolds and shifting alliances, identifications, and rivalries are formed.

As in any therapy with two or more people, subgroup alliances can impede or promote change. The therapeutic interventions are essential in keeping the group on a growth oriented course. Due to the importance of therapeutic interventions, ''how to and what type'' are paramount for the co-therapy pair to discuss before and during the life of the group. Any mobilization of a subgroup, constructive or destructive, is made overt by the therapists within the group process at some appropriate point.

The inherent subgroups basically have little to do with therapeutic interventions other than that the therapists were the creators of the group. In that sense they chose to put together people who obviously would have certain commonalities of which the therapists were aware. The alliances or rivalries that form after the group has begun have a great deal to do with both the therapeutic interventions and the content that emerges. To the extent that therapists guide and structure some of the content in the way of expectations and direct interventions, they could be said to guide and structure subgroupings.

9.2. Open and Closed Models

Our review of the literature indicates that MFGT treatment time varies from 12 sessions to several years. The latter occurred in the case of chronically ill psychotic patients who continued in aftercare (Lansky, Bley, McVey, & Brotman, 1978). The shorter-term groups were planned where adolescents and their families were involved. A contract for regular family attendance was more likely to be made in the short-term groups. Open-ended groups appeared more regularly in medical settings and were based on family availability during visits. The open-ended group is especially valuable in the institutional setting where the identified patients have a length of stay determined in part by hospital policy and insurance coverage. Since inpatient turnover is rapid, a group can be offered with very specific foci related to hospital stay and discharge planning. This is a task-oriented therapeutic structure that seems to benefit both the hospital and the patient/family. An open-ended group is different from a closed group extending over a longer period of time with a consistent population, as is more often the case in the outclient setting. This chapter focuses more directly on groups that are time-limited and closed.

The length of time we determine for time-limited but not necessarily short-term[7] MFGT can vary from a few weeks to several years, depending on goals and orientation. However, it is difficult to structure MFGT as we are suggesting in less than 20 sessions. We prefer a structure allowing a minimum of 30 sessions and a maximum of 60. We prefer a closed group structure in part because of the demands of MFGT. Having a

[7]For our purposes we are defining short-term as less than three months (basically 6 to 12 sessions).

defined end date helps members and therapists sustain and cope with the intense demands of the experience.

The use of a time structure in the MFGT setting, as in any therapeutic setting, with its beginning, middle, and end, has important applicable parallels to family life. When the co-therapeutic pair agree to use a time limited MFGT they take on the responsibility to make manifest each stage related to time. There has to be repetitive weaving together of time in the group's life with time in the families' lives.

9.3. Beginnings, Middles, and Endings

In any time-limited group the stages of beginning, middle, and end can be divided arithmetically according to stipulated length of the group. Approximately one-fourth of the time for beginning, one-half for a middle phase to develop, and one-fourth devoted to ending. Within each of these stages, there are certain universally accepted themes.

In the beginning process, reactions such as anxiety, development of trust, and fear of exposure are universal. This is true in all new psychotherapeutic situations and in MFGT it is equally or more pronounced. Whole families sit and face strange other families. The arena is one in which comparisons will be drawn, family secrets revealed, and "dirty laundry" aired before virtual strangers. Each person's secret family life will cease to be secret in that a small portion of the world now will be made aware of what previously was private within the nuclear family. In addition, realities that family members have known but never dared to speak among themselves now will be spoken before others. Many protective tribal and cultural rules break down in the MFGT context.

The co-therapeutic pair have the option of structuring the beginning phase of the group by making these issues overt or they can watch the issues surface symbolically. Given an active screening process that touched on potential beginning phenomena, it is possible to help the group as a whole and the families within the group recognize anticipated and unanticipated themes as they are played and replayed. For those themes of which the family is aware, the group process is like a well orchestrated symphony or concerto. The theme is stated in the beginning, that is, screening, and it is played and replayed in each of the subsequent movements, that is, phases. Having heard the major theme(s) stated in the beginning, it is apparent to most whenever it is reworked.

The ways in which the beginning reactions of anxiety, fear of exposure, and evolving trust surface in the group varies from situation to situation and the methods therapists employ can be equally varied. For instance, there can be discussion of how each family characteristically begins new tasks[8] and how individual members reflect or do not reflect this pattern. This type of process related to use of time binds the group members by virtue of its universal application (Schulman, Personal communications, 1971–1976; Laqueur, 1968). Some therapists will directly encourage group members to relate to this content or will themselves respond about the therapists' anxiety in beginning with a new group. Others will be less directive and will wait until a group member addresses the issue(s). Frequently, anxious displacement or projection will be utilized by certain subgroups. For example, the parents often begin to talk within the group about children. They reveal facts about the children, such as the "bad" things the specific children do and the angry responses evoked by the child's behavior. Both of these themes have an inherent blaming quality. Therapeutic interventions can shift the blaming and scapegoating system so that

[8]Do they venture forth and take risks in life or do they retire to their private grouping and remain more isolated?

the flow of the group is noticeably altered. Leichter and Schulman (1972) point out that this is done without tampering with the basic power-hierarchical structure in which parents have the ultimate authority over their children and therapists have the ultimate responsibility for the group. For instance, the therapists might comment that people in the group have begun to talk by describing their parent–child relationships. Therapists can inquire if there are other roles of importance that they fill in life. The purpose of the intervention is threefold: (1) to label group content as parent–child related, (2) to identify the content as blaming, and (3) to shift the focus from the blaming aspect to discussion of other roles. This can open up material related to husband–wife roles, individual feelings about self, and so forth. The therapists also can request that no group member reveal facts about another group member, but rather that each individual talk about him or herself. In these ways embarrassment is eased, individuation is underscored, and the message is conveyed that in this group there will be some equality and respect for children as well as adults.

Every intervention shifts and refocuses the group content so that different issues become overt. Also, every intervention the therapists make in trying to bring this about is powerful and therapists must be prepared to pick up the reverberations stemming from these interventions. Group members can be angry they were cut off and fallout has to be handled before the group can move on.

9.4. Middles

Once beginning phenomena have been recognized and discussed, the group can move into a middle or working phase. Time is spent in evaluating how well each family and each person within the family is progressing toward the accomplishment of goals carefully arrived at during the screening sessions. There can be exploration either structured or free form[9] about how families use time, where they get stuck en route to some desired goal, and how the individual family's old growth inhibiting patterns are being replicated within the group. The middle phase is used to free families from the stuck places in order that they move closer to stated goals. The same process should be implemented with each individual.

During the middle phase families and individuals do substantial therapeutic work, which includes a dramatic range of internal and external observations and changes. As a part of this middle process, goals are rediscussed and progress evaluated. A successful working group in this phase requires that the therapists edit the group content and comment on process. This therapeutic function in the middle phase differs from the strongly catalytic function in the beginning, because the group no longer needs the therapists to spur them on. They have long since jelled. Another function of the therapists at this middle stage is to move from the family focus to more of the individual issues within the family system. This is a good time to introduce exercises designed for the specific families. Sculpting, gestalt exercises, and so forth, are useful in freeing material that has remained caged.

> For instance, in the Greene family, described earlier, Jennifer, the oldest daughter, had remained peripheral in her involvement within the group. On many occasions the

[9]We are here defining structured as referring to purposefully exploring the issue rather than inferring from the group process.

therapists had attempted to make a connection with her. The leaders suggested in the middle phase of treatment that she sculpt her family. She arranged the family with parents facing, Naomi in the middle, and Gail attached to the mother. Jennifer positioned Naomi so that she, Naomi, was pushing the parents apart. When the therapists asked that Jennifer set the sculpture in motion, she ran frantically around the perimeter trying to keep her mother from falling backward, her father from falling out, and trying to keep Naomi from pushing them apart. When the exercise was completed, she was exhausted and burst into tears, recognizing for the first time that she asked for little from her family because they had little to give. The therapists pointed out that much energy was expended in the role she had assumed of holding family together and that it helped her remain an outsider. In a situation where the demands were great, her self-assigned job as the oldest child was to attempt the self-depleting task of keeping the nuclear family from falling apart. This exercise in the group was timed at a point where there was sufficient trust for her to participate.

The sculpting experience underscored the mechanisms at work in the basic family system and each person's deprivation. It made it possible for Jennifer actually to ''join'' the group and the family as a bona fide member for the first time. We view the ability to make good use of this exercise as related to timing and the way in which the subsequent material was handled by the co-therapists. The latter point enabled her to be a recipient of sustenance, some of which was given by other nurturing group members from other families (Mrs. Blue, mentioned earlier). During this middle phase, therapists actively encouraged identification across all life roles and stages.

9.4.1. Marathon Sessions in the Middle Phase of MFGT

It is extremely useful to plan a marathon session at or near the middle-middle segment of treatment. The marathon session can intensify the working phase and offer time for defenses to become less rigid. Early in our MFGT experience we began to utilize marathon sessions during the middle phase of a group. The sessions are held for one day, lasting from 10:00 A.M. to 5:00 P.M., usually on a Saturday or Sunday so that working members can attend. They are conducted outside of the regular agency group setting, most often in the home of one of the therapists. The decision always is dictated by available space and location. For private MFGT, marathon sessions can be held in a large office or home. A session is planned six to eight weeks in advance so that there will be enough notice for everyone to plan to attend. This early planning builds in a certain amount of excitement and apprehension related to a marathon's specialness and its unknowns. Members pay twice their weekly fee for the session and contribute a set amount of money for food. All food purchase and preparation is done by the therapists. We think that although families pay a fee for the therapy and provide money for the food, the therapists' role as the preparers of the food is important in that it gives members something special and tangible from the therapists. Therapists also contribute food money.

The work of the actual marathon is divided in half with a full lunch served during an hour-long middle break. The break is always a much needed respite for all, before the last segment of hard work. The introduction of gestalt techniques, sculpting exercises, and so forth, are particularly valuable in a marathon session where they serve as catalysts to intensify the process within an already intense session. For two to four weeks following the marathon, therapists need to address themselves to explicit feedback from the marathon experience. The marathon sessions are always intense, productive, and exhausting and can be attempted only by therapists who are well trained and not too frightened of the unknown or uncertain.

The middle phase of a time-limited group is a period when rich work is accomplished and, because of the hightened tempo, the ending phase seems to arrive more quickly than expected. Although the passage of time is commented upon and duly noted as the group progresses, the realization that only five to ten sessions remain comes as a surprise to most members. The therapists generally need to restate this fact several times in order to get a process started that makes the termination theme overt.

9.5. Termination in MFGT

In the beginning of the termination phase, the dynamics of ending will emerge fully if the therapists are active in making this content manifest. Termination is particularly difficult to focus because of the more intense resistances most of us have in anticipating, experiencing, and accepting loss. There is much room in this phase for drawing parallels to family life and the separation–individuation themes. The major dynamics to emerge during termination are: denial that ending time has come, anger with the therapists for causing the end, mourning for that which will cease to be and/or never was, and resolution by evaluating the group experience and moving forward.

We find that the natural stages that emerge during the ending phase of any time-limited group closely parallel the stages referred to by Elizabeth Kübler-Ross in *On Death and Dying* (1970). Although we have observed that the stages follow the basic order outlined by Kübler-Ross, the boundaries never are absolute. There are four major stages in the ending phase of time-limited groups and we will offer some examples of how they can be optimally utilized in the MFGT realm.

The tendency to deny the ending in all therapies occurs in MFGT and most often is signified by the group members continuing to discuss current content without acknowledging the ending date. Frequently, however, and not unexpectedly, the explicit or the underlying content has to do with themes of separation and loss. For instance, a mother might comment on her continuing difficulties with a young adult staying out late at night and threatening to leave home. The therapists can generalize from the theme of difficulty in separation for that family to the difficulty in the group of talking more directly about the impending group terminations. At a point where the therapists have successfully turned the group to thinking and talking about the group's end and terminations in life, it is not uncommon for the anger to emerge directly.

Recriminations toward the therapists are frequent and often revert to a blaming system, this time external to the family. Whereas in the middle phase of a group the transferential importance of the therapists is diminished, in the ending phase the group's need to reactivate discussion of the importance of the therapists is pronounced. Therapists can use the themes of anger toward "authorities" to underscore and dramatize issues of separation and individuation moving back and forth between the inherent need to separate in families and the need to separate from the group and significant others who have become important. All of the group members' transferences to authority figures are important. At the height of the group's anger with the therapists, there will be efforts to have the group extended, accusations that the therapists have failed to deliver a number of wished-for solutions, and charges that the therapists have failed to care enough. Unlike other time-limited groups where this type of projected blame recurs, the possibilities for spreading the blame around are greater so that not only therapists are confronted, but also transferential-authority others. Angry charges against significant others are explored in terms of the transferential meaning. Although we are significantly directive in helping this content become overt, other therapists utilize an indirect approach, thereby diminishing resistance.

Anger, of course, is not the sole emotion to emerge. There is relief that the ending has come and much ambivalence regarding the forces of change and sameness. When the group is able to live through the bombardment of anger, it is possible to connect members to their feelings of sorrow and loss. In the MFGT situation, many losses of significant family members are brought to mind and members can be encouraged to pinpoint others in the group who remind them of the special people in their lives, real and alive, deceased or wished for. Children learn more information about deceased relatives and their parents' relationships to these people. This is an extension of the intergenerational benefits that continue throughout the group. Children see their parents in more human light as having feelings of sadness and unfulfillment, just as they, themselves do. The universality of life's experiences which have been thematic throughout now are intensified. Within the life of the group each member has had the opportunity to work on evaluating his or her life in general through his or her life in the group. Families as units and as individuals move into an assessment of goals outlined in the beginning, redefined in the middle, and now finally realized or not realized in the ending. Because of the diverse population of the group, adults and children get a range and intensity of feedback from outside others that is not available in other therapies. In the course of the evaluation each family and each individual defines what they would like to do from this point forward after the group has terminated.

Some significant highlights relevant to the ending phase in MFGT as we conceive it are that: the therapist has the ultimate responsibility for focusing the end of the group; the difficulty for the therapists in focusing the end and the difficulty for the group in living through the end is the universal pain that separation and loss evoke; and that a time-limited group offers tremendous opportunities for comparisons with life.

10. Follow-up Sessions in MFGT

In the latter part of the ending phase of an MFT group we request of the group that they attend a one-time follow-up session six months after the group terminates. We acknowledge that the group in large part will be doing something for us in returning one time. The group is told that this is largely for our purposes although the group members sometimes get a great deal back through the evolving process. It is to be noted that the process is different from the ongoing group process because the solidifying oneness of the group is greatly diminished if not lost entirely. We do expect that families pay a fee at the follow-up.

In the follow-up sessions therapists learn from group members the ways in which they perceive future groups can be improved. Members are willing to offer feedback, hopefully improving the quality of future groups. We have found that after six months have elapsed people are more candid about the positive and negative value of the group and about themselves in relation to each other. The follow-up sessions help us observe the extent to which changes are or are not integrated or internalized. This follow-up also can provide an opportunity to offer a booster shot when a family or person is in a brief slump.

We are able to compare our assessments of family change and progress at the point of ending with the reality that we see after a time lapse. When we see that we have been in error in our ending recommendations we acknowledge this to the family and consider contracting for a further segment of treatment for one person, a marital couple, or the whole family.

We recognize that in presenting this framework for organizing and leading MFGT we sound as if nothing ever goes wrong. It might seem to the reader that if the format is mastered and implemented no group ever will fall apart, no family ever will drop out, no co-therapists ever will "divorce." This is far from true. These problems occur in all therapies and MFGT is no exception.

11. Final Thoughts on Structure, Time, and Process

We have attempted to provide a blueprint for the structure, the content-framework (largely fleshed out during the screening), and the process, which is woven throughout. If one thinks of MFGT from creation to completion, it conjures up a symphonic metaphor, where the final production/performance will achieve excellence only to the extent that the composer–conductor has memorized and integrated the form, timing, varied parts, and theme of the work. The composer–conductor always puts these variables together with care and attention to the parts as they contribute to the whole. When the trumpet sounds a wrong note, or the timing is off in the string section, the conductor has a concept of the whole work into which he or she can fit the unexpected parts. When during the termination phase a group member or family unit wants to focus quickly on "what next" before any other termination issues are discussed, the therapists know that this is out of place in the time-process frame and carefully helps put that content on hold until the time is right to work with it. In a sense we are stressing that although the structure of a group exists strongly as a formal reality, the content and process within that structure is always fluid and spontaneous and can vary almost without limit. We are not saying that the therapists use the structure or process to control in the sense of "impede," but rather that structure is used to organize and encourage the varied spontaneous content. The symphony is best concluded when the conductor is attentive to every detail from timing to the complex interweaving of many separate parts.

12. Final Thoughts

At the conclusion of each section we have considered some questions and implications for the future practice of MFGT. It is clear that published literature on out-client MFGT is limited quantitatively and that the application of newer family therapy techniques is not yet reflected adequately in the literature as it applies to MFGT. There is some beginning evaluation emerging on inter- and intrafamily communication patterns within MFGT, but again, little substantive conclusion.

Perhaps the lower status of both family and group therapy in the psychotherapeutic community influences the secondary role of MFGT; or conversely, perhaps the complex nature and requirements of MFGT always will relegate the modality to a less significant position. Whatever the reason for the limited practice of MFGT, it is our hope that this will undergo a change in the coming years.

ACKNOWLEDGMENTS

We wish to thank Florence Bass, Lois Goorwitz, Glenn Gritzer, Elsa Leichter, Nancy Sahlein, Gerda Schulman, and Anne Zweiman for their critical thinking in the preparation of this chapter.

13. References

Anthony, E. J. There and then and here and now. *International Journal of Group Psychotherapy*, 1975, *25*(2) 163–167.

Bell, J. E. A theoretical framework for family group therapy. In P. J. Guerin (Ed.), *Family therapy theory and practice*. New York: Gardner Press, 1976.

Bloch, D. A. Including the children in family therapy. In P. J. Guerin (Ed.), *Family therapy theory and practice*. New York: Gardner Press, 1976.

Bowen, M. Principles and techniques of multiple family therapy. In P. J. Guerin (Ed.), *Family therapy theory and practice*. New York: Gardner Press, 1976.

Cohen, C. I., & Corwin, J. A further application of balance theory to multiple family therapy. *International Journal of Group Psychotherapy*, 1978, *28*(2), 195–209.

Cooper, E. J. Beginning a group program in a general hospital. *Eastern Group Psychotherapy Society (Group JEGPS)*, July 1976, 6–9.

Davies, I. J., Ellinson, G., & Young, R. Therapy with a group of families in a psychiatric day center. *American Journal of Orthopsychiatry*, 1966, *6*, 134–146.

Donner, J., & Gamson, A. Experience with multifamily time limited out-patient group at a community psychiatric clinic. *Psychiatry*, 1968, *31*(2), 126–137.

Farley, J. E. Family separation—Individuation tolerance: A developmental conceptualization of the nuclear family. *Journal of Marital and Family Therapy*, January 1976, 61–66

Fieldstiel, N. D. Therapist or leader: Group and family therapy experiences. *Eastern Group Psychotherapy Society (Group JEGPS)*, 1980, *4*(3), 40–42.

Foley, V. D. Current leadership styles in family therapy. *Eastern Group Psychotherapy Society (Group JEGPS)*, 1980, *4*(1), 19–28.

Gilder, R., Buschman, P. R., Sitarz, A. L., Wolf, J. A. Group therapy with parents of children with leukemia. *American Journal of Psychotherapy*, 1978, *32*(2), 278–286.

Green, L. R., Abramowitz, S. I., Davidson, C. V., & Edwards, D. W. Gender, race, and referral to group psychotherapy: Further empirical evidence of countertransference. *International Journal of Group Psychotherapy*, 1980, *30*(3), 357–363.

Gritzer, P. H., & Bass, F. *Multiple family therapy groups: A unique experience*. Unpublished manuscript, 1976.

Gritzer, P. H., & Eckhaus, D. *The termination process in time-limited therapy groups*. Unpublished manuscript, November 1973.

Kimbro, E. L., Taschman, H. A., Wylie, H. W., & MacLennan, B. W. A multiple family group approach to some problems of adolescence. *International Journal of Group Psychotherapy* 1967, *17*, 18–24.

Kubler-Ross, E. *On death and dying*. New York: Macmillan, 1970.

Lansky, M. R., Bley, C. R., McVey, G. G., & Brotman, B. Multiple family groups at aftercare. *International Journal of Group Psychotherapy*, 1978, *28*, 211–224.

Laqueur, H. P. Multiple family therapy. In J. H. Masserman (Ed.), *Current psychiatric therapies* (Vol. 4). New York: Grune & Stratton, 1964.

Laqueur, H. P. General systems theory and MFT. In J. H. Masserman (Ed.) *Current psychiatric therapies* (Vol. 3). New York: Grune & Stratton, 1968.

Laqueur, H. P. Multiple family therapy. In P. J. Guerin, (Ed.), *Family theory and practice*. New York: Gardner Press, 1976.

Leichter, E. Group psychotherapy of married couples group. Some characteristic treatment dynamics. *International Journal of Group Psychotherapy*, 1962, *12*(2), 154–163.

Leichter, E., & Schulman, G. L. Emerging phenomena in MFGT. *International Journal of Group Psychotherapy*, 1968, *18*(1), 59–69.

Leichter, E., & Schulman, G. L. Interplay of group and family treatment: Techniques in MFGT. *International Journal of Group Psychotherapy*, 1972, *22*(2), 167–176.

Leichter, E., & Schulman, G. L. MFGT. A multidimensional approach. *Family Process,* 1974, *(13)*1, 167–175.

Leichter, E. Personal Communications, 1971–1978.

Lieberman, M. A. Problems in integrating traditional group therapies with new group forms. *International Journal of Group Psychotherapy,* 1977, *27*(1), 19–32.

Lonergan, E. C. Humanizing the hospital experience: Report of group program for medical patients in health and social work. *Health and Social Work,* 1980, 53–63.

Luber, R. F., & Wells, R. A. Structured short term multiple family therapy: An educational approach. *International Journal of Group Psychotherapy,* 1977, *27*(1), 43–58.

Lurie, A., & Ron, H. Multiple family group counselling of discharged schizophrenic young adults and their parents. *Social Psychiatry,* 1971, *6*(2), 88–92.

Lurie, A., & Ron, H. Family centered after care for young adults. *Hospital and Community Psychiatry,* August 1976, pp. 36–38.

MacLennan, B. W. Co-Therapy. *International Journal of Group Psychotherapy,* 1965, *15*(2), 154–166.

MacLennan, B. W. The personalities of group leaders: Implications for selection and training. *International Journal of Group Psychotherapy,* 1975, *25*(2), 177–183.

Mahler, M., Pine, F., & Bergman, A. *The psychological birth of the human infant, symbiosis and individuation.* New York: Basic Books, 1975.

McFarlane, W. R. Multiple family therapy in the psychiatric hospital. In, H. S. Harbin (Ed.), *Psychiatric hospitals and families.* New York: Spectrum, in press.

McFarlane, W. R. Personal communication, 1982.

McGee, T. F., & Schuman, B. N. The nature of the cotherapy relationship. *International Journal of Group Psychotherapy,* 1970, *2*(1), 25–36.

McGee, T. F. The triadic approach to supervision in group psychotherapy. *International Journal of Group Psychotherapy,* 1974, *24*(4), 471–476.

McGee, T. F. Transition in the cotherapy dyad: To wait or not to wait. *Eastern Group Psychotherapy Society (Group JEGPS),* 1980, *4*(1), 65–71.

Minuchin, S. *Families and family therapy.* Cambridge: Harvard University Press, 1974.

Paul, H. L., & Bloom, J. D. Multiple family therapy: Secrets and scapegoating in family crises. *International Journal of Group Psychotherapy,* 1978, *20*(1), 37–47.

Paulson, I., Burroughs, J. C., & Gelb, C. B. Cotherapy: What is the crux of the relationship? *International Journal of Group Psychotherapy,* 1976, *36*(2), 213–224.

Pellman, R., & Platt, R. Three families in search of a director. *American Journal of Orthopsychiatry,* 1974, *44,* 224–225.

Pasnau, R. O., Meyer, M. Davis, L. J., Loyd, R., & Kline, G. Coordinating group psychotherapy of children and parents. *International Journal of Group Psychotherapy,* 1976, *26*(1), 89–103.

Raasoch, J., & Laqueur, H. P. Learning multiple family therapy through simulated workshops. *Family Process,* 1979, *18,* 95–98.

Roth, B. E. Countertransference and the group therapists state of mind. *Eastern Group Psychotherapy Society (Group JEGPS),* 1981, *5*(1), 3–9.

Scheidlinger, S. The psychology of leadership revisited: An overview. *Eastern Group Psychotherapy Society (Group JEGPS),* 1980, *4*(1), 5–17.

Schulman, G. Multi-family group therapy—A not so new challenge!! Report of unpublisbed paper, November 1976.

Schulman, G. Personal Communications, 1971–1976.

Skynner, A. C. R. *Systems of family and marital psychotherapy.* New York: Brunner/Mazel, 1976.

Spiegel, D., & Yalom, I. D. A Support group for dying patients. *International Journal of Group Psychotherapy,* 1978, *28,* 233–244.

St. Luke's-Roosevelt Hospital Center (New York), Roosevelt Site, Department of Social Work. Index of 1980 Group Programs, pp. 1–25.

Strelnick, A. H. Multiple family therapy: A review of the literature. *Family Process,* 1977, *16,* 307–325.

Wellisch, D. K., Mosher, M. B., & Van Scoy, C. Management of family emotion stress: Family group therapy in a private oncology practice. *International Journal of Group Psychotherapy,* 1978, *28*(2), 225–231.

16

Co-therapy with Families

DAVID V. KEITH AND CARL A. WHITAKER

The practitioner of psychotherapy needs to balance the steady pressure between fulfilling the community's expectations, providing patients with an opportunity for growth, and keeping himself alive and creative. Co-therapy teaming has been vital in helping us to maintain a dynamic equilibrium between these three vectors. The term *co-therapy* denotes a number of different arrangements. Chiefly, it is the way that professional psychotherapists avoid, consciously or unconsciously, isolation. We use three methods of co-therapy:

1. The commonest type of arrangement and the focus of this paper is the professional and/or symbolic marriage of two therapists who intend to be present at all or most of the interviews.
2. Use of a consultant is another model. The therapist may invite another colleague in for a single or intermittent visit. The patient also may go off to see the consultant without the therapist (a visit to grandmother).
3. Another co-therapy model pictures a group of colleagues who meet on a regular basis to interview a family or discuss one or more treatment cases. The group may prefer a long-distance consultation with a speaker phone.

There are some other co-therapy methods that operate covertly:

1. A more symbolic form of co-therapy is the in-the-head ghost. This inevitable group includes a wide array of friends, teachers, therapists, parents, spouses, colleagues, teaching institutes, the women's movement, and the culture.
2. Family members may become co-therapists.

a. A common family co-therapist is the family square. These include the reasonable husband with his crazy symptomatic wife, the overadequate wife with the alcoholic spouse, or the complaining but patient, overfunctioning mother with her delinquent teenager. In psychotherapy work that is not family oriented, the square often manages to escape attending any therapy sessions except to give a special distorted brand of history, sometimes by telephone only.

DAVID V. KEITH and CARL A. WHITAKER • Department of Psychiatry, University of Wisconsin, Clinical Sciences Center, Madison, Wisconsin 53792.

b. In a family with children, the white knight becomes the co-therapist because he is able to give support to the therapists and espouse a psychological point of view. The white knight is the counterweight for the black sheep. He carries the virtues for the family. There are several problems connected to allowing the white knight to work as co-therapist. First, the white knight usually is impotent, and aligning with him gives the family the ability to be immune to the therapist. Second, the white knight has a functional job in the family. He is in training to be impersonal and isolated and the psychotherapist needs to interrupt that process rather than support it.

1. Co-therapy as Symbolic Marriage

In this process two therapists (or more) form a professional marriage in order to become a parent generation to the patient or family. Marriage is a metaphorical model that we use to understand the strengths and the complications of co-therapy.

In order to give perspective to the value that we place on co-therapy, you must first understand our psychotherapeutic methodology. Our work is experiential, growth-oriented, and proto-gestalt. We think of psychotherapy as moving at cross current to the culture. We do not plan to help people adapt better or to normalize themselves. We see the purpose of our therapy method as helping people to become more of themselves with the freedom to adapt or to differentiate.

We hold the idea that anxiety is required for family change and should be linked with esprit de corps (enthusiasm, devotion, and jealousy of the group honor). Among the combined strengths and problems of an anticultural therapy is that family system anxiety tends to be higher and thus the need for the co-therapist is much clearer, lest the single therapist be eaten up by the family.

Co-therapy is a way to provide mutual support for two professionals who are expanding their life experience by doing psychotherapy. Psychotherapy trainees expect to outgrow the need for co-therapists by learning to operate independently. This is an appropriate expectation if one is working with individuals, some kinds of groups, or some kinds of couples, but probably not for the family therapist. Once he or she gets into the unstructured terrain beyond the first three interviews one becomes too vulnerable. We do not think of co-therapy as training to work alone with families. Marriage is not a method of training to become a single parent.

Co-therapy team relationships, like marriage, are highly variable. The team may be the combination of two incomplete therapists to make a psychotherapeutic "I," or at the other end of the scale, a combination of two therapeutic "I's" to make a therapeutic "We." All degrees of differentiation are possible on this continuum. As a co-therapy relationship progresses along the scale, its therapeutic potential increases. So, although co-therapy can be of critical importance for beginners, we are most interested in it as an art and a means to augment the styles of mature therapists.

Our model for learning co-therapy matches our pattern for learning to become a family therapist. We suggest that the team begin work together by working with a couple. In this way the dynamics are not complicated by the biologic triangulation introduced by children. Next, treat a couples group; this helps the co-therapy team to become a couple among couples. They can find the freedom to enjoy and/or struggle with one another because the group is the therapist. Next, treat an individual with co-therapy (Whitaker & Warkentin, 1959). Then they are ready to work with a family. The more clinical situations that the team deals with the deeper the relationship and the more secure its members.

Although co-therapy may be *described* metaphorically, it is simultaneously an existential action metaphor in which the relationship between the therapists becomes one of the therapists and one of the patients. When treating a family with a mother, a father, and two children, there are five patients. The fifth patient is the family. When co-therapy is used, there are three therapists; the two individual therapists and the team, that is the relationship between them. Thus, a relationship system is used to treat a relationship system. The mechanism is not well understood, but a prototype is seen in the way that a marital relationship affects the development of children. This may be better understood if we draw a triangular model of the family in which each child has a relationship to each of the parents individually and to the marriage as well. Usually the level of the intimacy possible between co-therapists sets the level of intimacy between family members. Some orientations prefer the use of male/female co-therapy teams. More important than the heterosexual co-therapy match is the bilateral caring and/or respect between team members. For us, a growing, evolving, caring association between co-therapists has more therapeutic value than the simple blending of the sexes for political reasons.

2. Developing a Creative Co-therapy Relationship

Regardless of how the marriage begins, the partners have to do something about becoming a team. Sharing excitement or pleasure is certainly the best way. The pleasure of getting to know someone else or sharing ideas about the therapy are the ways we expand our own therapeutic potential.

It is inevitable that problems will arise in any co-therapy team. Sometimes a difficult treatment case forces the team into joining. The male therapist may feel that the wife is too pushy or that the husband is too passive. The woman co-therapist may worry that her partner does not notice how deeply disturbed the mother is. It is not the problems *per se* that are disruptive, but rather the unwillingness to recognize and discuss them that makes for trouble. Preferably, problems can be discussed in front of the family because it gives them a model for disagreement.

Goolishan, Sheeley, and Pulliam (1975) described four stages of development for co-therapy teams: (1) honeymoon, (2) pseudomutual, (3) conflict, and (4) resolution–maturity. Rice, Fey, and Kepecs (1972) did a study of co-therapy experiences among psychiatrists at the University of Wisconsin that indicated that therapists tended to value co-therapy initially and then to drift away from the use of the co-therapy model. Whitaker's (1972) discussion of the latter paper describes the failure or unwillingness to push for intimacy between co-therapists. The honeymoon stage may last five minutes to five visits, but when conflict arises it is important to struggle with the issues and to use the experience to better the therapeutic work. If the conflict remains covert, therapy may become dysfunctional and that defect may be reflected in the therapy itself or in the anxiety and discomfort of the co-therapists.

Any marriage as such is a complex, high voltage relationship that stimulates each partner's growth. When it goes awry, it has components that are destructive and crippling to each partner. This also is true of the co-therapy situation where therapists may find their therapeutic potential augmented by some partners but limited by others. Co-therapy, like marriage, generates a constant tension between the conflicting need for a perfect, single-minded union on the one hand, and complete, autonomous individuality on the other. The synthesis of this thesis–antithesis stress is the heart of growth in a marriage and also in a co-therapy relationship. It is the pressure that pushes toward divorce and expands creativity. Co-therapy, like marriage, reminds each therapist that individuality, like we-ness, is an illusion. Some are gratified by the reminder, others confused. Some find it bothersome, others are enraged.

Teaming develops most naturally in the debriefing after the therapy hour. It is like the parents' conference after the kids are in bed. The therapists share responses about the family, and review the interview process. Debriefing is most important (1) with less experienced therapists, (2) with people who have not worked together very much, (3) when the family is in a crisis, and (4) if a lot of affect has been mobilized in one or both therapists and has not been discharged during the hour. Debriefing also is important when approaching termination. Both experienced and inexperienced therapists should debrief at these times. It is a way of consolidating the professional marriage so that the children can leave comfortably.

Therapists who are expert in working together require less post-flight debriefing and almost no plan for the next time. They complement each other by moving in and out reciprocally. Like well-married parents, they have a way of *living* together that needs fewer seminars. A concern about "what is she doing?" is replaced by "I do not feel that I have to come between her and the kids. I trust her judgment and I know that she loves the kids as much as I do."

In professional colleague settings where one works closely with a co-therapist in a stressful or intimate situation, the co-therapy relationship may, however, be a threat to the therapists' real-life intimates. It is best then to keep this process in the working world and not have the confusion of much social overlap. It is bad judgment to come home from work and tell one's spouse about those emotional orgasms of the clinic hours.

Divorce has many damaging residuals. Our experience in supervision shows the same result when a co-therapy team goes haywire. One failure can leave both therapists allergic to further work as a co-therapist team. In backlash one even may acquire co-therapists such as the drug salesman, the American Psychiatric Association, or worst of all, the culture.

Since the family transmits and programs its members to conform to the culture, psychotherapy is anticultural. The psychotherapist who uses the culture as co-therapist must be suspect. Like the military psychiatrist, his first responsibility is to the larger system. He never is able to bring his whole self into the therapy. The co-therapy team is a buffer between the therapist and the culture, as the family buffers between the individual and the culture.

2.1. The Stress of the I and We

A standard rule in co-therapy is the acceptance of the "We" function by each "I" in the co-therapy team, whether there are 2 or 20. When a co-therapist speaks, he or she speaks for the "We." Each co-therapist, however, must be stable in refusing to triangulate. He or she may express doubts, for example, "I see it another way" or "It didn't seem that way to me." The therapist must accept the fact that each therapist has a contact with the family that is unique to that person and not available for monitoring by the co-therapist. There is no right, there is no wrong.

"Opposites attract" goes the old marital saw. But opposites can have a hard time making it without some common bonding if the family background produces a disruption. When the co-therapists' philosophical differences are too wide or not counterbalanced by interpersonal respect or sense of humor, there may be trouble. Differences should make for excitement and growth if the bond between the therapists is a strong one.

Most of us are inclined to save all discussion of differences for behind the scenes. That is, at times, appropriate, but it is best to discuss almost everything with the family present. The kids need to know about divorce so that their fantasies do not get too far out of line with reality. Working with a partner is difficult and sometimes adds complications, but it is not as bad as trying to do family therapy alone.

Some therapists conduct heated disputes in the presence of patients. A fight, however, might be difficult for inexperienced therapists in front of their patients, especially when the therapists have not established some kind of "We" beforehand. Yet, it is always true that the spontaneous affect carries with it the very risk that make therapeutic growth possible.

3. Standard Problems of Co-therapy

3.1. Role Rigidity

At best, any role should be available to either co-therapist. Personality style, experience, and training background limit the extent to which this is possible. The usefulness of co-therapy breaks down when the role expectations are pre-set and fixed. For example, use of male/female teams may be the optimal co-therapy arrangement, and good for public relations, but a fixed arrangement of this sort cheats the male therapist out of the opportunity to develop his mothering capacity. The real pitfall is not with the initial reality of the roles, but with subsequent role fixation (male/female, student/teacher, parent–child, nurturer–administrator, nurse–doctor) and the extent to which the roles cannot be altered or even discussed. It is like the father who absolutely will not change diapers or the wife who will not wrestle on the floor with the kids. It imposes a reality orientation and cancels out the "as if" component of family living.

Case Examples. A social worker and a psychiatrist were seeing a family with a psychotic adolescent. The social worker had little previous experience with psychosis and was staying on the periphery, deferring to the psychiatrist. The treatment was not going well. One day just before the interview, the psychiatrist described his anxiety to the social worker. During the following hour, the social worker came off the bench and made some important interventions and the hour proceeded very well. During the debriefing just after the hour, the psychiatrist remarked on how well the hour had gone. "What brought you alive?" "When you told me you were scared before the hour, I saw that you really were. I never knew that you *really* needed me."

Two experienced family therapists had a clumsy first interview with a big family. Near the end of the interview Dr. M. noted that they had been getting in each other's way. "Can you think of some way that we can avoid doing that?" Dr. Z. said, "Sure, I assume that it is mainly a timing problem. We are like a tennis doubles team who occasionally hit one another's racket." Within a couple of sessions they were working together smoothly.

3.2. Problem of Therapist Splitting by a Powerful Family

This problem has three facets: (1) one of the therapists overidentifies with the family or a family member and gets locked in; (2) projective identification where the family projects upon the therapist, he or she then buys into it and becomes the projection; (3) one therapist gets locked out—a WASP in a black family.

1. The overidentified therapist gets locked in and gratified by the family warmth or admiration. The other therapist may then become withdrawn. If the co-therapists are not working with some awareness of this process or do not value the bond between themselves, the rejected co-therapist may feel useless and leave. Ideologic splits that exist between therapists may be wedged further by the family. Splits between disciplines, splits in experience level, in interpersonal style, or in political connections are all dangerous. Therapists who are tentative about work with family systems may misinterpret the patients attempt to split the team as an indication to begin individual psychotherapy. It is better to increase the size of the group at points like this. Adding new family members or a therapeutic consultant can clear the air.

> **Case Example.** A family therapist was seeing a very disturbed family with an adolescent daughter as scapegoat. The therapist felt protective of the girl and was frightened by her suicidal threats. During the course of therapy the parents backed out and the adolescent was being seen in individual therapy. The woman therapist was uneasy about her patient's power and invited a male therapist in as a consultant. The patient became angry with the intruder and demanded that he leave. The female therapist acceded to the adolescent's wishes. Therapy had failed but the interviews continued as before; there was no change. The outlook is grim when the family takes over treatment planning.

2. Projective identification is a powerful process affected by families although it happens in any group process. Often, the major task of the family therapist is to disrupt the system of projections in the family and then to work through the turmoil precipitated by disrupting their comfortable paranoia. In order to stay the same, the family seduces the therapist into the system. In serious work with families there is no way to remain completely free of projections and still be therapeutic. If there are no projections, can there be any therapy? The therapist, however, needs to be free to leave his role and at his own initiative. Parenthetically any training center knows that family role-plays are a way to discover how systems produce roles. It is remarkably simple to play the role of a schizophrenic, of the angry withholding mother, or of the detached, bellicose father to fill the family psychodrama. The problem of projective identification is more than symbolic when treating a family system. The therapist should be alert when he or she experiences extreme anxiety, is suspicious of his or her own motives, overresponsible, angry or indifferent toward the family, or when there is a relationship that he or she hides from colleagues.

> **Case Example.** Two psychiatrists, experienced in family work, treated a family with six children where one of the adolescent sons had an acute schizophrenic reaction. The pair guided the family through the first psychotic experience to a satisfactory resolution. During the son's hospitalization the family developed a phobia about hospitals. Eight months later the son became psychotic again. The co-therapy team agreed with the family's wish to treat him outside of the hospital with daily family interviews. After the first week of psychotherapy, one of the therapists went on vacation. After he left both of the parents turned the parenting over to the remaining therapist; the more maternal one. Mother went off looking for a job and giving piano lessons while father devoted all of his energy to a play he was directing in a community theater. The therapist replaced the mother in the family and he had the postpsychotic depression after the son returned to college.

The projective identification process becomes a *real-life* problem when a dynamically important family member is absent; if, for example, the divorced mother is seen with the kids and the therapist becomes the father. The co-therapist is very important at such a time in protecting and retrieving her colleague. The therapist's role is to relate to the family as a whole. If he accepts a role as family member he is not therapeutic—merely supportive—a poor substitute.

3. One therapist is locked out. This situtation is most likely to occur when there is a cultural or religious difference. The family may divide at some natural split, for example, the faculty guy is in, the resident is locked out. The most common situation is when one co-therapist joins late and the family has already attached to the primary therapist. The late arrival is a step parent with all those dynamics. This sometimes can be changed by acknowledging the fact of the split, by having the outside therapist meet alone with the family, or by the inside therapist being clear that the new co-therapist outranks the family.

Case Example. An 18-year-old young man was referred by his family doctor after the young man had taken an overdose of aspirin at home. The family therapist saw them alone in the first interview because it was an emergency and he could not get a co-therapist. At the second interview one of the senior residents came in as a co-therapist. The family was casual about the suicide attempt. At the end of the interview when a time was to be set for a third interview the family agreed on a time but it was one that the co-therapist was unable to make. The therapist said that he would change the time to meet the co-therapist's schedule. The family agreed but the father objected to the inconvenience, stating that Dr. B. was his doctor and he did not think that a "student" should come first. Now it happened that the senior resident had longish hair and also carried a tooled leather male purse. The next day the father called back and left a message saying that he was canceling the interview and that Dr. B. could spend as much time as he wanted to with his friend with the purse. Dr. B. wrote the father a letter acknowledging the cancellation and adding that the father only proved Dr. B.'s point. You can not trust patients, so we need to stay true to our co-therapists.

3.3. Complications from Therapists' Projections onto the Patient Family

These projections may come from the therapist's family, his or her past, and from his or her own slivers of pathology. Often, without a co-therapist present, he or she is unable to identify these projections. The co-therapist functions as an early warning system.

Case Example. The therapist had seen a new family three times and felt overpowered. He asked a colleague to join him as a co-therapist. Five minutes after that co-therapy interview began, he sensed his problem. The free association stunned him. "She looks like my mother, she looks like my mother, she looks like my mother," ran through his head.

3.4. Temptation to Plan the Treatment Process

At times, working with families stimulates disturbing approach–avoidance conflicts in a therapist that can be more tolerable when a co-therapist is involved (of course, the co-therapist may evoke another set of approach–avoidance pushes). One way to deal with a multilayered anxiety is to develop a preinterview game plan. Such a strategy can be disastrous when therapists feel bound to it and do not have access to their own spontaneity. The attempt to preplan the hour is also a symptom of change in initiative. The therapists have assumed the magic role rather than insisting that the patients push for their own changes. They have started to behave as though they were really the parents. Usually, any game plan is just irrelevant because the family has moved on from where the preceding hour ended.

Evidences of maturity in a co-therapy pair include their ability to live with and enjoy the partner's creativity even though they may not understand everything the partner does. One partner may have a metaphorical thread that does not include the other therapist or one therapist may do therapy with an individual or a family subgroup (playing with the kids) that does not include the co-therapist.

> **Case Example.** One of the authors worked with a co-therapist who had a joke with the patient couple in which mayonnaise and Miracle Whip became a metaphor for assertiveness. It came out of some spontaneous conversation while the author was playing with the children. The joke recurred throughout the therapy with the family; however, the author never did understand its meaning or origin, nor did he feel the need to understand.

3.5. Problem of Creativity versus Clinical Responsibility

This split often shows up in co-therapy teams where one is creative and the other careful and responsible. These roles are necessary but need to be exchangeable between the partners. When therapy becomes growthful, it is a turn-on for both patients and therapists. We spoke earlier of the tension between this element of therapy and the balance imposed by clinical responsibility. When the therapy is static and not like play, the process often does not go anywhere and, in fact, becomes a way to keep things the same. The process is like the marriage between the obsessive and the hysteric. In the effort to change the other partner, the whole project may fail.

A productive marriage gives the partners the opportunity for more creativity. When the marriage breaks down, caution increases along with self-doubt and brings a fear of adventure lest one spouse suffer criticism from the other and/or the kids. All of these possibilities are present in the co-therapy team.

In his *Primer of Family Therapy,* John Sonne (1973) describes the metaphorolytic capacity of dysfunctional families. This is the means by which a family removes the fun and poetry from life. It is an anesthesizing process that envelops and deadens therapists. It is more hopeless when therapists do it to each other.

3.6. Co-therapists May Not Parent Each Other

Co-therapists must be peers. This is one key to keeping the therapy marriage alive. It is best illustrated in a family with children. One parent interferes with the other's parenting to say, "You are not strict enough," or, "You are too harsh." When suspicion arises in one partner about the way the other handles the children he must ask, "Does she care?" If she does, then all her pathology is interpersonal sharing. Losing one's temper, crying, feeling depressed, sarcasm, and acting silly are all flashes of pathology in which the therapist is as naked as he or she is able to be. The payoff is growth for the therapist and for the patients and a glimpse around the professional facade of the therapist. The discovery of the therapist's crumbly clay feet breaks up the boundary between good and bad, adequate and inadequate, healthy and pathologic, and facilitates therapeutic growth. We think this is also true in the training situation where the rookie teams with a pro. The use of co-therapy is an invaluable way to learn, but problems can arise with treatment if the student–teacher vector is too prominent in either direction. Although all vectors of the relationship cannot be balanced, there must be reciprocity in some of their number in order for the team to work well.

Case Example. A psychiatrist, with five years of experience as a family therapist, teamed with a woman psychologist who had no family therapy experience and three adolescent children of her own. The treatment case involved a family with four children, three teenagers and a 7-year-old. The psychiatrist knew a lot about families but not much about adolescents; the psychologist knew very little about family therapy but a lot about adolescent children. They taught each other.

We like co-therapy because it gives us a way, as therapists, to get more for ourselves. We assume that patients benefit from our growth. There are time and money constraints in the use of two professional therapists that cannot be ignored. It would be ideal to be able to work with a co-therapist in every treatment case. Where it is not possible, however, it is important to have a general atmosphere of co-therapy among a working group that allows an easy sharing of one's experiences, successes, and failures. There are some situations in which co-therapy is indispensable unless the therapist has heroic or messianic aspirations. These include work with families where there is a very disturbed member (psychosis), a VIP, a psychosomatic problem, or where there have been multiple psychotherapy failures.

4. The Co-therapist as Consultant

Our second method of co-therapy is the use of a consultant. Psychotherapy tradition has sanctified the therapist–patient relationship. Possibly the roots of this ritual secrecy reach back to the confessional where the sinful words were spoken by the sinner to the priest and God.

The illusion of secret confidences can inhibit effective psychotherapy. Physicians make liberal use of consultants, but psychotherapists are cautious about, and may never even think of, using a consultant. We think of our consultation patterns as co-therapy variants. In medicine the consultant is brought in because of (a) his or her specialized knowledge and what it adds to the management of a given patient; (b) in order to provide a second look at a primary physician's diagnosis (to be sure he or she has not missed anything); and (c) when the physician has lost his or her "objectivity" about a patient. We use consultants in our work with families for similar reasons, but the order of importance is reversed.

A psychotherapist is more likely to lose his or her objectivity somewhere between the middle of the first interview and the end of the second. The objectivity is gone when he or she begins to care about the family and also to worry about what might happen to them. Not only does the therapist lose objectivity, he or she also loses ability to dissociate from the family and then to rejoin. The therapist is very much like the single parent who is locked in with the children and cannot escape because there is no adult subgroup to join.

Because of the mass of dynamics that contribute to a given family's functioning, we may become too focused in the initial interview. A consultant can expand our point of view, as in the case below.

Finally, a consultant can be used because of specialized knowledge. It is valuable to have a black therapist in when seeing a black family. When a Catholic family is seen we try to get a priest as a consultant. When the wife is a feminist it is helpful to have a feminist therapist, or if the family is divorced a divorced therapist can be of immeasurable help.

The consultant comes in and the primary therapist reports to him or her and asks for a consult. Then the consultant reviews the history with the family. We have been impressed by the dramatic change in perspective that it usually brings.

In an ideal group practice arrangement, one should have a consultant in for the second interview with every family. For example, Keith would do the initial interview with the family alone and then Whitaker would come in for the second interview and vice versa.

Here is an example of how the consultant process works and then remains a ghost co-therapist in the continuing therapy.

> **Case Example.** The Winkle family included father, mother, 12-year-old son, and a 14-year-old daughter. They came in because father feared his daughter was predelinquent. The initial history revealed a good number of psychodynamics within the family pattern: father's years in the Army, mother's liberation efforts in the past few years, and daughter's capacity to wedge the two parents so that mother and daughter were in collusion against father. A colleague was invited in for the second interview. The story of the first interview was reported to him and he reviewed the history. He discovered that mother had recurrent depressions associated with her menstrual periods and usually spent one day each month in bed. He discovered that father had been drinking heavily for the last four years since his stepmother died and his father started running around with several younger women. Many of the people in their small town were complaining to him about his father. The co-therapist discovered that the grandmothers on both sides had died early so that father and mother were orphans when they married. He further found that father and mother had a heated struggle over religious differences. Father was brought up a Catholic. Mother was indifferent to religion and refused to raise the children Catholic.
>
> As soon as the consultant had finished his half-hour history taking, he and the primary therapist talked in front of the family about the situation, the multiple factors involved in the setting, about father's concern that mother's move for independence would leave him with nobody to lean on (a sad prospect for a dependent man), about the cynicism of the son who was becoming isolated from the rest of the family, and how mother was very concerned about the son. The consultant recommended ongoing family therapy with the primary therapist and agreed to return if either the family or the therapist felt he was needed. He estimated that the family therapy would be fairly brief, probably 15 to 20 interviews, and that the therapist would later be available for a brief recapitulation if that seemed needed.

In our usual pattern, co-therapy is thought of as the process of two therapists functioning symbolically as parents for the family. This does not demand that the two be present at every interview. The primary therapist (mother) is usually there full time. The consultant (stepfather) can come for only the first or second interview, then be on call by the therapist or at the request of the family. The consultant, like the father, functions with a unique capacity and freedom. He or she is not so deeply responsive, therefore can be more insightful. The anesthesia (security) for his or her confrontation or invasion of the family has been established by the primary therapist. The therapist also may invade, attack, support, or be creatively useful to the primary therapist within the interview setting. His or her administrative suggestions also can be very valuable. He or she may sense that the family is ready to end, that it is time to get the grandparents in, or that they seem to be making no progress and should give up and consider the therapeutic effort a failure.

The consultant also may be used later if there is an impasse. The process is similar to that described in the example of the Winkle family although the history review may have more to do with the therapy experience. At this point a component of the impasse is related to the therapist joining the family and participating in the obstruction of therapy. For example, the family may be worried about the possibility of father's death, but they are impassed around their fear of death. The therapist may become inhibited by this fear. The use of the consultant to the extended therapy may be fairly dramatic as is evidenced by the following case example which is also an action metaphor. A metaphor usually is thought of as a bit of poetic imagery. An action metaphor involves the whole person. Its impact is psychosomatic; it is not just an intellectual experience.

Case Example. Paula and Winthrop initiated therapy eight months after their baby was born. Both were brilliant, articulate professors in the Humanities. The baby had melted down their intellectualized living patterns and disrupted many of their early-marriage covert contracts. Their interpersonal manner had all the intimacy of William Buckley interviewing Dick Cavett. The interviews were witty and bright but sounded like lunch table conversation among literary critics. It was intimidating to the therapist and he was too shy to bring in a co-therapist lest he expose his insecurity and feelings of intellectual inadequacy.

The therapy went surprisingly well for five interviews, then bogged down. The therapist presumed that it was because he had fallen in love with this trio. Without warning he brought in a woman colleague as a consultant. The couple said nothing about her but seemed shocked. The consultant described what she saw in the family, which did not add significantly to the therapist's point of view. However, he noted as the interview was ending that he felt more lively and creative with them then he had during the course of treatment. At that point they decided to change the consultation into co-therapy.

The therapist's first notice that the control dynamics in the therapy had been disrupted was when Winthrop called in mid-week to check on the time of the next interview. Throughout the course of therapy their association had been casual and he had used the first name of the therapist. In this phone call he called him "Doctor." The next indication that the therapy temperature had been turned up came when Paula arrived first at the next interview. She tapped at the door as she entered saying, "friend and foe." When Winthrop arrived they said how angry they were about the co-therapist. It had been an intrusion on the therapeutic incest. Paula said that she had cried for three days following the consultation interview. Winthrop was angry and crisp and thought that the therapy should end. The consultant agreed with ending, putting it this way: The therapist and Winthrop are competing to be the wife's therapist and the therapist thought he would give up because Winthrop was able to see her for extended periods every day and the therapist could see her only for one hour a week.

Next, the consultant in an aside told the therapist a joke about a schizophrenic who wanted to learn how to have intercourse. Telling the joke consolidated the therapy team and set up the generation gap. The joke came off-the-wall and had implications for the couple and the therapist (which the therapist did not realize until two weeks later).

The therapist felt both anxious and excited during the interview. On the one hand it felt as if his move to introduce the co-therapist had been a double cross, but at the same time it shattered the symbiotic set and opened up all sorts of dynamics and fantasies. The presence of the co-therapist disrupted the couple's intellectual style. They were both smarter than the therapist and the therapist was easily intimidated by that intelligence to the point that it blocked his personhood.

This consultation provided a high intensity experiential metaphor that transcended their pseudogrown-up intellectualizing. Before starting therapy the couple's symbiosis had been heated up by the arrival of the baby. The success of the initial therapy lay in the fact that they had brought the therapist in to stabilize it. When the consultant came in she broke the symbiotic structure and the couple dropped into a primary-process basement of hunger, loneliness, deeper love, confusion, sadism, and anger. The impact was like a lightning bolt. It was dazzling and not entirely conscious.

5. The Professional Cuddle Group

This group of therapists meets regularly two hours each week to share experiences, ideas, talk over cases, and expand the conceptual component of their work. The group occasionally provides a kind of marital therapy for one team of co-therapists. One way to initiate a cuddle group is to have each member describe his or her own family tree by drawing a genogram on the blackboard and telling about the experiences of their family of origin; who the characters are and what life was like through the generations. We find this process helps to develop a cohesive group of colleagues and provides a way to start working as co-therapists by this profound way of knowing one another.

We have used the group in many ways. Sometimes we bring a family in for a single-interview consultation. On several occasions we have seen a family over an extended period of time. Therapy was done by the whole group and it was a rich experience. There have been times when a crisis with a family in therapy has tempted the therapist not to attend the group. We encourage them instead to bring the desperate situation into our group.

The cuddle group helps to maintain the therapeutic adequacy of its members. Even when they are good at what they do, therapists often are instinctive outsiders. The danger of being without a professional group is that we come to rely too heavily on patients for maintaining our self-esteem or we turn to real-life intimates and those relationships falter.

6. The Advantages of Co-therapy for Patients

Very little is said about the advantages of co-therapy for the patients. The consultant's presence does allow the family to be critical of either co-therapist without the danger of massive counterattack or loss of the therapist's love. The second therapist also provides extra support and protection. Although they sense the power of the twosome and that power may be frightening, it is reassuring. The family is less panicky about deteriorating into chaos when it has this twosome. Their breadth and flexibility serve as a subculture. The family or the couple usually try to split the therapeutic team into a "goody" and a "baddy" in much the same way children try to split their parents. Discovering the security that the therapists have with each other gives the family the freedom to belong to this suprafamily. Seeing that the two therapists are more crucial to each other than are the patients leaves the family free to end therapy when it is ready. They feel no need to pay back the emotional debt to the team as the team is secure.

The presence of the consultant as a ghost in the interviews makes it possible for the therapist never to be cornered in terms of administrative decisions since he or she always can say, "I need to talk to my consultant about it." The family members also are free to express their negative feelings during therapy because they can ask for the consultant. They thereby can express feelings they are not comfortable with in the dependent set of the usual therapeutic interview. The therapist also may say, "I'd rather talk to my consultant about that. We will arrive at a decision and I'll talk to you about that the next time and then if need be we can get him in for subsequent interviews." Finally, once one has dared to let someone else into his or her ongoing interviews, it becomes easier and easier to use a consultant for specific purposes. When in doubt, frightened, or one-down in the therapy situation, the consultant is available for a rescue operation, for reinforcement, or simply for an overview.

7. Conclusion

Co-therapy can take many forms, each of which are valuable to us in our work with families. Some factors are basic to making co-therapy work. First, the partners need to have an interest in co-therapy and recognize it not simply as a stop-gap but as a specialized technique in the art of psychotherapy. Second is the realization that the significant other is our colleague not the patient. Co-therapy keeps us from getting isolated and it makes our work as psychotherapists constantly exciting.

For some professionals co-therapy is not useful and may be viewed as ridiculous or an unnecessary complication. This may be true when family therapy is primarily a technique-oriented, problem-solving process. However, as the therapist becomes deeply involved with the family's living on a symbolic level and engages in an ever unique voyage with each family where his or her own growth is also an issue, co-therapy may become critical. A therapist's own growth is seen to be at issue when he or she finds him or herself asking, "What am I getting out of this?"

Behind those two parents—we mean therapists—is a mysterious third entity. It's called "they." Who is "they"? Nobody really knows, but whenever the chips are down one therapist or the other, or both, become victims to "they." No family who enters family therapy should be without a "they." The "they" consolidates the family into a "We" who usually succeed in proving the old cliché, "People know more than anybody."

8. References

Goolishan, H., Sheeley, M., & Pulliam, G. Developmental phases of cotherapy relationships and their effect on family systems. *Psychiatric Spectator*, 1975, *10* 4.

Rice, D. G., Fey, W., & Kepecs, J. Therapist experience and style as factors in co-therapy. *Family Process*, 1972, *11* 1–12.

Sonne, J. *A primer for family therapists*, Morristown, N.J.: The Thursday Press, 1973.

Whitaker, C. A longitudinal view of therapy styles where N = 1. *Family Process*, 1972, *11* 13–15.

Whitaker, C., & Warkentin, J. The involvement of the professional therapist. In A. Burton (Ed.), *Case studies in counseling and psychotherapy*, Prentice-Hall, 1959.

III

Special Problems and Issues

17

Therapy with Minority Families

JO-ANN M. RIVERA AND JANDYRA VELAZQUEZ

Clinicians increasingly are convinced of the central contribution of healthy, well integrated families to the life and identity of society and its members. A family is not merely a collection of people or aggregate of individual psyches occupying a particular physical and temporal space. Nor is it just a social group characterized by a common residence, economic cooperation, and reproduction. A family is a natural social system with a structure, development, and function that builds into a vast network of interpersonal relationships. It involves conscious and unconscious processes that provide its members with an identity and a historical continuity. Family systems provide the primary environment for growth, development of identity, and sense of belonging in the world. All its members, including adults, move in an evolutionary process, which challenges each member to new and different developmental tasks and roles. Family norms function to bind this unit in a common culture and boundary.

> Values provide the definitions of time dimension, contain concepts concerning the responsibility and worth of individual members of the family, point to certain commonly held life goals, impose a framework within which the pursuit of—and risks connected with—pleasure impulses take place, and involve a system of sanction. (Parad & Kaplan, 1966, p. 58)

Family boundaries must be managed so that within each group there is a sense of "I-ness" and "We-ness," promoting an individual and family integrity. The family boundary also must be semipermeable so that there is a balancing of the family system with the outside—community, society, world. Several levels of values influence the family structure, including individual values, family values, and societal values. The family unit holds certain values as a result of its cultural identification, its history, and the meshing of the individual values of its members. Society provides the extrafamilial environment and

JO-ANN M. RIVERA • Family Studies Section, Albert Einstein College of Medicine, Bronx Psychiatric Center, Bronx, New York 10461. **JANDYRA VELAZQUEZ** • Child, Adolescent, and Family Services. Fordham Tremont Community Mental Health Center, Bronx, New York 10457.

reference group for what the family ought to do and how it should behave. The family's positive identification as a functional unit is influenced by societal values and society's evaluation of the family as a growth-supporting unit.

The family must maintain enough flexibility in its boundaries to allow for a feedback exchange between itself and the larger societal system. Such an interlocking, interdependent, complementary relationship is necessary for the evolution and complex developmental progress of the individuals, the family's organization, and the societal system.

> The nature of ecology is such that the larger societal entity does much to shape the societal units within it. A group that reflects its values will find that the encompassing society complements and supports, in most spheres and levels, the formal and informal social organization the group requires for its development. (Aponte, 1976, p. 434)

The environment can be a support and a catalyst to family growth by providing nourishment to family esteem, normative affirmation, and social binding relationships through shared norms and values. If there is an overlap between the family's and society's expectations, role behaviors, meanings, values, and collective goals, the family's and its individual members' identity will be more unified. The disruption, loss, and/or absence of membership in support networks, which accompanies an inconsonant environment, presents the familial group with vulnerability in effective functioning (Caplan, 1974; Cassal, 1973).

We learn from the literature on migration that the orientation dissonance resulting from the mismatch between family and the environmental values triggers family ''disorganization'' and/or multiple symptoms that affect the family and its members for several generations. *Disorganized* is the label given in the literature for the process that the family goes through to achieve assimilation. We feel, however, that readers take it to have a negative connotation, that is, chaos, and therefore, take it to mean pathology. Instead, it needs to be viewed as a sociological process that is normal and congruent to assimilation. Minority families have been described as disorganized, impoverished, and chaotic groups, rather than seen as families in reorganization to a new environment and/or adaptation to loss of support.

For the conflict resolution of assimilation to take place, the family needs to reorganize around a new environment by compromising the family's identity. The degree of resolution of the dissonance depends on the degree of receptivity in the new environment to the different group, the degree of role discontinuities, the amount of pressure to cut off the old values and ways, and the space (economic, psychological, etc.) provided to become an integrative member of the new society. Even under the best circumstances, the migration process and the following process of dissonance ''disorganizes'' families.

In addition, the new environment can inhibit the family's capacity to function optimally and affect the process of reorganization through tribalism and scapegoating. These societal negative value judgments and prejudices are organized around and attached to perceived differences among the groups: color, ethnic origin, religion, and/or socioeconomic status. Symbolic meanings are attached to these differences which are subjectively experienced as danger. The person and/or group showing the difference is felt to be the invasive stranger(s) who threatens the security of others and brings conflict to a dynamic equilibrium.

What we are speaking of is a concatenation of events in which two groups, representing perceived manifest value differences, participate in a process of scapegoating that takes place at all levels of psychological experience—society, family, and individual. We are talking of a process that is real, abundant, intense, and far-reaching in its affects on society, the families, and the individuals. These attitudes and dislikes are irrational in that they are fixed, automatized, generalized, have cut off the corrective influences of the existing reality, and in fact alter the reality to make it consonant with this attitude (Ackerman, 1966). It is a process by which the group feels powerless and is placed in the throes of social disorder. It is this process that is at the *heart* of the minority experience.

In this chapter, the word *minority* is being utilized to mean those social groups who hold marginal social position due to membership in an assigned low-status subgroup (racial, ethnic, and/or socioeconomic) which often is seen at variance with societal expectations and values. Those members of the societal environment who are relegated to low status are at risk to social isolation, social marginality, and status inconsistency which will affect the adaptability, resources, and coping mechanisms available in the inter- and intrafamilial spheres. These families experience a disruption or arrest in the organizational cycle, disruption of family integration, and a reduction or loss of family integrity. It affects the family role relations within and between the family and its context. For the minority family, it becomes more difficult to assimilate, since they are relegated to the space of low status, placing and maintaining them on the periphery of societal boundaries. As such, the family's integrity is continuously pitted against the societal value system.

Culture and ethnicity play an important role in the formation of self-concept, development of family identity, and the development of a historical continuity (an experience of family immortality). American society emphasizes a melting pot philosophy and deemphasizes variations in norms and values from the dominant culture. The family's history and existential meaning becomes insignificant. Those groups in society that are manifestly most different from the dominant norms are given negative attributes. As will be seen in an example later, Hispanics hold values that are at variance with the Western value system, are viewed negatively by the dominant society, and are relegated to minority status in American society.

In the minority family, there is a drama of loyalty conflicts that impinges and influences the developing identity, self-esteem, and competence of the family and its members. The family must choose (consciously or unconsciously) which mores and norms of the majority society it will incorporate into its identity and functions. This clash of norms and values becomes maximized in minority families in that they have become ghettoized by choice or force and, therefore, places them in isolation and, in essence, powerless.

The process of conflict resolution and the means of coping within the matrix of changing patterns of interaction are central to family dynamics and health. Families have at their disposal various means by which to cope with conflict. They can re-people the group by eliminating a member or adding a new one. They can change the configuration of family role relationships through rigidification of boundaries and risk retardation of growth; through fluidification of roles, but internal identification and efficiency is reduced; through maintenance of the role and reduction of the intensity of the felt conflict (this device only temporarily brings equilibrium); through changing roles appropriate to family's and individual's development; and through a shift in alignments and splits within the group.

The minority family is vulnerable to replicating the process of tribalism within its family boundaries by developing splits that represent the family's identity, goals, and values and the competing dominant society's value representations. The emergence of such behaviors brings the extrafamilial system's prejudicial scapegoating[1] into the family system boundaries. The family reorganizes into alignments and splits around the scapegoating of a family member as a means to neutralize the perceived danger. For the minority family, the danger is the fear of discontinuity of family functioning and boundaries through society's assault on its prestige and values. What becomes manifestly evident is the split of the family group into competing emotional alliances.

1. Hispanics

The United States is populated by a large and rapidly growing Hispanic minority population. In 1978, the Hispanic population was 12,046,000, with a growth of 32.8% since 1970 (Fitzpatrick & Gurak, 1979). The Hispanic total does not include the population of Puerto Rico, which is estimated as 3.4 million, nor the undocumented or illegal Hispanic immigrants who have entered and live in the United States. Should large-scale migration continue, however, the Hispanic population will surpass the Black population as the United States's largest minority group. Internationally, this suggests that the United States will be the fourth largest Spanish-speaking nation in the world (Mexico, Spain, and Columbia being first, second, and third).

Hispanic is not a nationality but rather an adjective utilized to describe groups of different nationalities with commonalities in language, religion, history, and a Spanish cultural heritage. Although they share these characteristics, including a common identity as a minority, they are by no means one people. By their origins, folkways, local environments, distances (social and geographic), and points of geographic concentration in the world they also are different.

Economic and political conditions in the Hispanics' home countries and the hope of better lives have been the overwhelming factors that have motivated their migration to the United States. Hispanic migrants present a great range of color and, like Blacks, their presence is marked by discrimination. Such discrimination is further exacerbated by the Hispanic's tie to a native language and to an extended family system characteristic of rural, preindustrialized countries which sets him or her apart from Americans and the Western culture. Although Blacks and Hispanics *represent numerically no minority,* and America presents an open door, melting-pot ideology, they are still identified as minority by the nature of their differences in socioeconomic status, cultural values, and most significantly racial characteristics.

The Hispanic culture places much emphasis on the person (*personalismo*) (Fitzpatrick, 1976; Gillin, 1960; Padilla, 1958; Wells, 1969). Hispanics live in a world of intimate relationships. There is the belief in the value and singularity of every individual. This form of individualism focuses on the inner importance and uniqueness of each person. A person is measured by those qualities and behaviors that make him or her good and respected. Every person, no matter his or her position in life, should be respected. In a culture where one died in the social class in which one was born, self-worth could not be measured by one's competence in achieving status and/or material worth. If you do not respect a person you are violating his or her dignity.

[1]Prejudicial scapegoating is a mechanism introduced by N. Ackerman (1966) as a coping mechanism to internal changing interaction. In this chapter we are expanding the concept of prejudical scapegoating to include the process as a mirroring of the prejudices of an even larger group than the family, society.

A "vertical man" is one who has shame, honesty, humility, and dignity. Individuals must accept God's will stoically by resignation to their destiny. To complain about what has been dealt to you in life is degrading and unworthy of respect. To have shame is to be humble and of moral conviction. These are Christian virtues and they must be respected (Lauria, 1964).

Personalismo also is expressed in the resistance to form groups or to submit their individuality to an organization. Person-to-person relationships as well as a network of intimate personal relationships are supportive. Formalized systems are not seen as readily supportive, but as impersonal and mechanical in their forms of communications. In addition, Hispanics are most responsive to manifestations of personal respect and to styles of leadership that bring out the person rather than the platform or program.

The rules of respect are complex and very much reflected in the language. For example, a Hispanic child is expected to listen to his elders even if it is an older sibling with a minimal difference in age. It also is disrespectful to have direct eye contact with strangers, elders, and persons of authority (all adults are figures of authority). This behavior is expected especially of women and children.

Related to the aspect of personalismo is humanism. Man is also valued if he can combine impulses with the intellect. Due to the validation of respect and dignity, Hispanics avoid direct confrontation and respect repression of hostility. The best way to solve a dispute is to do it in good terms so that no one's feelings are hurt. Submissiveness, deference to others, and passivity are encouraged as the ultimate in civilized behavior, as opposed to the American value on aggressiveness.

Supporting the cultural values of personalismo is the role of *padrino* and the system of *compadrazgo* (co-parenthood). Usually the padrino (godparent) is a person in a higher position of the social structure who has a personal relationship to the person and can provide advocacy and support. The compadrazgo institution is a system of companion parent with the natural parents. They constitute a network of ritual kinship, as serious and important as that of the natural kinship, that provides economic assistance, emotional support, and personal education (Mintz & Wolf, 1950). These are special relationships which are influential and particularly powerful during periods of crisis.

Also associated with personalismo is *machismo,* literally maleness. It is a style of personal daring by which one faces challenge, danger, and threat with calm and self-possession. It is associated with sexual prowess, influence, and power over women, reflected in a vigorous romanticism and jealousy. It includes the belief that man is superior to woman. It also is seen as man's ability to protect his family and function as the "man" of the house. Machismo may be seen as the Puerto Rican's cultural expression of male chauvinism with a stronger emphasis on male virility (Mizio, 1974).

This perception of the world as consisting primarily of a network of personal relationships, whether among family members or friends, tends to take precedence over efficiency and the so-called good government of mainland Americans. As suggested by Zwerling, Alvarez, Batson, Carr, Parks, Peck, Shervington, and Tyler (1976), the social drama gets played out differently.

> Mainland Americans tend to subordinate the personal relationships to the demands of efficiency; eyes are on the efficient method or the democratic process to get the job done; the human coefficient is taken into account to make sure that efficiency is properly served. The Puerto Rican tends to subordinate the efficient method of the democratic process to the network of personal relationships. The American sees an efficient world in which you try to be considerate of the persons involved; the Puerto Rican sees a world of persons in which you try to be efficient. (p. 217)

The Hispanic places such a high value on individualism that he or she is motivated to safeguard the inner integrity of the individual against group pressure. Hispanics are fatalistic about their destiny. This quality leads to the acceptance of many events as inevitable and also softens the sense of personal guilt for failure. The popular song "Que sera, sera" ("What will be, will be") is a simple expression of this acceptance of fate as well as the expression "Si Dios quiere" ("If God wills it").

Because a person's life is subject to fate, luck plays an important role in the events that are to lead him or her to fulfillment of his or her destiny. Individuals may not be able to achieve their life goals if bad luck plagues them. The attitude is that while a person may try very hard to get ahead and be proper and good, he or she may be trapped by destiny or by bad luck. Illness, poor economic conditions, serious misbehavior of the children, and getting into trouble are due to causes beyond one's control, particularly when one knows he or she has been good. In the face of such events, a person may have to reach for supernatural explanations.

A person also must try to protect him or herself from the evil power of others and do something to change his or her fate and control the immediate solution. There are various rituals and charms, herbal water, appealing to saints and the Virgin Mary, and prayers used to cope and solve problems. Religion and ideas about the supernatural are not circumscribed within the boundaries of any particular church. They transgress into a variety of ideologies, which are not conflicting but coexist under the premise that all religions are good, important in training children, and for the purpose of understanding the nature of forces that are beyond control of the individual man (Padilla, 1958).

Hispanics emphasize the spiritual values of life, making their fundamental concerns not with this world but satisfaction of spiritual goals. Being is more important than doing or having. One has a sense of spirit and soul and they are much more important than the body and are intimately related to the person's value. The Hispanic's goal is to live in harmony with nature. To reach such harmony, the Hispanic expresses the willingness to sacrifice material satisfactions. In contrast, America's goals are to master the world rather than seeking the values of the spirit. America's emphasis is on domination, technological programming, and mastery of the physical universe.

2. The Family

Personalism is rooted in the family. The family has an essential role in the institutional character of Hispanic society. It is the family where primary relationships are formed. The family, therefore, is seen as an extension of the self and primary to all other activities and social action. Family unity is strong and family concepts extend far beyond the immediate union of father, mother, and child(ren). The family offers support, control, and protection. The family's welfare, unity, and honor are valued highly. There is a deep sense of commitment, obligation, and responsibility. The family is where there are strong emotional ties. As such, separations among Hispanics are cause for extreme grief. Mourning takes place within the family, within the person's community. Not only does one wear black, but one also must observe various prohibitions to social activity.

Traditionally, the Hispanic family structure has been an extended system where kinship ties are not only by blood and marriage but also include various ritualistic non-blood relatives (*compadrazgo, hijo de crianza, padrinos*). The extended family as described in the literature has alternated between that of a family with many relatives living together in one household and that of a nuclear family living alone but in a large kinship network. The Rogler and Hollingshead study (1975) described how the Puerto Rican family, for example, enmeshes its members in a system of help-giving exchanges crisscrossing blood and affinal relationships and geographic boundaries (i.e., from New York to Puerto Rico). In those countries, such as Cuba and Puerto Rico, where there is a large middle class and/or where migration has been high, there is a tendency for the structure to shift from an extended system to the more traditional American nuclear family. When families migrate to the United States, this shift becomes more pronounced, due in part to separations from relatives in their homelands but also to the different values and ways of life that lead to the isolation of nuclear families from others. Nuclear families take the same form as is presently seen in the United States. Besides, the mother/father/child(ren), one also finds in Hispanic nuclear families other compositions: (1) father/ mother/ child(ren)/ child(ren) of the spouse's other union, and (2) single-parent families, especially headed by females.

Consensual unions are quite common in several Hispanic groups, for example, Dominicans, although the trend is shifting toward legalized relationships. These relationships are bound by the same code of values as legalized unions and are not usually seen as improper. Children born of such unions carry their father's name. Another accepted practice is the transfer of children from one nuclear family to another within the extended system in times of crisis or identified need.

Another pattern of household organization and living is the joint families (*familia unida*). This household composition differs from the nuclear family in that there are two nuclear families under a single authority, who share living together on a common budget under the same roof as a single family unit. Usually it is three generations under the direction and authority of a grandparent. The married children and grandchildren are subordinate to the grandparent. In their ways of living, joint families promote the ideals of family unity. Family sentiment and obligations are encouraged to such an extent that an individual always can believe and feel that he or she can rely to the fullest on his or her own family. The joint family is a structure that expresses many of the ideal values of the Hispanic extended family. However, it is also a structure that leaves its members particularly open to the diverse conflicts that may exist in the context of the American culture. For those who live in such a unit, the conflicts of young with the old, of the American-born individual with Hispanic-oriented parents and of authority versus the various roles of subordination may be exacerbated (Padilla, 1958).

For migrant Hispanics, the pattern of close interpersonal relations and the recognition of obligations toward kin, although usually weakened by residence in the United States, operate to a great deal as special bonds that strengthen both relations with family in America and in their home country. This is particularly evident in Puerto Ricans, where transportation from the United States to Puerto Rico and back is facile. In contrast, among adults who have grown up in the United States, emphasis is on the nuclear family as an independent unit. Vivian Garrison's research (1972) in the South Bronx demonstrated that only 20% of the Puerto Rican households contained extended families. However, it also was found that 61% of these households interacted in an extended kinship network. In a later study, Vivian Garrison (1978) reports three-fourths (79%) lived either in an extended family household or had kin living in the immediate vicinity. It is apparent that, even with migration, it was uncommon for Puerto Rican women to be separated from all of their own kin.

Regardless of the composition of the household, social class, and levels of education, the Hispanic family traditionally has a patriarchal ideology with belief in male superiority and dominance (Mussen & Maldonado-Beytagh, 1969; Steward, 1966; Wolf, 1952). In reality, families are matrifocal. Father is manifestly the head of the household and in his absence his wife substitutes for him. Wife and children are expected to obey and respect his decisions. Informally, mother is holding the real power in the family. The marital subsystem is segregated and independent where each of the partners lead relatively independent lives in separate and distinct activities with different sets of people. The Hispanic wife counts on her own kin for basic support functions. Her husband provides advice, guidance, and approval as authority of the family. The Hispanic family expects a lineal hierarchical arrangement in locus of power, authority, and control.

The family plays a fundamental role in the governance of its members. There are mutually adjusted expectations, duties, and obligations to be performed by various members. These expected role functions are dominated by a double and complementary system of values that are gender confined—virginity and machismo. In virginity, not only is pureness implied but it also stresses ignorance in relation to sex. It structurally places woman in a restricted familial environment since her parents, siblings, and relatives are expected to secure her maximal pureness before marriage. Man, however, must assert his sexual prowess before and after marriage. The lives of parents are oriented toward their children: "*Lo mas que se quiere en este mundo, son los hijos*" ("What is loved most in this world, are children"). A good father expresses his love for his children by his control over their conduct and by presenting them with an example of a good person. The mother is the primary transmitter and reinforcer of these family values. This emphasis on the family as the center of the adult's obligations is cultivated from early childhood. The basic ideals of behavior to be imparted to a child by his family are respect, obedience, control of feelings of aggression, and fulfillment of duty appropriate to sex and age. Machismo and virginity are further reinforced in the differential training and evaluation of children. Since the good woman is expected to possess different qualities from the good man, these differences are stressed in every part of a child's life and are consistent with the double moral standard of the Latino value system. The end product of a boy should be a man of character, who is educated, likes to work hard, is responsible toward his parents in their old age, a good parent to his own children, respectful and respected, courageous but not troublesome, and a macho. Boys are accorded higher status and the relationship between mother and son, in particular, is very strong.

A girl is to grow into a modest and virtuous woman. She is to acquire an education in case it is necessary to work. She is to be able to care for her home and children. She is to be quiet, obedient, and faithful to her husband and help her parents in their old age. In contrast to the masculine role as associated with aggression, women are not to be aggressive by any means. Women use gossip as an indirect way to express aggression, with the content of the stories reflecting victimization of women and hostility toward men. It needs to be noted that although men are given less social strictures in expressing aggression, Hispanics value and reinforce inhibition of aggression in all members through providing social recognition for those who resolve a potentially hostile situation without aggression. Interdependency of parents and adult offspring are expected and normative in this culture group, generationally reinforcing a kinship system (Wolf, 1952).

There are pertinent clinical implications for the therapist who fails to maintain a level of cultural awareness. There is, for example, a very contrasting cultural process among Anglo-Saxons and Hispanics in reference to achieving individual autonomy. In the Anglo-Saxon culture, independence is defined as occurring and culminating in a psychological and physical moving away from the nuclear family. It usually is expected that young adults will leave home. In this modern nuclear family, there is a value placed on self-expression. The adolescent generally begins to utilize the extrafamilial environment, especially peers, to assist in the development of self-identity and independence. During this developmental period in the life of the adolescent and his or her family, the family has a secondary position of authority. Among Latins, in general, one never abdicates membership from one's family of origin. In the Hispanic family, there are authoritarian controls that modify autonomy, decrease self-expression, and reinforce interdependence. Within this framework, opportunities for individual expression and autonomy are reduced. The Hispanic adolescent is provided with a sense of belonging but any direction toward individual choices is viewed as disloyalty to the family.

Most mental health practitioners view independence in a manner consistent with the Western process of autonomy. Successful treatment often has been correlated with the independence of an individual and his family of procreation from his family of origin (Leichter & Mitchell, 1967). Such a conceptual difference in the expectations and the pathways toward autonomy presents both diagnostic and treatment considerations in the engagement of the Hispanic family and in identification of treatment goals. The application of white American norms of independence and self-sufficiency as developmental standards leads to a clash of value system between the therapist and the Hispanic family. The case[2] of Mrs. Rosario illustrates this point.

> Mrs. Rosario had lost her mother and contact with her father at a young age. In her young adult years she had moved to New York City with her two daughters. In New York, she married and had a boy and girl from this union. After a stormy relationship, Mr. Rosario left with their son. Soon thereafter, Mrs. Rosario's second daughter was referred for treatment for her acting out in school and cutting classes. In the interview, Mrs. Rosario attributed the daughter's problems to her, Mrs. Rosario, lacking family support and being without her family. She said, "I understand the children not wanting to do their best because they don't have a family to praise them and teach them the proper way to grow into an adult." Mrs. Rosario also expressed desires to die because she was a failure as a mother.
>
> The clinician prescribed antidepressants and recommended that she enter individual therapy because of loss of self-esteem. He communicated to her that cutting classes or acting out at school were very common among adolescents and it was adolescents' way of growing up. Mrs. Rosario thanked the clinician, took her drugs, but did not take the medication or return.
>
> The clinician had recommended individual treatment, coming from the position that the adolescent's behavior was a way of expressing autonomy. However, to Mrs. Rosario, respect for authority, repression of aggression, and continued dependence on the family as the primary authority are the more acceptable behavior. To Mrs. Rosario, her daughter's disrespectful behavior and her waning control were of the most concern. At a later date, when Mrs. Rosario was seen by another unit, she was engaged in treatment by working with her definition of the problem and her source of motivation. Family therapy is a modality that fits very well with Latin values. Mrs. Rosario and her daughters were seen by a family therapist who supported and encouraged the mother to

[2]In all case examples, identifying data have been altered to provide confidentiality to all parties.

> find her family members. The therapist joined the family in a co-parental role (similar to a compadrazgo), supporting the mother in her parental skills. When Mrs. Rosario found her father, he joined the meetings so that the therapist could assist in establishing him in the family. Once her daughter's "disrespectful" behaviors were curbed, Mrs. Rosario requested individual therapy sessions where she discussed her inadequate feelings in reference to parenting and the loss of her husband.

Another transcultural dilemma facing clinicians is the traditional psychotherapy model that describes motivation, self-will, and the ability to control one's behavior as prerequisite to behavior change in therapy. Latins believe in faith and outside sources as the cause of dysfunctional behavior. Thus, added to a cultural value system of interdependency on others, is the conflict of internal versus external dichotomy in the explanatory model of health/illness and treatment expectations.

> Mrs. Aponte is a 36-year-old woman, married, with three adolescent children. She sought treatment because of feelings of despair. She had strong feelings that something awful would happen. to her that day. She has had anxiety attacks since her husband's successful career terminated. Since then, she has attended the Catholic church daily, asking for forgiveness and help from God so her burden would be released.
>
> Mrs. Aponte describes her life as a series of fated misfortunes. She was very sure that her parents did not like her and singled her out as the parents' bad luck in their marital relationship. Whenever she questioned her parents about their treatment of her, they would tell her she was different from her sisters. She was told she was stubborn (*rebelde*) and brought bad luck (*mala suerte*). As her parents, they needed to prepare her future. She left home as a young adult and married a man who did not get the approval of her parents. They began their married life struggling. However, Mr. Aponte soon became a very successful businessman and the envy of her family. Three years later the husband's brother and business partner died. Her husband became severely depressed and abandoned the family. This necessitated Mrs. Aponte changing her life style drastically. She experienced the change in her life from husband to no husband, from house in suburb to small apartment in ghetto, from self-sufficiency to public assistance, as her fault. "Good things don't last."
>
> Several years later, Mr. and Mrs. Aponte reconciled. However, she is continuously afraid of being abandoned again. These fears are expressed in anxiety attacks, which on one occasion resulted in hospitalization, a diagnosis of depression, and medication. Notwithstanding, Mrs. Aponte has never taken any of the medication because all man-made substances are contrary to her philosophy of life: "Man cannot change one's destiny."
>
> Mrs. Aponte was referred for outpatient treatment. The therapist requested the family's participation in the assessment phase. Treatment was conducted with the marital couple. The husband agreed with the wife that they both had bad misfortunes of life and that the only good thing that has happened to them is their children. The therapist and Mr. and Mrs. Aponte agreed to the children not attending the family sessions. The therapist reinforced the locus of problem as within the marital subsystem. It was important for the therapist not to challenge their world view but to utilize Mr. and Mrs. Aponte's philosophy of life to facilitate trust and begin the process of bridging their philosophy of life to the view that one can negotiate differences in the intra- and extrafamilial environment.

For many minorities, the process of migration to the United States has meant not only the need to assimilate to a new environment, but also has carried with it the process of oppression. Rayna Rapp (1978, p. 294) has pointed out that the very ideology of family that has been important to the oppressed has been utilized to blame them for their own condition. The extended network has been historically used as a supportive and viable agent in the process of assimilation, providing the minority family with a range of unavailable societal resources and supports. The minority has used their families as a way to patch up tenuous relations to survival by extending their networks and highlighting their boundaries vis-à-vis dominant societal institutions.

In adapting to a new and nonreceptive environment, intra- and extrafamilial dissonance usually is expressed through heightened conflict in the marital/parental subsystem or between generations. These value conflicts surface as the length of time lived in the United States increases and the more discrepant are the values between the family and environment. In addition, situations of scapegoating and psychological processes related to minority status begin to increase symptoms of social and familial stress. In order to evaluate the adaptational capacity for any family, one must consider the family structure, cultural values, and social context in which they live.

3. Clinical Implications

Family system psychotherapy is geared to look at specific issues from the point of view of how these issues affect the relationships. In this sense, system therapy can be perceived by the therapist and conveyed to the client as an intervention to relieve or reduce the tensions and symptoms that bring the family to treatment. Family system shows results, especially in symptom relief. It encourages the therapist to "teach" the client the changes that are needed and how they are achieved. In this way, the dynamics of change remain in the family rather than in the therapist's office. This allows the family to invest the time needed for change by doing the therapeutic work outside the therapist's office and using the therapist's "couch" when time and money are available.

For the clinician, it gives him or her an approach that is cross-sectional and longitudinal. It allows for the examination of the family in relation to its interaction with other systems. As such, it provides the therapist with a view of the collective interacting forces that impinge on and influence the family boundary management. Viewing the family as an open system, which through its interaction with supraordinate systems can develop or stymie the family growth, it moves the therapist away from the polarities of normal versus abnormal or healthy versus pathogenic.

Family system thinking views psychotherapy as a social experience: the therapist is an active member of the therapeutic system. When the therapeutic system is viewed this way, the issue of value conflicts and value growth becomes a critical interaction in the assessment, engagement, and treatment of minority families. This is not a question of the therapist imposing or converting the family members to the therapist's value system. All therapists, however, have an operational definition of health and illness that derives not only from their professional training but from their participation in society. A clinician's value system reflects an orientation and judgments from within his or her family, culture, Western society, and professional affiliations. It becomes important for clinicians in their work with minority families to develop a sensitive level of awareness to differing value systems within cultures so that the meaning of human differences and corresponding clash of values is faced.

Minority families continuously are struggling to define and protect their boundaries while concomitantly increasing their resources for survival. It is important for the therapist with the family to make clear boundaries around each of the treatment subsystems and the treatment itself. Contrary to the occidental middle-class (professional) value system which places an emphasis on individual's self-determination to seek increases in scientific knowledge, in introspection, and in wisdom through assistance from extrafamilial systems, minorities utilize natural support systems as problem-solving institutions. Help from white, middle-class traditional institutions is mistrusted since they are seen as members of an oppressive society and often are experienced as incongruent to a minority's life experiences and belief systems. Many minority families bring to treatment a sense of resignation and fatalism in the face of poverty and sense of powerlessness (which is often seen clinically as compliance or hostility) to affect any change in their life condition. For the Hispanic and other minorities it is necessary to add to this a cultural value orientation of fatalism and supernatural causation as an integral part of the explanatory model of mental and emotional illness.

Regardless of the therapist's orientation, the theoretical frame of reference will need to change in order to bring this context into the treatment. The life experiences, cultural beliefs, and attitudes of the family must be nonjudgmentally explored and taken into account in the assessment, diagnosis, and treatment plan. There needs to be a fit between the family and the therapist as to the understanding and management of the symptoms, rather than the therapist viewing their attitudes toward illness and treatment as hopeless superstition and scientific unsophistication. Role expectations of both the recipient and provider of treatment have to be explored and clarified so that clinical issues of resistance, compliance, dependency, and duality responses to authority are dealt with in the contract phase. Historically, the minority's experience with authority is in the context of oppression, tribalism, and colonialism. For the minority family, the therapist and therapy become representations of society's authority, the family's sense of powerlessness, and conflict of values, beliefs, and behavioral norms.

There is an attitude issue from therapists that exacerbates the hostility symptom when therapists come from a preconcept of anger as a dysfunction in the family. The therapist thereby re-creates society's prejudices and stereotypes and places him or herself in the position of the receptor of all hostile feelings and responses. The ability of the therapist to deal directly with anger and hostility is particularly important in working with minority families whose hostility is tapped easily and at times generalized. They often anticipate therapy to be like other institutions: oppressive. If the therapist has difficulties in the recognition and expression of his or her own anger and prejudices and has the need for being a parent-like figure, he or she will recapitulate the perceived controlling environment of society. It is critical that, with the therapist's consent, the minority family expresses the hostility. For the therapist, it is of particular importance that he or she be cognizant of his or her feelings and values.

> For example, Mrs. Roberts came for a family evaluation session with her teenage daughter and small son. She seemed very angry and spoke loud. Every time the family therapist would ask a question, Mrs. Roberts would misunderstand or imply that it was done in an offensive manner. The therapist asked her to try to listen better and allow the children to answer their own questions. The mother commenced to speak in a more hostile tone of voice: "You're a jolly, witty lady, with a family picture showing that you have a man and kids. What do you know about pain? What do you know about living in the projects or dying to have the comfort of a man who wants to stay with you and give you a family?"

The therapist dealt with the confrontation by allowing Mrs. Roberts to focus on her feelings of being prejudged and categorized as an inadequate single parent by other institutions. The therapist depathologized the anger by giving recognition to the mother's struggle and the necessity to protect the family's identity against societal negative perceptions. Thereby, the therapist also gave license to the expression of anger and directed the treatment toward increasing mother's executive functioning.

Minority families carry with them hostility as a symptom of powerlessness. Powerlessness in that they are viewed by society and messaged that they are ineffective members; powerless in that they are not integrated members of the environment; and powerless to change that perception because in order to be able to do that they need to be integral members of society. In order to survive, many minority families move their individuals to a compromise solution resulting in an intellectualization of a sense of self, which in turn negates the identity conflict but moves them to a position that appears more integrative and allows for boundary cohesion. In essence, it shifts the identity conflict to the next generation but does not resolve the emotional issue of loyalty. Such a resolution is perceived by the minority subculture as a "selling out." Thus, for the minority individual and his or her family the drama of loyalty conflicts remains, but this time it is in isolation from the subgroup of origin.

The social organization and boundary management of the minority family is particularly vulnerable to weakening as a lack of environmental support and powerlessness associated with minority status. The minority family attempts to protect successfully its integrity and maintain its functioning by utilizing its internal resources, but at the expense of further isolation from societal structures and exhaustion of its members and its capacities for growth. Eventually, what clinically occurs is the burdening of an individual or a subsystem with less and less availability to meet the natural changing aspects of the family life within the new environment.

Families may engage their children as catalytic agents between societal systems and the family to negotiate the conflicting value operations. The children then will be permitted to accept the societal norms while at the same time encouraged to keep the traditional ones. In essence, the family replicates in reverse the double bind presented by society. The parental subsystem experiences a loss of structure in which the traditional line and function of authority was supported. It places the parental role in an adolescent position with the majority societal standard as the ultimate form of authority. For the family the child is ascribed the role of negotiating the external and by default the internal system. For example, among Hispanic families it is common to see children serve as translators and be kept from school to take the family to various social institutions (welfare, court, doctors, etc.). The family comes to depend on this individual for its own functioning with the extrafamilial environment. This role as mediator for the family is dysfunctional if the parental subsystem has abdicated its authority, thereby placing the child in the role of the executive power in the family. This role becomes burdensome for the individual and eventually places him or her in the role of scapegoat in the family. He or she gets to be viewed as the representative of the dominant value system and a traitor to the traditional values and, *ipso facto*, family. This alignment of family roles is contrary to the hierarchical structure of all families, regardless of culture and socioeconomic group.

The Gonzalez family brings this clinically to light.

> The identified patient, Juan, was referred for individual psychotherapy for antisocial behavior, which had brought him to the attention of various judicial authorities. During the evaluation phase, the family provided the following information: Mr. and Mrs. Gonzalez came from Cuba 25 years ago. The children, George (24) and Maritsa (22), and identified patient, Juan (19), were born in the United States. However, in the

first individual psychotherapy session, Juan said he was Portuguese. The two oldest children are married and live with Mr. and Mrs. Gonzalez and Juan in a two-family house, in a *familia unida* constellation.

The family unified around the perception that Juan was the problem. His antisocial behavior was seen as the major point of dissension in the family. During one of the meetings, the structural family issues surfaced, highlighting the primary dynamic in Juan's outcast role. Maritsa, quite angrily, said that "Juan says my parents are not his parents. My parents have worked very hard for all of us. This is how he repays them. I am sick and tired of him embarassing us. If he doesn't want to be a part of this family, then let it be so." Through historical and family roles exploration, it became apparent that Juan shares very little ethnic identity with his family of origin. The other siblings have negotiated successfully their independence and self-identity by maintaining a close allegiance to their parents' cultural roots. Difficulties between Juan and parents have relegated Maritsa and George into the position of surrogate parents to control Juan's unacceptable behaviors.

In this case, the therapist needed to utilize his position inside the family boundary to help modify this interactional process while continuing to move the family toward new information and resources. The therapist needed to use himself as a vehicle for providing new data—Juan as different from other family members in his identificatory allegiance—and at the same time support those members who were frightened by this change. The goal was to help each family member gain greater social competence and mastery which might result in alteration of family structure and increased flexibility. In particular, the therapist provided support to the parental subsystem to find new ways of providing executive power—moving Maritsa and George out of the failing disciplinary role and Mr. and Mrs. Gonzalez to negotiate Juan's participation in the family.

Another structural form in which an individual in the family becomes the linkage between the family and society is in the burdening of the family executive power so that distribution of power and effectiveness is only in this family member.

The pertinent history of the Jones family begins in the South with the death of Betty's grandmother. The oldest daughter, Millie, makes a deathbed promise to look after the family and at all cost to keep them together. When Betty's parents move to New York, they are quickly incorporated into the matriarchal community established by Millie. The promise continued to be a powerful covenant in this family's organization around major life events and crises when Betty decompensated and required treatment.

At this time, the clinical staff participated with Betty in viewing Millie as a culprit in Betty's illness. The treatment plan was geared toward eventual separation of Betty from her aunt by preparing her for an adult residence. Notwithstanding, years later, we were to see that this assessment of the system's dynamics and conflict forces was an underestimation of the various roles family members had viš-a-vis Millie. In the past three years, since last contact, Betty had been in and out of the hospital several times. Outside the hospital, she remained involved with an extensive family network. Mrs. Jones as the primary caretaker, maintained contact with the clinic, managed the household and financial affairs, and served as the stable and functioning center of Betty's and all other family members' lives. The family has had a myriad of social and economic problems that have increased in the past 10 years. More and more the family boundary had become insulated from the outside world. For herself, Mrs. Jones joined a new religious affiliation (Jehovah's Witness). Mrs. Jones came to the North in the hopes of bettering the lives of the various family members, but in reality things became worse. Mrs. Jones felt she had been alone in her struggle all along and that even those agencies, welfare and mental health, that have been involved in "helping" actually have added to the burden.

One is struck at first by the rigidity of the roles and family structure over many years. There is one central strong woman with numerous dependent individuals. Family members repeatedly seem ready to break apart but the elastic band of their dependency on Mrs. Jones is secure. The positive aspect of the structure is that the strength of the central figure has held a number of disorganized and problem-ridden units together for many years. Mrs. Millie Jones was providing the only life-supporting linkage to the extrafamilial environment. It was apparent that Mrs. Jones had been strained and burdened, so that the matriarchal structure had begun to falter.

Given Mrs. Jones's mistrust of social agencies, the therapists proceeded to work at forming a therapeutic alliance with her and engaging her in family treatment as a family individual needing new resources and relief from her matriarchal role. Her involvement with the Jehovah's Witnesses as a network providing her with support and self-esteem was reinforced. Given Mrs. Jones's central position in the family system, any shift in her role was expected to result in profound repercussions for all family members. Therefore, family meetings also focused on helping the others, especially Betty, to become part of other networks which would allow for a fixed independent distance for each one, as well as replace Mrs. Jones's role for them. This necessitated the therapists taking on roles of coordination and liaison to facilitate availability and support of these new resources.

In both these cases, the role of the therapists was to bring to the family greater control and synchrony within its boundaries and with the extrafamilial environment. As such, the family reinstitutes efficient utilization of power and of roles within its system, facilitating an image of self-worth. As an entry issue, it became important for the therapists to depathologize the symptom picture and to have an attitude that brought the family to a new experience—therapy supports the growth of families in its relationship to a difficult environment. As such the assessment process also involved a mapping of the relationship and interface of the family to the community and society as a whole. The families' coping mechanisms were not labeled as pathological or dysfunctional but viewed as the natural resources that are available to minorities and their families.

Arthur Brown (1980) has suggested another coping mechanism by which minorities deal with conflict of low status and attempt to protect self and family's identity boundaries. In order for a minority to achieve competency while at the same time maintaining dual membership, the individual needs to develop duality. *Duality* is a trait that grows out of the necessity of Blacks to maintain a double or twofold pattern of functioning in a culture that puts restraints on an individual's effort to assimilate and become a full-fledged equal member of a culture that makes demands on him or her and gives double messages regarding expectations and participation. Duality, to become a functional characteristic, has to be a spontaneous response. For example, a doorman who makes enough salary to qualify as middle class was required to act dumb, be called "boy," and tolerate being treated as lower class. In the Black community, however, he is respected.

The concept of duality has been discussed in reference to the Black minority groups. It is, however, a process of adaptation and assimilation that can be applicable to other minority groups. In this process, the minority person can be a member of the environment and maintain a balance between society's ambivalent messages and his or her sense of self. This brings the individual and the family into a dance in which the individual, family, community, and society orchestrate a functional complementary interaction.

These are issues to consider and explore when making an assessment of minority family functioning. Duality and contradictions can appear rampant in families who feel it is necessary to sustain in therapy the idea of assimilation. However, they also can mask the problem issues in the family. Duality appears as a reactive response although it sometimes is a sophisticated conscious manipulation and at other times a dysfunction and defense. These characteristics can be more readily confused in traditional individual therapy and direct toward a diagnosis of a psychosis since they may suggest a thought disorder, grandiosity, or even paranoia. In the case of dysfunctional defenses, duality and contradictions are issues that must be worked through before the problem issues can be dealt with. Once duality and contradictions are put in perspective they can be dropped and a differentiated self can emerge.

4. Summary

In family practice, it is important to take a system's perspective in order to understand the individual in the family and to understand the family in the context of the environment. Systems approach and network intervention are much more congruent with the experiences of minority families. These approaches bring to the therapist field how each of the subsystems interconnect and influence each other. For minority families, who are in the throes of oppression and low status, a systems perspective helps the therapist view the development and selection of coping patterns as an interaction between internal and external forces in the definition of family boundary. It permits the practitioner to deal with minority responses and family structure as different rather than as pathological. These are responses and a structure that attempt to make available more and stable resources for growth, but which also bring to their family functioning an issue of loyalty conflicts, duality, and tenuous management of boundaries. Understanding cultural differences, roles, value systems, history, and the context in which the "disorganized" behavior takes place very often can change the therapist's perception of the minority family. The therapist must not bring the life of oppression into the process of treatment, but the oppressive life experiences of the minority family must become an integral part of the treatment content in order to facilitate individual and family mastery.

5. References

Ackerman, N. *Treating the troubled family*. New York: Basic Books, 1966.

Aponte, H. Underorganization in the poor family. In P. J. Guerin (Ed.), *Family therapy theory and practice*. New York: Gardner Press, 1976.

Billingsley, A. & Giovannosi, J. M. *Children of the Storm*. New York: Harcourt Brace Jovanovich, 1972.

Billingsley, A. *Black families in white America*. London: Prentice-Hall International, 1968.

Brown, A. *Duality: The need to consider this characteristic when treating black families*. Center for Family Learning Conference, New York, March 22, 1980.

Bureau of Census, U.S. Department of Commerce. *The social and economic status of the black population in the U.S.A. A historical view 1970–1978*. Current Population Reports, Special Studies, No. 80.

Caplan, G. *Support systems and community mental health*. New York: Behavioral Publications, 1974.

Cassel, J. The relation of the urban environment to mental health: Implications for prevention. *Mount Sinai Journal of Medicine*, 1973, *40*, 539–550.

Fitzpatrick, J., & Gurak, D. *Hispanic inter-marriage in New York City: 1975*. Hispanic Research Center, New York, Monograph 2, 1979.

Fitzpatrick, J. The Puerto Rican family. In C. H. Mindel & R. W. Habenstein (Eds.), *Ethnic families in America*. New York: Elsevier, 1976.

Fitzpatrick, J. *Puerto Rican Americans: The meaning of migration to the mainland*. Englewood Cliffs, N.J.: Prentice-Hall, 1971.

Garrison, V. *Social networks, social change and mental health among migrants in a New York City slum.* Unpublished doctoral dissertation, Columbia University, 1972.

Garrison, V. Support systems of schizophrenic and non-schizophrenic Puerto Rican migrant women. *Schizophrenia Bulletin,* 1978, *4*(4), 561–596.

Gillin, J. Some signposts for policy. In R. N. Adams (Ed.), *Social change in Latin America today.* New York: Vintage, 1960.

Hill, R. B. *The strengths of black families.* New York: National Urban League, 1972.

Hill, R. B. *The illusion of black progress.* New York: National Urban League, 1978.

Lauria, A. "Respeto, Relajo," and interpersonal relations in Puerto Rico. *Anthropological Quarterly,* 1964, *37*(2), 53–67.

Leichter, H., & Mitchell, W. *Kinship and casework.* New York: Russell Sage Foundation, 1967.

Mindel, H., & Habenstein, R. W. *Ethnic families in America: Patterns and variations.* New York: Elsevier, 1976.

Mintz, S., & Wolf, E. An Analysis of ritual co-parenthood (compradrazgo). *Southwest Journal of Anthropology,* 1950, *6,* 341–368.

Mizio, E. Impact of external systems on the Puerto Rican family. *Social Casework,* February 1974, pp. 76–83.

Mussen, P., & Maldonado-Beytagh, L. A. Industrialization, childbearing practices and children's personality. *Journal of Genetic Psychology,* 1969, *115,* 195–216.

Padilla, E. *Up from Puerto Rico.* New York: Columbia University Press, 1958.

Parad, H., & Kaplan, G. A Framework for studying families in crisis. In H. Parad (Ed.), *Crisis intervention: Selected readings.* New York: Family Service Association of America, 1966.

Rapp, R. Family and class in contemporary America: Notes toward an understanding of ideology. *Science and Society,* 1978, *42*(3), 278–300.

Rogler, L., & Hollingshead, A. *Trapped: Families and schizophrenia.* New York: Wiley, 1975.

Steward, J. *The people of Puerto Rico.* Urbana: University of Illinois Press, 1966.

Wells, H. *The modernization of Puerto Rico.* Cambridge: Harvard University Press, 1969.

Wolf, K. L. Growing up and its price in three Puerto Rican subcultures. *Psychiatry,* 1952, *15,* 401–433.

Zwerling, I., Alvarez, R., Batson, R., Carr, A., Parks, P., Peck, H., Shervington, W., & Tyler, F. *Racism, elitism, professionalism.* New York: Jason Aronson, 1976.

18

Special Treatment Problems with the One-Parent Family

HARL H. YOUNG AND BONNIE M. RUTH

In America in the early 1970s, one out of every six children lived in a one-parent family (Bronfenbrenner, 1976). The divorce rate continues to spiral, with many urban center officials estimating that as many as one out of two marriages fail. With the coming of the women's movement, more and more women are choosing to have children outside of marriage. Men more frequently are seeking child custody. Women are entering the work force in greater numbers. There seems little question that the one-parent family is increasing at a sizable and accelerating rate. Death, more or less permanent separation, lengthy temporary work assignments in foreign countries, and parental abandonment are additional contributing reasons for greater numbers of one-parent families.

Clinicians who specialize in family treatment report that a significant proportion of their case loads are devoted to the one-parent family. Mental health center staff have been especially concerned about the burgeoning number of requests for services by these families in this era of economic constraints and unpredictability. Kalter (1977) studied the composition of the case load of a public outpatient clinic and determined that approximately one-third of the clients who were children came from "broken homes," one parent families in this case.

Curiously, the special problems and appropriate treatment strategies for this clinical population have been seriously neglected. Our rather comprehensive review of the literature yielded less than 50 titles referring specifically to the one-parent or single-parent family. This phenomenon has been referred to earlier by Brooks (1980). Major family theorists are surprisingly silent on these issues.

HARL H. YOUNG • School of Professional Psychology, University of Denver, Denver, Colorado 80208. BONNIE M. RUTH • Bonnie Ruth and Associates, Ltd., Lakewood Medical Center, Lakewood, Colorado 80215. (At the time this chapter was written Bonnie M. Ruth was affiliated with Rocky Mountain Rehabilitation Consultants, Denver, Colorado.)

The recently published, frequently cited *Handbook of Family Therapy* (Gurman & Kniskern, 1981) does not contain a special section on this area, and indeed does not have a listing for one or single-parent families in the index.[1] Most textbooks on psychotherapy make scant mention of the subject. Remarkably, only recently has there been a sudden increase in the literature (e.g., Visher & Visher, 1979; Katz, 1981) regarding step-families and their special difficulties.

Purposes of this brief chapter are to (a) focus attention on this neglected area, (b) begin the process of winnowing and narrowing of the unique and special difficulties of the one-parent family and the unusual challenges they pose for the clinician, (c) set forth some preliminary treatment considerations, and (d) make a plea for systematic research in this area.

1. Varieties of One-Parent Families

We have seen how one-parent families can be brought about by many different chains of events. The term is applied very broadly. It is used equally to refer to families that got that way by chance, by choice, and through no fault of their own. Moreover, families that begin with two parents and lose one along the way are commonly lumped with those that have always had just one parent. No differentiation is made whether a partner[2] is lost by choice or involuntarily. The literature contains no typology in widespread use. Researchers must be very cautious in generalizing from one group to another.

One schema is proposed by Billingsley and Giovannoni (1971). They suggest that four variables are critical: sex of parent remaining with the family, reason for only one partner (death, separation, divorce, never married), permanent or temporary absence, total or partial absence. Since research almost never has been carried out involving such specified subgroups, it is obvious that we must await further study before we may draw solid conclusions.

We strongly believe that families where there is only one parent, there never have been two parents, and there is no expectation of a second parent materializing are quite different compared with a similar family having a lost or absent parent. Children in the former families have not had to cope with the loss and/or change of the latter. Evidence, however, is meager one way or the other, and expert opinion differs (see, for example, Cline, 1977; Corkill, 1977; Rexford, 1976; Weiss, 1979). The Cline study set out to examine Minuchin's (1974) concept of enmeshment–disengagement. The results indicated that the one-parent families formed a different structure than comparable two-parent families (see Glasser & Navarre, 1965).

Because of our cultural traditions, it is tempting to think of two parents who are married and have children as having attained the most desirable state and a one-parent family as suffering a deficit, which may or may not be the case. Studies are urgently needed describing clinicians' observations and treatment outcomes with "one-parent-by-choice" clients. Special strengths of one-parent families should be identified and used as positive goals for newly single parents. These may include positive effects on children of a happier, more independent female role model.

[1]We have chosen the term *one-parent family* over single-parent family because of the confounding of number with marital status.

[2]The word *partner* is used in this chapter instead of spouse because of the increasingly common practice of couples living together.

Of course, the one-parent family that can be described as experiencing a deficit is the most common by far that clinicians see and about which most is known. In this chapter we will focus on the "deficit" family, but caution the reader against generalizing to other subgroups.

A particularly difficult subgroup with which to work is the one-parent, never married, not-by-choice group. These are typically very homely women (or handicapped, disfigured, or mentally retarded) who have illegitimate children repeatedly without being able to find someone to marry them. Families and friends often make referrals or bring these families directly to you for help.

The family psychotherapist soon learns that some familiar concepts in family theory do apply to the one-parent family. Ideas such as family homeostasis (Jackson, 1968), schism and skew (Lidz, 1968), rubber fence (Wynne, Ryckoff, Day, & Kirsch, 1958), and double bind (Bateson, Jackson, Haley, & Weakland, 1956) illustrate phenomena common to one-parent and traditional families alike. What is not clear is whether specific interventions arising from these conceptions can be reasonably expected to produce the same results when used in a different manner with a different group than one upon which they were originally derived. Henceforth, contemporary theorists should make a special effort to discuss the implications of their concepts and strategies for the one-parent family.

Having made the foregoing points, we may proceed to discuss what is unique or particularly characteristic of the one-parent family. Since the literature is virtually silent on these matters, we intend to be as practical and concrete as possible in order to be of maximum benefit to clinicians. We are aware that we are covering familiar territory for more sophisticated readers.

2. Special Problems of the One-Parent Family from a Deficit Model Viewpoint

The most readily apparent and the most complained about feature of the parent with a lost or absent partner is the stress overload due to the assumption of responsibilities of the absent partner. The departure of one's partner often occurs abruptly and with little notice for the assumption of massive new duties and activities. Activities may be unfamiliar; one must learn or relearn such exasperating matters as how to iron a shirt, providing instructions to workmen and repairmen, resetting a circuit breaker, what temperature to bake a casserole, or balancing a bank account. More seriously, newly single mothers often face a real and frightening poverty. Specters of dead-end employment or children poorly clothed or housed may loom large. Obviously, one person cannot adequately carry out the responsibilities formerly shared by two and the resulting frustration leads to feelings of being overwhelmed, anger at the injustice of being placed in such a position, and the like. Necessarily, compromises are made in investing one's time and energy. Priorities must be reconsidered and one's usual efficiency declines. Previously latent personal psychopathological tendencies may surface. Friends and relatives may be called upon, appropriately and inappropriately, to assume part of the load.

Even if a separation, divorce, or death was a bitter or angry occasion, after a period of time there often is a period of mourning, of regret, and of self-recrimination. There are fantasies of what might have been and anger over the loss. Thus, the clinician may see alternating depression and anger, which may or may not be displaced onto the child or other loved ones.

A particularly troublesome situation is one in which the remaining parent exploits the children in the service of his or her personal needs—for example, the mother who overly relies on the oldest daughter to take of the house and supervise the children, or who overly relies on the oldest son for her emotional support and male companionship needs: the so-called parental child and the parent-child marriage, respectively (see for example, Minuchin, 1974). In extreme form, parental exploitation can lead to profound neglect or child abuse in its many other forms, especially physical and verbal assault. In many states, therapists have specific legal obligations to report abuse in any form. It may be that the therapist should consider referral if he or she is unfamiliar with this familial syndrome. The number of treating agencies and other resources in this area are growing rapidly.

Almost inevitably, children find the absent parent situation a difficult one with which to cope. The circumstances are conducive to much dysfunctional communication. A child finds many opportunities for playing the parents against each other if the absent partner is accessible. If not, the youngster easily can fabricate a picture of the absent parent based on his or her needs of the moment. Moreover, the child distorts memories about and messages from the absent parent in the service of his or her immediate interactions with the present parent.

These communication difficulties are compounded by tendencies of both child and parent alternately to blame themselves and each other for the departure of the absent parent. Resulting guilt in each must be dealt with in some manner. If there are several children, the permutations of accusation and blame become staggering. Several older children who "gang up" on the remaining parent can be very intimidating.

Because the present parent often has been seriously hurt in many ways by the absent partner, it may be easy to disparage him or her. Sometimes sweeping generalizations are expressed about the inevitable failure of intimate relationships; "men are no good," "women are only out to get everything they can," "marriage is a terrible thing," and so forth. Such statements can be taken seriously by children and may complicate ongoing relationships with the absent parent and other adults. Moreover, if the present parent intends to enter another intimate relationship soon, then life can be made much more difficult for the incoming partner.

Some people find it surprising to learn that moving to a one-parent family status after a committed relationship involves a drastic change of identities, literally how one looks at and presents oneself. In addition, the requirements may seem ludicrous or paradoxical, for example, the woman who is a mother yet who is sexually available, or the career woman who is also a homemaker, or the man who is a corporate vice-president who cooks every night. This in itself may be perplexing.

Clinicians long have held the opinion that a youngster may "act out" the unacceptable impulses of his or her parents (see, for example, Satir, 1964). A corollary view is that the particular form of acting out behavior has symbolic meaning in relation to the nature of the conflicts between parent and child, or more likely the conflicts over which the parents may be struggling. Research data validating these hypotheses are nonexistent, but every experienced clinician has observed such processes.

One might think this process would be simplified in the case of the one-parent family because of the absence of one party. Such is not the case. Fantasy becomes distorted in the presence of ambiguity and the absence of opportunities to check out reality regarding the absent parent. Thus this process, already little understood, becomes more clouded. However, a reasonable hypothesis might be as follows: Given instigating circumstances, a youngster will act out the unacceptable impulses of either parent, depending on the length of the one-parent family's existence and which parent he or she may be angry at at the moment. If the history of the family is relatively short, it is more likely to be the absent parental impulses. If not, the behavior is more likely to involve more current issues between parent and young person, but is still expressed in unacceptable forms. A final wrinkle that makes this complex picture even more perplexing is the potential for the remaining parent to act out the unacceptable impulses of his or her own parents and thus continue his or her own adolescent rebellion.

The characteristics of the troubled one-parent family and some hypotheses concerning their development are presented above in terms typical of the clinical literature. Nowadays, more often than not, family oriented clinicians have moved toward conceptualizing the family in terms of systems theory (Von Bertalanffy, 1968; Miller, 1965; Steinglass, 1978). The same is true for those specializing in working with one-parent families. One observes a mother or father and one or more children engaged in constantly recycling struggles that none of them want but somehow cannot abandon. In addition, the struggles seem to be associated with some gratification for each and are reciprocally supportive of each other's destructive behavior. Some theorists have referred to this as "interlocking pathologies" (Ackerman, 1956). However framed in our thinking, there can be little doubt that the cyclic, reciprocally supporting, destructive patterns are readily recognizable and that traditional individual psychotherapy is likely to be superficially palliative since it addresses only one segment of the interactional pattern. A systems view seems considerably more fruitful.

3. Practical Treatment Issues

Practical and procedural problems with one-parent families can be especially trying, particularly if the family has only recently suffered the loss of an absent parent. Most often this is, of course, the father and most often also, the breadwinner. In this case, the mother may have a host of problems financially, as observed earlier. Health insurance may be expiring soon. Income may be diminishing markedly. Arrangements regarding housekeepers and baby-sitters may be a priority. All such issues contribute to the stress overload mentioned before. Among these issues is, of course, the question of who will pay you.

Very frequently, the present partner will make a bid for individual therapy initially, sometimes for him or herself or sometimes for a child or children, or both. In the absence of definitive knowledge about indications and contraindications, the best advice is as follows: If you recognize the cyclic pattern referred to earlier, then it is preferable to recommend family therapy. If the problem centers around internal individual conflict or is traceable to external factors (poor school conditions, or unsavory companions, for example), then individual treatment may be more appropriate. If the family members seem to be reasonably well adjusted and are responding primarily to the additional stress, then perhaps some supportive sessions both conjointly and individually may be in order to get them past a difficult time for all.

The required identity changes for the partner alone in the newly created one-parent family plus the markedly increased stress levels have significant implications for subsequent behavior. Finding a job or a new job or retraining for a better job or going back to school may be necessary. A switch from husband–breadwinner to single man–student or from wife–homemaker to single woman–apprentice can be uncommonly threatening and stressful. Competition for companionship and sexual partners can be very intense and the alternatives, such as withdrawal and aloneness or overinvestment in children, are not usually as gratifying or as wholesome. Such stressful events and behaviors often lead to such symptoms as mood swings, sleep disorders, extreme appetite variations, anxiety symptoms, and less predictable behavior generally. All of these may be reflected in erratic attendance, missed appointments, and a spotty payment record.

In trying to cope with the above pressures, the alone partner is caught in another difficult dilemma: how to balance (and do justice to) his or her needs versus those of the children. Some people try to be Superman or Superwoman and thus vow to do it all, but most of us have to make some very difficult choices. One easily can be too selfish or too martyrish. Outside guidance often is valuable to provide a moderating influence.

One of the problems most frequently encountered by the therapist specializing in one-parent families is the attempt by the parent in the group, wittingly or not, to engage you in fulfilling some of the functions of the absent partner. Some of this "pull" is of course natural to the circumstances, such as the provision of emotional support. However, expectations or maneuvers to pull for personal affection, doing favors, helping find a job, having lunch together, writing a letter of reference, running an errand, and the like may be questionable. Less subtle are those who make direct requests for seeing all the children in individual therapy, testifying in court in their behalf, providing explanations to employers for undue absences, and special financial considerations. The therapist must be aware that no matter what you do, you will be fulfilling some of these needs, and that may be appropriate. There may even be growth-promoting opportunities to reflect the impact a client may have on you. A therapist should, however, be wary because these gambits may involve diversionary tactics to keep attention away from problematic relationships in the family, or a bid (perhaps unwittingly) for you to replace the absent member of the dysfunctional family. A therapist often can feel "tugs" to join the characteristic, non-productive, cyclic style of functioning of a family in pain or seeking help.

4. Treatment Recommendations

The following are general strategies often applicable to the typical recently developed one-parent family seeking services. As we have seen, there are many sybtypes of one-parent families and these rough guidelines may have very limited scope and application.

An additional cautionary note: Most family therapists stress the necessity of maintaining an active, in-control, assertive, yet collaborative posture for family work. Those persons moving to family work from individual therapy most often have trouble adapting to this style. Traditionally, the individual therapist is quite passive (some would say "laid back" these days). This posture immediately leads to difficulties with families because of the therapist's vulnerability to being drawn into the family system and becoming a part of their characteristic style or being seen as withdrawn and uninvolved.

We have learned from our work with clients in crisis (Lindemann, 1944) that those who have suffered severe losses, perhaps abrupt and traumatic, appear stunned and lethargic, sometimes for a matter of days or weeks. Such persons may require gentle but firm direction in the conduct of their everyday affairs until recovery. For those who recently have lost an intimate partner, the situation is not greatly different. Empathic understanding and providing an opportunity for the person to express feelings and emotions about the traumatic events are especially important. But direct advice and firm direction may be equally so. In families where the absent partner departed long ago, presenting difficulties often are: conflicted relationships within the family, a member has encountered problems with an outside agency or peer group, or a youngster is having trouble relating to a parent's new romantic interest.

While the therapist is helping the person or family through the immediate crisis, it is important to put together a new support network or refurbish the old one as soon as possible. Consider calling on relatives and friends initially, but if necessary ask neighbors, clergy, fellow workers, teachers, and anyone who knows the family members well. Collaboration with the client on making full use of community resources can enhance progress and rapidity of movement in family treatment. Resources for specialized treatment (e.g., a child abuse or speech therapy clinic), Alcoholics Anonymous, plus the many other kinds of self-help groups, Legal Aid Society, homemaker services, visiting nurse programs, neighborhood babysitting co-ops, and Meals-on-Wheels are a few examples of possible assistance. Social, athletic, and civic organizations also can be helpful for leisure time activities and enhancing social skills.

Usually such massive outside mobilization is not necessary. What is critical is that family members realize that significant relationships may not have been jeopardized by the departure of a parent and that indeed opportunities may be opened for greater enrichment of existing relationships. Because of misunderstandings or prior problems arising from the views or activities of the absent partner, barriers which are now removed, it is sometimes possible to renew old friendships or neglected family ties. In general, reconnection to previously gratifying relationships is the overall goal. Within the extended family of the remaining parent often lie unexpressed sympathy, admiration, support, and encouragement. One such process of linking people back with their families has been described by Speck and Attneave (1973). The goal of the process is called retribalization, after a concept by Laing (1964).

When a parent departs, there is an inevitable blurring of family roles and responsibilities. Possible indecision by the remaining parent and confused expectations by the children are common. Therapeutic interventions during this phase should be consistent with whatever naturally occurring compensatory processes may be going on. The therapist should be an active collaborator in helping to ensure that the compensatory activities take a wholesome and constructive direction. For example, the oldest child of the same sex as the departed parent tends to take over some of the duties and responsibilities previously carried out by that parent. Since this can be a comfortable situation for both remaining parent and youngster, it is a good idea for the therapist to monitor such naturally occurring processes to ensure that one or the other party does not get exploited. In extreme cases, these processes can lead to such phenomena as the "parental child" (Minuchin, 1974) and "parent-child marriage," previously referred to. In such cases the therapist may need to intervene aggressively.

Family boundaries also may shift. For example, grandma or grandpa may come to live with the family in order to help with the children and the chores. This situation is fraught with similar potentially troublesome possibilities. Therapeutic interventions generally should be geared toward or at least be consistent with clarifying, establishing or reestablishing roles, responsibilities, and boundaries plus preserving the generational lines of power, influence, and authority.

Associated with role and boundary changes are often changes of job, neighborhood, city, and school which can be very disruptive of routine, rules, structure, and general stability. In spite of the disorganization and uproar, this is not the time for relaxing rules and discipline. In the absence of limits, children will press for the outer tolerances of behavior. With everything else to deal with, Mom or Dad may find that lenience at this time is almost always more trouble than it is worth. If the parent has difficulty with such activities as rule making and limit setting, then these must become vital parts of the treatment process. Anxiety and acting out behavior will diminish as routine is reorganized and everyone knows what is expected of them. Therapists should be prepared to take active roles in assisting family members to learn how to negotiate and carry out rules and responsibilities.

In a previous section we discussed the importance of the remaining parent developing the delicate art of balancing personal needs against those of the children. Here we want to point out the importance of letting the children know what to expect from the present parent and then educating them on what the parent expects of them in response. For example, if a woman says nothing to her children about having men in her life and she then abruptly has an overnight male guest, it is understandable that the children may be upset. Moreover, a woman should not be surprised to observe her child being rude to her guest. Therapists can furnish a valuable service by providing emphasis on and gentle reminders about keeping children informed about such crucial areas as opposite sex companionship and sexuality and parental expectations about their behavior in this regard. Detailed explanations are not required, but basic information exchange and expectation sharing can prevent much conflict and pain later, especially if Mom or Dad plans to enter a new relationship relatively soon. Amid new circumstances and high stress, new behaviors take some time to learn and proper allowance must be made in these areas.

Parents and therapists alike tend to be concerned about the impact on emotional development, psychosexual development, and personal adjustment of the child due to lack of exposure to adequate models of the opposite-sex parent. Current clinical wisdom suggests that there is adequate justification for this concern and the parent should make extra efforts, if necessary, in order to provide such experiences.

A related issue is whether a youngster is better off living with the same or opposite-sex parent, other things being equal. Santrock and Warshak (1979) compared 20 mother-awarded custody children with 20 father-awarded custody children. The findings indicated that youngsters residing with the opposite-sex parent were less well adjusted than their counterparts with same sex parents. Also, contact with additional adult caretakers was associated with positive social behaviors. Although these results cannot be considered definitive, they do attest to the importance of contact with adequate adult figures of both sexes outside the home.

5. Summary and Suggestions for Future Research

In this chapter we have discussed the varieties of one-parent families, noting that there is no widely accepted classification schema. We selected the most frequently observed sybtype of one-parent family, the so-called deficit model, and proceeded to describe some of the special problems of this group. Next we considered some practical treatment issues and made some suggestions regarding treatment of this special group. Suggestions for further study include the development of a classification schema about which some consensus can be mustered. We noted that contemporary theorists in the family therapy area simply have neglected consideration of the one-parent family and, for the most part, are silent on the applicability of their conceptions to this group. We urge writers to address these issues. Descriptive and empirical studies are sorely needed on the subtypes of one-parent families, especially on the "by choice–marriage-not-desired" variety. We are not aware of the development of a natural history of the one-parent family comparable to the published work on families generally. Such a developmental effort should be mounted. Which forms of family treatment work best for which subtypes is an area that is virtually untouched. Are certain subtypes more often associated with certain diagnoses of the identified patient? Does using co-therapists offer additional benefits with one-parent families? Are therapists of the same or opposite sex from the remaining parent more effective? What are the contraindications for family treatment for one-parent families? Are there contraindications for use of certain theoretical perspectives with certain family syndromes? What are the outer limits of the useful application of family treatment, especially with one-parent families?

We could go on and on. The work has barely begun. Systematic research in this field lags far behind practice and clinical folklore. Sensitive researchers and astute practitioners are critically needed. Their contributions will be most welcome.

6. References

Ackerman, N. Interlocking pathologies in family relationships. In S. Rado, & G. Daniels (Eds.), *Changing concepts in psychoanalytic medicine*. New York: Grune & Stratton, 1956.

Bateson, G., Jackson, D. D., Haley, J., & Weakland, J. H. Toward a theory of schizophrenia. *Behavioral Science*. 1956, *1*, 251–264.

Bronfenbrenner, U. Who cares for America's children? In V. C. Vaughan & T. B. Brazelton (Eds.), *The family—Can it be saved? Chicago: Year Book Medical Publishers, 1976.*

Bertalanffy, L. V. General system theory. New York: Braziller, 1968.

Billingsley, A., & Giovannoni, J. M. One-parent family. In R. Morris (Ed.), *Encyclopedia of social work* (Vol. 1) (16th issue). New York: National Association of Social Workers, 1971.

Brooks, P. E. *Family therapy with single parent families*. Unpublished doctoral dissertation, University of Denver, 1980.

Cline, B. J. A construct validity study of disengagement-enmeshment: Some individual, family, sociocultural correlates. *Dissertation Abstracts*, 1977, Vol. 38 235613.

Corkill, H. The solo parent home. *Delta*, 1977, *21*, 42–49.

Glasser, P., & Navarre, E. Structural problems of the one-parent family. *Journal of Social Issues*, 1965, *21* (1), 98–109.

Gurman, A. S. & Kniskern, D. P. *Handbook of family therapy*. New York: Brunner/Mazel, 1981.

Jackson, D. The question of family homeostasis. In D. Jackson (Ed.), *Communication, family, and marriage*. Palo Alto: Science and Behavior Books, 1968.

Kalter, N. Children of divorce in an outpatient psychiatric population. *American Journal of Orthopsychiatry*, 1977, *47*, 40–51.

Katz, L. *A Conceptual framework for understanding stepfamilies*. Unpublished doctoral dissertation, University of Denver, 1981.

Laing, R. D., & Esterson, A. *Sanity, madness and the family*. Baltimore: Penguin, 1964.

Lidz, T. Family organization and personality structure. In N. Bell & E. Vogel (Eds.), *A modern introduction to the family*. New York: Free Press, 1968.

Lindemann, E. Symptomatology and management of acute grief. *American Journal of Psychiatry*, 1944, *101*, 141–148.

Miller, J. G. Living systems: Basic concepts. *Behavioural Science*, 1965, *10*, 193–245.

Minuchin, S. *Families and family therapy*. Cambridge: Harvard Univeristy Press, 1974.

Rexford, M. Single mothers by choice: An exploratory study. *Dissertation Abstracts*, 1976, *37*, 934–B. Order #76–18, 122.

Santrock, J. W., & Warshak, R. Father custody and social development in boys and girls. *Journal of Social Issues*. 1979, *35*(4), 112–125.

Satir, V. *Conjoint family therapy. A guide to theory and technique*. Palo Alto: Science and Behavior Books, 1964.

Speck, R., & Attneave, C. *Family networks*. New York: Pantheon, 1973.

Steinglass, P. The conceptualization of marriage from a systems theory perspective. In T. Paolino & B. McCrady (Eds.), *Marriage and marital therapy*. New York: Brunner/Mazel, 1978.

Visher, E., & Visher, J. *Stepfamilies: A guide to working with stepparents and stepchildren*. New York: Brunner/Mazel, 1979.

Wynne, L., Ryckoff, I., Day, J., & Kirsch, S. Pseudomutuality in the family relations of schizophrenics. *Psychiatry*, 1958, *21*, 205.

Weiss, R. Growing up a little faster: The experience of growing up in a single-parent household. *Journal of Social Issues*, 1979, *35* (4), 97–111.

19

Treating Stepfamilies

LES KATZ AND SHARON STEIN

Stepfamilies are families in which either one or both partners in a remarriage have been previously married, with at least one of the partners having had children from that previous marriage. These families have also been referred to as blended, remarried, reconstituted, or second families. There has been a dramatic increase in the number of stepfamilies in our society, paralleling the high divorce rate. In fact, along with the nuclear family, and the single parent family, it is one of three major western world family forms, and comprises over 13 percent of all families with children under 18 in the United States (Visher & Visher, 1979, p. 4). In the past several years there has been a steady growth of both popular and professional interest in the stepfamily, rectifying a previous situation of virtual neglect (see Visher and Visher, 1978). The inclusion of a chapter on stepfamilies in this Handbook is one example of this new interest. The stereotyped views of the stepfamily as being inferior, and consisting of a "wicked" stepmother, or a "cruel" stepfather, and "neglected" stepchildren, is giving way to a broader understanding of the many unique features of this type of family form.

Despite considerable interest in the stepfamily, there are still significant gaps in our knowledge and in our ability to provide services for this type of family. Sager, Steer, Crohn, Rodstein, and Walker (1980) found five areas of lacunae of information regarding remarried families. These are:

> 1. A failure to develop theoretical constructs that deal with the Rem family. [Sager *et al.*, 1980 and Sager, Walker, Brown, Crohn, & Rodstein, 1981, use the term "Rem families" to describe the remarriage population—Rem families are a broader group than stepfamilies as defined here, for they include remarriages in which no children are involved.]
> 2. A lack of specific treatment approaches.
> 3. A lack of attention to the Rem therapist's attitudes and emotional reactions in their professional work.
> 4. A lack of work in the area of prevention of malfunction in the Rem family.
> 5. A lack of recognition of the positive effects of Rem on the lives of many adults and children. (p. 20)

To this list, we would add that there has been a lack of well designed research studies

---

LES KATZ • 2993 S. Peoria, Suite 302, Aurora, Colorado 80014. **SHARON STEIN** • Department of Behavioral Sciences, Children's Hospital, Denver, Colorado 80218.

that might add to our knowledge of stepfamilies (see K. N. Walker, Rogers, & Messinger, 1977, for a discussion of this problem).

In this chapter, we will provide a descriptive overview, a conceptual framework, and an approach to both assessment and treatment of the stepfamily.

1. Descriptive Features of Stepfamilies

There has been a tendency to view stepfamilies as a homeogeneous population and to refer to it as "The Stepfamily." Stepfamilies actually are a heterogeneous population, having certain structural characteristics in common, and are more aptly referred to as "Stepfamilies." The heterogeneous nature of these families is based on their variable life histories and composition. There are, in fact, numerous types of stepfamilies.

The thread that ties these varied family units together is certain characteristics that delineate them from other family forms. Adapting from a list developed by Visher and Visher (1979, p. 19), these characteristics can be summarized as follows:

1. There is a biological parent elsewhere (i.e., either the parent is dead, or most commonly, is divorced and living elsewhere).
2. Stepfamilies are families that form after the dissolution of a previous family unit. Virtually all family members have sustained a loss. This loss may be the actual loss of a spouse or parent through a death. More frequently what is lost is the previous family unit, although the relationships may survive in some altered form.
3. The relationship between the biological parent and his or her children predates the marriage.
4. There is a remarried marital couple in stepfamilies.
5. Children may be members of more than one household.
6. The stepparent is not legally related to his or her stepchildren (adoptions will change this legal relationship, but is a relatively uncommon situation, and of course, does not change the biological reality).

Visher and Visher (1979) have compared these characteristics to the characteristics of other family forms (intact, single parent, adoptive, and foster) and have noted that while other family forms may have some of these characteristics (for example, in single parent families there is a biological parent elsewhere), none have the combination of features seen in stepfamilies.

The unique characteristics of stepfamilies would lead one to hypothesize that these families have certain common features or ways of functioning that would distinguish them from other family forms. This hypothesis derives credence from a literature that often is overflowing with descriptions of the unique circumstances and problems of stepfamilies. These descriptions are gleaned primarily from self-report of members of stepfamilies or from clinical case vignettes, and consequently may be biased. In addition, no feature described can be a universal to all stepfamilies, and some characteristics of stepfamilies also may be common to other family forms. Despite these caveats, we believe that a summary of the descriptive features of stepfamilies taken from the literature are worth noting, for they provide the "meat" for the conceptual framework that follows. Table 1 is a summary of these features. (For references that detail these features in more depth, see, for example, Capaldi & McRae, 1979; Maddox, 1975; Roosevelt & Lofas, 1976; Visher & Visher, 1979).

Table 1. Some Common Features of Stepfamilies

A. Issues related to the previous marriage and family unit

1. The necessity of mourning the loss of the previous family unit.
2. The necessity of learning how to deal with an ex-spouse after marital ties have been severed.
3. The tendency to idealize the absent ex-spouse/biological parent (particularly likely if deceased).
4. The tendency to denigrate the absent ex-spouse/biological parent (more likely if divorced).
5. The tendency to fantasize the reconciliation of the marriage and previous family unit (particularly likely for children).
6. The tendency to ignore unresolved anger and guilt related to any or all of the above.

B. Issues related to the divorce and the single parenting experience

1. A necessity to enter the adversary legal system in order to establish custody, visitation, child support, and spousal support arrangements.
2. An adjustment to new circumstances, such as new job situation, living situation, or altered household management arrangement.
3. A sense of unresolved guilt or anger about the divorce. Children may continue to feel resentful or responsible for the divorce. Parents also may continue to feel responsible or resentful.
4. A feeling that the noncustodial parent is uninvolved and unwilling to help provide support to the family.
5. A feeling that the noncustodial parent is too involved and interfering in the single parent family.
6. Children are placed in the middle of parental battles.
7. Children are asked to take over many adult responsibilities.

C. Issues related to the remarriage

1. The role of the stepparent may be unclear with subsequent confusion concerning all roles in the family.
2. The lines of authority in the family may be unclear and results in confusion in areas such as discipline.
3. The expectations stepfamily members have for each other may be unrealistic in either a positive or negative direction.
4. The routines, rules, and traditions may be new and difficult to adjust to.
5. There may be disruption caused in the family resulting from the children shifting back and forth between two households.
6. There may be a sense of divided loyalty. Biological parents are divided between the children and their new spouse. Children are divided between their biological parents and their stepparent.
7. There may be a tendency to give children a great deal of power in the stepfamily because of fear they will gravitate to the other parent.
8. There may be a financial strain placed on the stepfamily as a result of the divorce and support settlement.
9. There may be a desire to create a "new" family and disregard the ex-spouse.
10. The previous divorce settlement may allow an ex-spouse to have too much control in the stepfamily.
11. Children may have the feeling that they are being left out of the new marital relationship, which may result in jealousy and resentment.
12. The issue of sexuality is more difficult as the married couple must develop their relationship in the presence of children. The incest barrier is weaker.
13. The family unit is not as emotionally close as an intact family.
14. The biological parent and the stepparent have different parenting histories and as a result may view the children differently. This may turn out to be viewed as an advantage or as a disadvantage by the family.
15. The fear of past failure may result in fear of failure in the new relationship.
16. Stepmothers are stereotyped as being "wicked" by other family members.
17. Stepfathers are stereotyped as being "abusive" by other family members.
18. Stepchildren are stereotyped as being "neglected" by other family members.

(*continued*)

Table 1 (*Continued*)

D. Issues related to society

1. There is a tendency for society to view stepfamilies negatively: "the wicked stepmother," "the cruel stepfather," "the neglected stepchildren."
2. There may be conflicts that result from issues with the extended family; lack of acceptance of the divorce and/or the remarriage, feeling left out of the new marriage, overprotection of the children, interfering with the forming of new relationships, too many relatives to deal with, etc.
3. The law may interfere with solidifying the stepfamily; divorce settlements are rigid and inflexible; stepparents have no legal rights; inheritance laws do not apply to steprelationships; legal relationships can interfere with emotional ties.
4. The tendency for societal convention to work against stepfamilies; the school system does not recognize stepparents; different last names are awkward; the tendency to mistake stepfamilies for other family forms.

2. A Conceptual Framework for Understanding Stepfamilies

Several writers have noted the need for the development of conceptual formulations applicable to the special characteristics of stepfamilies (Katz, 1981; Sager *et al.*, 1981; Visher & Visher, 1978). In this section on theory we will present a framework we have found useful in working with stepfamilies (Katz, 1980a; Katz, 1981; Katz & Zeiger, in press). Our method has been to adapt already existing family theory to the special characteristics of stepfamilies. In the following sections we will describe the stepfamily system and how it differs from the nuclear family system in terms of subsystems, boundaries, roles, and development.

2.1. The Stepfamily System

Stepfamilies have many similarities to other forms of families. Like all families they attempt to achieve the overall family tasks of "the socialization of the children and the stabilization of adult personalities" (Lewis, Beavers, Gossett, & Phillips, 1976, p. 2). The stepfamily is an interactive system with properties common to other interactive family systems. It is an entity greater than the sum of its individual parts. The system has a hierarchically organized structure and operates such that a change in any one part of the system will effect the rest of the system; a change in the system will activate mechanisms that attempt to bring the system back to its previous status quo (homeostasis); and changes come about, in part, as a result of changes in the developmental life cycle of the family.

The similarities of stepfamilies to other family forms does not alter its unique character. It is this unique character that we shall detail in the following sections, focusing on the composition, subsystem boundaries, roles, and development in these families.

2.2. The Composition of Stepfamilies

A stepfamily system is more complex than a nuclear family system. Nuclear family systems are composed of a single household unit consisting of a mother/wife, father/husband, and a varying number of children taking on the roles of son/brother and daughter/sister. This nuclear family system exists, of course, in the context of a fabric of larger social systems (i.e., extended family, neighborhoods, social and religious organizations, etc.), but the system itself usually is demarcated at the household level of interaction.

Stepfamily systems are organized differently than nuclear families. First, there are a varying number of households that comprise the system. The most common stepfamily system is a two household one where children live in one household (the custodial household) and visit the other household (the noncustodial household). There are times when a stepfamily system consists of only one household, as, for example, when one of the biological parents has died. There also are three or more household systems (an example of a three household system would be when two previously married parents remarry. The system would consist of each of the ex-spouses' households and a third household created by the remarriage). Since interactions take place between households, it is useful to conceptualize the households as being subsystems within the larger stepfamily system. By doing this we can avoid the common problems that arise when a remarried household is viewed as an entity unto itself and attempts are made to stabilize and integrate the remarried household in the same way that one would go about stabilizing and integrating a nuclear family.

An additional difference in composition between nuclear families and stepfamilies is that the composition in stepfamily households is quite varied from household to household, although it usually will consist of a biological parent, a stepparent, and a varying number of children who are either biological siblings, stepsiblings, or half-siblings to each other. As conceptualized here, a household in a stepfamily system could also consist of a single parent whose ex-spouse has remarried. The wide variations of compositional makeup within households in stepfamilies can be simplified somewhat if one thinks of types of household units within the system:

Type 1—a previously married woman with children marrying a man with no children
Type 2—a previously married man with children marrying a woman with no children
Type 3—a remarriage where both spouses have children from previous marriages
Type 4—a single parent with children whose ex-spouse has remarried

Within these four types there can be a number of factors that result in even more variation in stepfamily households. These factors would include variations in custodial status (mother custodial, father custodial, joint custody, divided custody where one parent has some children and the other parent has others, and changing custody); in the ages and number of children; in the number, if any, of children born into the stepfamily; in the previous marital status of the stepparent without children; and in the type of previous family status (divorced, spousal death, desertion, multiple divorces, unwed motherhood, etc.). Although each stepfamily must be evaluated regarding the impact of its constellation of variations on family members, it is strikingly clear that no stepfamily household has the familiar compositional structure seen in nuclear families, that is, mother, father, son, and daughter. This feature of stepfamily life results in a different structure of subsystem patterns and role relationships than is seen in nuclear families.

3. Subsystems

A family system "differentiates and carries out its functions through subsystems" (Minuchin, 1974, p. 52). A subsystem is composed of any subgroup in the system, including individuals, dyads, triads, and so on. The sanctity of the subsystem is protected by the boundaries, or invisible dividing line, that is established between the subsystem and the rest of the system. The "boundaries of a subsystem are the rules defining who participated and how" (Minuchin, 1974, p. 53). A clear subsystem boundary, preventing interference from other subsystems but allowing for contact with other family members, is necessary in order for a subsystem adaptively to fulfill its subsystem functions. It is this clear boundary, for example, that would allow a marital couple to continue developing a marital relationship despite potential interferences from children in the family. Disturbances in family functioning arise when boundaries are either inappropriately rigid, interfering with interaction across subsystems, or overly diffuse, decreasing distance and blurring boundaries.

3.1. Household Boundaries

Most stepfamilies must face the task of establishing a boundary between the households in their family system. K. Walker and Messinger (1979) have characterized boundary formation in stepfamilies as being more "permeable" than that seen in nuclear families. In a stepfamily "parental authority as well as economic subsistence may be shared" (K. Walker & Messinger, 1979, p. 186) between the households in the system. This results in a greater degree of interaction occurring outside the household boundaries than usually is seen in nuclear families.

Stepfamilies must adapt to the reality of this higher degree of interaction and this can be a slow, ongoing, and often unsuccessful process. One often hears complaints such as "I thought I divorced the man, but he's come back to haunt my present marriage" or, "When I married him, I had no idea I was marrying his ex-wife also." The interaction with the other household often is seen as destroying any attempts to create a new household.

From our perspective, the problem for a stepfamily household is not that another household exists. We have seen many families, in fact, who have turned this reality into an advantage resulting in growth for all family members. Rather, the problem for a stepfamily is finding a way to acknowledge the reality and to respond to this reality by establishing stable and clear household boundaries. We see several related components to this task:

1. First, the household must develop a realistic perspective on the extent of the involvement of the other household. How often, for example, will children be visiting their father? How much child support can be expected? If something comes up suddenly, can the other household be depended on to care for the children?

2. Second, the household subsystem must develop a realistic appraisal of the quality of the interaction with the other household and take steps to alter the interaction if it is destructive. Does, for example, the visitation arrangement place burdens on children that are beyond their capacity? Is the other household consistent in its monetary obligations to children? Does visitation or custody place children in unacceptable danger? Are interactions between ex-spouses destructive? This realistic appraisal is an extremely difficult one for a family to make because of the tendency to be overprotective of children and to see the influence of the other household in a negative light. The constructive alteration of destructive interaction can take many forms, from attempts at direct negotiation with the other household to offering support to children in their efforts to master the interaction to seeking legal changes.

3. Finally, the household unit must learn to adjust to some degree of shifting membership in the course of its life cycle. Children often move back and forth between households and this can result in families being uncertain as to who to include in their definition of family. Families who manage to define themselves as a stable family unit, and include children whose stay in the household may be only temporary seem to fare better than families who define the issue in terms of loyalty ("If you go live with your mom, that's it, you will no longer be a member of this family") or punishment ("If you don't shape up, I'm sending you to live with your dad"). When children want to move out precipitously to avoid some problem ("I'm moving to my dad's if you make me study any more") they are dealt with firmly but without any sense that their family membership is on the line.

The most adaptive stepfamilies, then, are those who establish a clear family boundary. They recognize that the other household unit interacts with their own and they develop a realistic evaluation of the extent and quality of this interaction. When interaction is destructive, they take steps to change this. In addition, they attempt to provide a stable sense of family despite shifting family membership during the course of the family life cycle. Obviously, adaptation requires both flexibility and a recognition that interaction outside the household may have a significant effect on family life.

Less adaptive stepfamilies either respond to the reality of interaction between households in too rigid a manner, attempting to cut off interaction with the other family, or too permeably, allowing the interaction to prevent them from developing a stable sense of themselves as a family.

A common rigid boundary solution may result in family members in one household acting as if they were a nuclear family. The importance of the other household is consistently denied. Relationships between households are nonexistent or antagonistic. Goldstein (1974) has described a type of remarried family he calls "pseudomutual" and these families appear to be similar to the ones we describe here. Expression of anger within the family, says Goldstein, "is too great a threat since the fear of facing family dissolution is always present" (p. 435). Children in these families often experience intense loyalty conflicts. If children maintain an interest in interacting with the other household they eventually are seen as traitors to the family and their continued membership in the household is in jeopardy. A variation of this nuclear family solution to boundary establishment are families that act as if they are single parent families. These families also deny the importance of the other household but in addition refuse to allow anyone else to play a role in their family system.

Families who establish boundaries too permeably may result in their looking either like a large extended family or in not looking like a family unit at all. Some families attempt to deal with the reality of interaction by becoming too cooperative. Ex-spouses attempt to become good friends, and authority and decision making often are shared in a cooperative manner. The cooperative atmosphere in these families obscures the fact that the spouses have dissolved their marriage and that family members have sustained the loss of a family unit. Stepparents often become frustrated by the high degree of interaction in the family and become the symptom bearers of the family. Other families deal with the reality of interaction by giving up on any effort to establish a family identity. They often rather quickly find themselves dissolving their new family units, thus heaping loss on top of previous loss.

3.2. Boundaries in Other Subsystems

The complexity of a stepfamily system results in a greater number of possible subsystems than is seen in a nuclear family. Although some of these subsystems can be expected to have a high degree of interaction within their boundaries, others, like the subsystem consisting of two stepparents in a system where both ex-spouses have remarried, can be expected to have little interaction. Although there are numerous possible subsystem alignments based on combinations of old and new family ties, it is useful to focus on the boundaries established in three specific subsystems in the family. These are: (1) remarried couple, (2) custodial parent and children, and (3) divorced couple. We think of these subsystems as the "power" subsystems in the family. Attempts to work with problems in other subsystems in the family often will fail unless the power subsystems are included in the work. Changes in the power system often will result in changes in other subsystems in the family. When evaluating a family, we attempt to get a reading on the clarity of the boundaries of these subsystems.

In the remarried couple subsystem we want to know if the couple has been able to establish a marital relationship despite the presence of children in the family. Remarried couples often do not have the opportunity of getting to know each other before having children and this can interfere with their ability to work out a stable marital contract. The success of the remarriage is, of course, dependent on the couple's ability to establish a workable marriage. In addition, the couple simultaneously has to negotiate a parental relationship. Both custodial parent and stepparent must begin to define their roles with children. Some of the pitfalls for a remarried couple involve establishing too rigid or too permeable boundaries. When the boundaries are too rigid, the couple often invests a great deal of energy into the marriage at the expense of their parenting tasks. Either the children are not given the attention they need or they are handled inconsistently. The stepparent, for example, may vacillate in his or her involvement with the children, sometimes becoming actively involved, sometimes angrily resenting the presence of children. When the boundaries are established too permeably, the couple either invests a great deal of energy in being parents at the expense of their marital task work, or they do not invest energy in either. Couples may spend endless hours discussing what to do about the children, how to have them be part of the family, how to deal with the ex-spouse, and so forth, all the while ignoring that they are more than just parents. When they do focus on their marriage, they often begin to face fears that they may not be able to succeed as marital partners.

In the custodial parent and children subsystem we are interested in whether this subsystem has both maintained stable ties throughout the alterations in their family structure and, in addition, have allowed for new members to become active in their lives. Rigid subsystem coalitions will result in maintaining stability at the expense of the continuation of other old relationships or the development of new relationships. Often this subsystem will breach generational boundaries as children begin to play adult roles in the family. The permeable boundary solutions will result in the stability of the relationship being interrupted. Children often feel they have to fend for themselves. Parents often feel in a bind between their own needs and their children's needs, seeing these as mutually exclusive and choosing their own needs more often than not.

In the divorced couple subsystem we want to see if the ex-spouses have been able to separate out their parental and marital role functions. If they have, they can act in the best interests of their children. If they establish too rigid boundaries, they will cut off interaction as parents or interact in an antagonistic manner. Children usually will suffer for their parent's inability to negotiate. If they establish too permeable boundaries, they often will use their continued parental relationship as an excuse to stay married to each other. There may be repeated attempts at reconciliation. Children may be used as pawns in their parents' interactions or themselves may be active in trying to keep the parents together.

Difficulties in establishing boundaries in any of the power subsystems will result in either an inordinate amount of power being held by one of the subsystems at the expense of other subsystems or there being a power "vacuum" in the family, which often results in one of the nonpower subsystems, such as the children, taking power in the family. The therapeutic goal is to work toward a "balance of power" in the family. Strategically, whoever holds the actual power in the system needs to be attended to. As the therapist works toward changing the power structure in the family, he or she more and more enlists the aid of and reinforces the need for the three power subsystems to establish clear boundaries.

4. Roles in a Stepfamily

We define family roles as those defining how individuals participate in family life. As used here, roles are the boundaries individuals establish. Dysfunction occurs when roles are established too rigidly or too permeably.

Several writers have commented on the ambiguity of the steprole and the difficulties stepparents have in enacting a role within the family (Draughon, 1975; Fast & Cain, 1966; Goldstein, 1974; K. Walker & Messinger, 1979). Goldstein says that the most dramatic problem seen in stepfamilies is the "stepparent being frozen out of his role." In fact, our observation is that all roles in the stepfamily have a potential for becoming ambiguous and conflict laden and that the stepparenting role is just the most obvious to the observer.

In the process of moving from the nuclear family, to postdivorce family, to stepfamily, all family roles often undergo some dramatic changes. As soon as a family moves out of a nuclear family setting, they lose a set of well defined roles. Even though societal definitions of nuclear family roles are changing, there is an institutionalized standard by which to measure these changes. The basic roles in the nuclear family are the reciprocal, paired, and hierarchically organized roles of husband/father, wife/mother, daughter/sister, and son/brother, and functions become elaborated from these basic roles.

When a family moves from nuclear family to single parent family, they lose only one of these role relationships established in the nuclear family, that of the husband/wife. Every other role in the family, however, undergoes some alteration. The "part-time" father role, for example, is much different from the "full-time" father role (see Wallerstein & Kelly, 1980, for an investigation of this role). The role of the custodial parent also changes significantly.

When the family moves again from single parent family to remarriage they lose no roles, although the existing roles again are altered by the remarriage. In addition, the stepfamily adds the following roles: (1) a new husband–wife role relationship, (2) a new stepparent–biological parental role relationship, and (3) new stepparent–stepchildren role relationships.

(More complex stepfamily systems will add even more role relationships, such as stepsibling roles, or if both ex-spouses remarry, two stepparenting roles. In "blended" families, parents are biological parents to some children and stepparents to others.)

The altered and added roles in the stepfamily can become a source of confusion and conflict for all members. Valued role functions can become lost in the evolution from one family unit to another, and the additional member may be seen not as adding anything to the family, but rather, as taking something away.

As our knowledge of stepfamilies has increased, more attention has been given to analyzing and clarifying the roles in the stepfamily, particularly the role of the stepparent. K. Walker and Messinger (1979), for example, have suggested that although roles in a nuclear family are ascribed, that is, assigned without reference to innate ability, steprelationships need to be achieved, that is, left open to be filled through competition and individual effort. Turner's (1962) concept of "role making" has been applied to roles in stepfamilies (Aldous, 1974; K. Walker & Messinger, 1979). This concept proposes that in situations where there are few guidelines, family members need to "make" their roles. "Interaction patterns have to be worked out through a fumbling process requiring the participating partners to determine how to get along with a minimum of disagreement and conflict" (Aldous, 1978, p. 233).

To this analysis of role relationships in the stepfamily we would add the following:

1. The concept of role making can be extended to all role relationships in a stepfamily system. The entire system has undergone change, and the entire system is experiencing some sense of role ambiguity and lack of guidelines as to how to proceed. It is just as accurate, for example, to say that the noncustodial parent is learning to make a role and that this role has aspects that need to be achieved, as it is to say that this is the case for the stepparent.

2. The role of stepparent, although needing to be achieved to a certain degree, also has an ascribed aspect to it. The very name *stepparent* implies some type of parental role function and has some parental demand characteristics. As one stepparent noted when discussing his role, "At first, I saw myself as a friend and roommate to these kids, but I don't remember ever having to tell my roommates to be in bed by 9:00 P.M."

We have found it useful, therefore, to talk of the primary and secondary importance of role relationships. The role relationships formed in a nuclear family are primary need meeting relationships. They are both primary and ascribed. The step role relationships are not based on this primary relationship, but are an "instant" relationship based on two adults' decision to marry. They are secondary to the biological family's relationships, but still are ascribed. Over time, as step relationships develop, a primary relationship may be achieved, or the relationship may remain secondary. (The biological relationships may go the other way. They always will be ascribed relationships but may move from primary to secondary. This process normally occurs in development, as children individuate and develop relationships outside the home, but it also can occur because one or both biological parents withdraw their involvement.)

3. In evaluating stepfamilies, it is important to assess how the role ambiguity and conflict is being negotiated. Some families, for example, as Goldstein suggests, may "freeze" out the steprole. Others may define the role in too permeable fashion, giving it a primary ascribed significance perhaps at the same time as they are "freezing" out the noncustodial parent.

5. A Developmental Model of Stepfamilies

The developmental approach to the family studies the stages a family travels through in the course of its family life cycle (Aldous, 1978; Duvall, 1977; Solomon, 1973). The stages coincide with the important life events of the family. Solomon (1973), for example, proposed a five-stage model around the family life events of (1) the marriage, (2) the birth of children and subsequent child rearing, (3) the individuation of family members, (4) the actual departure of children, and (5) the integration of loss. Each change of life event forces certain structural and interactional alterations in family life, and consequently presents family members with a number of tasks to resolve. Successful resolution results in growth-producing changes for a family, while failure at resolution results in maladaptive, growth-inhibiting patterns.

The developmental approach to the family has been applied primarily to the orderly unfolding of development as seen in the nuclear family and rarely to variant family forms. A developmental model of the stepfamily must incorporate the major life cycle events of that type of family organization into a developmental scheme. These life events are much different than the life events seen in a nuclear family and these differences produce different stages and different task work for a stepfamily.

A stepfamily's altered life history, like its structural complexity results in a number of features that are not present in a nuclear family. These features are:

1. There are always *overlapping stages of development* in a stepfamily because there are children present who predate the marriage. The individuation of children in a stepfamily always is occurring simultaneously with other stages of development. Developmental stages in a nuclear family (Solomon, 1973), on the other hand, tend to unfold sequentially. The overlapping development in a stepfamily produces both a higher potential for interference in children's individuation and a potential for interference in the integration of the stepfamily. A common example of this is seen in newly formed stepfamilies with adolescents. The adolescent is striving to separate from the family at the same time that the family is attempting to consolidate as a family unit. The family consolidation often is perceived by adolescents as a threat to their strivings for independence and the adolescent may respond to this threat by attempting to disrupt any efforts of the family to consolidate. The rest of the family may perceive the adolescent as the reason for their difficulty in consolidating and may step up efforts either to bring the adolescent closer into the family (thus further threatening the individuation strivings) or to push him or her out of the family (thus causing the adolescent to separate prematurely).

2. Within the stepfamily system, there usually are at least *two separate households, each involved in its own family development*. When the two households are at different stages of development, stress and conflict within the entire stepfamily system may result, and cause problems for all members of the stepfamily. A common example of this occurs when one ex-spouse has resolved the loss of the first marriage, and remarries, while the other ex-spouse continues to hope for reconciliation. The ex-spouse who has not resolved the loss of the marriage may attempt somehow to re-create the old family homeostasis by disrupting the other spouse's attempts to consolidate in a new marriage. The children frequently become the focus of these attempts as increasingly destructive interactions with the children lead the remarried parent to focus more attention on the children and ex-spouse and less attention on the new relationship.

3. The life events in a stepfamily tend to produce more *dramatic structural changes* than those seen in a nuclear family. Nuclear family development tends to unfold more gradually than stepfamily development. For example, Solomon (1973), in discussing the individuation stage, states that "many families slide through this stage of development with little or no awareness of the difficulties involved until the first child reaches adoles-

cence'' (p. 185). Contrast this with some of the major life events of a stepfamily. A divorce, for example, is ''often characterized by a disequilibrium approaching severe disorganization. For many families, this process extends over several years'' (Kelly & Wallerstein, 1976, p. 22). A remarriage is also a time of dramatic structural change. The ''initial adjustment period can be a crisis time ripe for the onset of symptoms and the danger of pathological structural formation'' (Whiteside & Auerbach, 1978, p. 275).

4. Stepfamilies tend to have a *greater load of task work* at each stage of development than nuclear families. Stepfamilies, in other words, often have more issues to resolve than nuclear families. These extra tasks often require more energy over a longer time period than task resolution in a nuclear family.

Since stepfamilies are a heterogeneous group, there are wide variations in the life history and structural characteristics of individual stepfamilies. This results in a broad variety of developmental task work among stepfamilies. In fact, it would be more accurate to stage several developmental models of stepfamilies. For example, a family that sustains

Table 2. The Developmental Stages of the Stepfamily

Stage 1. The single-parent headed household
- Tasks:
  1. Relinquishment of investment in the previous family unit
  2. Renegotiation of the relationships altered by the family dissolution
  3. Establishing a single-parent headed household

Stage 2. The remarriage
- Tasks:
  1. Relinquishment task work:
     - (a) Relinquishment of the exclusive nature of the gratifications received in the single parent family
  2. Investment task work:
     - (a) Establishment of clear family boundaries and roles

Stage 3. The birth of the first child into the stepfamily and subsequent child rearing
- Tasks:
  1. Further development and enhancement of the relationships established at Stage 2
  2. Development of the new roles of:
     - (a) Parents to biological child
     - (b) Half-siblings to child

Stage 4. Individuation in the stepfamily
- Task:
  To allow for appropriate individuation of family members despite potential interferences due to family dissolution and family formation taskwork

Stage 5. The actual departure of the children
- Task:
  Allowing children to depart from 2 households and to leave appropriately both biological and stepparents

Stage 6. The integration of the losses
- Tasks:
  1. Resolution of losses
  2. Resolution of variant family life history

a death has different task work than one that survives a divorce, and a family consisting of two sets of children has different task work than one where there is only one set of children. The developmental model staged here will focus primarily on the most common type of stepfamily household unit, the remarriage of a divorced custodial mother to a man who becomes a stepfather at the remarriage. A six-stage model is proposed. These stages follow the life events of (1) divorce, (2) remarriage, (3) birth of children, (4) individuation, (5) departure of children, and (6) the period of the "empty nest."

5.1. Stage 1: The Single Parent-Headed Household

The life event at this stage is the divorce of a marital couple. The family unit becomes a single parent headed household (this term is used instead of single parent family, which seems to imply the existence of only one parent). There are three tasks at this stage: (1) relinquishment of investment in the previous family unit; (2) renegotiating the relationships altered by the divorce; and (3) establishment of a single-parent headed household.

5.1.1. Relinquishment of Investment

The task involves relinquishing investment in the previous family unit, in effect mourning the loss of a family and the sense of identity derived from being a member in that family. The relationships as they existed in that family unit must be mourned. Family members often experience extended feelings of sadness, anger, and disbelief in response to the loss (Toomin, 1974). The sense of loss may be independent of the reality of the previous family experience (Wallerstein & Kelly, 1976). Individual family members will show variations in their response to loss, but each family member will have the same task of relinquishing his or her investment. Children, in particular, may have profound difficulties in resolving the loss.

5.1.2. Renegotiating the Relationships Altered by the Divorce

After a divorce, family members are faced with the difficult task of renegotiating old ties under new circumstances. Ex-spouses have the task of terminating their marital relationship while maintaining their parental relationship. The noncustodial father and his children have the task of maintaining their relationship in an unfamiliar environment. The custodial mother and her children have the task of maintaining their relationship while adjusting to their altered roles in a single-parent headed household. (Section 5.1.3. contains a fuller discussion of this task.)

Successful resolution of this task does not necessarily entail a continuation of pre-divorce relationships. Rather, it is to develop a realistic appraisal of the existing post-divorce relationship. When both parents continue their involvement, they are able to differentiate their needs from their children's and deal flexibly with the new reality. Children often are allowed relatively free access to both parents (Wallerstein & Kelly, 1976). Often, of course, the ideal resolution is not possible, but a successful resolution still can be attained. For example, one of the parents may be destructive to the children (i.e., abusive or unable to care for them). What may be needed is for the other family members to recognize the deficit in the relationship and respond appropriately to this. On the other hand, after a divorce some parents may begin to become more constructively involved with their children than they were prior to the divorce (Wallerstein & Kelly, 1980). The task in this case would be to allow this involvement to occur. Of central importance for a family is not so much the reality of their circumstances as the manner or process by which the reality is evaluated and negotiated (Marotz-Baden, Adams, Bueche, Munro, & Munro, 1979).

5.1.3. Establishing a Single Parent-Headed Household

The actual management of a single parent-headed household is closely related to the altered relationships. The family unit must reorganize its "domestic and economic responsibilities and its system of affectional and emotional support. Authority shifts are common. Discipline and other socialization practices become primarily the task of the custodial parent" (Marotz-Baden *et al.*, 1979, p. 8). The adjustments often entail "a reduction in the tasks performed and/or a reduction in adequacy of performance, or (seeking) external assistance" (Glasser & Navare, 1965, p. 651).

If a family is able to establish a relatively stable and secure single parent household, there is a greater likelihood that the family will be able to resolve their other task work at this stage. If, as is often the case, the family has to make compromises (i.e., financial disturbances, forced moves, parental absence without the provision of a consistent caretaker, etc.) that threaten the sense of security of its members, the likelihood of having the resources available to deal with other task work is reduced.

5.2. Stage 2: The Remarriage

There are two tasks at this stage. (1) Relinquishing the exclusive nature of the relationships in the single parent headed household and, (2) investing in the new stepfamily unit.

5.2.1. Relinquishment Task Work

The new roles developed after a divorce may become highly valued. At the remarriage these roles are disrupted. Children who either had, or had fantasized, that they had, a very special relationship with their mother may experience a double loss. First, they feel that they have lost their parent to an intruder in the family and may then experience this as an abandonment. Even if the mother actually had been involved with other men throughout the postdivorce period, the child may have fantasized an exclusive relationship and the actual remarriage often disrupts the fantasy. Second, the children may feel that the role functions they filled after the divorce, such as homemaker, rule enforcer, nurturer, and so forth are being taken over either by the stepparent or by the custodial parent who now has time and a desire to fulfill these functions.

The custodial parent may experience a similar loss. The ways in which she had become accustomed to managing her household will change to some degree with the addition of a new family member. In addition, she may respond to her children's loss with a feeling of guilt. She may feel caught in a bind between her desires for investing in her new marriage, and, as a result of her sense of guilt, a desire to maintain the old relationships with children. Another factor often overlooked is that members of the extended family may have moved into the family system after a divorce and performed valuable role functions. They too may feel displaced at the remarriage and may resist the changes.

5.2.2. Investment Task Work

The investment or family formation task work in a stepfamily is much more complex and difficult to achieve than family formation task work in a nuclear family. It involves (1) the establishment of clear family boundaries and (2) the establishment of functional, clearly defined family roles.

How cathected family members become to the new family depends on the complex interplay of a number of interrelated factors. These factors speak to, once again, the heterogeneity of stepfamily, as well as to the individualized approach each stepfamily must take in forming their family. The factors include:

1. The ages of the children at the time of the remarriage. As a rule of thumb, younger children will invest more easily and more appropriately in a stepfamily then older children. Adolescent children, in their need to separate from the family unit, appropriately may place some distance between themselves and the stepfamily investment task work.
2. The nature of the involvement of the noncustodial parent. The rule of thumb here is that if the father has negotiated a constructive, postdivorce relationship with his children, the children have more energy freed to invest in the stepfamily, irrespective of the amount of time they spend away from the stepfamily visiting their father. If the postdivorce involvement is destructive, the children will experience conflict and have less energy to invest in the stepfamily. If the father is uninvolved with the children postdivorce, the energy available for the new family depends on the process in which the family has handled this noninvolvement. A destructive handling results in conflict.
3. The nature of the involvement of the custodial parent. Again, if the postdivorce relationships are constructive, more energy is available for new relationships. If the post divorce relationships were overly close, with children highly invested in new roles or overly distant, with children unable to feel any sense of security from the mother, less energy is available for new relationships.
4. The desire of the stepfather to become involved in new relationships with children. The stepfather may define his role in such a way as to preclude meaningful involvement with the children. This may or may not be part of the contract with his wife.

Other factors that are important in investment in the new family are: the sex of the children; the number of children; the acceptance by the extended family of the new marriage; and the ability of the marital couple to consolidate as a couple.

5.3. Stage 3: The Birth of the First Child into the Stepfamily and Subsequent Child Rearing

The task for the stepfamily at this stage is twofold. First, it must further solidify the relationships established during Stage 2. Second, it must begin to develop new family roles. The marital couple are now the biological parents of a child. The children in the family now have a half-sibling. Problems can arise when the birth is used to avoid remarriage task resolution and becomes an attempt either to cement tenuously established stepfamily relationships ("The baby will bring us all closer together") or to give up on establishing these relationships ("Since the old family isn't working, let's give up on it and start a new one").

The new child brings to the forefront the issue of sense of belongingness in the stepfamily. The already existing children from a previous marriage may feel that there is no place for them in this new family. The custodial mother may feel torn between her ties to old and new families. The stepfather may be tempted to relinquish the frustrating step role for the hoped for gratification of the biological parent role.

5.4. Stage 4: Individuation in the Stepfamily

Solomon (1973) has conceptualized individuation as requiring family members to redefine and modify their roles with each other. "Parental expectations and demands of the child must allow for individuation and progressive independent functioning. At the same time, their development must be syntonic with the child's own wishes for himself" (p. 185).

The complex interplay of stepfamily life events and the developmental capacities of the individuals involved all affect individuation in the stepfamily. There is a potential for either enhancement of or interference with individuation strivings. Interference will take the form of either premature separation or extended dependency.

The potential for enhancement of individuation is conceptualized around the task work required in the single parent and remarried families. For example, parents and children involved in a single-parent household often are required to take on more responsibility and to work harder at negotiating relationships. A remarriage can stimulate opportunities for more varied experiences and the development of new and valuable relationships. The redefinition and modification of family roles becomes a more obvious and urgent task in stepfamilies than in nuclear families because of the more dramatic shifts in family organization. Families have to work much harder at their task work and this process can be beneficial for the problem-solving and task-resolution abilities of all family members. This may also result in more flexibility among individual family members.

The potential for interference in individuation is perhaps a more apparent outcome in stepfamilies. The complex and confusing task work can overwhelm the capacities of family members. The more disruptive the life events, the more energy is required to cope with the life event and the less energy there is to deal with individuation task work. Children's developmental capacities may be overwhelmed by the task work required in divorce and remarriage. At certain stages of development children may be at higher risk for developing problems after a parental divorce or remarriage. Although all children seem to have difficulties with a divorce experience, there are marked differences between age groups regarding how overwhelmed the children become, how adaptive they are in responding to the loss, how extended their difficulties are, and what psychological issues are touched off by the divorce (Heatherington, 1979; Kelly & Wallerstein, 1976; Wallerstein & Kelly, 1974a, 1974b, 1976).

A particularly difficult problem for children is the potential for a life event, such as a family dissolution or a remarriage, to come at a time when their own needs are developmentally in opposition to these family developments. A child who is struggling with separation anxiety will have tremendous problems with a family dissolution, while an individuating adolescent will have considerable difficulties with a stepfamily unit attempting to deal with family formation issues. Any life event of the stepfamily has the potential for intensifying children's issues around such factors as separation, object constancy, guilt, sexuality, aggression, self-esteem, loyalty, and competition. Regression to earlier stable points of functioning (i.e., extended dependency) is one common attempt to master the situation. Progression to areas not yet mastered (i.e., premature individuation) can be another reaction. If parents react to their own difficulties by holding on too long or letting go too soon, these patterns are intensified for children.

The same potential either for enhancement or for interference with growth and development also can be seen in the adult members of the stepfamily. New experiences in the single parent family and new relationships in a remarriage often serve as a counterbalance to earlier unrewarding experiences and self-doubts or as a reinforcement of these issues. A parent freed from the demands of a dysfunctional marital relationship may begin to respond more appropriately to the needs of children. If, however the parent is overloaded with task work, he or she may respond less appropriately to the children. A stepparent's growth may be enhanced if he or she is able appropriately to establish a role or interfered with if consistently frozen out of a role in the family.

5.5. Stage 5: The Actual Departure of the Children

The task work at this stage involves

> relinquishing the primary nature of the gratification involved in the roles of parent and child and the assumption of the more secondary gratification of parents and separated adult. . . . The family members who have separated must seek need-satisfactions from their peer group from which their mate will be selected. The parents must modify their demands and expectations so as to permit this to occur. This invariably necessitates the existence of a stabilized marital relationship that can tolerate an increased need meeting investment as each child departs. (Solomon, 1973, p. 186)

Stepfamily task work differs from nuclear family task work in two respects:

1. The children often are departing from two different households and need to relinquish primary gratifications from both. In addition, children must relinquish the secondary gratifications involved in the step-relationship or the achieved primary relationship with the stepparent.

2. There may be differential feelings about the departure. A stepparent who has not shared the bulk of the gradual development of children will naturally feel different about a loss than a biological parent who has participated in that entire development. The marital couple may experience feelings that are out of "sync." The biological parent may be reworking or reviewing the parenting role and the stepparent may feel left out of this process.

5.6. Stage 6: The Integration of the Loss

The tasks for the stepfamily at this stage are similar to those in the nuclear family. As conceived by Solomon (1973), relationships to

> children are significant but hopefully individuated and separated. The task involved here is the resolution of the losses in economic, social and physical functioning that are experienced by either or both marital partners. . . . The dynamics of this stage tend to follow our traditional conceptualizations about the need to grieve over loss, actual or fantasized, before realistic investment in future functioning is possible. (p. 187)

This stage also involves individuated children assuming the caretaking responsibilities for parents when this is necessary.

The differences between stepfamilies and nuclear families at this stage are:

1. The stepparent and biological parent may have significant differences in response to the loss of this stage. Since the stepparent has not participated in the total development of children, his or her mourning work will differ from that of the biological parent. The task would be for each of the marital partners to allow the other to mourn their own losses, cognizant of the differences in meaning attached to the loss.

2. The integration task work includes reassessing the life history of the family members. The family dissolution, the single parenting, the remarriage, and so forth are looked at from the perspective of old age of the marital couple and adulthood of the children.

3. Another difference may be in the complications that arise in the relationship with individuated children. Since the noncustodial parent also may be involved with individuated children and their families, there may be complications involved for all concerned. For example, there may be up to four grandparents on just one side of the family interested in continuing relationships with grandchildren (grandparents and step-grandparents). This may cause additional task work for all of the families involved.

6. Stability and Change in the Stepfamily System

Nuclear families are distinguished by the "special sense of solidarity that separates the domestic unit from the surrounding community" (Shorter, 1975, p. 205). This stability contributes to the operation of maintenance forces in a nuclear family. Its members may be able to separate and individuate in an atmosphere of stability and continuity with a strong sense of having a buffer between the family unit and the often chaotic world outside the family. Yet, this stability also can result in a family focusing on maintenance at the expense of adaptation to change. In fact, a common criticism of the nuclear family form has been that it has become too isolated and is unable to respond to current social realities. The "death" of the nuclear family may come about because it has become too limited, too isolated, and too structured to provide its members the flexibility necessary for living in an everchanging technological society.

Stepfamilies, on the other hand, are families born as a result of change. The family structure has been altered dramatically in the course of its life cycle. In fact, stepfamily life often consists of a repetitive series of losing and gaining members, symbolized most dramatically by the movement of children back and forth between divorced parents. Change is omnipresent in a stepfamily.

The stepfamily, then, can be conceptualized as living in a state of crisis, if we define crisis as a normative response to change. The advantage of this is that there are ongoing opportunities to improve family functioning. Family members have the opportunity to experience a variety of relationships, roles, and rules. Positive new experiences can provide a constructive counterbalance to previously negative experiences. The demands of stepfamily life may result in family members increasing their flexibility and their range of possible responses, thus becoming better prepared to respond to new challenges.

The negative side is perhaps a more obvious outcome. The problem often is twofold. First, there can be a lack of stabilizing forces in the family. In its series of changes the family fails to maintain any order and family functioning becomes chaotic. Second, the chaos is destructive. The family's response to change results in a kind of snowballing of negative interactions. Subsystem coalitions may develop in opposition to one another and each interaction between them is a reinforcement of the previous negative interactions and leads to further amplification of the problems. These patterns are all too common between households in the system and result in a problem much larger, more powerful and more destructive than any of its component parts. This view may be quite dystonic for individuals within the system and result in significant loss of self esteem. It may lead to faulty assessment by therapists (see sections on assessment and treatment) who judge the family to be more dysfunctional than it is, and consequently intervene inappropriately or are fearful of becoming involved at all. Two ex-spouses, for example, divorce because of long-standing marital dissatisfaction. She saw him as an uncaring manipulator. He saw her as overly dependent. The postdivorce interactions not only reinforced these mutual perceptions but also the intensity of investment in maintaining them. During their marriage, the couple had some ways to counter temporarily these perceptions - they would talk and make up, have relative periods of calm, be able to see positive traits in each other. After they divorced these counter mechanisms all but disappeared and the couple was left only with increasing suspicion and hostility toward each other. This pattern of increasing amplification of negative perceptions also often can be seen in the relationship between households.

In the previously mentioned example both ex-spouses remarry and the child becomes a member of these new households. The relationship between the ex-spouses continues in the previous postdivorce amplified negative pattern. It is exacerbated even further by the lack of communication, except through the child, whose own fears are rising in proportion to the perceived distortions of the parents. Due to fear of the anger the child reports to the custodial household that discipline he received while visiting the other household was harsh and inappropriate. This resulted in legal and social agencies becoming involved in the investigation of otherwise quite adequate and appropriate parents. This led to increased guilt for the child, and subsequent acting out behavior, requiring the involvement of school authorities. This pattern of increased amplification of negative perceptions resulted in involving systems outside the stepfamily, that as individuals, and individual subsystems, would never have required services. The resolution resided in working with both households together to stop the negative amplification, restore previous perceptions of positive traits and facilitate a more realistic view via direct communication.

Ultimately the lack of homeostatic mechanisms and the propensity toward destructive amplification of deviation in the family results in many stepfamilies being at high risk for continuing dysfunction and ultimately repeated family dissolution. The therapeutic task is to help build stability into the system, to interfere with the destructive amplification, and to use the ongoing family crisis as an opportunity to improve family functioning.

7. A Typology of Stepfamily Functioning

Stepfamilies already have been classified in this chapter according to how they establish family boundaries and how far they have progressed in their family life cycle. In addition, we find it useful to classify them according to their level of organization. Following Beavers (1977), we place families along a continuum in one of three levels of organization. The "severely dysfunctional" families are extremely chaotic, have poorly established boundaries, and repeatedly breach generational boundaries. The "midrange" families are more effective, but are rigidly organized and poorly adapted to change. "Healthy" families are more flexible, have clear boundaries, and enjoy family interactions. Beavers goes on to discuss two distinct styles of interaction at the various levels of organization. Utilizing the work of Stierlin (1972), Beavers says families have either centrifugal patterns that propel members outside the family unit to get needs met, or centripetal patterns that contain need meeting to within the family. These patterns are similar to Minuchin's concepts of disengaged (i.e., centrifugal) and enmeshed (i.e., centripetal) boundaries. The more dysfunctional families generally show one style of interaction, while mixed patterns are more possible in higher levels of organization. We tend to think of five types of stepfamily households.

7.1. Severely Dysfunctional—Centrifugal

These families do not appear to be families at all. There usually is little sense of family identity. Family members often are in some kind of legal difficulties. Family members come and go, and once someone leaves the family he or she is either not heard from again or their involvement is minimal. The stepparent is often one of a series of temporary parental figures who pass through the family. Children have a sense of vagueness regarding parental figures. Physical and sexual abuse may be common in these families. Treatment of these families is very difficult. It usually entails working with other agencies and may involve placement of children. Attempts at solidifying the custodial parent–children subsystem sometimes are successful. In addition, stepparents sometimes want to help change the disengaged patterns in the family and can be used as allies in working with the family, although the danger is that they then will be labeled as the family problem.

7.2. Midrange—Centrifugal

This is a fairly common type of stepfamily. It may be that somewhat isolated patterns began with the dissolved nuclear family (and in fact was a centrally contributing factor to the divorce) and just continue in the stepfamily. The dramatic life changes in stepfamilies may reinforce a more distant style of interaction and distrust of getting needs met within the stepfamily. In addition, if children are older and are involved with both biological parents, there may be less of a desire to create a close family unit. Stepparents often have a limited role in the family. Treatment of these families would need to depend on what the cause of the rigid boundaries is and how much of a problem it is for family members. It may be important to strengthen certain subsystems in the family such as the remarried couple while dispelling the myth that this should be one big happy family. On the other hand, it may be that patterns in the stepfamily are simply repetitions of earlier patterns and the family experiences some sense of pain about this. Then the work may entail trying to get the family to open up their boundaries and allow new relationships to develop gradually. In addition, it would be important to help these families work through old experiences and losses before they can move into new relationships. The advantage of a stepfamily system is that some interaction with the other household and/or the presence of the stepparent may keep the family in some pain and they may be more accessible to intervention.

7.3. Healthy Families

These families have established clear boundaries. Subsystems function in a complementary rather than an oppositional manner. There is a role for the stepparent. These families adapt to new challenges. If they come for treatment there usually is some crisis that momentarily has stymied the family. Crises usually are resolved quickly.

7.4. Midrange—Centripetal

This is a fairly common type of stepfamily. They often attempt to become too close, too soon. These families usually establish a rigid boundary with the other household and act like a nuclear family. The treatment strategy usually is to encourage the stepparent to enter the system more gradually, to allow children to develop some appropriate relationship with their other biological parent, and to begin to discuss the fears behind the family need to be overly close.

7.5. Severely Dysfunctional—Centripetal

These families are an extreme of the midrange centripetal family. They are quite suspicious of outside intervention. Children have a very difficult time growing up and usually several members of the family will have severe individual psychopathology. Communication in the family is chaotic and generational boundaries are very weak. Treatment usually is of long duration and may involve repeated psychiatric hospitalizations of some family members.

Obtaining an overall impression of the level and style of family functioning allows the therapist to develop prognostic hypotheses as well as general treatment approaches.

8. Assessment and Treatment

8.1. Assessment

When a stepfamily comes for treatment, they are usually having difficulties managing some aspect of stepfamily life. The presenting problems can be quite varied. They range from direct expressions of concern that the family is having problems related to being a stepfamily, to a series of more indirect complaints of psychological, physical, social, educational, and/or legal dysfunctions. In the assessment process we are attempting to form hypotheses regarding the connection between the presenting problem, the family's structural patterns and the adequacy of their developmental task resolution. The presenting problem is seen as a consequence and expression of a stepfamily systemic dysfunction.

In the assessment phase of treatment, we are interested in gathering information about the details of stepfamily structure and development. Essentially, the data collection could be organized around two central questions: (1) "What is the reality of your family situation?" and (2) "How well have you adapted to this reality?" More dysfunctional stepfamilies deny or attempt to alter in some fundamental manner, the reality of their family situation. They may, for example, refuse to allow an ex-spouse to have involvement with the children, and require children to call stepparents "mom" or "dad." Pained, but functional stepfamilies, can readily acknowledge the reality of their family situation, but have considerable difficulty adapting to it. These families have a limited and rigid repertoire of overreactive or underreactive responses to problems which arise in stepfamily life. The most functional stepfamilies can both accept their family circumstances, and respond flexibly to any problematic events which arise in the course of stepfamily life. Table 3 is a summary of the types of questions we find useful in our attempt to formulate hypotheses about the adaptation of the stepfamily that comes to us.

The therapist will begin to develop a "diagnosis" of the family dysfunction during the assessment process. A family, for example, might come to treatment with the follow-

Table 3. Assessment Interview

A. The presenting problem

1. Get a detailed description of the presenting problem-nature of problem, extent, duration, precipitating events, etc.
2. How is the family affected by the problem? Who in the family is affected?
3. Does the family understand the problem to be connected to problems in the stepfamily? If so, what do they see as the connection? If not, what do they see the problem related to, if anything?

B. The composition of the family

1. Find out, in some detail, the composition of the stepfamily, system (Use of a genogram is often helpful).
2. How comfortable does the family seem in talking about ex-spouses, steprelationships, extended family, etc?

C. Two (or more) households

1. How are interactions with the other household negotiated and managed? How much interaction is there?
2. What are the custodial, visitation, and financial arrangements between the households?
3. How much does the presenting family know about the other household? Do the kids talk about their experiences with the other household? To what extent?
4. Do the parents in the 2 households talk to each other about the children? Who is involved in these talks? How often do they take place? How do the talks turn out? How do the ex-spouses get along?
5. Begin to make a determination as to how the relationships between the two families relates to the presenting problem. Find out how the family feels about the possibility of therapist involvement with the other household—their response to this question usually reinforces ideas about how the boundaries are established between the two households.

D. The remarriage

1. How long has the couple been married? How many times has each been married?
2. How does the couple describe their marriage? Begin to look for indications of difficulties in communication, parenting, intimacy, finances, division of household tasks, etc.
3. Does the couple experience stepfamily life as an interference in the development of their relationship? Begin to determine if the demands of the stepfamily are, in reality, interfering, or if the demands are being used to avoid addressing marital issues.

E. The biological parent/child(ren) relationships

1. What is the relationship between parent and child like? Find out what this subsystem does together and they do with other members of the family.
2. How has the relationship changed over the past several years, as the family moved from nuclear to single to remarried family? Are there indications of unresolved developmental issues in the family?
3. Has this subsystem retained some sense of identity while, at the same time, allowed for new relationships in the stepfamily to develop? Have they tended to maintain a tie at the expense of the new relationships, or developed new relationships at the expense of the tie?

F. The step relationships

1. What role does the stepparent play in the family? What role do they want to have in the family? Are they allowed, encouraged, forced, prohibited, etc. from playing the role they would like?
2. How does the marital couple negotiate the type of role the stepparent plays? How much does the stepparent participate in child rearing, discipline, limit setting, etc. in the family? Does the couple agree about the value of this involvement?
3. How do children see the stepparent(s)? (Intrusive, helpful, demanding, uninvolved, etc.)? Is a relationship with the stepparent desired, feared, denied, defended against, etc?
4. If there are stepbrother and stepsister, halfbrother and halfsister relationships in the family, evaluate these in terms of closeness, distance, rivalry, sexuality, etc.

ing presentation: "Our daughter's life is being ruined by her father. She gets sick everytime she has to visit him. We wanted to go to court to eliminate visitation but our lawyer suggested we see you first. We'd like her to be able to have a relationship with her father, but not if he keeps treating her like this." The therapist, after gathering more information about the presenting problem, the current visitation arrangements, the history of the divorce and remarriage, and after observing family interactions, may develop the following initial formulation: "This is a pained (or midrange) family. They have few resources to deal adaptively with the presenting problem. This household unit has established its boundaries with the other household in a rigid fashion, cutting off interaction. Within its household boundaries it would like to define itself as a nuclear family. Developmentally, the family has not yet resolved the previous divorce and family members continue, in one form or another, to play out unresolved issues. In addition, the remarried couple seems to be focusing their attention on the daughter and ex-spouse, thus avoiding focusing on their own relationship. The girl is caught in the middle of the adults inability to resolve issues, while at the same time insuring, through her getting the family to focus on her psychosomatic symptoms, the continuation of the single parent headed household, thereby preventing adequate investment in the new family.

Assessment, then, is essentially the process of formulating a family's presenting problem in terms of their structural and developmental characteristics. We develop ideas about the level of organization (healthy, midrange, severely dysfunctional), the style of interaction (distant or close), the boundary establishment between households (rigid or permeable), some of the central struggles of the subsystems of the family, and the unresolved developmental issues in the family. It is from this assessment that we begin to formulate our treatment strategy.

During the course of our assessment, we actively engage the family, or the part of the family we are seeing, in the assessment process. As the family begins to talk about and organize the data, they often begin to gain a new appreciation of the type of family they belong to. Suddenly, they can begin to frame their own symptomotology in light of the stepfamily system dysfunctions as they become more aware of them. Comments such as "No wonder I felt so badly," or "It never felt right to talk about these things, but I always had a sense that something was wrong," are common. Assessment then becomes an active educational and treatment process for the family involved in it. At the same time when families become anxious when we begin to ask questions about the entire stepfamily system, and indicate that they do not understand it has to do with the presenting symptom, the response becomes a valuable part of our assessment.

8.2. Treatment

8.2.1. Who Should Treat Stepfamilies?

Working with stepfamilies requires a tolerance of ambiguity and uncertainty on the part of the therapist. Stepfamilies are complex family units; therefore the work with stepfamilies is also complex. We find it necessary to change directions quickly, see various subsystems at various times during the course of treatment, and attempt to bring together family members who often do not want to be in the same room together. Just as there are few guidelines for the stepfamily to follow in its attempt to become a functioning family unit, there are few guidelines for the therapist to follow in treating stepfamilies. Each stepfamily will bring some unique factors into treatment with them, each requiring some variation in technique on the part of the therapist. The therapist needs to be prepared to be flexible in his/her approach.

Therapists need to have a grounding in family systems theory and technique. They must understand the special characteristics of stepfamilies. They should have an understanding of the effects of divorce on children, and how these interact with the normal developmental task work of children. They must have an appreciation of the interaction between stepfamily structure and the dynamics of the individuals in the family.

It has been our observation that several types of therapeutic approaches are less effective in work with stepfamilies. First, are a group of therapists who do not seem to have an understanding of the characteristics of stepfamilies. Their own values or ideas about families are often based on ideas about nuclear families, and they have difficulty in conceptualizing stepfamily processes, and thus misunderstand the data they collect. For some therapists, increasing their appreciation of stepfamily structure and dynamics is all that is necessary for them to become more effective with stepfamilies. Others may have to explore their basic value judgments about families and the "optimal" family experience before they can begin to take a less judgmental stance with stepfamilies. Second, are a group of therapists who work primarily with individuals in the stepfamily in individual treatment. There may be a tendency for the therapist to view dysfunctions of the individual as primarily an internal process; rather than an expression, at least in part, of the stresses of stepfamily task resolution. If the therapists can begin to develop an appreciation of the interplay between individual dynamics and stepfamily system, we believe that they can work more effectively with individuals in the system. Finally, are a group of therapists who seem overidentified with the stepfamily. These therapists tend to place a great deal of emphasis on society's misunderstanding and mistreatment of the stepfamily, and focus on the normative, healthy aspects of the stepfamily experience. While this educational approach can be very useful, these therapists may be prone to overlook the need to treat specific systemic dysfunctions in individual stepfamily systems, and sometimes reinforce a family's desire to avoid correcting these problems by reassuring them that society, and not the family, has a problem.

Since stepfamilies can be so complex, it is often useful to work with a co-therapist. Sometimes this means working together, in the same room, with a family; at other times, each therapist will work with different subsystems in the family. We are a married couple involved in a stepfamily, and we have usually found that this works to our advantage in working with stepfamilies. However, we certainly do not feel that either being a marital couple, or being involved in a stepfamily, is a requirement for working effectively with stepfamilies. Either, in fact, can be a disadvantage if the couple begins to overidentify with the stepfamilies they see.

8.2.2. Decision Making: Whom to Treat

The decision of whom to see in the stepfamily system can be a complex one. When, for example, should the entire family be seen? Are there contraindications to seeing both households in a stepfamily system? When is marital treatment indicated? What are the indications for individual therapy for members of stepfamilies? When should the course of treatment be changed, such as moving from marital to family treatment? Is it possible to start treatment with one household, and then, after an alliance has formed, bring in the other household? Should stepparents always be included, or are there times when only the ex-spouses should get together to negotiate issues in "the best interests of their children"?

Our own approach is to base our decisions about whom to treat in part on our assessment of the case, and in part, on the basis of the desires and circumstances of the family. We do not always recommend that the entire stepfamily system come in for treatment, and, in fact, feel that, in certain cases, there are contraindications to doing this. Our general feeling is that the treatment needs of the family may change during the course of treatment, and we leave the door open to changing directions in terms of what we do and who we see as treatment progresses. The risk we take in following this approach is the potential of having the family perceive us as being aligned with one subsystem in the family, and to view our attempts to include them later with some suspicion. This is a danger even when we have evaluated the entire stepfamily system in the assessment phase of treatment, and then recommend that one subsystem be worked with initially, and then other subsystems be included later. From our point of view the disadvantages are far outweighed by the advantages we see in basing our decision of whom to see on our assessment of the problems.

No matter who we decide to see in the family, we are always cognizant of the fact that they are only one part of a larger, interconnected system. We are aware that changes in any one subsystem usually has an effect on the rest of the system, and we can anticipate certain countermeasures on the part of the rest of the system in an attempt to bring the system back into some type of equilibrium.

Our approach allows us to see any of the subsystems in the stepfamily system when we feel that this is indicated. Usually the most common subsystems seen are (1) one household unit in the system, (2) the marital couple of one household, (3) the custodial parent and some or all children, (4) all of the adults in the family, including the ex-spouses and each of their respective new spouses, and (5) particular individuals in the family. At times we will see various combinations of these subsystems separately until we feel that they can benefit from coming together. Following are a series of guidelines used to make decisions about who to see in the family and why:

1. Generally, *members of more than one household are seen together when the children have developed symptomatology which seems related to the establishment of rigid boundaries between households,* resulting in a lack of interaction between the households, or in antagonistic interaction between the households. In addition, if both ex-spouses have remarried, the remarriages of both should have enough stability to not be threatened by attempts to improve the interaction between the households.

Case 1. A remarried woman and her husband were referred because of the woman's increasing concern that her ex-spouse was mistreating their two children, particularly their son, who was 12 years old. She had noticed a bruise on her son's arm after one visit, and neither of the children would talk about what had happened. Both children had been having increasing difficulties in school, and both were failing several classes. Her 14 year old daughter seemed sullen and depressed. The mother had called her attorney to see if visitation with the father could be stopped, or if he could be evaluated to see if he was abusing her children. After an evaluation by social services of the husband revealed that he was not an abusive father, and that the boy's bruise was related to a fight he had with his sister, the case was referred for family treatment. The mother was initially quite distressed, feeling that the social service agency had been fooled by her ex-husband, who "can really pull the wool over someone's eyes. He deceived me throughout our marriage." The divorce had occurred seven years previously, and both ex-spouses had been remarried for over four years. Each had children from their new marriages. During the seven years since their divorce the two ex-spouses had few interactions. The two sets of couples were interviewed separately. Both couples were stable in the remarriages, so treatment involving having both couples meet together was recommended. Separate meetings with the couples were used to help lay groundrules for meeting together (emphasizing the goal of working in the best interests of the children), to emphasize to both sides the importance of having the stepparents involved, since both played significant parenting roles, and to talk about each sides fears about getting together. The conjoint meetings began to dispel the fears each had, as they saw that the other parents were struggling with the same parenting issues as they were. They began to see how the children were using the lack of communication between them as a way to manipulate each set of parents. They were astonished to see that each household came up with strikingly similar solutions to problems with kids. The presence of the stepparents provided a useful, and often more objective perspective on some of the problems the children were having. The two couples began to talk about parenting strategies, and about ways to open up communication between the two households. The ex-spouses were able to put aside long standing animosities toward each other in order to work toward problem solving between them. Each indicated that they realized that the other was significant in the lives of their children, and that they did not want their own feelings to interfere in the relationships with the children. Interestingly, both couples reported that the children were quite curious about the sessions the parents were attending. The parents reported that they were beginning to handle the complaints about the other parents in a different manner, and felt that the ways that the children had in raising their anxiety about the job the other household was doing, were no longer able to work. The children seemed relieved, and both began to have improved performances at school. The sullenness of the daughter was no longer seen as a problem. Once the couples were satisfied that they had established better ways of communicating about the children, they decided to terminate the joint sessions, with the understanding that if this communication broke down in the future, they would come back for further help.

2. Generally, *members of more than one household are not seen conjointly when the children have developed symptomatology which seems related to the establishment of permeable boundaries between the households.*

Case 2. A couple came to treatment at the insistence of the stepmother who was becoming increasingly distressed about their relationship with his ex-wife. She felt that she and her husband were unable to have a relationship with each other, and she was contemplating leaving her husband, even though she felt that he was very important to her and her own two children from a previous marriage. The divorced wife was calling their house four or five times a day for advice about numerous problems she would experience during the day. The ex-wife belonged to the same church as the couple, and would sit with them at church. On several occasions the ex-wife engaged the new wife in discussions about the sexual performance of the husband. The two households were within walking distance of each other. The two children experienced severe disturbances manifested by psychotic episodes in the 5 year old girl, and the aggressive behavior on the part of the 9 year old boy. Both seemed confused about which was their primary household, and what names to call their parents. This became even more confused as the biological mother had remarried two other times since the divorce of their biological parents, and she told the children that neither of them were actually fathered by the man they thought to be their father. The husband in this case also had a desire to change the relationship with his ex-wife, but experienced guilt of psychotic proportions whenever he contemplated making these moves (the husband had a history of individual treatment for a schizophrenic disorder. Psychotic episodes were common around separations and loss). The treatment strategy in this case was to begin to help the couple establish a boundary with the other household. Despite the severe dysfunctions in this family, the couple gradually moved toward more appropriate limit setting with the ex-wife. This work was gradual, because any attempts to move quickly in the direction of putting a boundary between the two households led to an increase in the psychotic delusions on the part of the husband in response to the angry retaliatory moves by his ex-wife. The marital couple was able to agree that the current type of involvement with the ex-wife was destructive for them and for the children. They also realized that moves away would cause increased anger from the ex-wife and increased disturbances in the children. They decided that this was the necessary, and ultimately less destructive course to take. The family began to limit phone and social contact. They joined another church. Eventually, they moved to another part of town. Each move resulted in a stronger bond between the couple, and an increased ability to anticipate, and respond to the manifestations of psychopathology in the children. After extensive treatment, the psychiatric disturbances of the children diminished as they were able to respond to the increased stability of the couple. The biological mother was able, after considerable expression of anger, to develop a fragile, but growing alliance with the individual therapist of one of the children. She used this to replace the loss of the relationship with the husband. The therapist was gradually able to help the mother utilize slightly more appropriate parenting skills with her children, and was used as a sounding board when she was angry with the other household. In this case the therapists consistently denied attempts of the divorced husband and wife to meet together to "talk about all of our problems," feeling that this would only reinforce the already overly permeable boundaries in the family.

3. Generally, *members of two households will not be seen conjointly when the potential risks in doing so appear to outweigh the benefits.* This is often a judgement call in which the dysfunction between households, and its negative effect on children, has to be weighed against a dysfunction within one of the households. This is often the case *when one of the marital relationships appears to be quite tenuous.* In these cases, the family dilemma of having multiple, but conflicting problems, is one that is discussed openly with the couple. The importance of a stable relationship in meeting the challenges of stepfamily life is emphasized. Usually, the other side of the ambivalence of working on the marital relationship involves a sense of guilt, often on both the biological and stepparent's part regarding the difficulties one or more of the children are having. The couple has a difficult bind to work out. If they attend to their marriage, they fear that they are damaging the children. If they attend to their children, and problems between households, they are unable to deal effectively with the problem, because of their inability to negotiate a workable marital relationship. Particular care should be taken not to involve an ex-spouse in parental negotiations when there appears to be some continuing ties between the ex-spouses which can further threaten and destabilize the marital relationship.

4. Generally, *members of more than one household will not be seen conjointly when the children do not seem to be manifesting difficulties which have as their source problems of household boundary establishment.* Often the source of problems for children will be related to either problems within one or both households, or to unresolved developmental problems not currently being maintained by the system.

Case 3. A family consisting of father, stepmother, and 14 year old girl, came to treatment with the following presenting problem: At times, the girl was not cooperative around the house and seemed withdrawn and depressed. The couple went back and forth feeling angry with her because of her passive noncompliance, and feeling sadness because they recognized that her behavior often coincided with interactions with her biological mother. The biological mother was a severely depressed woman who had been repeatedly hospitalized for chronic depression and treated with a variety of medications and shock therapy. She had a long standing drug abuse problem. The mother moved in and out of town, and when she was in town would call her daughter, promise her a variety of things, but then fail to show up for scheduled meeting times. The family had struggled with how much contact to allow the mother, but, on the advice of their lawyer, had never stopped regularly arranged visitation agreements. Over the years, when the mother was in town, she would have the girl, then in latency, for periods ranging from a weekend, to as long as several weeks duration during the summer. Her care of the girl was inconsistent, and often neglectful. There were times when she would not get up until 3 or 4 in the afternoon, and the girl would be faced with having to take care of herself all day. The mother had always made the girl promise not to talk to her father about her visits.

The stepfamily unit itself was a stable family unit and the girl had a positive, trusting relationship with the stepmother. The family had difficulties expressing feelings, and in knowing how to help the girl with her obvious depression around contact with the mother. The father, in particular, had difficulties with this, and this was compounded by his desire not to "bad mouth" the biological mother, even though he had strong concerns about her ability to care for the daughter.

The treatment in this case involved engaging the family in the process of sharing their sadness, and in learning to help the girl with her particular difficulties in interacting with her mother. After sharing their own guilt about allowing the mother as much visitation as they did over the years, they began to more directly empathize with the girl, and help her out of her dilemmas with the mother. The girl was able to begin to share her sense of aloneness when with the mother, and get help sorting out that she was not responsible for the mother's problems. The girl, with the family's help, was able to engage in a mourning process, and to come to grips with the reality of her biological mother. The bond with the stepmother became further solidified, and the lines of communication with her father opened up considerably, to the delight of both. The girl's moods and behavior improved significantly.

5. Generally, *subsystems in the family will be seen when there are particular tasks that that subsystem needs to resolve, independent of the rest of the family.* The two most common subsystems seen in treatment are the marital couple subsystem, and the subsystem consisting of a biological parent and his/her children.

A. A *marital couple* is seen when the marital relationship is easily disrupted by tbe stresses involved in forming a stepfamily, and/or when the couple avoids attending to issues arising in the marriage by focusing primarily on issues which arise in the stepfamily. Besides the usual assessment of marital issues around intimacy and sexuality, communication, division of labor, etc., the therapist should look for specific indications that the couple is experiencing stepfamily life as an interference in the development of their relationship.

When a couple cannot seem to attend to their marriage primarily because of the stresses involved in stepparenting, and the disruptions involved in interacting with an ex-spouse, the initial work should focus on problem solving around how the couple can begin to develop ways to "draw a line around" their relationship, and insulate themselves, to some degree, from the disruptions they have repeatedly responded to. Often, the work will involve exploring with the couple the reasons they so easily allow themselves to be drawn into conflict in the family. For the biological parent, this may be connected to a sense of guilt about putting their children through the divorce and remarriage process, and a defensive overresponding to problems which arise. For a stepparent, it may involve unrealistic expectations about what they would be able to accomplish in the new family, and/or a defensive overinvolvement as a reaction to their resentment about the problems which arise in the family.

When a couple attends to problems in the family primarily as a result of their fears of focusing on their marriage, the initial work often involves a gradual reframing of the problem. Stepfamily issues are framed in terms of their effects on the couple, and the process by which they work together on the problem. Parenting and stepfamily system issues usually evolve gradually into marital issues. The work then involves exploring their fears in the marriage. For the previously married spouse, there is usually some fear of repeated failure, and a fear of becoming involved in the same type of dysfunctional marital interaction patterns as existed in a prior marriage. For the previously unmarried spouse, there may be a fear that they will not live up to the expectations of the other spouse, both in the parenting and marital spheres, and/or that their inexperience puts them at some disadvantage with their more experienced spouse.

Usually, couples present a mixture of the two types of problems discussed. They find the realities of stepfamily life to interfere in their ability to attend to their marriage, yet use this reality as a way to avoid exploring their fears in the marriage.

B. A *biological parent and his/her children* are seen when this subsystem has unresolved issues from the past unrelated to events in the stepfamily and/or when the events in the stepfamily begin to interfere in the ability of the subsystem to maintain a stable tie.

There are many times a stepfamily is formed prior to the resolution of previous developmental issues. There has not been an ability, desire, and/or opportunity to share feelings, perceptions, distortions, and so forth, regarding the common history of the family. In addition, the lack of task resolution interferes in the ability of the family to adapt to the new stepfamily. Treatment often proceeds more rapidly when this subsystem is seen alone, as the presence of new family members may more easily allow the issue to be sidestepped. Common issues discussed are feelings about the previous divorce, disruptions in the parent/child relationship during the separation and post divorce periods, and the fears of further disruptions of the relationship.

Closely related to the unresolved developmental issues, is the tendency in some families for this subsystem to begin to lose its identity in the larger stepfamily system. This is often seen in families where there is some spoken or unspoken pressure for family members to bond together as if they were a nuclear family. Treatment often focuses on the need of the subsystem to retain an important bond despite the involvement of other family members. The subsystem may be instructed to do things together independently of the rest of the family. This may stimulate issues related to the family's need to attempt to make a nuclear family, with the source of this attempt often related to avoid past pain by "starting over."

6. Generally, *when a stepfamily household is having problems in integrating as a family unit, it is recommended that the entire household unit become the unit of treatment.* The presenting problem is often a steprelationship conflict, whether it be stepparent/stepchildren, stepsibling, or stepsibling/halfsibling conflicts. It is, of source, important to evaluate for the source of the manifest problem. The steprelationship conflict often serves as a cover for other unresolved problems in the family. When this is the case, the course of the problem needs to be treated, and less emphasis is placed on the manifest expression of the problem.

When the therapist is satisfied that the steprelation issues are the manifestation of investment difficulties in the stepfamily household unit, all members of the household unit are asked to participate in the treatment. Steprelationship problems are conceptualized as a family problem, and not simply as an interactive problem between steprelations. The biological parent is usually a significant factor in the development of a steprelationship problem. The biological parent is involved in negotiations with both children (the parent/child subsystem) and spouse (the marital subsystem) in determining how involved the spouse will be with children, and how free children will be to develop a relationship with stepparents and other stepchildren in the family. The biological parent may then become the "power broker" in the family,determining who can have how much power in the family. The other family members, baving some ambivalence about forming relationships with each other, may attempt to give the biological parent power, even when the parent desires to allow relationships to develop in the family.

Case 4. A mother, stepfather, and 10 year old son came to treatment hoping to get an evaluation of the son. The boy had developed some rather severe obsessive-compulsive rituals, spending hours eating dinner or getting undressed at night. Whenever asked a question, he would pause for a long period of time, and then, with great difficulty, stutter out an answer. The family had been together for 5 years. The mother had divorced her first husband when the boy was 2, and the boy visited the father, who lived in another state, every summer. The couple was alarmed about the symptoms of the boy, but also angry at his withdrawal and refusal to participate in family life. The mother was particularly concerned about the stepfather's difficulty in forming a relationship with the boy, feeling that her son would benefit from a relationship with her husband. She was fearful that the son would become like his father, who was a withdrawn and noncommunicative man, and hoped he could begin to identify with her second husband, who was quite verbal and communicative. The stepfather agreed that he and his stepson had a poor relationship, but attributed this to his close attachment to his mother.

Assessment of the family made it clear that all family members participated in both the development of the symptom and in the maintenance of the family structure in which the symptom developed. The mother wanted the son to develop a relationship with the stepfather, but also feared that he might be hurt in the relationship. She gave out conflicting messages to the son about whether he could have a relationship or not. In the same way she encouraged the husband to have a relationship, but to do it in a way that reduced her anxiety. The husband, for his part, wanted to please the wife, but sensed that whenever he attempted to do something with the son, that it wouldn't live up to her standards. The son was trapped between the conflicting messages of "Have a relationship", "Don't have a relationship", and became paralyzed and angry. He attempted to draw his mother in to the same type of close relationship they had prior to the marriage, as a way out of the dilemma. At the same time, he clearly wanted to have a relationship with the stepfather. Interestingly, the stepfather and son both reported having a good relationship when the mother was not present.

When the family was able to begin to understand each's ambivalence and could talk about the binds each of them experienced, gradual progress was made toward establishing a stepfather/stepson relationship. The mother realized that in order for the son to develop a relationship with the stepfather, her own relationship with both son and husband would need to change. The father also realized this and moved to more of an equal partner status with his wife. The son began to free up and gave up both stuttering and the bulk of the obsessive-compulsive behavior. He continued to struggle with giving up a close tie with his mother, but was able to verbalize this, and stopped attempting to pull his mother back into an infantile relationship with him.

7. Generally, *individuals in a stepfamily are seen in individual psychotherapy under the following circumstances:*

A. When an individual is struggling with issues quite independent of whatever is going on in the stepfamily. This should be evaluated carefully, because a wide range of presenting problems can be expressions of stepfamily dysfunction.

B. When one family member is seeking treatment and the rest of the family refuses treatment. Often, the treatment involves helping the individual sort out their own individual issues from the family's need to make the individual the problem. The question "What do you want to do about your family's refusal to involve themselves in treatment?" needs to be raised.

C. Individuals are seen when some trauma occurring during the course of development of the family, has overwhelmed one particular individual's capacity to overcome the trauma. An example of this would be when a child has had a parent die at a particularly vulnerable age, and cannot seem to attach to new members of the family. Ideally, the family is used adjunctively, both as a support to the individual member, but also to help other family member their own unresolved, but less devastating responses to the loss.

D. An individual is seen when that individual becomes symptomatic as a result of preexisting psychological conflicts that are "stirred up" by stresses in the stepfamily, and when the therapist ascertains that the rest of the family is not invested and/or able to work on these problems within the context of family treatment.

The structure of the stepfamily system can lend itself, in many ways, to family member's individual dysfunctional dynamics becoming exacerbated and repeatedly enacted in stepfamily life. Incompletely resolved issues such as sense of identity and belonging, masochistic savior fantasies, abuse and neglect scenarios, and so forth, take root in the ambiguous stepfamily soil. The family structure is often unclear enough that it becomes like a projective test for family members. Incidents in the family become "proof" for the vulnerable individual that they are not wanted, that they are doomed to fail, that they are inadequate, second best, unloved, and so on.

It can be helpful to an individual in the stepfamily to get a better perspective on the source of the internal conflict. The person can then begin to sort out internal vulnerability from external stresses and respond more effectively to both. Interactive patterns within the system can be broken when the individual stops enacting their side of the process.

8. In a broader sense, *whom the therapist sees in treatment is dependent, in part, on the therapist's prioritizing of the structural and developmental problems in the family.* An ex-spouse not being included in treatment when a remarried couple's relationship is tenuous (see Guideline 3) is but one example of this process. The therapist needs to formulate a strategy based on what problems are determined to be of higher priority than others, and this will result in not only decisions about whom to see, but also, on what material to address when the therapist is meeting with a family.

The questions in prioritizing problems are "What problem or problems have to be focused on first before we can proceed to other issues?," "What problems *can* wait?," "What problems *have to* wait given the vulnerability of the system?," and "What problems are best left unaddressed?" Problems that prevent stability in the family or that tend to threaten whatever stability the family has achieved usually are of top priority.

Families with overly permeable boundaries, for example, are unable to form a family identity, and so the first therapeutic task in these families is to help them to establish a boundary that would allow them to develop relationships with each other. The work on developmental problems usually has to wait until there is some stable forces in the family, or the work will simply overwhelm the family and add to the instability in the system.

Prioritizing a family's problems with the family can be particularly useful for the family. Stepfamilies who seek treatment often are feeling overwhelmed by the heavy load of task work they must face. The prioritizing lends some sense of stability to the family as they begin to develop a way to sort out their problems.

8.2.3. Treatment Modalities with Stepfamilies

In addition to stepfamily system, household unit, marital, parent/child, and individual treatment approaches, there are several other modalities that may be used to particular advantage with stepfamilies. These are:

Couples' Groups. These are marital couple psychotherapy groups, the members of which are all involved in remarriages. They are open ended groups of four or five couples. Issues generally revolve around all of the areas spelled out in this chapter, with the main focus around parenting issues and marital difficulties in the context of stepfamily life. Generally, couples who have mastered some of the initial taskwork of stepfamily life and are struggling with role, boundary, and intimacy issues connected primarily with the remarriage are most appropriate for this type of group.

Educational Groups. These are time limited groups for couples, with the focus on providing information for families involved in remarriages. Almost all families can benefit from education about what to expect in a stepfamily. The more adaptive families may need only education. Other families may use the information to better understand what their difficulties are and to formulate better their need for treatment. The educational groups usually focus on a different theme at every session. Common themes are "surviving the divorce," "mourning losses," "new rules/old rules," "being a stepparent," "dealing with children," "having children of our own," and so on. Sharing common problems can be therapeutic to a family and reassures them that they are not alone in their struggles.

Parent Counseling. Parents often are confused about what is "normal" and what is "abnormal" behavior in a stepfamily. They often are at a loss as to how to deal with some common problems that arise in a stepfamily, but would never be at issue in a nuclear family, such as handling children's refusal to go to visit the other parent, threats of living with the other parent, and refusal to accept discipline from a stepparent. Providing counseling to help parents sort out what is an expectable developmental struggle for a child and what is a reaction to unusual strains in the system is often useful to a couple. Learning how to be a parent in a stepfamily can require a somewhat different set of skills than parenting in a nuclear family. Parent counseling also can be a way to begin to explore how the couple works with each other to make decisions and can be a useful tool in opening up broader issues of the remarried couple's marital relationship and the rules governing it.

Stepfamily Mediation. Whenever ex-spouses are asked to meet to resolve issues in the "best interests of the children," it is useful to conceptualize this as a mediational process, and not as a psychotherapy process. The contract involves working on the goal of removing the impediments that prevent parents from working effectively in the best interests of their children. With the groundrules clearly spelled out, it is easier for parents and therapists to avoid delving into unresolved emotional issues of a divorced couple. At the same time, it is important to allow parents to work at accepting the reality of their stepfamily system. The importance of both households is emphasized, the needs of all adults to work together in their children's best interest, and the interdependency of the system, are all factors which are emphasized during the course of a stepfamily mediation.

Whenever there are stepparents involved in the family system, it is important to attempt to involve them in the mediation work. At times, someone in the family will make a bid to exclude them from sessions. This is usually based on some resistance to accepting the reality of stepfamily structure and the importance of the stepparent in family life. Once exploring the reasons someone in the family wants to exclude the stepparent, the therapist emphasizes their importance in family life, and the need to include them in all parental discussions.

Stepfamily mediation is most effective with, as previously discussed, families who have established rigid boundaries between households. A subgroup who can respond positively to mediation are families who struggle ineffectively with a previously established divorce settlement that no longer fits the current needs of family members in their new circumstances. The old settlements may become a roadblock to further development in the family (see Katz, 1982).

9. Conclusion

The treatment of a stepfamily requires that the therapist have a clear understanding of stepfamily structure, dynamics, and development. The therapist must be able to help the family acknowledge, gain an appreciation for, and begin to develop flexible adaptations to a complex family system.

In working with a stepfamily, the therapist, like the family, is often required to tolerate a high degree of frustration, and sense of uncertainty. Stepfamilies often report that they have a sense that their own family life is out of their control, and that they are dependent on the whims of ex-spouses, unsympathetic legal systems, and unsupportive support systems. Basic issues of what is a family, what is a parent, and what is a home, are ones that are raised repeatedly in stepfamilies. A family's attempts to problem solve can meet with seemingly unsolvable dilemmas, and stirs up in them basic doubts about their adequacy to deal with everyday problems.

The therapist must be able to enter the stepfamily system, and attempt to develop a feasible treatment strategy that addresses the multiple layers of dysfunction often seen in stepfamilies. Without an understanding of the stepfamily system, and the ability to properly "diagnose" a stepfamily's presenting problem in terms of its particular structural and developmental characteristics, the therapist is unable to be effective with the stepfamily. Treatment procedes more effectively when the therapist develops the conceptual skills necessary to appreciate the complexity of stepfamily life.

10. References

Aldous, J. The making of family roles and family change. *The Family Coordinator,* 1974, *23,* 231–235.
Aldous, J. *Family careers: Developmental change in families.* New York: Wiley, 1978.
Beavers, W. R. *Psychotherapy and growth: A family systems perspective.* New York: Brunner/Mazel, 1977.
Capaldi, F., & McRae, B. *Stepfamilies: A cooperative responsibility.* Viewpoints Vision Books, 1979.

Draughon, M. Stepmother's model of identification in relation to mourning in the child. *Psychological Reports,* 1975, *36(1),* 183–189.

Duvall, E. *Marriage and family development.* Philadelphia: Lippincott, 1977.

Fast, I., & Cain, A. The stepparent role: Potential for disturbances in family functioning. *American Journal of Orthopsychiatry,* 1966, *36,* 485–491.

Glasser, P., & Navarre, E. Structural problems of the one-parent family. *Journal of Social Issues,* 1965, *21,* 98–109.

Goldstein, H. Reconstituted families: The second marriage and its children. *Psychiatric Quarterly,* 1974, *48,* 433–440.

Heatherington, M. Divorce: A child's perspective. *American Psychologist,* 1979, *34,* 851–858.

Hoffman, L. *Foundations of family therapy: A conceptual framework for systems change.* New York: Basic Books, 1981.

Katz, L. *A conceptual model for understanding stepfamilies.* Unpublished doctoral thesis, 1980. (a)

Katz, L. Adult development in a stepfamily. Unpublished paper, 1980. (b)

Katz, L. Stepfamilies: A family systems perspective. In *7th annual child custody* workshop handbook. Denver, Co.: National Center for Continuing Legal Education, Inc., 1982.

Katz, L., & Zeiger, C. Stepfamilies. In R. Hinds & W. Wittlin (Eds.), *Child custody for the lawyer, judge, and mental health professions: An interdisciplinary approach.* New York: Irvington Press, in press.

Kelly, J., & Wallerstein, J. The effects of parental divorce: Experiences of the child in early latency. *American Journal of Orthopsychiatry,* 1976, *46,* 20–32.

Lewis, J., Beavers, W. R., Gossett, J., & Phillips, V. *No single thread: Psychological health in family systems.* New York: Brunner/Mazel, 1976.

Maddox, B. *The half parent.* New York: Evans, 1975.

Marotz-Baden, R., Adams, G., Bueche, N., Munro, B., & Munro, G. Family form or family process? Reconsidering the deficit family model approach. *The Family Coordinator,* 1979, *28,* 5–14.

Minuchin, S. *Families and family therapy.* Cambridge: Harvard University Press, 1974.

Roosevelt, R., & Lofas, J. *Living in step: A remarriage manual for parents and children.* New York: McGraw-Hill, 1976.

Sager, C., Steer, H., Crohn H., Rodstein, E., & Walker, E. Remarriage revisited. *Family and Child Mental Health Journal,* 1980, *6,* 19–33.

Sager, C., Walker, E., Brown, H., Crohn, H., & Rodstein, E. Improving functioning of the remarried family system. *Journal of Marital and Family Therapy,* 1981, *7,* 3–13.

Shorter, E. *The making of the modern family.* New York: Basic Books, 1975.

Solomon, M. A developmental, conceptual premise for family therapy. *Family Process,* 1973, *12,* 179–188.

Stierlin, H. *Separating parents and adolescents.* New York: Quadrangle/New York Times, 1972.

Toomin, M. K. The child of divorce. In R. Hardy & J. Cull (Eds), *Therapeutic needs of the family.* Springfield, Ill.: Charles C Thomas, 1974.

Turner, R. Role taking: Process vs. Conformity. In A. Rose (Ed.), *Human behavior and social process.* Boston: Houghton Mifflin, 1962.

Visher, E., & Visher J. Common problems of stepparents and their spouses. *American Journal of Orthopsychiatry,* 1978, *48*(2), 252–262.

Visher, E., & Visher, J. *Stepfamilies: A guide to working with stepparents and stepchildren.* New York: Brunner/Mazel, 1979.

Walker, K., & Messinger, L. Remarriage after divorce: Dissolution and reconstruction of family boundaries. *Family Process,* 1979, *18,* 185–192.

Walker, K. N., Rogers, J., & Messinger, L. Remarriage after divorce: A review. *Social Casework,* 1977, *58,* 276–285.

Wallerstein, J., & Kelly, J. The effects of parental divorce: Experiences of the preschool child. *Journal of the American Academy of Child Psychiatry,* 1974, *14,* 600–616. (a)

Wallerstein, J., & Kelly, J. The effects of parental divorce: The adolescent experience. In A. Koupernik (Ed.), *The child in his family.* New York: Wiley, 1974. (b)

Wallerstein, J., & Kelly, J. The effects of parental divorce: Experiences of the child in later latency. *American Journal of Orthopsychiatry,* 1976, *46,* 256–269.

Wallerstein J., & Kelly, J. Effects of divorce on the visiting father-child relationship. *American Journal of Psychiatry,* 1980, *137*(12), 1534–1538.

Whiteside, M., & Auerbach, L. Can the daughter of my father's new wife be my sister?: Families of remarriage in family therapy. *Journal of Divorce,* 1978, *1*(3), 271–283.

20

Sex Therapy for Couples

RUTH E. CLIFFORD AND ROBERT C. KOLODNY

Therapy for sexual dysfunctions or dissatisfactions has existed at least since the advent of psychoanalysis. Traditionally, lengthy treatment and broad-based personality change were seen as prerequisites for reversal of these symptoms. More recently, in the 1950s and 1960s, briefer treatments that specifically addressed the target sexual complaints developed. Behavior therapy (see Annon, 1974; Wolpe, 1958), cognitive therapy, (e.g., Ellis, 1968) and family therapy (e.g., Sager, 1976) all made strides in this area, working sometimes with individuals and sometimes with couples, or indeed larger family units. Masters and Johnson's publication in 1970 of *Human Sexual Inadequacy* sparked much wider acceptance of the value of dealing with both partners when sexual dysfunction or dissatisfaction is the complaint. This chapter gives an overview of the current status of therapy for couples[1] with sexual problems, emphasizing the Masters and Johnson approach but also discussing contributions of other leading sex therapists as these vary from, and often deliberately modify, the Masters and Johnson model.

Two types of sexual problems are considered in this chapter: sexual dysfunctions, which involve impaired physiological arousal or orgasm, and sexual dissatisfactions, which cover a wider range of problems not specifically associated with impairment of the sexual reflexes. Examples of the latter category include fear or guilt concerning otherwise desired sexual behaviors and conflicts between partners about some aspect of their sexual interaction such as timing, setting, types of activity, or frequency. Also under the heading of sexual dissatisfaction would be problems commonly termed "desire phase disorders." These include sexual aversion and inhibited sexual desire.

Why sex therapy for *couples?* Although no well designed research to date demonstrates the superiority of couple over individual therapy for sexual problems, there are a number of reasons to expect advantages from the couple approach in a large percentage of

[1]For the purpose of this chapter a "couple" will be considered as a heterosexual marriage, and examples of therapy will be presented within that framework. The reader should know, however, that most of these same principles apply in working with homosexual couples, unmarried couples, and to a somewhat lesser degree, with individuals using surrogate partners.

RUTH E. CLIFFORD • Department of Psychiatry & Behavioral Sciences, Stanford University School of Medicine, Stanford, California 94305. **ROBERT C. KOLODNY** • Masters and Johnson Institute, 24 S. Kingshighway, St. Louis, Missouri 63108.

cases. In terms of assessment, taking histories from two sexual partners separately often reveals vital information that would not have been available from one partner only. For example, one impression may be gained of an individual's motivation to change by asking the person directly. Quite another may unfold in the partner's description of that person's behavior and remarks while applying for therapy and on the way to the first visit. Interviewing the partner can add materially to the therapist's understanding of a problem's development. When she was not orgasmic, for instance, did he try so hard to give her an orgasm that she felt under a spotlight and thus even less free to let go? Or, if he lost his erection, did she start pretending to not be interested in sex to protect him from feeling inadequate?

Masters and Johnson state that "there is no such thing as an uninvolved partner," which means that the existence of a sexual problem has an effect not only on the dysfunctional individual but also on the partner, and the partner's reaction, often well intended, can in fact perpetuate and even aggravate the problem. An important part of therapy is to highlight this dynamic so that as one individual changes his or her attitudes and expectations the other is fully informed and understands how his or her own attitudes and expectations need to readjust. The chances of backsliding due to inadvertent partner reactions are thus reduced. In some cases, as systems theory teaches us, partners actually may be invested in each other's difficulties. A good history with the "asymptomatic" partner may alert the therapist to this possibility, allowing attention to that person's own insecurities as therapy moves along. Finally, some partners react to their spouses' dysfunctions by developing sexual symptoms of their own. Such a development is not uncommon in, for instance, partners of women with vaginismus, who may develop impotence. Therapeutic contact with only the "identified patient" may miss the important contribution of secondary dysfunction in the partner in maintaining the presenting problem.

A final prefatory word: All of the treatment methods described in this chapter have been reported to be highly effective in work with series of cases. The number of cases and the duration of follow-up varies tremendously. Few of these approaches have been subjected to rigorous evaluation in comparison to no-treatment or placebo control groups or compared systematically with one another. Where meaningful comparisons have been carried out, those results will be noted in the text. Recent overviews of the effectiveness of sex therapy, with couples as well as individuals, have been thoughtfully presented by Marks (1981), Schumacher (1977), Stuart and Hammond (1980), and Wright, Perreault, and Mathieu (1977), along with astute comments regarding theoretical and methodological issues. All agree that these methods show promise but that more attention to diagnostic and evaluation strategies is needed. Interested readers are referred to the above reviews for a detailed examination of the effectiveness question.

1. Concepts of Sex Therapy

At the outset, it is important to recognize that sex therapy is a form of psychotherapy that deals principally, but not exclusively, with sexual problems. Like other forms of psychotherapy, sex therapy begins in a diagnostic, data-building phase and proceeds to a series of interventions individualized to suit the dynamics of each case. Some modalities of sex therapy, such as the Masters and Johnson approach, tend to be directive rather than interpretive, but almost all practitioners of sex therapy to some extent help clients obtain insight into the factors maintaining their problems as part of the process. Here, we will review some of the core concepts of sex therapy that are applicable to the vast majority of cases.

1.1. Sex as a Natural Function

Social learning is clearly a major influence on human sexual behavior. However, as Masters and Johnson repeatedly have emphasized (e.g., 1972, 1976), the physiological events of sexual response are natural reflex functions that do not require training. One illustration of this fact is that vaginal lubrication and penile erection are commonly observed in newborn infants. In addition, it is well documented that during sleep healthy adults exhibit these reflex signs of sexual arousal in a regular cycle and also can experience orgasm. The fact that sex is subject to the impact of thoughts and emotions during the waking state is quite similar to the ways in which other natural functions such as breathing or bowel or bladder function also are influenced by these processes.

This perspective has implications for the way in which sexual dysfunctions arise as well as for their treatment. In some cases, cultural expectations subvert the naturalness of sexual function. For instance, the common notion that a male should be instantly aroused at the drop of a bra imposes a performance criterion that may trigger anxiety; the anxiety (either on the part of the male, who is worried he is not "measuring up," or on the part of the woman, who may become concerned about her own attractiveness or her ability to arouse her partner) often tends to dampen sexual response further. In other cases, too much thinking about sexual techniques (or too much goal orientation) becomes an obstacle to natural sexual function. In general, attempts to force sexual response usually make the desired response more elusive.

Therapy for sexual dysfunctions, in Masters and Johnson's view, is more a matter of removing the factors that impede functioning than of specifically teaching how to respond. Although an important part of sex therapy is education to undo learned misconceptions about sex, the physiological events of sexual response themselves usually only require being allowed to surface. Although this may be a complex process employing a number of strategies to reduce anxiety, dissipate guilt, foster intimacy, and repair self-esteem, "teaching" the "how-to's" of sex rarely is effective.

1.2. Performance Fears and Spectatoring

One of the signal achievements of Masters and Johnson's early work on sex therapy was pinpointing the nearly universal existence of performance fears as a major roadblock to sexual response and satisfaction. Anxieties about the adequacy of one's sexual performance may arise in a number of different ways. For instance, sexual activity with a new partner commonly provokes a degree of anticipatory anxiety that relates to both unfamiliarity with the partner's style and preferences and to uncertainty about the partner's expectations. As another example, performance fears often follow an episode construed as "failure" and, as these fears mount or accumulate before the next sexual encounter, they often turn into self-fulfilling prophecies.

The primary reason for this is that performance anxieties typically tend to distract people from savoring the erotic and interpersonal components of a sexual situation while they instead focus on observing and evaluating their own response. The ostensible purpose of this so-called spectator's role is to alleviate anxiety by checking to see that everything is proceeding smoothly, but the actual result is that the diminished spontaneity and involvement have negative repercussions that magnify, rather than lessen, performance fears. This triggers a fear-spectatoring-greater fear cycle that eventually becomes contagious, so that the partner joins in the anxious vigil and intimacy and spontaneity are reduced even more. Thus, what may have begun as an individual problem typically becomes the couple's problem. Because of the tenaciousness of this spectatoring cycle, a large part of sex therapy often is devoted to strategies for anxiety reduction and helping the couple attend to the erotic stimuli in their interaction in a fashion that frees them from the need to rate each episode as "success" or "failure."

1.3. Sensate Focus

One means employed by most sex therapists to reduce anxiety and to create a relaxed framework of intimacy in which the naturalness of sexual function can emerge is a series of touching experiences devised by Masters and Johnson (1970) as "sensate focus" (see Hartman & Fithian, 1974, and Kaplan, 1974, for variations). Beginning on the first day with an explicit ban on *sexual* touching, that is, with the breasts and genitals "off-limits," the couple progresses to including genital touching, mutual (simultaneous) touching, genital-to-genital touching in the female astride position without penile insertion, and penile-vaginal containment. These stages serve merely as a point of departure in tailoring suggestions to each couple's specific needs. The emphasis throughout is on awareness of physical sensations without either the need to work toward a goal, to respond in a particular manner, or to evaluate the experience in terms of specific performance criteria. Secondarily, the sensate focus exercises provide a matrix in which couples can improve their nonverbal communication skills.

Sensate focus has a variety of purposes that vary to some extent depending on the specific problem(s) being treated. It can help couples break out of old patterns of trying to touch in the "right" way, which may have become stultifying for both people. It provides an opportunity for sensations to take on an erotic quality and accumulate within a session and even from day to day. Freedom from having to go on to intercourse or orgasm can allow earlier stages of sexual involvement to emerge more readily. Sensate focus also can serve to desensitize anxiety connected with having to perform or with touching or being touched in certain areas or certain ways. Perhaps of equal importance, it can establish or regenerate a sense of closeness and acceptance in the couple where fears and/or hostilities have caused them to avoid contact.

Sensate focus opportunities can surface emotions and lead to insights about previously mystifying inhibitions. For instance, a woman kneeling over her husband may find herself pounding on his chest and then burst into tears. She may then realize the depth of her anger at him, which she may have denied up to that point. Finally, sensate focus can serve as a diagnostic tool. In some couples it has been so long since they last had a sexual encounter that the therapists may not know until they have interacted for several days just what types of difficulties may emerge. In addition, because many people's recall of their past sexual experiences is somewhat hazy and overgeneralized, discussing specific details of a sensate focus session gives the therapists a more accurate means of assessing the quality and dynamics of the couple's interaction.

1.4. The Role of Communication

Communication, the exchange of information between a sender and a receiver, receives tremendous emphasis in most couples' sex therapy. The basis for this approach is the intimate connection between sexual response and satisfaction and the ability to express emotions and desires, both in the sexual arena and in the relationship at large (Masters & Johnson, 1970, 1975).

Communication skills include both verbal and nonverbal modalities. Both forms depend on a fundamental state of openness and trust between the partners, what Masters and Johnson call vulnerability (Masters & Johnson, 1975). Since just the opposite state exists in many cases at the outset of therapy, practice in communication usually is started at a very basic level.

The process of enhancing verbal communication skills commences with the device of representing one's self in simple sentences starting with the pronoun "I" to convey immediate feelings and wishes. Judgment of these feelings is avoided; rather, any differences in needs are negotiated through a search for mutually acceptable alternatives or, when this is impossible or impractical, using the guiding principle of going in the direction of the person whose need is greatest as long as this does not involve hurting the other partner. The couple discovers in the initial phases much that may have been lost or never realized in their ability to enjoy and trust each other. They can respect each other's moods, try new activities, and support each other through difficult times. As they progress, more loaded areas may be opened up for discussion. The couple may be able to share deeper feelings of fear as well as hope and positive feelings toward each other. Long held secrets may be aired and seen in less threatening perspective. Areas that before were extremely conflicted, such as how one person deals with the children, or decisions about job hours, or whether one person is willing to try oral-genital sex, become topics for calmer and friendly exploration. In addition, skills for accurately *receiving* messages as well as sending them are emphasized. Since any information may be garbled unwittingly by the receiver's listening bias, both spouses are instructed to check out how their messages were interpreted if they get an untoward or unexpected response. Nonverbal communication is developed through various suggestions in the context of sensate focus. The quality of touch, body movement, posture, sounds, and hand signals all can be used in addition to words to convey preferences. In addition, a whole kaleidoscope of emotions may be expressed: relaxation, excitement, discomfort, humor, forcefulness, tenderness, and joy. Greater spontaneity unfolds as each person feels freer to initiate new types of play without censure from the other. As the physical relationship is enhanced, it draws more and more attention from spectatoring activity, allowing more sexual response to take place.

2. Format

2.1. Frequency of Sessions

Some sex therapy is conducted in a once-a-week format for the convenience of both couples and therapists. Many optimistic reports of this format have been published (see, e.g., Bancroft, 1975; Kaplan, 1974; Lobitz & LoPiccolo, 1972; McCarthy, 1973). However, Masters and Johnson (1970) inaugurated a new, rapid-treatment approach with daily sessions over a two-week time period. Many sex therapists today offer a compromise format, with two or three sessions a week or a choice of formats stressing the advantages of the rapid-treatment model.

The advantages of daily therapy sessions are that: (1) an intensive approach tends to focus attention on the relationship with a minimum of distractions, enhancing intimacy and communication; (2) couples have an opportunity to get rather immediate, day-by-day feedback from the therapists, which minimizes the chance of maladaptive "mistakes" becoming entrenched, while producing ample opportunity for positive reinforcement of newly developed skills; and (3) a cumulative therapeutic momentum can build up which materially improves self-esteem and may even increase client motivation by showing that rapid change is attainable.

2.2. One Therapist versus Dual Sex Therapy Teams

Most sex therapy, like marital therapy, is conducted by one therapist, usually because paying two therapists is prohibitive for most people. In many cases, using one versus two therapists probably makes little difference in outcome (see, e.g., Mathews, Whitehead, Hackmann, Julier, Bancroft, Gath, & Shaw, 1976). However, a dual-sex co-therapist team working well together may make a difference when extreme hostilities exist between partners and the likelihood of being accused of taking sides is greatest. This danger is substantially reduced when there are a male and female therapist, each committed to representing the same-sex client (Masters & Johnson, 1970). In working with a heterosexual couple this means clarifying the same sex spouse's needs, what he or she means when talking, and how he or she interprets whatever is being said by the other three people present. The relationship is the patient (Masters & Johnson, 1970), so that the same sex therapist continually asks, "How does this individual go about getting what he or she wants in the relationship? How does that affect what he or she gets?" Each therapist can model good communication by actively representing the attitudes and subjective sexual feelings of the same sex, while deferring to the opposite sex in their own domain of expertise. The divergence of male and female inner experiences is acknowledged and respected by the therapists, and the clients are encouraged to follow suit in their communication. For instance, a woman may say she is satisfied although she did not have an orgasm, which her partner discounts until the female co-therapist validates the experience.

2.3. History Taking

Histories in couple sex therapy usually are done with each spouse separately. At Masters & Johnson Institute an extensive history is taken from the same-sex partner in the morning and a supplemental "cross-sex" history from the partner in the afternoon. Besides gathering information on experiences and attitudes, the history has several other purposes. One is to establish some confidence on the part of the client in the therapist's expertise and nonjudgmentalism. By his or her choice of unloaded words, unruffled reaction to information, and demonstrated sophistication with slang and socially condemned lifestyles, the therapist conveys a commitment to work within the values of the client, rather than impose his or her own. A second purpose is to allow the individual a chance to share the information that they wish kept confidential from the spouse. Finally, the histories sometimes reveal major contradictions between the material from each spouse. The cross-sex history gives a chance to explore these further.

3. Etiological Factors in Sexual Dysfunction

Lacking definitive longitudinal studies that might clearly demonstrate the variety of factors that cause sexual problems, intelligent guesses about etiology are presently based principally on the assessment of clinical populations. Although most clinicians have found that a majority of cases reveal a predominant psychosocial etiology, previous estimates of organic causes in only 5% to 10% of cases of sexual dysfunction are now being revised upward on the basis of increasingly sophisticated diagnostic testing procedures (Schumacher & Lloyd, 1981; Spark, White, & Connolly, 1980; Wagner & Green, 1981).

At the same time, it should be recognized that selected cases with a major organic component to their etiology nevertheless may respond well to sex therapy, particularly when fears of performance, misinformation, and diminished self-esteem perpetuate or magnify the sexual problem(s). Thus, although impotence in diabetic men often is irreversible, in a series of 45 cases treated with sex therapy at the Masters & Johnson Institute after determining that no significant neuropathy or vascular disease was present, 84.4% had successful reversal of their sexual difficulties.

3.1. Evaluating for Organic Factors

In order to assess possible organic factors in cases of sexual dysfunction, a competent medical history and physical examination along with appropriate laboratory testing is required. Although a detailed discussion of these procedures is beyond the scope of this chapter,[2] a few brief comments are in order. Supplementing the baseline laboratory studies useful in obtaining a general health profile (e.g., blood counts, a biochemistry screening profile, a urinalysis, a check for syphilis, and assessment of relevant endocrine status), several tests recently have emerged as potentially useful in a substantial number of cases. Monitoring nocturnal penile tumescence (NPT) patterns in a sleep research laboratory provides a helpful screening test with about an 85% accuracy rate for determining whether impotence is organic or psychogenic. When regular sleep-associated erections are found, it is highly unlikely that an organic problem exists; conversely, when no nocturnal tumescence occurs or when nocturnal erections are weak or only of brief duration, the likelihood of an organic problem is greater and further, more sophisticated diagnostic testing is in order. For example, doppler (ultrasound) measurement of penile blood pressure and blood flow is useful to assess the vascular component of male sexual function, and measurement of serum testosterone and prolactin is useful to assess the hormonal component of male sexual function. Regrettably, fewer advances have been made to date in testing for organic conditions causing female sexual dysfunction.

3.2. Psychosocial Evaluation

3.2.1. Psychopathology

Information about possible psychopathology is gathered most often in sex therapy by interviews with the two clients and in some clinical settings also by psychological tests such as the MMPI. At Masters & Johnson Institute we rely on a clinical judgment of the person from his or her interview—intellectual capacity, reported psychological symptoms, presence of contradictory or bizarre material, moodiness, defensive style with the therapist—as well as on the spouse's report of that person's response to stress, and when available, a psychological evaluation sent by a referring psychotherapist. At MJI, according to a study done in 1970 by Maurice and Guze, one-quarter of dysfunctional men and one-third of dysfunctional women in therapy had psychopathology that was diagnosable

[2]Interested readers are referred to the *Textbook of Sexual Medicine* by Kolodny, Masters and Johnson (1979) for detailed information in this area.

according to a conservative set of criteria. According to data collected between 1971 and 1979, 8% of our sex therapy clients have had a diagnosable psychiatric disorder, while about 30% had clearcut psychopathology that did not fit the criteria for a particular diagnosis (Kolodny, 1981).

Certain types of psychopathology preclude doing sex therapy, for instance active psychosis or extreme obsessiveness which prevent much attention to information or reality testing. Kaplan (1974) states that depression always should be treated before sex therapy is undertaken. However, most couples motivated enough to seek sex therapy are experiencing considerable anxiety, depression, and/or hostility (see Derogatis, Meyer, & King, 1981). These states may not have caused the original difficulties but resulted from them and in the process may have aggravated the sexual problems. Our experience is that they usually can be treated successfully. A study by Clement and Pfafflin (1980) substantiates the positive effect that sex therapy can have on the depression and aggression of sex therapy clients.

A good understanding of a person's intelligence, cognitive flexibility, sensitivity to authoritative instructions and feedback, and defense styles can help prevent unnecessary crises and funnel therapeutic efforts in the most useful direction. For instance, in talking with an intellectualizing person, posing more closed-ended questions and interpreting the wordy, analytic style as a means of detaching oneself from sensory experience may be useful. Other common defenses that may be addressed in sex therapy are repression, projection, rationalization, somaticization, and displacement.

3.2.2. Prior Psychotherapy

Many sex therapy clients have received prior psychotherapy, either as couples or individually. At Masters & Johnson Institute, among couples seen between 1971 and 1977, 86% included at least one member who had undergone prior psychotherapy. Sex therapists need to be aware of the content, both what was welcomed and what was rejected, of former therapy. This information sometimes can be mobilized to serve the client's current goals. Therapists also need to be sensitive to the transference and/or countertransference dynamics in other therapy experiences. If a client worships a therapist back home, we are careful to minimize any sense of competition with the mentor: to celebrate that person's competence and emphasize our desire to cooperate with him or her during the follow-up period. On the other hand, a client who believes he or she was seduced or mistreated by a former therapist understandably will be on guard and needs appropriate support. Finally, if the couple has undergone sex therapy before, the current therapists need to be forewarned about what similar suggestions were given and why that therapy is believed to have failed. Every effort should be made to avoid prior pitfalls and to convey a sense of freshness, at least of context and timing, even when similar suggestions are made.

3.2.3. Relationship Issues

More often than individual psychopathology, relationship difficulties have etiologic significance for sex problems. Of course, sexual problems also have an impact on even good relationships, so that a vicious cycle can develop. Sexual fears can lead to avoidance of sex, causing the spouse to feel rejected, frustrated, hurt, and eventually angry. If these reactions are shared, the fearful individual may react defensively, and frequent arguments over trivial matters may result. Alternatively, he or she may turn to drinking or "workaholism'' to escape expanding pressures in the relationship, which may lead the spouse to take a lover. It is easy to see how so many couples entering sex therapy are on the brink of divorce.

One relationship problem that frequently leads to sexual difficulties is a pronounced dominant-submissive dynamic in individual roles. Typically, this takes the form of male and female sex-role stereotypes presenting as a full-blown double-standard relationship. Some among such couples are comfortable and integrated with these roles at little expense to their self-esteem and manage to function well within their constraints. But for many, the inequities of such a relationship take a high toll sexually. Often, the woman feels too helpless and unsophisticated about sex to take any self-responsibility and passively waits for her partner to provide what she might need. The man, equally handicapped by his role expectations, frequently tries to fix his wife's problem and becomes increasingly weary and frustrated. He may push for more frequent contact (feeding her growing aversion to sex), or he may turn to another partner to assuage his hurt feelings, ending up feeling guilty. Even if he holds the traditional double-standard belief that extramarital sex is his male prerogative, his wife may be deeply offended by his behavior, leading to discord, depression, or retaliation in kind.

Another relationship issue that commonly leads to sexual dysfunction is lack of communication skills to resolve conflicts through negotiation. Poor conflict management is a common marital problem which can undermine sexual functioning in numerous ways. For instance, some couples are terrified of facing disagreements of any kind, so that these are masked but rankle under the surface. Building resentment may cause lowered sexual excitement in one or both spouses. Other couples argue viciously, and wounds persist as growing mistrust and even fear. Especially if there is physical abuse, the victim may become phobic to the abuser's touch. Sex therapy may be largely devoted to teaching simple, practical devices for resolving disagreements constructively.

Although conflict resolution is a necessary part of a good marital relationship, by itself it results in a purely businesslike partnership, not conducive to long-term sexual functioning. The missing aspect is intimacy, a sense of bondedness and abiding acceptance by the other person. Emotional sharing is an essential ingredient of intimacy, but may be inhibited in various ways. For instance, role-playing may prohibit sharing "weak" feelings: hurt, fear, confusion. The "macho" male plays such a role as does the rescuer of either sex. Some individuals are simply too narcissistic to be interested in another person beyond exploiting them for their own needs at the moment. They do not have any concept of the solace that confiding in an accepting human being can provide, so they do not ask for it or offer it. Their attention span for any topic other than themselves is minimal. They approach decision making purely on a unilateral basis. They have minimal capacity for vicariously appreciating another person's pleasure and therefore are not very motivated to cooperate with feedback on what pleases the spouse. They may be rapid ejaculators or lack desire for sex with the spouse, preferring masturbation. The spouses of these individuals often report feeling lonely and complain of anorgasmia or lack of afterplay. They may be angry or resigned. Sex therapy may make some progress if the narcissistic person can be shown what he or she stands to gain, and if the spouse's expectations are minimal and he or she has plenty of other social resources.

Lack of commitment is another relationship issue that frequently lies at the heart of sexual problems. For example, with a partner threatening divorce (meaning it or not), the client who wants to stay in the marriage may try to use sex to keep the spouse. His or her desperate sexual advances may turn the partner off completely. Or the person may try too hard to perform well, with the opposite effect. In another scenario, one spouse is discovered having an extramarital affair and may find that lingering distrust of the partner damages his or her sexual attraction and response to that person. Even the suspicion that the spouse wants to leave the relationship or has been unfaithful can manifest as sexual conflict, lack of desire, or dysfunction.

Finally, there are cases where sexual problems simply reflect an overall dislike of the partner, ranging from indifference to loathing. The dislike may be related to something specific, for example, the physical appearance of the spouse, or very general, so that every aspect of the spouse is objectionable. These relationships tend to be marked by panoramic hostility that must be defused early in therapy if good results are to be obtained.

3.3. Sexual Experiences

Certain types of sexual experiences, especially early in a person's life, can be important etiologically. One dramatic example is in cases of premature ejaculation, where ejaculating rapidly often seems to be conditioned in the first few sexual encounters. The key factor is whether for any reason there is a premium on ejaculating quickly (Masters & Johnson, 1970). The female might be in pain and encouraging the male to finish quickly. The prostitute might hurry one man so that she can service more customers per hour, or the couple may be surreptitiously having intercourse in a parked car, hurrying in order to finish before the police discover them.

Traumatic sexual experiences either in the developmental years or later on also can set the stage for sexual problems. Rape, incest, molestation, or other unpleasant sexual encounters may inhibit sexual functioning even with a loved partner and not uncommonly lead to sexual aversion, a phobic attitude toward sex. In these circumstances, the traumatized individual is doubly victimized: first, by the impact of the traumatic experience (in both its physical and psychological dimensions); later, by lingering guilt, fear, diminished self-esteem, anger, and sense of helplessness.

Sexual interaction with a dysfunctional partner also can promote dysfunction. Many women with rapidly ejaculating husbands are nonorgasmic, at least in coitus, and may blame themselves for being unresponsive. With a wife who is vaginismic, many men become impotent due to ignorance, frustration, or guilt. Dyspareunia in either partner can be distressing to the other and cause lessened desire and/or arousal. Finally, sexual experiences with a partner who is pressuring one to perform, either belligerently or more subtly, typically leads to further problems. Thus, a premature ejaculator may become impotent, or a nonorgasmic woman may become sexually aversive due to the cascading effects of their partner's pressuring.

3.3.1. Affective Factors

Fears about performance already have been mentioned as central to many cases of sexual dysfunction. Other sexually related anxieties also can play an etiological role, such as anxiety about becoming accidentally pregnant. Less often, various phobias may inhibit sexual enjoyment: phobias toward semen, the vagina, venereal disease, and so forth. Sexual anxiety also is commonly related to body-image problems, which include concerns ranging from obesity to worries about genital appearance. Apart from specifically sexual anxieties, general stress and anxiousness in one's life also can reduce sexual satisfaction.

Any type of guilt can take a toll on a couple's sexual relationship. Cheating oneself out of sexual pleasure or abstaining from sex altogether can be a means of expiation for having done wrong. If the guilt relates to sexual fantasies or behavior specifically, it in itself can constitute a presenting complaint.

As mentioned earlier, one of the notorious reasons for inhibited sexual desire is depression. Associated with depression is frequently a chronic low level of self-esteem. Another reason, probably more common but less often officially recognized, is boredom. Sex can become routinized for genuinely uncreative people, but books full of ideas for experimentation abound. A more likely cause of sexual boredom is inhibitions about trying new things that may be perceived as ''kinky,'' ''perverted,'' or ''sinful.''

3.3.2. Cognitive Factors

Lack of information about sex is to some extent implicated in almost every couple in sex therapy, more so among the elderly but not exempting young couples. Many a nonorgasmic woman is misinformed about the location of her clitoris or how it can be overstimulated to the point of numbness (Masters & Johnson, 1966). Many a husband of such a woman believes the best stimulation for her is provided by fast, deep thrusting in the vagina. Many couples expect the penis to become instantly erect at the onset of touching and to remain completely hard until after ejaculation. The list of misconceptions is endless.

Beyond simple misinformation, negative attitudes toward sex often are at the heart of sexual problems. Religious teaching frequently has been blamed for these attitudes, but obviously much depends on the emphasis in teaching, on the parental example given, and on the individual's susceptibility to such messages. Many antisexual concepts are an integral part of our secular culture today. The ''uncleanness'' of the female genitals is stressed in advertising for vaginal deodorants and we have a profound ambivalence toward pleasure and play to the extent that these are seen as opposed to work, productivity, and responsibility.

Finally, sexual fantasies can be problematic in themselves for the individual who feels guilty about them or frightened by their presence. A person who experiences unwanted imagery of blood and violence when sexually aroused may prefer to cut off sexual feelings altogether. Another fantasy-related problem exists when one specific socially unacceptable object constitutes the total range of a person's desires, as is true for fetishists, pedophiles, and other paraphiliacs. If they act on their desires they are likely to encounter rejection by their spouses and trouble with the law. For such people, response to an adult partner may be minimal or unsatisfying.

3.4. A Concluding Word about Etiology

In this brief review of relevant etiologic factors, we wish to stress the fact that in many cases, there is not a clear-cut dichotomization of organic and psychosocial vectors. Our sexual responses and sexual feelings are governed by a complex—and as yet incompletely understood—interaction among physiological, psychological, and social elements. Ideally, sex therapy should include attention to these component parts throughout its course. With this point in mind, we will now turn our attention to the treatment of sexual problems.

4. Beginning Treatment: the Roundtable and Beyond

When the couple first meets with both therapists after history-taking and physical examinations to hear their feedback, a vital point in therapy has arrived. Masters and Johnson named this session the "roundtable" to suggest the four-way gathering (1970). It has several purposes. First, the nature of the problem to be addressed is defined. If unrealistic or contradictory goals have been presented, the therapists need to restructure the therapeutic aims into a workable mutual contract. If none is feasible, therapy generally would be halted at that point (Kolodny, Masters, & Johnson, 1979), perhaps accompanied by referral to another form of therapy. Second, the roundtable offers a summary of the etiological factors that appear relevant for the presenting complaints (Masters & Johnson, 1970). Even when the original reason for the problem's first occurrence has not been determined, this need not be a barrier to treatment. The therapists may offer an educated guess or confess their perplexity with the qualification that knowing the original cause is less important than recognizing the current factors maintaining the problem. Having a reasonable explanation for a frequently mystifying situation can be a source of comfort and reduce some of the paralyzing dread, guilt, and anger of couples at the onset of therapy. Third, a beginning is made in educating the couple about how to resolve their difficulties. Obviously the specific content will depend on the case. Besides discussing the concepts outlined earlier, such as sex as a natural function and the double standard, some typical areas introduced in the roundtable might include:

- Cultural expectations placed on sex, especially the concept that "sex" consists of an end-point (intercourse with simultaneous orgasms), whereas all other touching, looking, and words of affection have no sexual significance themselves except as "foreplay" to that end (Masters & Johnson, 1970)
- Adopting an attitude of starting fresh; not allowing past experience to predict what will happen now or in the future, or past hurts to infect the present (Kolodny *et al.*, 1979)
- Helping each client understand the concept of responsibility for self, meaning that one is to take active measures to cope with any feelings that are uncomfortable (e.g., anxiety or boredom) rather than wallow in them or expect the spouse to automatically provide a solution (Kolodny *et al.*, 1979)
- Pointing out that sex can serve many needs, including procreation, tension release, and ego-building; in a committed relationship it also can be a rewarding form of intimate communication, subject to the same principles as nonsexual communication and frequently interacting with the state of the couple's communication outside sex (Masters and Johnson, 1970)
- Accepting that feelings, one's own and one's partner's, are facts of the moment and not subject to blame or praise, though they may be perceived as comfortable or uncomfortable (Kolodny *et al.*, 1979)
- The concept of self-representation; capitalizing on each person's self-awareness by sharing his or her own feelings and desires without fear of deliberate hurt or manipulation, trusting that disagreements will be honestly negotiated in the best interest of the relationship (Kolodny *et al.*, 1979)

Fourth, and at least as important as the information given in the roundtable, is establishing the role of the therapists, through explanation and then demonstration. The therapists must convey a personally objective attitude to both clients, with neither being blamed or favored (Masters & Johnson, 1970). Usually even destructive behavior can be explained as a reaction to feelings and circumstances for which the person is not directly responsible. Although the tone of feedback will vary from extremely supportive to extremely confrontive, every step must serve what this couple needs in order to obtain their stated objectives, uncontaminated (insofar as humanly possible) by the therapists' personal reactions, and the clients must be repeatedly reassured of that intent.

Also in relation to their perceived roles, the therapists need to explain that little will be accomplished if the couple expects them to perform magic or do something to them that solves their problems. They are merely catalysts to the couple's progress. The clients' role is an active one of sharing their concerns, answering questions, and carrying out suggested activities in good faith. The gains that they take home will be largely a function of their conviction that they know how to handle difficulties themselves, which will come from seeing it in practice.

The remainder of therapy consists largely of applying the concepts presented in the roundtable to specific incidents that develop on a daily basis. For instance, a couple may have an argument. The way they handle it, whether they resolve it or escalate, and its effect on sensate focus that day becomes a microcosm of the issues of the couple more generally. From daily reports of the clients' activities and reactions, the therapists learn where there are gaps of information, areas of emotional discomfort, or other issues needing attention at that point. Repeated patterns of problems can be interpreted as resistances and held up for the couple's scrutiny. Most sex therapists are probably somewhat eclectic in practice, whatever their theoretical alliances, and interventions may include education, relabeling, *in vivo* desensitization, nondirective support, paradoxical techniques, depth psychoanalytic interpretations, and confrontation of deliberate sabotage, to mention just a few.

5. Treatment

We will now turn to discussing treatments for specific sexual problems. We will first consider sexual dysfunctions, female and male, and then sexual dissatisfactions, including desire disorders and selected other commonly presented complaints. A final section will describe a few special issues sex therapists frequently are faced with in their practice.

As a preface to this section the reader should note that it would be impossible to describe here all the facets of the treatment of any one category of distress. The etiological factors are compounded in unique ways in every couple. Further, in our experience at Masters & Johnson Institute, more and more cases are presenting with multiple distresses, requiring delicate balancing of attention to them all and sensitive timing of interventions. Finally, no attempt is made here to elaborate on possible medical approaches.

6. Female Sexual Dysfunctions

6.1. Vaginismus

Vaginismus is a relatively rare female dysfunction that involves involuntary spasm of the muscles or the perineum and outer third of the vagina. This is a reflex response to vaginal penetration, or the anticipation of penetration, due to fear of pain or injury. In its mildest forms it is experienced as tightening and pressure, making entry by a penis, finger, or speculum somewhat difficult. In more severe cases, penetration is painful and virtually impossible. Thus, cases of vaginismus often present as unconsummated marriages. The woman with vaginismus is sometimes anorgasmic, but frequently she reaches orgasm easily with external manipulation or minimal insertion of the penis.

Occasionally vaginismus is related to physical causes: for example, as a consequence of dyspareunia, current or past, or steroid starvation associated with aging and minimal sexual continuity. More often, psychogenic causes are involved. Often, there is a background of severe social conditioning of fear of sex: expectations are inculcated by family members and peers that intercourse will be painful, that one easily can be hurt by sex, that pregnancy is dangerous and childbirth hellish. The genitals are mysterious, dirty, and untouchable. Frequently, the woman has shied away from using tampons and may have extremely negative attitudes toward her menstrual periods. Attempts to use vaginal contraceptives are painful and frequently impossible. Pelvic exams are avoided. If one is necessary, it may have to be done with the woman under general anesthesia. Vaginismus also may be secondary to rape, to a traumatic initial pelvic exam, or to repeated experience with a male partner with sexual dysfunction. If the man repeatedly loses his erection or ejaculates upon attempted penetration, the woman may associate this social trauma with vaginal entry and react involuntarily with this symptom. Treatment of the male dysfunction usually will not reverse the vaginismus without specific attention to the latter.

Vaginismus may be suspected from the history as just outlined, but the diagnosis only can be established definitely by pelvic exam. In the exam the woman is reassured that no attempt will be made to insert a speculum. She is told what the physician is going to do at each step, and that she will have the ability to slow down or halt the exam at any time. Under these circumstances, even when the woman permits a physician to place a finger at the vaginal entrance or just inside, the reflexive tightening of the perineum and outlet is visible. A first step in therapy involves showing first her (with a mirror) and then her partner the response. It is important they both understand what it is: that she is not anatomically abnormal, nor is the spasm a voluntary refusal of entry. This can be a highly enlightening experience for the couple, who may have complained of dyspareunia, impotence, or an impenetrable hymen, but have had no idea of the real nature of their problem.

Treating vaginismus includes specific measures to recondition the vaginal muscles. This reprogramming is accomplished by the use of graduated plastic dilators, or by some therapists, fingers (Kaplan, 1974), which the woman inserts at her own pace into her vagina. The last point is an essential part of the treatment; the woman is less tense when she has control over the penetration, and she learns that she can help her body cooperate with her in allowing vaginal entry. The dilators typically are introduced to the woman following the roundtable. (For discussion of specific details, see Kolodny, Masters, and Johnson, 1979.) In some types of therapy, relaxation training is used as a preliminary to this step (Cooper, 1969).

A female therapist or co-therapist can be extremely helpful in this situation. Her credibility as a woman allows her to educate, coach, and encourage the client, with some degree of positive transference developing. The potential danger of an erotic transference to the opposite-sex therapist, which might interfere with the marital relationship, is minimized.

Depending on the severity of the vaginismus, the therapist may introduce additional, larger dilators every day or two until the woman comfortably can insert a size that matches that of the erect penis. She generally is asked to insert the smaller one first, leave it in place for about 10 to 15 minutes, and then remove it and insert the next size. This exercise is done several times daily. As a larger size dilator is given to her, the woman is asked to return the smaller of the two she has been using, so that she does not collect several at a time and become traumatized by seeing the range in sizes.

Therapy in cases of vaginismus involves work with the husband as well. He is often rather inhibited, sexually naive, and may come from a social background equally as repressive as his wife's (Kolodny *et al.*, 1979). Education about the problem, the female's genital anatomy, and sexual functioning all are relevant for him to reduce his timidity and unfamiliarity with his wife's body. As his approach to her becomes less tentative, he is less likely to take responsibility for her and becomes more sexually secure himself. Having him insert and play with the dilators in his wife's vagina (under her guidance) after she has used them herself for several days can expedite this confidence and her trust.

Sensate focus is conducted with an emphasis on building mutual trust and communication, greater spontaneity, and greater responsivity for both partners. At the point where the largest dilator has been successfully used, the couple should be ready to insert the penis gently within the context of nondemand play together. From the female-superior position, the woman conducts the penis into her vagina at her own pace, using careful instructions from the female therapist about angle and sufficient artificial lubrication.

Like all sex therapy couples, those presenting with vaginismus have their own marital problems, fears, and issues of low self-esteem. Therapy must address these areas with psychotherapy and work on communication if the reversal of vaginismus is to be lasting and meaningful to the couple. In some cases, the woman moves on rapidly to developing feelings of sexual pleasure from the penis in her vagina. In other cases, these feelings may not develop without further help; however, sometimes the couple says their only goal is conception, in which case the therapists respect the values of their clients at that time.

6.2. Anorgasmia

Difficulties in attaining orgasm are the commonest form of female sexual dysfunction seen by sex therapists. A variety of patterns of female anorgasmia have been recognized, leading to the following classification schema: *primary anorgasmia* refers to women who have never been orgasmic; *secondary anorgasmia* refers to women who previously experienced orgasm but do not do so currently; *random anorgasmia* describes women who have been orgasmic with various types of sexual stimulation but rarely; and *situational anorgasmia* refers to women orgasmic by some type of stimulation but desiring to reach orgasm in another way. *Coital anorgasmia,* or lack of orgasm during intercourse, is the commonest form of situational anorgasmia, but occasionally clinicians encounter *masturbatory anorgasmia:* namely, women who experience orgasms with intercourse but not with self-stimulation and who desire this latter form of response.

The etiology of anorgasmia is wide ranging. Although organic factors such as diabetes, hypothyroidism, multiple sclerosis, and alcoholism or drug abuse are known to be involved occasionally, these conditions seem to constitute only a small fraction of cases. Generally, anorgasmic women seen in therapy are physically healthy, and psychosocial elements seem to be the causative key. One frequently hears from the anorgasmic female a history of training in the traditional female role. The belief that men are the sexually active partner while women's role is to restrain them (at least until marriage) can be difficult to shake off just because marriage has occurred. Passivity in women may be highly valued, so that the anorgasmic woman may feel terrified of initiating steps to help herself. Even when she does, she may attribute the results to her partner's behavior or to chance and fail to maintain her new behavior.

In addition to the relational, affective, and cognitive factors described already, anorgasmia can result from the woman fearing what might happen if she lets go enough to reach orgasm. She may be afraid of feeling out of control; of losing physical control in general so that she will be incontinent, have convulsions, or black out; of looking ugly; or of becoming a "bad woman," perhaps a "nymphomaniac."

The approach to treating female anorgasmia typically begins by conveying permission for the woman to be a sexually responsive person. Therapists usually cannot accomplish this successfully unless their attitudes and their verbalizations express the idea that it is both acceptable and desirable to be female *and* sexual, which encompasses having pleasure and being able to play. Because of the sheer volume of cultural and familial messages to the contrary, such permission-giving needs to be frequent and emphatic to penetrate beyond mere intellectual understanding, and the value of this reorientation must be consistently reinforced as therapy progresses.

A prime consideration in therapy for anorgasmia, especially when situations with the spouse are involved, is the quality of the marital relationship (Chapman, 1968; Masters & Johnson, 1970; McGovern, Stewart, & LoPiccolo, 1975). If a women feels she is going to be monitored, evaluated, and criticized every time she tries something new to her, she very likely will be self-conscious and inhibited. The same result can come from the more superficially benign system where the woman is assumed, as a female, not to have the competence to know what she wants for herself. The man steps in as a chivalrous helper and discounts her input. A woman's performance fears will be aggravated if she feels her husband expects her to be orgasmic at a particular time, or in every sexual opportunity. A couple who is in a power struggle deliberately may deny one another's sexual requests, so that communication of desires is simply an exercise in frustration. Frequent arguments with unresolved anger can infect the couple's sexual play for hours or even years. Resentments may or may not be acknowledged, even to oneself, but often are expressed by withholding total sexual involvement. Deceit and commitment problems also are frequently found in couples with situationally anorgasmic wives. In such cases the therapists' job is to improve the couple's communication skills, neutralize old resentments by stressing a here-and-now viewpoint, and help the couple negotiate solutions to ongoing conflicts. These strategies are a means of helping the woman feel as secure and emotionally close to her husband as possible, supported by his affection and reduced irritation in the relationship. The couple's capacity to generate excitement, romance, and intrigue together also is tapped in accordance with their sexual value system so as to combat boredom and routine.

Performance fears are addressed first by presenting the therapeutic concepts discussed earlier. In particular, the notion that sex is a natural function is put forth and applied especially to an awareness that orgasm cannot be willed or forced. The pressure to have an orgasm whenever the male does is countered by suggesting, for example, that sexual function, like digestion, works better when each individual can respect his or her own level of appetite. Within this framework the couple is educated about sexual response with a particular emphasis on female sexual anatomy and physiology. Discussing such information ensures that, for example, both spouses understand where the woman's clitoris is and its role in sexual response. Among the myths dispelled are the concepts that direct stimulation of the clitoris is most preferred by females, and that intercourse must be performed in a position where the penis rubs directly against the clitoris to satisfy the woman.

As in the treatment of any form of sexual dysfunction, sensate focus plays a central role in anxiety reduction. The simple experience of being touched in a leisurely way can be physically relaxing. In its early stages, because intercourse and even genital touching are prohibited, the experience is less goal-directed, so that there are fewer expectations that could create performance concerns. Gradual progression of touching suggestions provides a context for desensitization. Anxiety is further curtailed by coping strategies that can be used by the woman. For instance, during touching sessions she is encouraged to express her fears to her mate, and he is to adopt a calmly accepting attitude; this process usually dissipates her anxiety somewhat.

The next component of therapy for anorgasmia is to increase positive and potentially erotic input. Not uncommonly the therapist will be told by the woman, "I don't feel anything." What this generally means is that she does not feel what she expects she should. Tactile appreciation begins in sensate focus with slowing the pace, focusing one's attention, and noticing whatever sensations do come in, of any intensity or quality. As she becomes aroused, the same principle applies: experiencing sensations moment by moment and communicating her desires for experimentation or continuing what feels good.

The experience of sensate focus can be extended to touching things in a sensual way in the course of the woman's daily activities, for example, noticing the texture of the blankets on the bed as she smooths them or feeling the petals of a rose in the park. In addition, the woman may take opportunities to touch her own body in an exploratory fashion. Many primarily anorgasmic women have never masturbated and therefore may not know much about their sensations and what might please them tactilely. They also may have some discomfort about their bodies, especially the genitals, that inhibits them when with their husbands. At Masters & Johnson Institute, self-stimulation is suggested to increase the woman's self-knowledge and comfort with her body, but not necessarily to lead to orgasm (Kolodny *et al.*, 1979). It would not, however, be introduced for clients whose moral values are opposed to it. Some sex therapy programs for couples include several specific steps for primary anorgasmic women to learn to masturbate to orgasm prior to sensate focus with a partner (LoPiccolo & Lobitz, 1972; Miller & Brockway, 1972). After the client locates the areas that feel pleasurable, she spends lengthy sessions stimulating those areas with her hand, or if necessary an electric vibrator. Once orgasm has occurred, she masturbates in her partner's presence, then shows him how to provide similar stimulation and then combines that with simultaneous intercourse. The therapeutic advantage of including "directed masturbation" within a couple's therapy program for primarily anorgasmic women was experimentally demonstrated by Riley and Riley (1978).

Enhancing other psychological dimensions besides the tactile may be necessary for many women to become orgasmic with their husbands. All the senses can contribute to their level of arousal. The woman can increase her visual input by having some light in the room, even using colored light bulbs or flickering candles to add atmosphere. In the auditory sphere, both spouses can be encouraged to make sounds during play; background music also can be used. Gustatory and olfactory stimulation can be appreciated through kissing and oral play anywhere on the partner's body. With a little creativity and the freedom to offer spontaneous suggestions, the couple can bring novel stimuli into their interaction, for example, honey, whipped cream, or scented oils.

Sexual fantasies can provide further erotic input for the woman. A few individuals actually may have no preexisting fantasies and may need exposure to a variety of themes commonly used by females. Probably more often the client simply needs permission or active suggestion to enjoy the fantasies she already has. Since the majority of women apparently fantasize during intercourse with their husbands, even in healthy relationships (Hariton & Singer, 1974), the client can be assured that she is not abnormal if she does likewise. Her husband may be present during discussions of the wife's fantasies to the extent that he can be nonjudgmental and unthreatened by them. The intention of the therapist(s) is not to diminish the woman's involvement in the interaction but to enhance it unobtrusively.

Treating coital anorgasmia involves applying all the above principles to the specific context of the penis in the vagina. Education includes an understanding of the natural potential of the vagina for taking in sensations. The fact that there are more nerve endings in the outer third of the vagina is explained to encourage the woman to explore thrusting patterns that vary in depth, contrary to the cultural notion that the best stimulation always comes from deep penetration. The couple is instructed in using positions comfortably, such as female superior and lateral (Masters & Johnson, 1970), where the woman has maximum freedom of movement for exploring sensations. Sensate focus with penile insertion is approached in the same nongoal-oriented manner of earlier touching sessions, with attention to whatever sensations are experienced, free of expectations. The woman is given responsibility for inserting the penis when she chooses and the option of removing it at any point and of reinserting it if she wishes. Play with the external genitals can precede, alternate with, or occur simultaneously with penile-vaginal thrusting (Kaplan, 1974; Kolodny *et al.* 1979; LoPiccolo & Lobitz, 1972).

Masturbation can be used as an adjunct to couple's sensate focus for coitally, not just primarily anorgasmic women. A. M. Zeiss, Rosen, and Zeiss (1977) describe an approach where masturbation, usually via manipulation of the external genitalia, is made to more closely mimic the coital situation. The woman uses a dildo to explore sensations within her vagina and includes intercourse in her fantasies. Applying the principles of conditioning, the dildo is at first inserted just prior to orgasm, and then gradually earlier in the course of excitement. Thus, the woman fades out external manipulation and relies more and more on intravaginal stimulation for orgasm. The last step is to insert the husband's penis using the same conditioning strategy. Annon (1971) reports a procedure using a similar rationale in which the woman gradually modifies her masturbatory fantasies or the position she uses when masturbating so that they approximate a real-life intercourse situation with the husband.

Clearly, if her husband ejaculates very quickly, a woman's chances of becoming orgasmic during intercourse are small. The couple actually may have developed habit patterns in trying to cope with rapid ejaculation that only exacerbate the woman's problems in responding. For instance, they may move to penile insertion the minute the penis is sufficiently hard and then engage in frantic thrusting to speed the woman up. Such a mistimed and mechanical interaction hardly is conducive to her being orgasmic. Or they may thrust very cautiously, stopping every few thrusts. Again, this places extreme limitations on what the woman can experience for herself. Effective therapy for such couples must include treatment of the premature ejaculation before coital orgasm is a realistic possibility for the woman.

7. Male Sexual Dysfunction

7.1. Impotence

Among male dysfunctions the most common presenting complaint at Masters & Johnson Institute is impotence, the inability to attain or maintain an erection sufficient for coitus. Masters and Johnson (1970) distinguish between *primary impotence,* where the man has been dysfunctional from his first coital attempt on, and *secondary impotence,* which has its onset after some period of normal erectile functioning. The latter is by far the more prevalent.

The male with primary impotence is likely to present with considerably impaired self-esteem and ineffectuality in interpersonal relationships. Probably this type of personality is in part the result of long-standing sexual difficulties, but such an individual is also a product of some of the same influence that fostered the impotence to begin with. For instance, a long-term sexual relationship with the mother is occasionally found in the childhood and adolescence of such cases. Extreme dominance by one parent or the other may be involved, often expressed through rigorous religious asceticism largely directed against sexual feelings and exploration. Some of these individuals are restricted to homosocial contacts and develop sexual interest exclusively in males, which is seen as less sinful and avoids the risk of pregnancy. Gender identity itself may be ambivalent. Thus, homosexuality can be involved in primary impotence cases. However, this does not mean that most men with impotence are homosexual or that all homosexual men are incapable of functioning sexually with females. Sometimes the crucial etiological event in cases of primary impotence is a traumatic first coital experience. Finally, an indeterminate number of men with primary impotence suffer from an organic impairment such as Klinefelter's syndrome or spina bifida.

Secondary impotence is known to occur as a result of many diseases, injuries, and medications (see Kolodny *et al.* 1979, for an extended discussion). However, as already mentioned, even when organic pathology is found psychogenic influences usually compound the problem. Virtually all the individual and marital factors cited in the general discussion earlier can have a bearing on erectile function. Even one episode of erectile failure, whether because of overindulgence in alcohol, fatigue, or some other transient factor can set the stage for performance fears to grow (Masters & Johnson, 1970).

Therapy for impotence depends to some extent on the specific etiology of the case and on the theoretical approach of the therapists. However, the general model of treatment focuses on re-education and behavior strategies for coping with performance anxieties and relationship problems (Apfelbaum, 1977; Cooper, 1969; Kolodny *et al.,* 1979).

Much of the therapy is designed to convince the couple that neither partner can make an erection happen by love, will, or physical effort when the man is overcome by fear and pressure. However, when pressure to perform is lessened, erection often will occur spontaneously with erotic stimulation. Naturally, the degree of erection will wax and wane to some extent throughout play. Many impotent men take the first sign of diminished penile rigidity to mean that they are "losing" their erection, which immediately translates into a fear that they will not be able to regain it. To counter this, at the time of sensate focus that includes genital play, the wife can be instructed to play with the penis, but to deliberately move away from it if a firm erection occurs, allowing it to subside before she resumes. The couple then has a chance to see that "lost" erections are not gone forever.

Progress early in therapy depends less on demonstrating "successful performance" than on using whatever the couple reports from their sensate focus experiences to help the man be aware of and acknowledge to his wife his performance fears. Acknowledgment is usually the first step toward circumventing these fears. It is important that the woman not be judgmental toward her husband because he is fearful. The therapist(s) can explain that the male's worries about sexual performance are deeper and more profound than a woman might guess from her own experience. If the therapist (or one of the co-therapists) is a woman, she can model an accepting response particularly effectively. It should be made clear to the woman that compassion does not obligate her to protect or coddle her husband. Rather, each partner has responsibility for him or herself. His principal responsibilities are to approach sexual play in a nongoal-oriented fashion and to articulate his performance concerns when they occur. He may then be instructed to focus his attention on one part of the partner's body—to become "lost" in the touch—since sensual involvement can reduce the cognitive component that typically fuels anxiety. The woman's principal responsibility simply is to involve herself in the situation for whatever she can get out of the experience without imposing any expectations on what "should" be happening for either partner. The therapist(s) need to stress that the touching sessions can be a positive experience whatever the engorgement of the penis might be, so that both partners can turn from their anxious spectatoring to more rewarding pursuits. For instance, the woman might straddle her partner and use his penis, regardless of the degree of hardness, to stimulate her own genitals, with the specific prohibition against inserting it into her vagina. As she becomes more aroused, her husband can attend to her response rather than his own concerns.

Therapy for impotence also frequently involves a great deal of attention to aspects of communication outside the sexual domain. If the man is intimidated by women and his wife in particular, the couple may need to learn a more egalitarian style of interaction so that he gains self-respect and she respects him more as well. Gains in general assertiveness often are reflected in the man's sexual functioning. The woman usually can be helped to see that she benefits not only sexually but also in sharing more daily responsibilities and emotional closeness.

In most cases of impotence, including those of long duration, this general approach will lead to a dramatic improvement in erectile function in fairly short order. Some men, however, find that attempts at coitus present a threat to their newly found sexual confidence and revert to a pattern of spectatoring that results in rapid detumescence either at "the moment of truth"—that is, just as insertion is attempted—or shortly after penetration. This dilemma is likely to be even more problematic in cases where this mimics the pattern of impotence before therapy was started, since the man is likely to feel that "I'm right back where I started."

Therapists can deal with this situation in several ways. First, they can present instructions for initial attempts at penile insertion in such a way that it is made clear that "I'm not telling you to go home to have intercourse; I'm simply suggesting that you extend the scope of the sensate focus to now include feeling the penis within the vagina." Second, they openly can anticipate the possibility that the man may have problems obtaining or maintaining an erection, stressing that: (1) this is not a sign of "failure" or of a poor prognosis; (2) the same strategies that have worked before for dealing with anxiety and spectatoring can be applied here; and (3) even if problems occur, this can be a valuable learning opportunity. Third, by instructing the wife to be in charge of both deciding when to insert and doing the actual insertion, the man can be relieved of some unnecessary responsibilities that are often distractions to his erotic involvement. In the small percentage of cases where these approaches do not circumvent the problem at this stage in therapy, other individualized approaches—such as encouraging the use of erotic imagery or recommending changes in coital position—often can be used to advantage. Finally, the possibility should not be overlooked that some men have a vested interest in maintaining their dysfunctional status, requiring more in-depth attention to both the individual psychodynamics and dyadic meanings of the situation.

7.2. Premature Ejaculation

There has been considerable difficulty in devising a universally applicable definition of premature ejaculation (e.g., Kaplan, 1974; Masters & Johnson, 1970; Perelman, 1980). DSM–III suggests that premature ejactulation can be diagnosed when "ejaculation occurs before the individual wishes it, because of recurrent and persistent absence of reasonable voluntary control." Whatever operational criteria are applied, it is quite clear that premature ejaculation is both a common condition (probably the most common dysfunction in the general population) and one that is marked by considerable variability in how it affects the individual and the relationship. Some men and their partners are not troubled at all by this pattern; more typically, however, the reaction ranges from one of simple sexual frustration to being the cause of significant marital discord. Similarly, premature ejaculation can range from a pattern wherein the male ejaculates after a minute or two of coital containment to more virulent forms where ejaculation occurs with the first few penile thrusts, at the moment of attempted insertion, or even earlier. The man may try to delay his ejaculation by distracting himself with boring arithmetic problems or pain from biting his tongue. Not only is this means ineffective, but it has the danger of cognitively cutting off so much stimulation that impotence results. His partner may try to reduce the amount of playing she does with him, with the same effect. Other maneuvers on her part, described under the section on anorgasmia, only prevent *her* from responding. Eventually, the couple may avoid each other physically altogether rather than provoke another frustrating sexual encounter. The woman may interpret her spouse's rapid ejaculation as a deliberate means of hurting her; thus hostility and defensiveness can infect the entire marriage.

There do seem to be a few couples where male hostility *is* involved in his choosing not to use his ability to control his ejaculation. In such cases, the pattern would have an onset sometime after a period of effective ejaculatory control. Much more often one sees men who have been premature ejaculators since their first few sexual encounters. As described earlier (see Etiological Factors), rapidity of ejaculation seems to be a conditioned response developed in situations where speed is desirable for any reason. A final etiological consideration would be coital frequency. The longer the interval between coital episodes, the more likely the male is to ejaculate prematurely. It is plain that a couple that avoids sex except on rare occasions because of anger, overwork, or other sexual difficulties may compound their difficulties with ejaculatory control.

Treatment first involves reducing the man's guilt and the woman's anger, to the extent that both apply. In the typical couple, authoritative information is given that the premature ejaculation is an involuntary reflex that was conditioned sometime in the past, perhaps even before this relationship began. In the roundtable the self-defeating strategies of both people are outlined and the hope of more effective techniques is offered in their place. Since anxiety about ejaculating usually exacerbates the problem, sensate focus is introduced to allow mutual pleasure with ejaculation irrelevant at first. As the woman learns to take responsibility for herself in the touching sessions, she can allow her own responsiveness, which has very likely been dampened by repeated frustration, to blossom once more.

Once some harmony and comfort in touching has been established, the couple is given instructions on use of the squeeze technique (Masters & Johnson, 1970). This method of reconditioning the timing of the ejaculatory reflex is used most effectively by the woman. If she is initially reluctant to try this out, the therapist can explain that her participation is as much for herself as for her partner. As Masters and Johnson prescribe the squeeze, it is administered in a dorsal-ventral plane at the coronal ridge of the penis. It is used at random intervals throughout play, not only when the man, feeling his excitement climbing toward the point of ejaculatory inevitability, requests it. The degree of pressure is reduced when the penis is less hard. The squeeze lasts for three to four seconds, which the woman counts silently, and is then abruptly released; touching then continues elsewhere on the man's body. (The couple is told in advance that a partial loss of erection may accompany the squeeze.) Six squeezes within every 15 minutes on the average are sufficient. If the male wishes to ejaculate thereafter, he may go ahead. After a day of familiarization, the female is encouraged to make squeezing a natural and automatic part of the touching experience which does not distract her from her own enjoyment.

When the couple reaches the stage of intercourse, intromission is immediately preceded by a squeeze and followed by quiet containment in the vagina for several seconds; then the penis is removed, squeezed again, and reinserted. Thrusting is minimal for a day or two and then gradually increased. At this point a modification of the squeeze which can be applied by either partner during coitus is introduced: the basilar squeeze (Kolodny *et al.*, 1979). Pressure is applied for three seconds at the base of the penis, dorsal to ventral, while the woman can continue moving as she likes. The basilar squeeze is intended only to supplement, not to replace, the earlier coronal squeeze, which is to be used during genital play several times a week for three to six months in order for reprogramming of the ejaculatory reflex to be complete. On some occasions during that period, the man still may ejaculate accidentally before the couple wishes; this has no prognostic significance.

Positions that enhance ejaculatory control are advised during the early stages of the reprogramming process. These especially include positions where the man is lying on his back. Gradually, various other positions may be allowed, such as the couple on their sides or rear-entry. The male superior position is reserved for late in the reconditioning period. The number of squeezes also is gradually reduced.

An alternate method to the squeeze was reported by Semans in 1956: the stop–start technique. In this approach, used quite successfully by Kaplan (1974) and others, the woman stimulates her husband's penis until he is nearly at the point of ejaculatory inevitability. He then signals her, and she stops stroking his penis until the urgency of his need to ejaculate subsides. Then she resumes, and the process is repeated several times. After that he may go ahead and ejaculate if he desires. Zilbergeld (1978) suggests that the stop–start can be applied to oneself during masturbation as well. In some cases where the squeeze technique is ineffective, the stop–start technique produces the desired results, and vice versa.

Although the squeeze technique is essential to the treatment of premature ejaculation, it should be stressed that it is best integrated into a process of psychotherapy that includes careful attention to interpersonal dynamics, communication skills, and residual areas of conflict. Failure to attend to these issues may result in situations of continuing relationship deterioration despite improvement in sexual functioning.

7.3. Ejaculatory Incompetence

This dysfunction, also known as retarded ejaculation[3] or ejaculatory impotence (Munjack & Kanno, 1979), is defined as the male's inability to ejaculate during vaginal containment. It does not include retrograde ejaculation, which releases semen into the bladder instead of out through the penis. Occasionally ejaculatory incompetence is preceded by a period of normal ejaculatory functioning. In such cases of secondary ejaculatory incompetence, the etiology may reside in resentment or ambivalence toward the spouse, in use of drugs such as guanethidine which impair the sympathetic nervous system's response, in injury to the spinal cord, or in some traumatic event (Kolodny *et al.*, 1979). For instance, a man may walk in unexpectedly on his wife who is having intercourse with another man, and the husband may glimpse semen at her vaginal opening. He subsequently may associate that sight with her vagina being soiled, tainted, or an otherwise unsavory receptacle for his own ejaculate. More commonly, however, the dysfunction is primary. Its antecedents seem to be parental attitudes, often religiously based, toward the genitals as dirty, females as unclean and evil, and masturbation as unhealthy. There may be terror of pregnancy or venereal disease. Homosexuality also may be present. In a minority of cases the man not only cannot ejaculate into his wife's vagina, but also never may have ejaculated at all except in wet dreams. Where even those ejaculatory outlets are lacking, the possibility of congenital abnormalities of the genitourinary system should be investigated (Kolodny *et al.*, 1979).

Diagnosis involves ruling out any possible voluntary motivation—avoiding consummating an unwanted marriage, or sabotaging the wife's attempts to conceive. If there were such a dynamic, the couple probably would need basic marriage counseling alone. However, after months or years of voluntarily holding back ejaculation, the man may have conditioned himself so well that it may not be possible even when he has changed his mind (Masters & Johnson, 1970). In that case, sex therapy is indicated.

Treatment consists of circumventing or reducing whatever roadblocks to functioning are identified for the couple. Much attention usually needs to be devoted to the wife's attitudes. On the one hand she may be angry at what she assumes to be a deliberate withholding by her spouse, especially if she wants children. She may participate little in sex or criticize her husband so that he develops fears about performance in terms of ejaculating. On the other hand she may feel inadequate as a lover. Communication between partners can be enhanced so that the man conveys effectively what he might find stimulating and so that she willingly cooperates. Indeed, a large part of her role usually involves applying prolonged and vigorous stroking of the penis to maximize physical input for the male.

Generally sensate focus is utilized to establish ejaculation as a response in the partner's presence and then gradually to approach the situation of vaginal containment, desensitizing fears, and disinhibiting the ejaculatory reflex along the way. Typical would be the couple who begin with the man stimulating himself to ejaculation with his wife nearby, then partially involved in stimulating him with her hand on or under his, and then with her completely taking over in touching him. A next step might be that when he signals reaching ejaculatory inevitability, she inserts his penis into her vagina, or at least

[3]At the Masters & Johnson Institute, we prefer to use the term *retarded ejaculation* to refer only to cases where ejaculation occurs only after prolonged periods of stimulation; in a sense, this disorder is the opposite of premature ejaculation.

allows some of his semen to spurt onto her external genitals. At that point the inhibition frequently seems to be overcome. After a few more positive experiences, with the penis inserted progressively sooner before ejaculation, the couple usually will have established the necessary confidence to complete therapy (Kolodny *et al.*, 1979).

Apfelbaum (1980) contends that the male who does not ejaculate with his wife but has no trouble doing so by himself is the victim of lack of desire for sex with a partner but manages to have automatic erections in spite of not being aroused. The therapist's task is to encourage the man to express his dissatisfactions and fears so that these can become accessible to treatment.

With those individuals whose ejaculations are limited to wet dreams, therapy may include sensate focus outside of the partner's presence, just as is done with primary anorgasmia for females. The man can attend solely to his own physical touch and sexual imagery and allow sensations to accumulate. When he first ejaculates, he can allay fears of pain, losing control, and so forth and also gain a frame of reference for the experience.

8. Problems of Either Sex

8.1. Dyspareunia

Pain during penile–vaginal insertion may occur for both men and women, though it is seen far more commonly in the latter. Organic causes are frequently found, for example pelvic adhesions, estrogen deficiency, or endometriosis. These are multitudinous and beyond the scope of this chapter; the reader is referred to Kolodny, Masters, and Johnson's *Textbook of Sexual Medicine* (1979). Some dyspareunia may be caused by sexual practices such as inserting the penis at an angle straight into the female's pelvis instead of toward her coccyx, or moving to intercourse without sufficient lubrication. Although pain during intercourse for females often is diagnosed as purely psychogenic, a more adequate pelvic examination by a knowledgeable, experienced physician may detect physical factors such as hymeneal tags or improperly healed episiotomies. However, medically treating dyspareunia may not be sufficient to restore a satisfactory sex life with a couple who have lingering anxieties about the possibility of pain. In addition, an unknown percentage of individuals appear to have no organic basis for their discomfort and may be somaticizing emotional unease about any aspect of sex. Both of these latter groups may need sex therapy, directed to their particular concerns (Lazarus, 1980).

8.2. Sexual Aversion

Sexual anxiety long has been recognized as a concommittant of anorgasmia and impotence and treated by such behavior therapy techniques as systematic desensitization (see, e.g., Friedman, 1968; Lazarus, 1963). Masters and Johnson (in Kolodny *et al.*, 1979) described the entity of phobic reactions to sex independent of sexual dysfunction, giving it the name *sexual aversion*. The manifestations of this phobia can be either physiological reactions (such as nausea, palpitations, and profuse sweating) or psychological feelings of fear, panic, freezing, or disgust and avoidance of sex as well as of any type of closeness that could lead to sex. The aversive person does not necessarily recognize that he or she fears saying "I love you" because it might lead to a sexual overture by the partner. Aversion may be particular to the spouse or more general. It may be primary or secondary, though usually the latter; and it occurs in both males and females, more so among the latter.

Developmental antecedents of sexual aversion are sexual traumas during childhood or adolescence, such as rape or forced incest; severe body image or self-esteem problems about, for example, late puberty, hirsutism, or clumsiness; or an unwanted pregnancy, especially if it was treated as a catastrophe in the person's social milieu.

In adulthood a common etiological pattern is that anxiety evolves slowly in the face of relentless pressure by the spouse to have intercourse much more frequently than desired, or in certain places, at certain times, and in certain ways that are objectionable to the person. Pressure may be conveyed directly, through angry outbursts or punishment by the spouse. It also may come across more subtly, when the spouse performs favors and then is disappointed when sex is not offered in payment. If the individual exercises the privilege of saying no, the spouse may become increasingly hostile and/or manipulative, so that communication deteriorates into a vicious cycle. Eventually the aversive person may try to please by guessing the spouse's expectations and so put him or herself under pressure even when it is not intended by the partner.

Psychopathology of various kinds may be seen in some aversive individuals, including phobias about sex-related matters such as pregnancy and sexually transmitted diseases as well as general timidity that can expand into agoraphobia. Depression and obsessive-compulsiveness also are seen. Sexual orientation may be a conflict or, rarely, the person may be a paraphiliac.

Treatment begins by giving both spouses a clear understanding of the etiological factors behind the behavior of each of them in reaction to their past experiences and to each other. Sensate focus is then introduced as a means of *in vivo* systematic desensitization of anxiety. For it to be effective in this context, the nonaversive spouse is exhorted to allow the partner to control the timing, duration, and content of physical contact until late in therapy. Any attempt to be manipulative or induce guilt in the spouse is confronted. Touching begins at whatever stage is most comfortable for that aversive person—possibly with some clothes on, or away from the bedroom. Each step is gradual but may evoke some degree of fear. The aversive person is challenged to take responsibility for self by acknowledging the anxiety and doing something to reduce it without withdrawing from contact altogether (Kolodny *et al.*, 1979).

As therapy proceeds, anxiety usually will not appear with equal intensity with each new step. More time may need to be spent at some stages than others, for example, when genitals are added to the areas to be touched. As fear subsides, the emphasis of sensate focus can be shifted to attending to incoming sensations and communicating with the spouse or partner. Verbal communication in the couple, especially the resolution of power struggles, receives attention as well. Finally, the factors contributing to the nonaversive spouse's tendency to pressure can be identified and resolved and bypassed. For instance, a man may have an explosive personality style that keeps his wife on edge, fearing his next outburst, which sometimes involves his breaking things. He may be motivated to learn some temper-control strategies, not just for the sake of their sex life but for his own self-growth. Although in most cases extinguishing the sexual phobia allows natural sexual feelings and functioning to spring forth spontaneously, in other cases extinguishing the phobia leaves a person who is unafraid but still uninterested in sex and in need of specific enhancement techniques to help them build a positive repertoire of avenues to sex arousal.

8.3. Inhibited Sexual Desire

Inhibited sexual desire has been identified as a common sexual problem for both males and females (Frank, Anderson, & Rubenstein, 1978; Kaplan, 1979; Kolodny *et al.*,

1979; Lief, 1977). Also known as low libido, this distress may come about as secondary to a sexual dysfunction or may occur in a completely functional individual. Its primary manifestation is impaired sexual receptivity or initiatory behavior; the degree of arousal that occurs once sexual interaction is underway is a separate matter. Inhibited sexual desire may exist in relation to just the spouse or more generally.

Unlike sexual aversion, inhibited sexual desire can be caused by quite a number of organic problems, such as alcoholism, anemia, and pituitary insufficiency (see Kolodny *et al.*, 1979). Inhibited sexual desire also may result from sexual traumas such as rape, affective factors, low self-esteem, obsessiveness, environmental stresses, and conflicts about intimacy. If the person is inhibited by such matters as sexual odors, or visited by disturbing imagery when aroused, he or she may avoid getting interested in sex. In addition to such individual factors, relational issues are common in these cases. If the spouse is considered boring, sexually unappealing, or deceitful, inhibited sexual desire can develop. Or there may be a power struggle, perhaps about a particular form of sexual activity such as oral–genital sex. Inhibited sexual desire can be a weapon in that struggle.

Education about sexual desire and initiation is a main focus of treatment. The point is stressed that libido can be facilitated in a variety of ways, through relationship enhancement, resolution of interpersonal conflicts, and adding interest and variety to the couple's sexual repertoire. Stultifying patterns of initiation according to sex role expectations are made more flexible. Fantasy also may come into play as a spice to the interaction.

Throughout therapy the effects of one person's sexual desire on the other spouse are examined and reinterpreted. When one's spouse is disinterested in sex, it is easy to feel personally rejected and then react to the feeling of hurt. One's sexual needs may seem to increase until they are nearly insatiable. It is important that both partners realize that this level of need is exaggerated by not knowing how long it will be until the next opportunity. Some sex therapists make suggestions in order to moderate this high level of sexual desire while increasing the degree of desire of the inhibited partner (Zilbergeld & Ellison, 1980).

The couple is encouraged to experiment with casual affection and sensual touching when not initially aroused, to see that desire can evolve when it has a chance. Options are created for handling situations where one spouse is sexually desirous and the other not, such as masturbating while being held. If there are fears about sexual performance, these are dealt with in much the same way as in the cases of dysfunction with libido unimpaired.

9. Concluding Comments

Although space limitations preclude a detailed discussion of the many complexities that sex therapy cases present, it is important to emphasize that a good sex therapist must be a competent clinician across a broad range of areas. Nowhere is this more apparent than in the need for sex therapists to deal effectively with client resistance, a problem that repeatedly tests the mettle of even the most skillful psychotherapist. Clients commonly "forget" instructions, bypass limits set by their therapists (particularly those that involve prohibitions of sexual activity early in tbe course of therapy), verbally attack their therapist(s), and in numerous other ways demonstrate subtle and overt reluctance to change or to accept the structure of the therapeutic process. Implicit in these situations is a need for clients to understand that what they are doing may sabotage therapy and to come to terms with the underlying dynamics, such as fear of success, wanting to drive a spouse away, or wanting to gain retribution. Dealing with resistance in sex therapy has been discussed concisely by Munjack and Oziel (1978), Kaplan (1979), and Weissberg and Levay (1981).

Other complicating elements that affect many sex therapy cases include: the cultural milieu in which the clients have been raised and in which they currently live; the matrix of religious beliefs that influence each person's sexual values; the family constellation, including problems with children, in-laws, siblings, or other relatives, as well as the nature of the family support system; socioeconomic factors; health considerations; and a host of therapy-related issues, including issues of confidentiality, transference, and countertransference. This amalgam of potential complexities often demands great care on the part of the therapists to separate the wheat from the chaff and to address directly the pressure points in each case.

Despite these complexities, sex therapy has enjoyed considerable success over the last decade. Most clients can be helped in finding sexual satisfaction with brief therapy, and the high level of acceptance of this therapy mode by the general public probably mirrors the general effectiveness. However, it is important to realize that sex therapy offers few "instant cures" and that, like all forms of psychotherapy, it depends in the final analysis on a good therapeutic alliance between a competent, sensitive therapist and a motivated client.

10. References

Annon, J. S. The therapeutic use of masturbation in the treatment of sexual disorders. Paper presented at Association for the Advancement of Behavior Therapy, Washington, D.C., 1971.

Annon, J. S. *Behavioral treatment of sexual problems* (Vols. 1 & 2). Honolulu: Kapiolani Health Services, 1974.

Apfelbaum, B. A contribution to the development of the behavioral–analytic sex therapy model. *Journal of Sex and Marital Therapy*, 1977, *3*, 84–94.

Apfelbaum, B. The diagnosis and treatment of retarded ejaculation. In S. R. Leiblum & L. A. Pervin (Eds.), *Principles and practice of sex therapy*. New York: Guilford Press, 1980.

Bancroft, J. H. The Masters & Johnson approach in a National Health Service setting. *British Journal of Sexual Medicine*, 1975, *1*, 6–10.

Barlow, D. H., & Abel, G. G. Sexual deviation. In W. E. Craighead, A. E. Kazdin, & M. J. Mahoney (Eds.), *Behavior modification principles, issues and applications*. Boston: Houghton Mifflin, 1976.

Chapman, J. D. Frigidity: Rapid treatment by reciprocal inhibition. *Journal of the American Osteopathic Association*, 1968, *67*, 871–878.

Clement, U., & Pfafflin, F. Changes in personality scores among couples subsequent to sex therapy. *Archives of Sexual Behavior*, 1980, *9*, 235–244.

Clifford, R. E. Development of masturbation in college women. *Archives of Sexual Behavior*, 1978, *7*, 559–573.

Cooper, A. J. An innovation in the "behavioral" treatment of a case of non-consummation due to vaginismus. *British Journal of Psychiatry*, 1969, *115*, 721–722.

Derogatis, L. R., Meyer, J. K., & King, K. M. Psychopathology in individuals with sexual dysfunction. *American Journal of Psychiatry*, 1981, *138*, 757–763.

Ellis, A. *The art & science of love*. New York: Lyle Stuart, 1968.

Frank, E., Anderson, C., & Rubenstein, D. Frequency of sexual dysfunction in "normal" couples. *New England Journal of Medicine*, 1978, *299*, 111–115.

Friedman, D. The treatment of impotence by brevital–relaxation therapy. *Behavior Research and Therapy*, 1968, *6*, 257–261.

Hariton, E. B., & Singer, J. L. Women's fantasies during sexual intercourse: Normative and theoretical implications. *Journal of Consulting and Clinical Psychology*, 1974, *42*(3), 313–322.

Hartman, W. E. & Fithian, M. A. *Treatment of sexual dysfunction*. New York: Aronson, 1974.

Kaplan, H. S. *The new sex therapy*. New York: Brunner/Mazel, 1974.

Kaplan, H. S. *Disorders of sexual desire*. New York: Brunner/Mazel, 1979.

Kaplan, H. S., Kohl, R. N., Pomeroy, W. B., Offit, A. K., & Hogan, B. Group treatment of premature ejaculation. *Archives of Sexual Behavior*, 1974, *3*(5), 443–452.

Kolodny, R. C., Masters, W. H., & Johnson, V. E. *Textbook of sexual medicine*. Boston: Little, Brown, 1979.

Lazarus, A. A. The treatment of chronic frigidity by systematic desensitization. *Journal of Nervous and Mental Disease*, 1963, *136*, 272–278.

Lazarus, A. A. Psychological treatment of dyspareunia. In S. R. Leiblum & L. A. Pervin (Eds.), *Principles and practice of sex therapy*. New York: Guilford Press, 1980.

Leiblum, S. R., Rosen, R. C., & Pierce, D. Group treatment format: Mixed sexual dysfunctions. *Archives of Sexual Behavior*, 1976, *5*(4), 313–322.

Lief, H. Inhibited sexual desire. *Medical Aspects of Human Sexuality*, 1977, *11* (7), 94–95.

LoPiccolo, J., & Lobitz, W. C. The role of masturbation in the treatment of orgasmic dysfunction. *Archives of Sexual Behavior*, 1972, *2*, 163–171.

Marks, I. M. Review of behavioral psychotherapy: II. Sexual disorders. *American Journal of Psychiatry*, 1981, *138*(6), 750–756.

Masters, W. H., & Johnson, V. E. *Human sexual inadequacy*. Boston: Little, Brown, 1970.

Masters, W. H., & Johnson, V. E. Sex as a natural function. Paper presented at AMA meeting, San Francisco, June 1972.

Masters, W. H., & Johnson, V. E. *The pleasure bond*. Boston: Little, Brown, 1975.

Masters, W. H., & Johnson, V. E. Principles of the new sex therapy. *American Journal of Psychiatry*, 1976, *133*, 548–554.

Mathews, A., Bancroft, J., Whitehead, A., Hackmann, A., Julier, D., Bancroft, J., Gath, D., & Shaw, P. The behavioral treatment of sexual inadequacy: A comparative study. *Behaviour Research and Therapy*, 1976, *14*, 427–436.

Maurice, W. L., & Guze, S. B. Sexual dysfunction and associated psychiatric disorders. *Comprehensive Psychiatry*, 1970, *11*, 539–543.

McCarthy, B. W. A modification of Masters and Johnson sex therapy model in a clinical setting. *Psychotherapy: Theory, research and practice*, 1973, *10*(4), 290–294.

McGovern, K. B., Stewart, R. C., & LoPiccolo, J. Secondary orgasmic dysfunction: I. Analysis and strategies for treatment. *Archives of Sexual Behavior*, 1975, *4*, 265–275.

Miller, V., & Brockway, J. Commonalities and differences in the treatment of 2 cases of primary orgasmic dysfunction. Unpublished paper, University of Oregon, 1972.

Munjack, D. J., & Kanno, P. H. Retarded ejaculation: A review. *Archives of Sexual Behavior*, 1979, *8*(2), 139–150.

Munjack, D. J., & Oziel, L. J. Resistance in the behavioral treatment of sexual dysfunctions. *Journal of Sex and Marital Therapy*, 1978, *4*(2), 122–138.

Riley, A. J. & Riley, E. J. A controlled study to evaluate directed masturbation in the management of primary orgasmic failure in women. *British Journal of Psychiatry*, 1978, *133*, 404–409.

Sager, C. *Marriage contracts and couple therapy*. New York: Brunner/Mazel, 1976.

Schumacher, S. Effectiveness of sex therapy. In R. Gemme & C. C. Wheeler (Eds.), *Progress in sexology*. New York: Plenum Press, 1977.

Schumacher, S., & Lloyd, C. W. Physiological and psychological factors in impotence. *Journal of Sex Research*, 1981, *17*, 40–53.

Schwartz, M. F., Bauman, J., & Masters, W. H. Hyperprolactinemia and sexual function in men. Paper presented at SSTAR, New York, 1981.

Semans, J. H. Premature ejaculation: A new approach. *Southern Medical Journal*, 1956, *49*, 353–357.

Snyder, A., LoPiccolo, L., & LoPiccolo, J. Secondary orgasmic dysfunction. II. Case study. *Archives of Sexual Behavior*, 1975, *4*, 277–283.

Spark, R. F., White, R. A., & Connolly, P. B. Impotence is not always psychogenic. *Journal of the American Medical Association*, 1980, *243*, 750–755.

Stuart, F. M., & Hammond, D. C. Sex therapy. In R. B. Stuart (Ed.), *Helping couples change*. New York: Guilford Press, 1980.

Wagner, G., & Green, R. *Impotence: Physiological, psychological, surgical diagnosis and treatment*. New York: Plenum Press, 1981.

Weissberg, J. H., & Levay, A. N. The role of resistance in sex therapy. *Journal of Sex and Marital Therapy*, 1981, *7*(2), 125–130.

Wolpe, J. *Psychotherapy by reciprocal inhibition*. Palo Alto, Calif.: Stanford University Press, 1958.

Wright, J., Perreault, R., & Mathieu, M. The treatment of sexual dysfunction. *Archives of General Psychiatry*, 1977, *34*, 881–890.

Yulis, S. Generalization of therapeutic gain in the treatment of premature ejaculation. *Behavior Therapy*, 1976, *7*, 355–358.

Zeiss, A. M., Rosen, G. M., & Zeiss, R. A. Orgasm during intercourse: A treatment strategy for women. *Journal of Consulting and Clinical Psychology*, 1977, *45*, 891–895.

Zeiss, R. Self-directed treatment for premature ejaculation. *Journal of Consulting and Clinical Psychology*, 1978, *46*(6), 1234–1241.

Zilbergeld, B. *Male sexuality*. Boston: Little, Brown, 1978.

Zilbergeld, B., & Ellison, C. R. Desire discrepancies and arousal problems in sex therapy. In S. R. Leiblum & L. A. Pervin (Eds.), *Principles and practice of sex therapy*. New York: Guilford Press, 1980.

21

Arbitration of Family Disputes

ROBERT HENLEY WOODY

Many people have difficulty handling the ups and downs of everyday family life. Herrman, McKenry, and Weber (1979) point out:

> People are typically "reluctant decision makers." They try to avoid conflict and decisions over which there is little control or decisions with possible negative effects. Divorcing parties have not been able to manage family conflict successfully in the past, otherwise divorce would not be imminent. (p. 17)

These unmanageable conflicts, however, are not confined to divorcing couples. They can plague all the adults and children throughout any family with significant disputes.

Due to their special expertise in dealing with family problems, marriage and family therapists are being called upon to serve in a mediation and/or arbitration role. This may cause some therapists to experience consternation. On one hand there is a wish to be helpful in any reasonable manner; but on the other, the legal arena seems somewhat foreign to the therapy room and the directive nature of mediation/arbitration seems to contradict some of the revered tenets of therapy.

This chapter is intended to clarify how the marriage and family therapist can attain consonance between arbitration and therapy. The posture of courts vis-à-vis family disputes will lead to consideration of arbitration and psychological frameworks, and guidelines will be offered for being a family dispute arbitrator.

1. The Posture of the Courts

The sanctity of marital and familial privacy has led the court to avoid intervening in family disputes unless clear-cut legal issues are involved. For example, if a father and mother were in dispute over whether their child should go to a public or a private school, the court would not accept the case; however, if they were divorcing and educational

ROBERT HENLEY WOODY • Department of Psychology, University of Nebraska at Omaha, Omaha, Nebraska 68182.

placement were an issue in deciding the custody, the court likely would resolve the question. This reluctance to expand court services to family disputes has left many people groping, often unsuccessfully, for solutions. The court's reluctance is especially common when decisions about childrearing are involved.

The courts have been aware of the faulty decision making for childrearing within families, but have refused to enter into familial disputes unless the "moral, mental and physical conditions are so bad as to seriously affect the health or morals of children" (Sisson, 1936, p. 285). The essential rationale of the court is:

> If we should hold that equity has jurisdiction . . . such holding will open wide the gates for settlement in equity of all sorts and varieties of intimate family disputes concerning the upbringing of children. . . . Never has the court put itself in the place of the parents and interposed its judgment as to the course which otherwise amicable parents should pursue in discharging their parental duty. (Kilgrow, 1959, p. 888)

Brieland and Lemmon (1977) conclude that this isolation from family disputes is guided by two principles: "Notwithstanding all their faults and mistakes parents will generally be more successful in caring for their children than strangers or agencies of the state, and the emotional ties between parent and child should be respected regardless of whether the child might enjoy both better care and more material advantages under the care of someone else" (p. 223).

To ease reliance on the court system and to facilitate family living, the American Arbitration Association (1979) has initiated the Family Dispute Services program of mediation and arbitration. Spencer and Zammit (1979) indicate a four-stage intervention objective:

> first, "conciliation," to assist husbands and wives in resolving marital problems, with a view towards their remaining together; second, "mediation," to assist separated parties in amicably arriving at the terms of a separation agreement; third, "reference" of those items upon which the parties cannot agree following mediation to a referee for final and binding determination (really "interest arbitration" by another name); and finally, "arbitration" of disputes arising under separation agreements. (p. 112)

As Spencer and Zammit acknowledge, the rules and procedures for the Family Dispute Services are patterned after the Commercial Rules used in labor arbitration, but have adaptations to better accommodate the uniqueness of family relations, such as meeting the best interests of child (e.g., the arbitrator may meet with the child *in camera* and may obtain professional expert opinions).

Reliance on an arbitrator for decision making has undeniable benefits for labor relations, but in the arena of family disputes, there are other considerations, namely of a psychological nature, that raise the possibility of deleterious effects. That is, the therapeutic objectives of essentially every school or theory of psychotherapy have the axiom of *effective self-responsibility*. In other words, a universally accepted criterion of mental health is that the person be able to exercise self-determination, to be responsible for the outcomes of his or her behavior, and to "own" his or her life's patterns. For example, extensive research has documented that "internalizers" (those who accept self-responsibility for outcomes) will be far superior in a myriad of measures of health than "externalizers," who attribute outcomes to the actions of others, chance, or bad luck (Lefcourt, 1976; Phares, 1976). Although conciliation and mediation (and possibly reference) easily could allow the individual to retain self-responsibility, arbitration places the decision making on a third party. Given the possibility of adverse psychological effects from this transfer of responsibility, the thesis question is: *How can family dispute arbitration further mental health objectives?*

2. Arbitration Framework

Arbitration in family disputes is supported by the Uniform Marriage and Divorce Act, wherein Section 306 accepts parties forming separation agreements that the court will uphold (unless they are unconscionable or tread upon sacrosanct court discretion, such as the *parens patrae* jurisdiction for safeguarding the best interests of the child): "While agreements to arbitrate financial and property matters are fully enforceable, this is not so with respect to matters involving children" (Spencer & Zammit, 1979, p. 116).

This endorsement and increased social awareness of the contractual nature of marital relationships have led many couples to prepare prenuptial agreements (which may or may not eventually be enforced by a court), and it seems more and more common for arbitration to be called for. On the other hand, there has been, to date, minimal dependence on the American Arbitration Association's formal Family Dispute Services program,[1] albeit that cases are appearing that report use of an arbitrator.

To establish a definition for arbitration, as is necessary for an analysis of the psychological considerations, the major goals for family dispute arbitration should be highlighted. Herrman, McKenry, and Weber (1979) explain:

> The major goal is to assist the parties to be rational and responsible enough to cooperate in making compromises acceptable to all. Successful mediation and arbitration is based upon open communication, the equalization of power, decreased dependency, and impartial conflict resolution of those issues not directly resolved by the parties. (p. 19)

There seems to be at least tangential recognition of the need to keep the parties responsible. This is manifested, presumably, by the parties exercising their freedom of choice in selecting the decision-making arbitrator. As Spencer and Zammit (1979) state:

> The ability to choose the arbitrator is necessary to the realization of the value of family autonomy, precisely that element which is absent from court litigation. It permits the parties to choose an arbitrator who shares their values, a parent surrogate who attempts to make the decision that they would make absent their present hostility. Indeed, this traditional advantage of arbitration is one which should be enhanced, to the point where the courts can no longer credibly claim to be in the best position to judge a child's interests. (p. 119)

Regardless of the freedom of choice procedure, reservations remain about the negative psychological concomitants of allowing any third party to be the decision maker, unless it is a legal issue in the court, for another person.

The four stages of the Family Dispute Services program, as previously described, allow for other than total third-party decision making, that is, through conciliation, mediation, and to a lesser extent, reference. Here, there would be little dissonance between arbitrators and the courts; there is a present emphasis on keeping matrimonial questions out of court (Strelecki, 1980) and relying instead upon conciliation services,

[1]Note that Spencer and Zammit (1979) report "while the number of marital disputes actually arbitrated at the AAA has been relatively small, it is probable that the number of separation agreements providing for arbitration of disputes arising thereunder is by no means insignificant" (p. 112). A personal communication (May 30, 1980) with Charles H. Bridge, Jr., AAA Regional Director in Chicago, supports that the flow of cases to the national offices has been slow.

including marriage and family counseling, divorce counseling, mediation of family conflicts, and custody and visitation evaluations, to name but a few areas (Barteau, 1980).

From a psychological point of view, there is a critical distinction between conciliation and mediation versus arbitration:

> Under mediation the parties use the services of a trained mediator in an effort to arrive at their own agreement. In the case of arbitration, a decision is made *for* the parties by a designated arbitrator. (Pickrell & Bendheim, 1980, p. 27)

Thus, in mediation, but not arbitration necessarily, the parties are personally involved in the derivation of solutions. The mediator merely facilitates their efforts in decision making; he or she does not act as the decision maker *per se*. As Stulberg (1980) describes it:

> Throughout all the meetings, the mediator works to keep the couple's energies constructive by transmitting information and creating new lines of communication. In an effort to move toward agreement, the mediator promotes cooperation, helps the couple to save face as individuals, and uses the concept of reality testing to separate the couple's wants and needs. (p. 5).

The purpose of mediation is consonant with the therapeutic goal of self-responsibility. Gleason (1980) states:

> People are more likely to adhere to arrangements that they have helped to formulate. Most important for the parties involved in a successful mediation, all leave the courtroom with some pride in having resolved their problem themselves. They have not engaged their adversary before a judge and lost . . . it provides an opportunity to work out a problem, to exercise humanity, to explore the nature of fairness. (p. 579)

And Stulberg (198C) adds, "When mediation is used to work out a separation or dissolution agreement the agreements are more durable and there is less friction over compliance . . . misunderstandings are kept to a minimum" (p. 5). Despite this seeming alignment with the goals of therapy, Pickrell and Bendheim (1980) caution, "The mediators will not function as attorneys or therapists, however, but as mediators . . . a mediator who is a marriage counselor must remember that he is not functioning in his traditional role, but strictly as a mediator" (p. 28). This is sound advice since, to date, becoming a mediator is not predicated upon professional training as a counselor or therapist. On the other hand, without such training, the potential to maximize therapeutic effects during the mediation may be sacrificed.

None of the foregoing is intended to denigrate the use of arbitration for family disputes. On the contrary, there is ample evidence that many persons, for their own welfare, need the competencies of an arbitrator. The challenge, therefore, is to consider how arbitration can be made more efficacious, while at the same time promoting healthful psychological results for the parties. This stance leads to the proper psychological framework for dispute resolution.

3. Psychological Framework

Matters brought to the arbitrator signal that the parties have experienced stress, dissension, and/or hostility to the point that they believe their personal resources are inadequate to cope with the decision-making processes; therefore, they turn to the arbitrator for a solution. These dynamics suggest that family dispute arbitration should draw upon the plethora of research on "crisis management." Stated differently, the need for family dispute arbitration signifies a need to resolve a crisis, and there is much behavioral science research on this form of intervention.

According to Dixon (1979), a "crisis" represents "a functionally debilitating mental state resulting from the individual's reaction to some event perceived to be so dangerous that it leaves him or her feeling helpless and unable to cope effectively by usual methods" (p. 10). Ewing (1978) adds that professional intervening has "the intention of assisting individuals or families to modify personal characteristics such as feelings, attitudes, and behaviors that are judged to be maladaptive or maladjustive" (p. 7).

Often the person's past success or failure with coping with problems will preordain subsequent problem-solving attempts, but whatever the response to a crisis, it is highly individualized according to the psychosocial needs of that person: "The idiosyncratic meaning of a precipitating event can only be found in the person's own reality, which houses his or her personal feelings, goals, expectations, and values, all determined by specific life experiences" (Dixon, 1979, p. 11).

Crisis appears to be predicated on a need to reestablish emotional homeostasis. Caplan (1964) provides a crisis theory based on emotional homeostasis that supports a four-phase model: (1) Initially, habitual coping measures are called forth by the threat to the person's needs (there is increased tension), in hopes of solving the difficulty and restoring emotional equilibrium (regaining an organism that is comfortably free from tension). (2) If these efforts are ineffective for halting the increase in tension, emotional upset leads to disorganization and trial-and-error efforts to resolve the problems and to regain mastery of the emotional state. (3) If the problem-solving efforts are still unsuccessful, escalating tension stimulates the mobilization of emergency and novel coping devices. (4) If the problem cannot be eliminated and/or the tension cannot be significantly alleviated, there will be a breakdown of the personality organization. Throughout the sequence, the specific goal is emotional homeostasis. Therefore, a goal of family dispute arbitration should be to help the parties regain emotional equilibrium.

Probably the foremost psychological effect of crisis is the danger to self-esteem. This is especially critical in family disputes where the very existence of the family is being tested; as Whitlock (1978) states: "An *emotional* or *psychological* crisis generally involves a *loss* or *threat of loss* or a *radical change* in one's relationship with oneself or with some significant other person or situation" (p. 3). Certainly these are the conditions within matters brought to family dispute arbitration.

Whitlock (1978) refers to situations or conditions that significantly diminish human possibilities, such as divorce, as "contractive" crises. He points out that the extent of loss will depend upon personal maturity and the sociocultural milieu, and he warns:

> A temporary diminishing of self-esteem in a crisis is a significant loss that affects a person at a level of depth, and it must be recognized and accepted. If the mechanism of denial is utilized, the result may be the development of physical or emotional disorders. Recognizing, accepting, and learning to cope with a temporary loss of self-esteem will enable a person to mobilize his or her inner resources. (p. 116)

Needless to say, the arbitrator is in a position to help the parties cope with a loss of self-esteem as part of the family dispute arbitration processes. Specific guidelines for fulfilling this duty will be presented shortly.

It is important to realize that family disputes are not limited to impacting upon an individual or just the adults. As distinct from labor disputes (at least conceptually), family disputes have connections to a complex human system, namely the family. Dixon (1979) states:

> The concept of the family as a system implies that a change in one member brings about a corresponding change in the rest of the system, in this case the other members. Each member has

> a different role and function. The quality of the functioning of the overall system depends on the functioning of the largest subsystem. In the case of the family, this is the marital pair. The marriage is the heart of the family, and all other subsystems revolve around it. It is the basis for understanding the interaction of its members. The family system also develops rules and procedures to keep it organized and to guide it in fulfilling its purpose and functions. There are dynamic forces, emotional exchanges, that govern the emotional and affectional atmosphere of the family. (p. 161)

When external or internal events debilitate the family system, its members will have feelings of helplessness and be less able to function effectively: "Although in a family crisis each member is affected individually and each member's method of coping varies, it is the threat to total family functioning that is the major focus" (Dixon, 1979, p. 162). The message for the arbitrator is to recognize that all family members are experiencing various emotions and attempting to cope with these in different ways.

4. Guidelines for the Arbitrator

Given the unique nature of family disputes, such as the profound emotional effects throughout the family system, the arbitrator must assume duties that may not be within the traditional labor-oriented arbitration model. Family dispute arbitration depends upon a blend of arbitration *per se* and marriage and family therapy.

The uniqueness of family dispute arbitration makes it likely that many family dispute issues can be handled best by a team approach, that is, an arbitrator and a therapist coordinating their efforts. The marriage and family therapist who is serving as an arbitrator might well find it impedes the therapeutic process to try to wear two hats (i.e., be both an arbitrator and a therapist), and the team concept should be considered instead.

Most basically, the arbitration task involves helping the parties (and family members) identify, understand, and master the psychological tasks created by the stressful situation that led them into arbitration (Lindemann, 1944). A technical frame of reference may be found in Ewing's (1978) guidelines that crisis intervention be brief, be extended to the whole family, not be limited to an isolated problem (discussions could go beyond the arbitration issues), emphasize the present (the parties need to learn to deal with the here and now in order to gain more adaptive mechanisms for future coping), be reality oriented, put the professional (the arbitrator) in what might be a "nontraditional" role, and prepare the parties for any further treatment that might be needed.

If specialized skills are involved, they do not necessarily go beyond the interviewing required for human services of any nature. Consider the four steps that Whitlock (1978) believes to be useful for coping with the loss of self-esteem in a crisis. The first step requires listening to the pain and assisting with the intense feelings (e.g., anxiety, anger, guilt, and despair). Making contact with the feelings and their defense mechanisms facilitates accepting the loss as a reality. Second, there is a need to explore past coping methods and to understand the reasons for their current ineffectiveness. Third, it is necessary to explore alternative ways of "experiencing a sense of success or self-fulfillment and reestablishing a feeling of self-esteem" (p. 130). Fourth and finally, there needs to be an opening of communication channels with significant others, such as might enhance emotional support systems that can assist the person's maintenance of self-esteem. To be sure, there probably are some nontherapist arbitrators who would find it difficult to offer these services, such as dealing effectively with feelings, but it seems safe to say that they would have similar trouble handling any interpersonal conditions within any kind of arbitration. Stated differently, the services necessary for crisis management in arbitration mandate effective interpersonal skills for interviewing. If these skills are lacking in any form of arbitration, the benefits will be diminished. This mandate, obviously, issues an invitation to marriage and family therapists to apply their specialized skills in mediation and arbitration.

As discussed previously, family dispute arbitration should be concerned with the total family system. Dixon's (1979) strategy is to determine the "nuclear problem" and identify the family's potential through analysis of the family's communication processes and interactions, and then move to assessment and evaluation of the family structure and functioning (e.g., the degree of debilitation, functional areas affected, areas of weakness, sources of strength, etc.). This assessment will enhance the family's ability to attain self-understanding, to plan, and to implement other treatment that may be needed. Again, the specialized training possessed by the marriage and family therapist should be adequate for carrying out this assessment function.

The handling of the emotional component of family dispute arbitration requires more a frame of reference than a repertoire of skills. Therefore, it seems appropriate to put forth an overview of the steps that the parties (and family members) will go through in crisis resolution. Hansell (1976) posits a seven-step strategy: First, there is the discovery of the "challenging event" (this must preface any problem solving). Second, the nature of the challenging event should be identified (i.e., defining the predicament and reconnoitering the conditions therein). Third, consideration is given to possibilities for action (as would facilitate self-esteem). Fourth, acceptance of a possibility requires linking it to an attractive future (if an option for action is implemented, there should be a reasonable prediction of success). Fifth, encouragement should be used to maintain perseverance in a selected course of action (i.e., taking action according to the selected, success-directed plan). Sixth, results of efforts should be evaluated, with the understanding that other options may have to be exercised. And seventh, the adaptational sequence should be replaced with a return to the usual (pre-crisis) behavior patterns (and this should be done as soon as is realistically feasible). The strategy should be congruent with arbitration objectives, as well as promoting crisis resolution.

At no point in crisis management is there a depreciation of the parties' responsibility for decision making. The healthful goal of self-responsibility is ever present and is complemented by the assistance offered. This nexus between self-responsibility and crisis resolution must be honored in family dispute arbitration. It is a critical dimension of mental health, and to accord to it a lesser status is to jeopardize the well-being of the entire family system. This self-responsibility creates the much needed consonance between arbitration and therapy. That is, arbitration need not contradict therapeutic growth.

5. Conclusion

It seems incontrovertible that arbitration fills a contemporary social need. At the same time, there is reason to believe that the arbitrator should attend to psychological factors. In family dispute arbitration, as distinct from certain other kinds of arbitral disputes, special attention should be devoted to cultivating healthful conditions within the person's affects. As pointed out, the stress associated with the arbitration issues can be a harbinger of both physical and mental problems.

A key to psychological health is self-responsibility. The reliance on an arbitrator for reaching a decision creates a risk of self-defeating reactions, such as a loss of self-esteem, more so than such related options as conciliations (with its emphasis upon counseling) and mediation (with its emphasis upon negotiating), each of which facilitates but does not perform the actual decision making. This fact would support that, in a sense, arbitration should be a "court of last resort," to be used only when the other options, particularly mediation, have failed and/or when it seems clear that the parties have depleted their psychological resources and that catastrophic breakdown of their functioning is probable unless someone, that is, an arbitrator, is willing and able to assume authority for making their family decisions for them.

The emotional dimensions involved in family dispute arbitration require expert attention, as possessed by marriage and family therapists. What is needed is a frame of reference that acknowledges that the arbitration processes must go beyond data collection and decision making. As delineated above, there are numerous strategies that can and should be used when the parties are engaged in a crisis situation (which is typically the case when an arbitrator has been called upon for decision making). The focus must reach into the total family system; the arbitrator must consider the needs of all persons affected and attempt to integrate them into the family dispute arbitration as much as is possible.

The chief objective of family dispute resolution should be to cultivate improved coping skills within the family. This requires far more than a simple solution to a present problem. Although it would be illogical to advocate "therapy" in the arbitration, there surely will be therapeutic-like effects through crisis management and resolution. Beyond the actual decision, a desired outcome for family dispute arbitration is to prepare the parties and their family members for effective self-responsibility in their later family life. By adhering to this approach, the thesis question, "How can family dispute arbitration further mental health objectives?" can find a definite answer.

6. References

American Arbitration Association. *Family dispute services* (brochure). New York: American Arbitration Association, 1979.

Barteau, B. How to create a conciliation court. *Family Advocate,* 1980, *2*(4), 6–7, 34.

Brieland, D., & Lemmon, J. *Social work and the law.* St. Paul: West, 1977.

Capland, G. *Principles of preventive psychiatry.* New York: Basic Books, 1964.

Dixon, S. L. *Working with people in crisis.* St. Louis: Mosby, 1979.

Ewing, C. P. *Crisis intervention as psychotherapy.* New York: Oxford University Press, 1978.

Gleason, A. L. Humanities as mediators: An experiment in the courts of Maine. *American Bar Association Journal,* 1980, *66,* 576–579.

Hansell, N., IV. *The person-in-distress: On the biosocial dynamics of adaptation.* New York: Human Sciences, 1976.

Herrman, M. S., McKenry, P. C., & Weber, R. E. Mediation and arbitration applied to family conflict resolution: The divorce settlement. *Arbitration Journal,* 1979, *34,* 17–21.

Kilgrow v. *Kilgrow,* 268 Ala. 475, 107 So.2d 885 (1959).

Lefcourt, H. M. *Locus of control.* Hillsdale, N.J.: Lawrence Erlbaum, 1976.

Lindemann, E. Symptomatology and management of acute grief. *American Journal of Psychiatry,* 1944, *101,* 141–148.

Phares, E. J. *Locus of control in personality.* Morristown, N.J.: General Learning Press, 1976.

Pickrell, R. W., & Bendheim, A. L. Family disputes mediation—A new service for lawyers and their clients. *Barrister,* 1980, *7,* 27–28.

Sisson v. *Sisson,* 271 N.Y. 285, 2 N.E.2d 660 (1936).

Spencer, J. M., & Zammit, J. P. Reflections on arbitration under the Family Dispute Services. *Arbitration Journal,* 1979, *32,* 11–12.

Strelecki, J. Keeping it out of court. *Family Advocate,* 1980, *2*(4), 2–3, 34–35.

Stulberg, M. C. When three is not a crowd. *Family Advocate,* 1980, *2*(4), 4–5.

Whitlock, G. E. *Understanding and coping with real-life crises.* Monterey, Calif.: Brooks/Cole, 1978.

22

Community Homes as Hospital Alternatives for Youth in Crisis

BRYAN D. BROOK AND PAULA WALKER

There is increasing stress upon community mental health centers to be involved with and provide 24-hour care for children and adolescents. Much of this pressure results from the trend to deinstitutionalize patients and to also avert psychiatric hospitalizations via alternative community settings. Since its inception, Southwest Denver Community Mental Health Center, Inc., has adopted the philosophy of keeping severely disturbed persons in natural environments rather than institutional care (Brook, 1973; Brook, Cortes, March, & Stirling, 1976; Brook, Kirby, & Vollman, 1976; Polak & Kirby, 1976). During the past three years, prehospital community alternative homes have expanded from treatment of adults to diversion of seriously disturbed adolescents and children from psychiatric hospitalization. One pointed view regarding treatment outcome of adolescents stipulates that:

> Traditionally, the treatment of choice for severely disturbed and hard to manage psychotic children has involved institutional placement. . . . However, clinical observation suggests that institutionalization frequently has a disruptive effect on childrens' emotional and intellectual development. (Flomenhaft, 1974)

Southwest Denver's alternative home system seeks to maintain distressed youth in their own community and build upon existing support and family structures as part of its comprehensive community mental health center programs.

1. Historical Background

The Children and Youth program of Southwest Denver Community Mental Health Center received a federal runaway grant in June 1974 to assist with the rapidly growing national crisis of runaway youth. A foster home alternative program soon was started on a pilot basis modeled after the center's adult alternative community home network (Brook, *et al.*, 1976). This program worked with youth in small family settings instead of institu-

BRYAN D. BROOK and PAULA WALKER • 3185 South Dahlia Street, Denver, Colorado 80222.

tions and provided them with both therapy and assistance to restructure their lives. The approach integrated the entire array of community mental health center services with environmental benefits of foster-care homes. Consequently, this program has evolved to include the wide range of children and adolescents who might profit from clinical services and transitional foster care. Thus, youth who are frequently placed in a psychiatric hospital or juvenile detention center are either seen as outpatients in their own home with key persons in their social system or transferred to one of the center's alternative family homes.

The stay with a family in their own community has provided a more relevant baseline for assessment of social functioning than adaptation to an institutional environment. In addition, family members and other key persons also are involved in sessions whenever feasible, which utilizes resources in a youth's social network. Financial cutbacks of many state hospitals have decreased inpatient beds and sufficient hospital staff, thus creating tremendous impact on the demand for community based services. Such austerity and national trend of treatment in the least restrictive environment have stimulated creative development of community options that may meet client needs more economically and effectively.

2. Alternative Home Treatment

Southwest Denver Community Mental Health employs a community philosophy of social systems intervention with alternative foster homes that replaces most of the need for institutional placement of youth. If intervention in a youth's natural setting still warrants therapeutic separation, alternative homes are used for short stay assessment and treatment. The homes are similar to foster homes and receive reimbursement for services, but are administered by the center as an integral part of Southwest Denver Mental Health's overall treatment resources. Each treatment plan is tailored to minimize the level of environmental disruption and built upon existing support structures. A timely and structured separation of a child and parents during an emotional crisis has been favorably regarded as one useful strategy.

> A short period of carefully structured separation at a time of crisis may be a valuable diagnostic tool in permitting a more intensive and extensive evaluation of intrinsic problems in the child and family. (Rose & Sonis, 1959, p. 412)

The study showed that providing at least partial relief to a destructive cycle between parent and child has therapeutic merit. It allows separation in order for the family to reorganize themselves constructively for future family living and to test their capacities to support each other or accept their incapacity to do so. The authors contend that children are not always best off in their own families and that realistic separations are not inevitably traumatic.

At Southwest Denver Community Mental Health the emphasis is on timely and constructive separations with specified goals with persons in the youth's social system taking responsibility for their part in the crisis. Thus, families may not just refer their children and step out of the picture, since their involvement is essential whether a youth returns home or is placed elsewhere.

> Short term separation of parents and child in selected areas can allow movement which might not occur under other circumstances. (Laybourne & Miller, 1962, p. 598)

Changes frequently occur with the family system when a youth has been temporarily removed from the home. Therapeutic involvement of parents may help a family reorganize, discourage the development of chronic pathology, and minimize a closing of ranks by taking over the youth's normal family functions. This approach also discourages leaving a youth out of his family's future plans by "setting him aside" while it offers opportunity for a smoother reintegration into his family or another community setting. Institutional care frequently tends to encourage social regression and serves to complicate effective rehabilitation of a youth's former role in his family and community life (Flomenhaft, 1974).

Therapeutic separation of a child from his home becomes necessary for a multitude of reasons ranging from a youth's constant disruptive behavior to a psychotic youth needing medication, stabilization, and evaluation. D. W. Winnicott (1958) writes of challenging an acutely psychotic child by placing the burden of the treatment on the family and treating him at home. However, he comments positively on the use of foster care with adoptive parents combined with case management.

3. Alternative Home Screening and Operations

Home sponsors chosen for the program are from the southwest Denver community. They are interested individuals, couples, or families who have stable community residence. Potential sponsors are screened regarding certain criteria such as: acceptance of others, impact of added stress with commitment from all, imposition of personal values, and willingness to follow treatment goals as part of a team. Careful screening minimizes those wanting treatment or just what appears to be "easy money." Screening takes place in a prospect's home and includes all family members to evaluate how the program might affect each of their lives and the family as a unit. This becomes crucial when there are children at home who would be sharing their parents. It also includes review of a prospect's parenting history and experiences plus other child-care issues.

Consequently, Southwest Denver Mental Health has been certified as a child placement agency to license its own foster homes using state licensing procedures based on a unique partnership with Colorado's State Social Services Department. The homes are licensed as short stay foster homes and integrated into the center's alternative resources for evaluation and treatment of youth for three months. Southwest Denver Mental Health is reimbursed for the majority of its foster placements by Colorado Social Services, who also refer youth from the southwest Denver area for short term placement and therapy. The alternative youth home program seeks to strengthen continuity of care while providing the therapist a wider range of protective environments.

Youth alternative homes also differ from state administered foster care homes in that center staff coordinators work with each home to resolve problems, liaison with a youth's therapist, and monitor the home sponsor's needs. Home coordinators also assist with keeping open staff communication lines that minimize client and family manipulations. Therefore, coordinators have an essential role in the development of each home as a center resource.

Home sponsors have another support structure via bimonthly meetings with other youth and adult home sponsors to discuss various common concerns. The center also negotiates a personal services contract with sponsors regarding salary, mileage, vacation, sick leave, and yearly cost of living increases. A 30-day paid mental health vacation is required for all sponsors to decrease the risk of program burn out. In addition, home coordinators provide informal rest periods following a very stressful client or some personal life crisis of the sponsor.

Homes are on 24-hour availability which permits crisis admissions during weekends and at night. During off hours, medical coverage is provided by a physician at Fort Logan State Hospital who examines a youth's physical and mental status, assesses medications, and writes an admission order to the foster home. Workday admissions are seen by the center's psychiatrist with a physical examination provided under contract by a neighborhood health center.

A sponsor family expects a youth to participate as a family member by helping with their room, dishes, and so forth. Whenever possible a youth continues in the same school program and maintains prior healthy friendships via passes. Rules, visits, and consequences for certain behavior are examples of areas covered under a client's negotiated plan. Schools have cooperated by allowing clients to stay in their school of origin while they are temporarily living out of that district. They also keep therapists and sponsors aware of a youth's school participation. When there are difficulties with attendance and academic performance, special monitoring is set up with schools and more individualized programs are developed. Sometimes youth not only attend school but also find part-time jobs. Clients generally are seen daily by their therapist for their first week to enhance the transition process. Family therapy sessions are held both during and following alternative foster home placement. Center volunteers assist youth in becoming better acquainted with community resources by providing transportation through a big brother/sister involvement. Volunteers also help sponsors when they provide youth sitting which gives sponsors a break by getting away during a particular placement.

4. Summary and Conclusion

The youth alternative home network is built on trust and open communication between sponsors, therapists, and home coordinators. The therapist's primary concern is to the client, while the home coordinator, although concerned with the client's treatment, mainly is focused on the sponsor's needs and responses. This unique model of integrating youth foster homes into a community mental health center provides clients with a needed noninstitutional evaluation and treatment option. It also may assist a youth in acquiring skills needed for emancipation and independent living. Hopefully, other community mental health programs will explore prehospital family alternatives within their own clinical services and communities as an additional avenue of treatment for children and adolescents.

5. References

Brook, B. Crisis hostel: An alternative to psychiatric hospitalization for emergency patients. *Hospital and Community Psychiatry*. 1973, *24*, 621–624.

Brook, B., Cortes, M., March, R., & Stirling, M. S. Community families as alternatives in psychiatric hospital intensive care. *Hospital and Community Psychiatry*. 1976, *27* (3), 195–198.

Brook, B., Kirby, M., & Vollman, R. Crisis hostel: An alternative to the acute psychiatric ward. In H. J. Parad (Ed.), *Emergency and disaster management*. Bowie, Md.: Charles Press, 1976.

Flomenhaft, K. Outcome of treatment for adolescents. *Adolescence*, 1974, *9*, 57–66.

Freud, A. *Psychoanalytic treatment of children* (trans. N. Proctor-Gregg). London: Image, 1941.

Laybourne, P. C., & Miller, H. C. Pediatric hospitalization of psychiatric patients: Diagnostic and therapeutic implications. *American Journal of Orthopsychiatry*, 1962, *32*, 596–603.

Polak, P., & Kirby, M. A model to replace psychiatric hospitals. *Journal of Nervous and Mental Disease*, 1976, *162* (1), 13–21.

Rose, J., & Sonis, M. The use of separation as a diagnostic measure in the parent–child emotional crisis. *American Journal of Psychiatry*, 1959, *116*, 409–415.

Shirley, H. F. *Pediatric psychiatry*. Cambridge, Mass.: Harvard University Press, 1963.

Winnicott, D. W. A case managed at home. In *Collected papers*. New York: Basic Books, 1958, 118–126.

23

Issues of Divorce in Family Therapy

STANLEY N. COHEN AND F. NOLAN JONES

As we enter the mid-1980s, it should come as no surprise that divorce, or marital dissolution as it is now commonly called, has become a "fact of life" in American society. The upsurge in the use of divorce as a means out of a dissatisfying marriage has been dramatic over the past 20 years. The number of divorces stood at 413,000 in 1962, and it doubled 10 years later. Since 1975, over one million divorces have been recorded annually (National Center for Health Statistics, 1981).

Although the annual number of divorces is expected to increase gradually during the next several years, the divorce rate appears to be stabilizing. Between 1966 and 1976, the rate rose steeply, doubling from 2.5 to 5.0 divorces per thousand population. Since 1976 the rise in the rate has leveled off at 5.3 for 1979 and 1980.

The number of children whose parents divorce also has risen sharply over the past 15 years. Bane (1976) estimated that between 20 and 30% of those born during the 1970s will see their parents dissolve their marriage, and if annulments and separations are considered, the figures rise to between 23 and 35%.

High marital disruption rates have come to be accepted as a part of contemporary life in the United States. At the same time, there is long-standing concern about the traumatic consequences of divorce, particularly on the well-being of children. Specifically, children who experience divorce generally are perceived to be more prone to social and personal problems than those who live in intact families.

1. Overview of Research Findings

The prevailing concern about how children are affected by the divorce of their parents has been a major topic of studies dealing with marital disruption. Early psychologically oriented research (Despert, 1953; McDermott, 1968, 1970, Westman, 1972) gener-

STANLEY N. COHEN • Department of Psychiatry, The Oregon Health Sciences University, Portland, Oregon 97201. F. NOLAN JONES • Clackamas County Family Court Service, Oregon City, Oregon 97045.

ally highlighted the trauma of divorce on the emotional development of children. The implication of findings from studies of this sort pointed to an expectation that children experiencing divorce would be subject to more emotional and developmental risks than children living in two-parent households. It should be noted that such studies typically based their findings on clinically derived samples, were retrospective in design, and did not assess children from intact family circumstances.

The works of Wallerstein and Kelley (1974, 1975, 1976, 1980) and Heatherington (1979; Heatherington & Cox, 1976) are recent psychologically oriented research efforts that have added to our understanding of how divorce impacts on the lives of children. Both were longitudinal studies, and Heatherington's had the added dimension of a matched group of children living in intact families.

The Wallerstein and Kelly study basically is a 5-year clinical analysis of 60 divorcing parents and their 131 minor children. The age range of the children was from 1 to 22. The families were selected nonrandomly, were primarily Caucasian, and middle class. Data were gathered from both of the parents and children at the time of the divorce or separation, one year, and five years after the event.

Heatherington and her colleagues conducted a 2-year study of preschool children (1976). The sample included 24 boys and 24 girls from divorcing circumstances who were matched on several attributes with an identical group of children living with both of their parents. The study subjects were described as Caucasian, middle class, and from families whose annual incomes averaged $22,000. Interviews, self-reports, and standardized measures were used to collect data two months, one year, and two years after the divorce. The findings of both of these research efforts are similar in many respects about the impact of divorce on children. The following is a summary of the salient points of these studies:

1. Divorce can best be understood in the context of a critical event that creates varied degrees of stress for both parents and their children.
2. Divorcing families go through a process of disorganization and reorganization of family interaction and functioning, that may take anywhere from two to three years.
3. The first year of the dissolution was found to be the most stressful for all the children and a majority of the parents.
4. The quality of the intra- and interparental functioning is a key factor governing the direction of the developmental and emotional well-being of the children.
5. The ability of older children to maintain their developmental stride is related to the degree to which parents are able to control their needs to derive emotional and social support from their children (Wallerstein & Kelly, 1980).
6. The continued involvement of the children with both parents is of primary psychological importance.

Early studies by sociologists (Bowerman & Irish, 1962; Kotch, 1961; Russell, 1957) found children from intact families scoring higher in emotional adjustment and having better relations with their parents than those from divorcing circumstances. But, when divorced and intact family samples were controlled for economic status, significant differences were not found between the children in school achievement, personal, and social adjustment (Burchinal, 1964; Thomes, 1968).

Sociologists also have studied the relationship of children's adjustment to family structure and family conflict. Two research efforts are relevant: In his retrospective study of high school-aged children, Nye (1957) not only compared children from intact and divorced families, but also controlled for "unhappy/happy" homes. His findings showed that children from both happy and unhappy divorced circumstances were less prone to psychosomatic illness and delinquent behavior and had better relations with their parents than children from unhappy intact homes. There also were no significant differences in school adjustment.

The effects of family conflict and family structure on the self-concept of children were studied by Raschke and Raschke (1979). The investigators conclude that the study findings:

> lend support to the proposition that children are not adversely affected by living in a single parent family, but that family conflict and/or parental unhappiness can be detrimental at least to self concept which also is a measure of social and personal adjustment. (p. 373)

The previously cited Wallerstein and Kelly (1980) study concluded that their findings provided no supporting evidence for the argument that divorce "is overall better for children than an unhappy marriage, or, for its opposite argument that living within an unhappy marriage is by and large more beneficial or detrimental than living in the divorced family" (p. 306).

Speculating about the apparent contradictory conclusions derived from the studies in question is not within the scope of this chapter. What is clear, however, is that the findings of studies on the impact of divorce as it reflects on the adjustment of children have been equivocal. In a recent publication it has been suggested that further research on the negative aspect of divorce is not warranted. Rather, the research question should address what it is about divorce that troubles children (Longfellow, 1979).

2. Divorce and Families

For better or worse, we reluctantly have come to accept the social reality of high divorce rates. If we have not experienced it personally, we have been witness to friends and relatives who more often than not have had to make profound adjustments in their family relationships when changing from an intact situation to one of separation and ultimately divorce. For all of its apparent discomfort and difficulty, most adults and children who have experienced divorce appear to make a satisfactory adjustment to changes in their living and personal circumstances.

Regardless of its prevalence, however, divorce somehow continues to be perceived as being particularly noxious and repugnant. Why the continued antipathy? The question obviously is a complex one and probably cannot be answered completely. However, the writers believe that divorce is viewed negatively because it is perceived to threaten fundamental, and to a large degree, inviolate conceptions Americans have come to have about the ideal family system. Such attitudes are deeply rooted in the fabric of our society dating back to Colonial days, and have been reinforced continually throughout our history.

Historical studies have shown that since our beginnings as a nation, the predominant and preferred family has been nuclear in structure, primarily child centered, and private in its decision making about family matters (Bane, 1976).

A belief commonly held by most Americans is that the family requires unconditional and permanent bonds between its members for its survival. Historically, and up to the present time, marriage has been defined as a lifelong commitment between two adults that typically involves maintaining a household and raising children. In other words, marital and parental relationships are thought to be one and the same. Simply stated, if your marriage dissolves or ends, so does your family.

Beliefs regarding the idealized American family obviously have not been reflected in the social reality of both our past and present history. This is particularly true about marital disruption in the lives of children. Interestingly enough, and apparently not readily known, the proportion of children affected by loss of a parent by death as compared to divorce has stayed approximately the same until most recently. Yet it is almost as if most people believe that marital disruption is a recent event and an artifact of our contemporary world. In this sense there is an unrealistic and nostalgic yearning for an earlier time when family life has been incorrectly viewed as being intact, stable, and lifelong in duration.

Obviously, when family life is viewed from a historical perspective it becomes clear that large members of children always have lived in single parent households as a result of marital disruption. In the past the major disrupter was death, now it is divorce. Curiously enough, marital disruption through death and its impact on children appears to have been more easily accepted than is disruption through divorce.

The perceived synonymity between marriage and family, as described earlier, carries over to commonly held conceptions about divorce. What results is a belief that divorce breaks up families rather than dissolves marriages, which is one of its major functions.

Although the law provides the overwhelming majority of divorcing parents with an opportunity to maintain parental relationships with each other and their children, a common perception frequently persists—namely, that their activities with each other have terminated. This view primarily is the result of divorcing couples thinking of their spousal and parental roles as being synonymous rather than distinct from each other. This misinterpretation of the intent of the law also is amplified by the adversarial nature by which divorce is processed through the courts, particularly if situations are contested or unresolved.

An additional misconception about divorce is that it is viewed as a permanent status rather than a condition subject to change. Such a notion carries with it a vision of disillusionment with marriage. Divorce also is thought generally to result in ever increasing numbers of minor children who permanently will be growing up in a single parent household.

Yet the patterns of remarriage rates are very high. This suggests that people are not discarding marriage as an institution, but rather the partner to whom they are married. The important point here is that a large portion of children from single parent homes eventually will live in a two parent household. There are, of course, instances when divorce will result in a permanent status for the parent living with the children, who has not remarried. Research findings dealing with the impact of single parenthood on a child's development are often contradictory. Regardless of one's belief about the desirability of two parent versus single parent families, the fact remains that most children (77%) continue to live in two parent households (1981).

The divorced parent not living in the household often believes he (and it usually is the father) has no role in the parenting of the children. This attitude apparently stems directly from a misconception that family life can occur only when the parents are living together. The fact is that parenting relationships are not intended to be terminated by divorce. Indeed the laws explicitly emphasize a reordering of parental and parent–child relations, the intent being to secure access to the child by the out-of-home parent. At the same time, the manner in which parenting responsibilities are to be shared during and after divorce have been clouded by the way family law has categorized the role of divorced parents in custodial and noncustodial terms. What is of particular concern to many noncustodial parents is that they have no legal basis to be involved in the lives of their children except on a limited basis. Recent changes in family law, for example, joint custody, have clarified and provided a legal basis by which both parents have the opportunity to participate in decisions related to the rearing of their children.

In summary, the ideal American family is one that is intact, nuclear, and child centered. This ideal is deeply imbedded in the cultural fabric of our society going back to colonial days. Family life also has been romanticized as a life-long commitment between two adults with no distinction having been made regarding the functional differences between marital and parental relationships and the implications of disruption to family members when a divorce occurs.

Analyses of the historical realities point out that marital disruption always has been a fact to be faced by parents and their children. It appears that marital disruption resulting from the death of a spouse has been culturally acceptable and viewed as an uncontrollable event. On the other hand, divorce, the current major disrupter of marriage, seems to be viewed as putting the institution of the family at risk and sustains particular concerns about the welfare of children. Consequently, when challenged by events such as increasing divorce rates, the family as an institution is viewed as if it is in serious jeopardy. In a sense, this perception contributes to a commonly held belief that divorce is "bad" for everyone, and children in particular.

2.1. The Divorce Process

The divorce process essentially involves two phases that have been described by Brown (1976) and Kressel and Deutsch (1977). The first phase focuses on spouses individually and/or collectively considering divorce and ultimately deciding to end the marriage. The second, or settlement phase, centers on couples deciding how to restructure their family relationships and resolve financial and property issues. The former relates to custody and visitation arrangements, and the latter to child and/or spousal support, property, and other financial matters.

Divorce is the legal means by which marriages are dissolved and settlements are approved. Attorneys, therefore, are the professional most frequently consulted by divorcing spouses. The stance or manner in which attorneys view their role varies. In a recent survey the data suggest that the crucial determinant insofar as the divorce outcome is concerned rests on the relationship between the two attorneys representing the spouses (Kressel, Lopez-Morillas, Weinglass, & Deutsch, 1978). The extent to which attorneys can work together in a collaborative fashion can influence and control adversarial aspects of the legal process that often impede and/or delay a satisfactory settlement of the issues needing resolution. Clearly, the attorney's role is of paramount importance in the divorcing process since clients usually rely heavily upon their advice and advocacy.

2.2. Decision to Divorce

Ambivalence toward the divorce by either or both spouses should be considered a major obstacle impeding the decision to end the marriage. The degree of ambiguity each feels, along with their lack of congruence about the areas that have created conflicting emotions, frequently contribute to a motivational unevenness between a couple that confounds the decision to divorce.

A major contributing element to the unevenness between spouses is often individual and collective reflections and sometimes nostalgic images of their "family album." In this context, both positive and negative factors about the marriage are considered when husbands and wives take into account their ultimate and permanent separation from each other. In a sense, reevaluations of one's marriage are assessed from both an emotional and a pragmatic perspective.

The ambivalance individuals or couples feel when divorce is being considered has been described by Levinger (1979). He defines conflicting emotions of couples as positive attractions, negative barriers, and alternative attractions. Positive attractions and negative barriers are viewed as those forces that move an individual toward or away from a marital relationship.

Illustrative and pertinent examples of positive attractions to remaining in the marriage include intra- and inter-reevaluations of the

1. Personal and physical characteristics of one's spouse
2. Advantage(s) of maintaining an intact two-parent relationship
3. Benefit(s) of sustaining kinship and friendship relations that have been developed as a result of the marriage
4. Economic value of maintaining an intact family

Examples of negative barriers to ending a marriage include reflections of the

1. Personal and social loneliness
2. Burden of being a single parent
3. Loss of daily contact with one's children
4. Response from parents and friends
5. Negative experience of friends and relatives who have divorced
6. Religious constraints
7. Reduction of income and/or wealth

Levinger points out that even when positive attractions are low, and barriers offer minimal restraint, alternative attractions must be perceived if the marital relationship is to end. Alternative attractions are those opportunities thought to provide personal and/or social experiences not perceived to be available in the marriage.

Examples of alternative attractions include: (1) economic independence, (2) a sense of freedom and new opportunity, and (3) interest in another person.

Weiss (1975) explains the ambivalence married people feel when contemplating separation and divorce as a function of the conflicted emotions resulting from a perception of a gradual erosion of love and persistence of emotional attachment to one's spouse. The persistence of attachment seems to be a major factor in sustaining both intra- and interpersonal ambivalance toward separation and divorce.

Feelings of ambivalence within and between spouses considering an end to their marriage may linger for some time. As divorce is perceived as a more viable alternative than the marriage, positive attractions are reevaluated as to their importance. At the same time, negative barriers and the emotional bonds of attachment decrease, as one or both spouses reassess their situation in the context of living apart from each other. When divorce is decided upon by at least one of the parties, there is a gradual movement toward internally resolving the issues associated with negative barriers to separation, as well as a diminishment of the emotional attachment to the other spouse.

Once at least one spouse has decided in favor of divorce, an unevenness of motivation can be expected to exist between the spouses. This condition not only can obstruct mutual decision making, but often creates the potential for additional conflict arising from one spouse's wish to pursue a divorce while the other does not. It is this disparity of motivation in wanting to end the marriage that is pivotal in the ability of couples to negotiate the second or settlement phase successfully. Although there are instances where a decision may result in a reconciliation, the focus of this chapter is to describe the dynamics associated with those who eventually divorce.

2.3. The Settlement Phase

With the decision to divorce having been made, the task of restructuring of family relationships and resolution of economic issues begins, often at an uneven pace because of the reasons mentioned previously.

In the restructuring of family relationships, distinctions must be made between those circumstances that are primarily marital in nature, and those that involve children. Distinguishing between marital and parental roles among divorcing couples is important because of perceptions often held that divorce terminates both relationships. This is in contrast to the reality of divorce which ends the marriage, and modifies parental and parent–child relationships. What is crucial for couples to accept is the fact that their continued involvement with each other as divorced parents is a reality if they both intend to be involved with their children.

In divorcing situations where children are involved, aspects of family relationships that need to be addressed are:

1. With whom and under what circumstances the children will live
2. How the parent not living with the children maintains contact with them
3. The degree of parental involvement in the rearing of their children
4. Consideration of the children's wishes and concerns about living circumstances

The resolution of financial issues accompanying restructuring of family relationships includes:

1. Income for the children's basic living and health needs and short and long-term educational expenses (child support)
2. Income to the spouses who may require additional short-term or fixed resources to maintain and/or improve their living circumstances (spousal support)
3. Division of family related assets such as the home, furniture, automobiles, and other personal belongings
4. Division of other real property, stocks, bonds, savings, economic business interests, and retirement benefits
5. Consideration of income tax consequences for each party

2.4. Summary of Divorcing Process

The ability of couples to respond cooperatively to the inevitable changes and dislocations inherent in the divorcing process is related to the emotional acceptance of the reality of the dissolution of the marriage. The emotional "letting go" of the marital relationship is considered a major element in the settlement and resolution of the divorce. Often, the emotions involved in acceptance of the divorce are like a roller coaster. At times there seems to be movement on the part of both spouses to deal with the emotions necessary in "unhooking" from each other. On the other hand, there may be periods of time when mutual acceptance of the divorce seems impossible. Both the decision and subsequent settlement are difficult transactions for the majority of divorcing persons and frequently take a considerable period of time to complete. The first year following a divorce generally is considered to be the most stressful time for family members.

3. Implications for Therapy

Most people agree that, at best, the transition from intactness to separation and ultimately divorce is a difficult course for family members to traverse. The degree of difficulty is largely contingent on the unevenness of spousal motivation to end the marriage and the individual emotional responses to varied economic, personal, and social dislocations resulting from separation and divorce. Nonetheless, the vast majority of divorcing couples and families appear to make the transition without outside help from marriage and family therapists. Couples who have experienced serious marital and family problems and where one or both spouses have considered divorce as an alternative to staying in the marriage typically are experiencing ambivalence and symptoms of distress. Clearly here the emphasis in therapy is in facilitating the couple's abilities to decide whether they want to continue or end their marital relationship. Couples in this category should be defined as being in the first or decision-making phase of the divorcing process. The direction of the treatment will take either the form of marital therapy if the decision is made to reconcile, or divorce therapy if marital dissolution is the course of action taken.

While speculations (Wallerstein & Kelly, 1980) have been made about the importance of providing professional help to those in the throes of divorce, there seems to be no substantive evidence to suggest therapy is needed for all such families.

The majority of divorcing couples who are seen by marriage and family therapists appear to fall into three general types. Couples who are undecided about continuing their marriage represent one type frequently seen by therapists. Another can be described as marriages in which a divorce has been decided upon by at least one of the spouses. The third general type encountered frequently in therapy are couples who clearly disagree with each other about dissolving their marriage. These kinds of couples can be characterized by:

1. Their degree of mutuality about getting a divorce
2. Their individual goals in seeking therapy
3. Motivational circumstances prompting them to contact a therapist

The comments that follow highlight the importance of assessing each couple in the context of these attributes before proceeding with therapy. This form of assessment can minimize the confusion inherent in dealing with couples who may have differing agendas that have brought them to therapy. Each case may represent a different stage of the divorcing process which in turn will determine the type of intervention provided.

Most therapists experienced in working with divorcing couples agree that those who have achieved a degree of consensus to end their marriage generally make the task of the therapist less arduous than with spouses who disagree about divorce. Although there may be varied degrees of mutuality about ending the marriage, couples of this sort typically are ready to begin the settlement phase of the divorcing process. As Brown (1976) points out:

> In a mutually agreed upon divorce, the role of the counselor is relatively simple, whether working with one spouse or the couple. Tasks are more likely to be straightforward matters involving plans for dissolution, custody, living arrangements, trade-off and the like, and less related to feelings of loss, rejection, or trauma. (p. 415)

The most challenging situations therapists encounter are those where couples are in disagreement about ending the marriage. Typically, one spouse has made the decision to divorce, while the other wants to continue the relationship. The emotions associated with the lack of mutuality between the spouses often is coupled with each person presenting different goals for which treatment and help is sought, for example, reconciliation versus divorce. Conditions of this sort are viewed as impeding and delaying the ability of couples to complete constructively the restructuring or settlement phase of the divorce. As Kressel and Deutsch (1977) have reported in their survey of professional therapists: "The single most frequently cited predictor of a difficult divorce was one spouse's eagerness to end the marriage coupled with reluctance to do so on the part of the other" (p 423).

The ambiance generated by divorce often prompts spouses (individually or collectively) to seek help for contradictory reasons. Therapists can anticipate that couples using their services may be highly motivated and desirous of assistance in resolving their problems. On the other hand, therapy can be sought primarily upon the advise of legal counsel or because of a judicial referral or court order. In cases of this sort, one or both spouses often contact therapists for reasons of compliance rather than due to individual interest and motivation.

Therapists also should be aware of situations in which the motivation for seeking help is based primarily on a perceived threat that could result in a social, personal, or economic loss. For example, a divorce may be initiated to signal a warning to the other spouse of the seriousness of the marital or family situation. Another circumstance could be grave concern over being disadvantaged around financial and property issues. Social embarrassment about an impending divorce is yet another example.

When divorce becomes a reality, all family members must face a series of economic, personal, and social changes in their lives. The circumstances imposed by the fact of marital dissolution are that it proceeds independently of the wishes of those family members unwilling to or disinclined to divorce. In other words, for whatever reason(s), persons not wanting a divorce are "dragged into something" they are powerless to reverse. Such an event sets up varied sets of resistance that, until resolved, cloud reality and obstruct the development of parental cooperation, considered necessary for children successfully to negotiate a satisfactory adjustment to the structural and interpersonal changes imposed upon them.

Two issues of divorce are of paramount importance for a constructive resolution of the settlement or restructuring phases of the process. The first is coming to grips with the fact that the marital relationship is ending. Typically the emotional attachments and unresolved feelings ending the relationship by the resistent spouse interfere with accomplishing the tasks related to the restructuring of family relationships. Spousal resistance in accepting the reality of the divorce can inhibit the ability of parents to make cooperative decisions thought to be so necessary, particularly for the well-being of the children.

Redefining their obligations and responsibilities as divorcing parents is the second issue that needs to be addressed by spouses ending their marriage. The following are consided particularly important:

1. Telling the children about the divorce, and preparing them for the anticipated shifts and changes
2. Providing an opportunity for the children to express their concerns, fears, and, when appropriate, desires about with whom and where they will be living
3. Parents deciding on the living arrangements for the children, including where and with whom

4. Deciding the manner and degree of involvement each parent will have with the children
5. Determining the level of interparental involvement in the rearing of the children
6. Reaching decisions about how the distribution of family financial resources, including economic support, meets the needs of the family

Therapists should be reminded that parents, rather than children, initiate divorce proceedings. In this context most children are asked to adjust to changes in the life-styles made for them, rather than with them. This suggests that children generally are spectators who "sit on the sidelines" as the drama of their parents' divorce unfolds. In this sense they are benign participants in the important decisions being made about where and with whom they are to live during and after divorce. Thus the active role of children in making decisions important in the restructuring of their family, school, peer, and kinship relationships is negligible.

Although the transition from family intactness to divorce is difficult and stressful, most individuals make the adjustment without seeking help from professional therapists. Those who do contact therapists typically are couples who have decided to divorce, those who are having serious problems but are indecisive about ending the marriage, and cases where one spouse wants to pursue a divorce while the other wishes to continue the marriage relationship.

Coming to terms with the fact that the marriage is ending and a redefinition of obligations and responsibilities as divorcing parents are two important issues for a constructive resolution of the settlement phase of the divorce process. Once the decision to divorce has been made, the parents are considered to be the primary decision makers regarding the restructuring of family relationships.

4. Issues for Therapists

4.1. Diagnosis

Individuals and couples who seek the services of marriage and family therapists require an extensive assessment of their individual and conjoint feelings about the marital situation. Determining the extent to which each spouse is committed to a divorce as an alternative to their marriage is crucial because it determines the course of treatment.

The fact that divorce is being contemplated does not necessarily mean that a marital dissolution will in fact take place. It is important to note that in the early stages of marital unhappiness divorce often is considered in a speculative and private sense by the spouse who has felt uneasy, frustrated, or disappointed about the way the marriage has evolved. Often such ruminations have been going on for some time and may not be known by the other spouse. Emotional feelings of marital dissatisfaction often then escalate with divorce frequently being used as a threat to the other spouse if the marriage does not improve. On the other hand, one or both marital partners clearly may be committed to a divorce as a course of action he or she individually or collectively wishes to pursue.

The examples mentioned represent a continuum of feelings and states of readiness a therapist can anticipate when seeing individuals or couples having marital problems. It highlights the need for a careful diagnosis of the marital and family issues prior to undertaking a course of therapy.

4.2. Unevenness of Motivation to Divorce

The legal characteristics of divorce are such that agreement between spouses is not required for an action to be filed. This frequently is the state of affairs therapists encounter in their practice. As mentioned previously, the unevenness of motivation to divorce represents one of the most difficult problems faced by therapists. Aside from the emotionality, stress, and anxiety generated within the resistant spouse, motivational unevenness creates an impediment to a constructive resolution of the divorcing process.

4.3. The Role of the Therapist

When marital dissolution becomes a reality, therapists are faced with a dilemma over the degree to which they should become involved in negotiating the terms of the divorce settlement. The traditional role of therapists' activity with their clients has been viewed as ending when the emotional and psychological issues have been addressed and, hopefully resolved. At the same time issues of the settlement of divorce, for example, custody, visitation, child support, and the like, in and of themselves are emotionally laden. An increasing number of therapists have come to recognize the importance of facilitating agreements regarding the complete settlement of the terms of the divorce.

In many respects when emotional and practical matters pertaining to divorce are undertaken, the therapist's role takes on the characteristics of a mediator—a term being used increasingly for this type of intervention. In this sense, the intervention goes beyond helping the individual or couple deal with the emotions of the divorce. An increasing number of therapists who have worked extensively with divorcing families in this manner see their role as mediating agreements between the spouses about custody, visitation, child and/or spousal support, and distribution of property and other family finances.

4.4. Working with Attorneys

The preceding comments bring into focus another issue therapists encounter when dealing with divorcing families. Unlike other marital couples or families who are seen by or seek the service of therapists, divorcing spouses usually have employed an attorney. Lawyers obviously play a pivotal role in the divorcing process. Here is a situation where each professional is committed to serving his or her clients, but typically the methods of resolution of the issues frequently are in contradiction to the other.

Therapists and attorneys traditionally have viewed each other's work with suspicion, and to a large degree ignorance. Until very recently, collaboration and interdisciplinary cooperation on a case has been minimal at best.

Family therapists have not been trained in the workings of the law related to divorce. Similarly, attorneys have viewed therapists as having a limited value in the resolution and settlement of a divorce. This is particularly true in the practical areas of settlement such as custody, visitation, child support and the like. The lack of collegial contact between both professionals has sustained misperceptions about the value of working closely together in divorce cases.

More recently, therapists and attorneys have begun to work more closely together. This probably is due to the prevalence of divorce, changes in family law, and a growing awareness of the advantages of an interdisciplinary approach to working with divorcing families. Consequently, a growing number of therapists and attorneys are developing interdisciplinary strategies that show promise for ways that may contribute to positive resolutions of divorce.

4.5. Objectivity

Maintaining a mutual stance is considered by most experienced divorce oriented therapists to be crucial in helping couples negotiate the emotional and structural changes they inevitably will encounter during their divorce. Pressures by clients who may be looking for support regarding decisions to end their marriage, holding on to the relationship, wanting custody, and so forth can lead inadvertently to what may be viewed as coalitions between therapist and one spouse against the other.

The consequences of perceived coalitions can and often do hamper the therapist's effectiveness, whether in the decision-making or settlement phase of the divorcing process. The outcome resulting from a perception by one or both spouses of a coalition often leads to resistance in reaching important mutual decisions, and in some instances may terminate the therapy itself.

On the other hand, assuming a posture of objectivity does not imply the therapist is without a point of view about divorce, the decisions being made by the client, and issues regarding the children. What is important is that the situations producing conflict so frequently encountered during the therapy require neutrality if there is to be a successful facilitation of both the negotiation and resolution of the divorce.

4.6. The Children

When dealing with matters pertaining to the children, it is important to understand what it is about the divorce of their parents that is troublesome to them. Efforts should be focused on assisting the parents to understand the importance of helping their children adjust to the myriad of events that accompany the shift from a two parent to a single parent household.

These remarks are not intended to convey the idea that all children who experience divorce must be seen by the therapist. On the contrary, therapists should focus their efforts with the parents, because they ultimately are the decision makers about the events to which their children must adjust. This is particularly true in those cases involving young children.

Probably the most critical factor that creates undue stress for the children is being put in a position of being a pawn or "bargaining chip" during the divorce. Such occurrences are not infrequent, particularly if spousal conflict is high and the unevenness of motivation to divorce is a continuing unresolved problem. Illustrative examples of the above behavior that the therapist can expect to encounter are parents making disparaging remarks against the other in front of the children, fostering a coalition with the children against the other parent, verbal and physical altercations that are witnessed or heard by the children, using the children as messengers, and holding children out as a reward in exchange for a child support, financial, or property settlement that favors one spouse over the other.

Providing a means by which an equitable custody and visitation agreement can be negotiated is another task for the therapist. This may include talking with the children privately and/or with their parents with the aim being to ascertain their preferences with regard to custody, living arrangements, and the nature of involvement with each parent.

There are of course times when children should be seen individually, together, and with the parents by the therapist. The need for sessions of this sort is occasioned by children exhibiting emotional distress as reported by the parents, a desire for parents to talk with their children with assistance from the therapist, and a need for children to have social support from the therapist when they wish to share feelings with their parents in a secure atmosphere.

Finally, some comments should be made about the educative and support role the therapist can play that has a beneficial impact on both parents and their children. Parents and their children typically are confused, anxious, and apprehensive about how divorce will impact on them personally and as a family. Parents frequently are concerned about how their children will fare following the divorce. The degree to which the therapist is knowledgeable about factors associated with children's adjustment to divorce offers an opportunity to provide realistic encouragement and support when it is most needed.

Other concerns frequently expressed by spouses relate to their personal circumstances. Examples include loneliness, insecurity about the future, and meeting new friends. Again, a therapist who intends to work with divorcing families should be aware of community resources and support networks that all too frequently are unknown to divorcing spouses.

Almost every study dealing with divorce has provided data that points to a direct relationship between the psychological well-being of divorcing parents and the adjustment of their children. This is particularly true for the parent who is the primary caretaker. Therefore the therapy logically should be directed toward the adults so they can better cope with the events associated with the crisis of divorce.

5. Summary

Objectively, diagnosis of the marital situation, unevenness of motivation to divorce, role of the therapist, and working with attorneys have been identified as key areas deserving special attention by therapists when intervening with divorcing families. The importance of these factors relate to the nature and characteristics of the divorce process.

Therapists who work with divorcing families deal with the emotional problems occasioned by divorce. In addition, they may be called upon or elect to function as a mediator of the practical issues related to the divorce settlement.

Although children are of central concern, the primary focus of treatment is directed toward the parents. This is because they are primarily responsible for the decisions affecting the children's living circumstances during and after divorce. In addition, parental adjustment has a direct bearing on how the children will respond to the divorce.

6. References

Bane, M. J. *Here to stay: American families in the twentieth century*. New York: Basic Books, 1976.

Bowerman, C. L., & Irish, D. P. Some relationships of step-children to their parents. *Marriage and Family Living*, 1962, *24*, 113–128.

Brown, E. M. Divorce counseling. In D. H. Olson (Ed.), *Treating relationships*. Lake Mills, Iowa: Graphic Publishing, 1976.

Burchinal, L. G. Characteristics of adolescents from unbroken, broken, and reconstituted families. *Journal of Marriage and the Family*, 1964, *26*, 44–51.

Despert, J. L. *Children of divorce*. Garden City, New York: Doubleday, 1953.

Hetherington, E. M. Divorce: A child's perspective. *American Psychologist*, 1979, *34*, 851–858.

Hetherington, E. M., & Cox, R. Divorced fathers. *Family Coordinator*, 1976, *25*, 417–428.

Koch, M. Anxiety in pre-school children. *Merrill Palmer Quarterly*, 1961, *7*, 225–231.

Kressel, K., & Deutsch, M. Divorce therapy: An indepth survey of therapists views. *Family Process*, 1977, *16*, 413–443.

Kressel, K., Lopez-Morillas, M., Weinglass, J., & Deutsch, M. Professional intervention in divorce: The views of lawyers, psychotherapists, and the clergy. *Journal of Divorce*, 1978, *2*, 119–155.

Levinger, G. A social psychological perspective on marital dissolution. In G. Levinger & O. C. Moles (Eds.), *Divorce and separation: Context, causes, and consequences*. New York: Basic Books, 1979.

Longfellow, C. Divorce in context: Its impact on children. In G. Levinger & O. C. Moles (Eds.), *Divorce and separation: Context, causes, and consequences*. New York: Basic Books, 1979.

McDermott, J. F. Parental divorce in early childhood. *American Journal of Psychiatry*, 1968, *124*, 1424–1432.

McDermott, J. F. Divorce and its psychiatric sequelae in children. *Archives of General Psychiatry*, 1970, *23*, 421–427.

National Center for Health Statistics. Annual summary of births, deaths, marriages, and divorces, 1980. Monthly vital statistics report, *29*:13, Washington D.C.: U.S. Government Printing Office, 1981.

Nye, I. Child adjustment in broken and in unhappy, unbroken homes. *Marriage and Family Living*, 1957, *19*, 356–361.

Raschke, H. J., & Raschke, V. R. Family conflict and childrens self-concepts: A comparison of intact and single parent families. *Journal of Marriage and the Family*, 1979, *41*, 367–374.

Russell, I. L. Behavior problems of children from broken and intact homes. *Journal of Marriage and the Family*, 1957, *27*, 124–129.

Thomes, M. M. Children with absent fathers. *Journal of Marriage and the Family*, 1968, *30*, 89–96.

United States Bureau of the Census, Current population reports, Series P-60, No. 365, Marital status and living arrangements. Washington D.C.: U.S. Government Printing Office, 1981.

Wallerstein, J. S., & Kelly, J. B. The effects of parental divorce: The adolescent experience. In A. Koupernik (Ed.), *The child in his family: Children at a psychiatric risk* (Vol. 3). New York: Wiley, 1974.

Wallerstein, J. S., & Kelly, J. B. The effects of parental divorce: Experiences of the preschool child. *Journal of the American Academy of Child Psychiatry*, 1975, *14*, 600–616.

Wallerstein, J. S., & Kelly, J. B. The effects of parental divorce: Experiences of children in later latency. *American Journal of Orthospsychiatry*, 1976, *46*, 256–269.

Wallerstein, J. S., & Kelly, J. B. Divorce counseling: A community service for families in the midst of divorce. *American Journal of Orthopsychiatry*, 1977, *47*, 23–29.

Wallerstein, J. S., & Kelly, J. B. *Surviving the breakup: How children and parents cope with divorce*. New York: Basic Books, 1980.

Weiss, R. *Marital separation*. New York: Rand, 1971.

Westman, J. D. The role of child psychiatry in divorce. *Archives of General Psychiatry*, 1972, *23*, 416–420.

Author Index

Subject Index

CRITICAL ISSUES IN PSYCHIATRY
Series Editor: Sherwyn M. Woods, M.D., Ph.D.

MARITAL THERAPY

A COMBINED PSYCHODYNAMIC – BEHAVIORAL APPROACH

R. Taylor Segraves

University of Chicago, Chicago, Illinois

In this excellent volume, three commonly held assumptions about marital therapy are questioned: that psychodynamic and behavioral approaches are irreconcilable; that individual and marital therapies are distinctly separate therapeutic modalities; and that the subtleties of marital therapy seriously limit the usefulness of empirically based models. With an extensive clinical background and a broad understanding of many different modalities, Dr. Segraves presents here a fresh, empirically based approach to the treatment of marital problems.

Features:

- In-depth discussion of marital discord and its relationship to psychiatric disability
- A scholarly review of different theoretical schools and their applications in marital therapy
- A new therapeutic model integrating the psychodynamic and behavioral approaches
- A description of the clinical ramifications of this model and an extensive case study illustrating its use

314 pp., illus., 1982, ISBN 0-306-40936-4

Made in the USA
Monee, IL
13 September 2026

62976978R00280